ACSM'S ESSENTIALS OF SPORTS MEDICINE

ESSENTIALS OF SPORTS MEDICINE

Edited by

Robert E. Sallis, MD, FAAFP
Director of Research, Family Medicine Residency and Kaiser Permanente/SPORT Fellowship Programs
Kaiser Permanente Medical Center
Team Physician, Pomona College
Fontana, California

Ferdy Massimino, MD, MPH, FACSM
Clinical Practice Guideline Implementation and Clinical Education, Regional Occupational Health
Emergency Medicine/Sports Medicine
The Permanente Medical Group, Inc.
Oakland, California

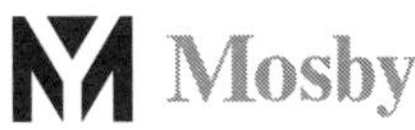

St. Louis Baltimore Boston
Carlsbad Chicago Naples New York Philadelphia Portland
London Madrid Mexico City Singapore Sydney Tokyo Toronto Wiesbaden

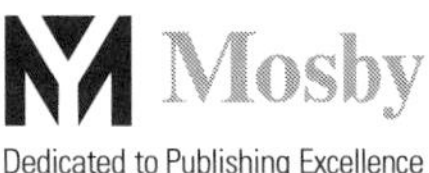

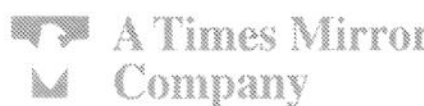

Vice President and Publisher: Anne S. Patterson
Editor: Robert Hurley
Developmental Editor: Lauranne Billus
Editorial Assistant: Marla Sussman
Project Manager: Linda Clarke
Production Editor: Jennifer Harper
Designer: Carolyn O'Brien
Manufacturing Supervisor: Andrew Christensen
Cover Photo: Philip and Karen Smith/Tony Stone Images
ACSM Group Publisher: D. Mark Robertson

Printed in the United States of America
Composition by Compset
Printing/binding by Malloy Lithographing, Inc.

Mosby–Year Book, Inc.
11830 Westline Industrial Drive
St. Louis, Missouri 63146

Library of Congress Cataloging-in-Publication Data

Essentials of Sports Medicine / edited by Robert Sallis, Ferdy Massimino.
p. cm.
Companion v. to: ACSM'S Sports Medicine Review / edited by Robert Sallis, Ferdy Massimino, Murray Allen. c1996.
Includes bibliographical references and index.
ISBN 0-8151-0157-0 (alk. paper)
1. Sports medicine. I. Sallis, Robert. II. Massimino, Ferdy. III. Allen, Murray. IV. ACSM'S Sports Medicine Review.
[DNLM: 1. Sports Medicine. 2. Athletic Injuries. QT 261 E78 1996]
RC1210.E782 1996
617.1'027—dc20
DNLM/DLC
for Library of Congress 96-6180
CIP

98 99 00 01 / 9 8 7 6 5 4 3

CONTRIBUTORS

Murray E. Allen, MD
Consultant, Musculoskeletal-Sports Medicine
Chief Examiner in Sports Medicine, American Academy Sports Physicians
Chief Examiner in Sports Medicine, CAQ Board Review Course
American College Sports Medicine
North Vancouver, British Columbia
CANADA

David V. Anderson, MD
Director, Orthopaedic Sports Medicine
Kaiser Permanente/SPORT Fellowship Program
Clinical Instructor, Loma Linda University, Medical School
Fontana, California

Raul Artal, MD, FACSM
Professor and Chairman, Department of Obstetrics and Gynecology
SUNY Health Science Center
Syracuse and Crous Irving Memorial Hospital
Syracuse, New York

Evan S. Bass, MD
Department of Family Medicine and Sports Medicine
Kaiser Permanente
Gardena, California

Mark E. Batt, MB, BChir, MRCGP, Dip Sports Med
Senior Lecturer/Honorary Consultant in Sports Medicine
University of Nottingham
Centre for Sports Medicine
Department of Orthopaedic & Accident Surgery
University Hospital, Queen's Medical Centre
Nottingham, United Kingdom

David E.J. Bazzo, MD
Assistant Clinical Professor of Family Medicine
University of California, San Diego
Clinical Director, UCSD Medical Group
San Diego, California

Mark D. Bracker, MD
Associate Clinical Professor
University of California, San Diego
San Diego, California

Philip J. Buckenmeyer, MD
University Instructional Specialist
Research Director, Women's Wellness Center
SUNY Health Science Center/Dept of OB/GYN
Syracuse, New York

Walter L. Calmbach, MD
Assistant Professor
University of Texas Health Science Center
Director, Family Practice Sports Medicine Fellowship
Department of Family Practice
University Hospital
San Antonio, Texas

Robert C. Cantu, MA, MD, FACS, FACSM
Medical Director, National Center for Catastrophic Sports Injury Research
Chapel Hill, North Carolina
Chief, Neurosurgery Service
Director, Service of Sports Medicine
Emerson Hospital
Concord, Massachusetts

C. Mark Chassay, MD
Graduate, Kaiser Permanenta/SPORT Fellowship Program and Team Physician, The University of Texas
Department of Intercollegiate Athletics for Women
Austin, Texas

Andrew J. Cole, MD, FACSM
Clinical Assistant Professor, Department of Physical Medicine and Rehabilitation
Clinical Assistant Professor, Department of Physical Therapy
University of Texas Southwestern Medical Center
Director, Spine Rehabilitation Services
Baylor University Medical Center
Department of Physical Medicine and Rehabilitation, Tom Landry Sports Medicine and Research Center
Dallas, Texas

Ellen J. Coleman, MA, MPH, RD
Nutrition Consultant
The Sport Clinic
Riverside, California

Mitchell W. Craib, PhD
Professor of Sports Studies
Guilford College
Greensboro, North Carolina

Robert J. Dimeff, MD
Medical Director, Section of Sports Medicine
Department of Orthopaedic Surgery
Cleveland Clinic Foundation
Clinical Professor, Family Practice
Case Western Reserve University
Cleveland, Ohio
Associate Professor, Department of Family Medicine
The Ohio State University
Columbus, Ohio

E. Randy Eichner, MD, FACSM
Professor of Medicine, University of Oklahoma Health Sciences Center
University Hospital and VAMC
Oklahoma City, Oklahoma

Wade F. Exum, MD, MBA
Preceptor, USOG/Glaxo Pharm. D. Fellowship
USOG Director of Drug Control Administration
Olympic Training Center
Colorado Springs, Colorado

Allen C. Felix, MD
Instructor, Kaiser Permanente/SPORT Fellowship Program
Family Physician, The SPORT Clinic
Riverside, California

Karl B. Fields, MD
Associate Professor, Dept of Family Medicine
Director Family Practice Resident
Moses Cone Health System
Greensboro, North Carolina

James G. Garrick, MD, FACSM
Director, Center for Sports Medicine
Saint Francis Memorial Hospital
San Francisco, California

Peter G. Gerbino, II, MD
Assistant Professor of Orthopaedic Surgery
University of Cincinnati
Division of Sports Medicine
Cincinnati, Ohio

Thomas J. Gill, MD
Clinical Fellow, Harvard Medical School
Department of Orthopedic Surgery
Massachusetts General Hospital
Boston, Massachusetts

Jorge Gomez, MD
Assistant Professor
Department of Pediatrics
University of Texas Health Science Center
Team Physician, San Antonio Pumas
University Hospital
San Antonio, Texas

Gary A. Green, MD, FACSM
Clinical Assistant Professor
University of California, Los Angeles, Division of Family Medicine
Assistant Team Physician, UCLA Intercollegiate Athletics
UCLA Medical Center
Los Angeles, California

Sally S. Harris, MD, MPH
Stanford University Team Physician
Pediatrician and Sports Medicine Specialist
Palo Alto Medical Clinic
Palo Alto, California

Stanley A. Herring, MD, FACSM
Clinical Associate Professor, Department of Rehabilitation Medicine
Clinical Associate Professor, Department of Orthopaedics
University of Washington
Puget Sound Sports and Spine Physicians
Seattle, Washington

Greg Hoeksema, MD
Clinical Staff, University of California, San Diego
Head, Marine Corps Recruit Depot Medical Clinic
Director, Sports Medicine Clinic
Naval Medical Center
San Diego, California

David O. Hough, MD, FACSM
Professor, Family Practice
Director, Sports Medicine
Head Team Physician, Michigan State University
East Lansing, Michigan

Jeffrey A. Housner, MD
Clinical Instructor and Sports Medicine Fellow
University of California, Los Angeles, Division of Family Medicine
UCLA Center for Health Sciences
Los Angeles, California

Michael D. Jackson, MD
Midwest Rehabilitation Physicians
Golden Valley, Michigan

Mimi D. Johnson, MD, FACSM
Clinical Assistant Professor, Division of Adolescent Medicine
Department of Pediatrics
Assistant Team Physician, University of Washington
Seattle, Washington
Washington Sports Medicine
Kirkland, Washington

Robert J. Johnson, MD, FACSM
Director, Primary Care Sports Medicine
Department of Family Practice, Hennepin County Medical Center
Family Medical Center
Minneapolis, Minnesota

Kirk Jones, MS, ATC
Associate Professor, Physical Education
Pomona College
NATA, ACSM
Claremont, California

Todd Jorgenson, MD
Graduate, Kaiser Permanente/SPORT Fellowship Program
Kaiser Permanente Medical Center
Fontana, California

W. Benjamin Kibler, MD, FACSM
Medical Director
Lexington Clinic Sports Medicine Center
Lexington, Kentucky

William D. Knopp, MD
Director of Sports Medicine, MacNeal F.P. Residency Program
MacNeal Hospital/Rush Medical School
Clinical Faculty, MacNeal Hospital
Berwyn, Illinois

Robert L. Kronisch, MD
Staff Physician
Sports Medicine Consultant, Student Health Service
San Jose State University
San Jose, California

Ferdy Massimino, MD, MPH, FACSM
Clinical Practice Guideline Implementation and Clinical Education, Regional Occupational Health Emergency Medicine/Sports Medicine
The Permanente Medical Group, Inc.
Oakland, California

Angus M. McBryde, Jr., MD
Professor and Chairman
The Medical University of South Carolina
Department of Orthopaedic Surgery
Division of Sports Medicine
Charleston, South Carolina

Roger L. McCoy, II, MD
Team Physician
Arizona State University
Family Practice/Sports Medicine
Arizona Orthopedics and Sports Medicine Specialists Sportsclub
Phoenix, Arizona

Douglas B. McKeag, MD, MS, FACSM
Formerly: Professor of Family Practice
Coordinator of Sports Medicine, Michigan State University Family Practice
East Lansing, Michigan
Currently: Professor and Vice Chairman Family Medicine and
Orthopaedic Surgery
Director of Primary Care Sports Medicine
Musculoskeletal Institute
University of Pittsburgh Medical Center
Pittsburgh, Pennsylvania

Lyle J. Micheli, MD, FACSM
Associate Clinical Professor of Orthopaedic Surgery
Harvard Medical School
Director, Division of Sports Medicine
Children's Hospital
Boston, Massachusetts

James L. Moeller, MD
Assistant Professor of Orthopaedic Surgery
Primary Care Sports Medicine
Department of Orthopaedics
University of Pittsburgh
Pittsburgh, Pennsylvania

James M. Moriarity, MD
Physician, University Health Services
University of Notre Dame
Notre Dame, Indiana

Aurelia Nattiv, MD
Assistant Clinical Professor
UCLA, Division of Family Medicine
Department of Orthopaedic Surgery
Assistant Team Physician, UCLA
Los Angeles, California

Steven R. Neish, MD, FACSM
Assistant Professor of Pediatrics
University of Colorado
Pediatric Cardiologist
Fitzsimons Army Medical Center
Aurora, Colorado

Andrew W. Nichols, MD, FACSM
Associate Professor, Department of Family Practice and Community Health
John A. Burns School of Medicine, University of Hawaii at Manoa
Team Physician
University of Hawaii at Manoa
Honolulu, Hawaii

Carol L. Otis, MD, FACSM
Adjunct Assistant Professor, Internal Medicine
Director, Specialty Clinics
University of California, Los Angeles, Student Health Services
Los Angeles, California

William Parham, PhD, ABPP
Associate Director, Clinical and COPE Services
UCLA, Student Psychological Services
Los Angeles, California

Herbert G. Parris, MD
Assistant Clinical Professor
University of Colorado School of Medicine
Teaching Faculty
St. Joseph Hospital Family Practice Residency Program
St. Joseph Hospital
The Denver Center for Sports/Family Medicine
Denver, Colorado

Peter B. Raven, PhD, FACSM
Professor and Chair
Department of Physiology
University of North Texas Health Science Center
Fort Worth, Texas

Troy Reese, PharmD
Resident Pharmacist
United States Olympic Committee
Colorado Springs, Colorado

E. Lee Rice, DO, FACSM
Clinical Professor of Family Practice & Sports Medicine
College of Osteopathic of the Pacific
Pomona, California
Assistant Clinical Professor, University of California San Diego School of Medicine
Department of Community and Family Medicine
San Diego Sports Medicine, Orthopaedics and Family Health Center
San Diego, California

Brent S.E. Rich, MD, ATC
Team Physician, Arizona State University
Private Practice, Arizona Orthopaedic and Sports Medicine Specialists
Phoenix, Arizona

David B. Richards, MD
Orthopedic Surgeon and Sports Medicine Physician
Lexington Clinic Sports Medicine Center
Lexington, Kentucky

Michael E. Robinson, MD
Primary Care Sports Medicine, Department of Orthopedics
The Permanente Medical Group
Team Physician, United States Water Polo
Sacramento, California

Aaron L. Rubin, MD, FACSM
Director, Kaiser Permanente/SPORT Fellowship Program and Team Physician, Rubidoux High School
University of California, Riverside
Partner and Staff Physician, Department of Family Medicine
Kaiser Permanente Medical Center
Fontana, California

Anthony J. Saglimbeni, MD
Fellow, Primary Care Sports Medicine
Family and Preventive Medicine
University of California, San Diego
Clinical Instructor
University of California, San Diego Medical Center
San Diego, California

Robert E. Sallis, MD, FAAFP
Director of Research, Family Medicine Residency and Kaiser Permanente/SPORT Fellowship Programs
Kaiser Permanente Medical Center
Team Physician, Pomona College
Fontana, California

Warren Scott, MD
Clinical Instructor of Surgery
Stanford University Medical Center
Chief, Sports Medicine
Departments of Orthopedics and Emergency Medicine
Kaiser Permanente Medical Center
Santa Clara, California

Lauren M. Simon, MD, MPH
Assistant Professor of Family Medicine
Loma Linda University School of Medicine
Director, Sports Medicine Program
Loma Linda University Family Practice Residency Program
Loma Linda, California

Stephen M. Simons, MD, FACSM
Associate Clinical Professor, Family Medicine
Indiana University
Associate Director, Family Practice Residency
Saint Joseph's Medical Center
South Bend, Indiana

Angela D. Smith, MD, FACSM
Assistant Professor of Orthopaedics
Case Western Reserve University School of Medicine
University Hospitals
Cleveland, Ohio

Edward D. Snell, MD
Assistant Professor
Medical College of Pennsylvania and Hahnemann University
Primary Care Sports Medicine
Allegheny Orthopaedic Associates/Allegheny General-Duquesne
University Sports Medicine Institute
Allegheny General Hospital
Pittsburgh, Pennsylvania

Steven D. Stahle, MD
Associate Professor
St. Louis University School of Medicine
Director of Sports Medicine
Deaconess Health System
Family Medicine, Dept. Deaconess Hospital
St. Louis, Missouri

Jeffrey L. Tanji, MD
Associate Professor and Associate Director, Residency Program
Director, Sports Medicine Program
University of California, Davis, Medical Center
Sacramento, California

Suzanne M. Tanner, MD, FACSM
Assistant Professor, Department of Orthopedics and Pediatrics
University of Colorado Health Sciences Center
Director, Adolescent Sports Medicine
The Denver Children's Hospital
Denver, Colorado

Steven P. Van Camp, MD, FACSM
Professor, College of Professional Studies
San Diego State University
Assistant Clinical Professor, Department of Pathology
University of California, San Diego, School of Medicine
Alvarado Medical Group
San Diego, California

Craig Wargon, DPM
Diplomate American Board of Podiatric Surgery
Residency Director, Kaiser, Santa Clara
Kaiser Permanente
Santa Clara, California

J. Michael Wieting, DO, Med
Instructor, Department of Physical Medicine and Rehabilitation
Michigan State University — College of Osteopathic Medicine
Staff Physiatrist
Michigan State University Sports Medicine Center
Michigan Capital Medical Center
East Lansing, Michigan

Carl Winfield, MD
Staff Physician, Division of Sports Medicine
Naval Hospital
Camp Lejeune, North Carolina

Robert A. Wiswell, MD
Associate Professor, Department of Exercise Sciences
University of Southern California
Los Angeles, California

PREFACE

The cornerstone for the delivery of quality health care today is the primary care physician. This reality is especially true in sports medicine, which encompasses a wide variety of disciplines. Although no single practitioner can provide all the care needed by an athlete, athletes do require a broadly trained physician as their point of first contact with the health care system. This physician should be able to care for most of the sports related problems they encounter and effectively arrange and manage consultative care when needed.

This role is nothing new for the primary care physician. Virtually all primary care physicians practicing today are confronted with a sick or injured athlete on a regular basis. A major portion of the field of sports medicine is really nothing more than the primary care of athletes. That is not to say that athletes do not at times require specialized expertise. A primary care physician with additional training in sports medicine can fill a vital role in caring for athletes, whether as a team physician or by seeing patients in a sports medicine clinic.

The American Board of Medical Specialties has defined the field of sports medicine as a broad area of health care that includes:

1. Exercise as an essential component of health care throughout life;
2. Medical management and supervision of recreational and competitive athletes and all others who exercise; and
3. Exercise for prevention and treatment of disease and injury.

Based on this broad definition, a sports medicine physician should have a wide scope of training. For this reason, the major primary care specialties (family medicine, internal medicine, pediatrics, and emergency medicine) developed an examination to recognize competence in sports medicine. Passing this examination, which was first given in 1993, confers a Certificate of Added Qualifications (CAQ) in sports medicine. To sit for this examination, physicians must hold board certification in one of these primary care specialties, and must have completed a one year fellowship in sports medicine. A practice eligibility pathway is available through the 1999 examination.

The origins of this book began with a board review course for the first CAQ examination in sports medicine. This course was conceived and organized by my co-editor, Dr. Ferdy Massimino, and sponsored by the American College of Sports Medicine (ACSM). It ranks as one of the College's most ambitious and broad based education efforts. This conference brought together a vast array of sports medicine experts from across the nation to cover the entire range of primary care sports medicine topics, and lasted 5½ days while encompassing over 50 hours of lecture time. The entire course was filmed by CME Video and released as a 27-tape, comprehensive review of sports medicine. A similar course was staged in conjunction with the American Academy of Family Physicians (AAFP) before the 1995 CAQ examination.

ACSM's Essentials of Sports Medicine has sprung from the massive syllabus that accompanied these conferences. Most of the topics and many of the speakers from these conferences are represented here. Most authors are primary care physicians who are leaders in the practice and teaching of sports medicine across the country. Numerous specialists, well known for their care of athletes, have contributed to this book as well. All have a strong background in understanding the needs of and providing relevant information for primary care sports medicine physicians.

Essentials of Sports Medicine is divided into 3 sections and consists of 82 chapters. The first 31 chapters cover medical topics relevant to the athlete. The next 42 chapters deal with musculoskeletal topics as they relate to the athlete. The final 9 chapters cover sports-specific topics and include an integrated discussion of important medical and musculoskeletal problems unique to athletes who compete in these sports. All chapters are done in outline format to facilitate easy study as well as to provide a rapid reference source.

Although this book was initially conceived as review material for the CAQ examination in sports medicine, its appeal will be much broader than that. It should be of great benefit to any physician who wants a comprehensive review of or easy reference to sports medicine. It should also be useful to residents (whether in primary care, orthopedics, or physiatry) who need a focused study guide to accompany rotations in sports medicine.

The companion text to this book is titled *ACSM's Sports Medicine Review.* Like *Essentials,* it originated from both the ACSM and AAFP review courses. Both of these courses included a daily mock board exam over the topics covered by the previous day's speakers. These examinations were graded each day and course participants were able to compare their scores with those of others taking the course.

Many of these questions, as well as numerous new ones, have been incorporated into the companion review text. With each question is a paragraph long answer explaining each of the choices. These questions correspond to the chapters in *Essentials* and highlight the important points of each chapter. These books should be used in combination and together provide an outstanding means of education and self assessment.

The education of primary care physicians is of vital importance to the American College of Sports Medicine. I believe the primary care physician is "where the rubber meets the road" in sports medicine. After the vast cadre of ACSM researchers and specialists advance sports medicine, the primary care physician takes this information and puts it into practice. Without well trained and receptive primary caregivers, the full benefit of the advances in sports medicine the College cultivates would not be realized. Our goal has been to help bridge this gap between new advances in sports medicine and their implementation.

I hope you will find both these books useful in your sports medicine endeavors.

Robert Sallis, MD
Rancho Cucamonga, CA
1996

ACKNOWLEDGMENTS

On behalf of Dr. Massimino and myself, there are a number of people to thank who were instrumental in getting this project completed. First and foremost are the physicians and scientists who contributed their manuscripts. We would also like to thank Mark Robertson at ACSM for his ongoing support and assistance. David Hough MD, Angela Smith MD, and Bob Cantu MD, provided support in developing the book's table of contents, and with suggesting authors. Thanks to Della Mundy and her crew at Kaiser Medical Editing for all their help as well. We also need to acknowledge our spouses Kathy Sallis and Sherry Massimino, along with our wonderful families, who make everything worthwhile.

I also need to thank my old friend Bret Miller in Mosby Sales for putting me in touch with Bob Hurley and his incredible editorial staff. Over the past year or more, I have very much enjoyed working with Lauranne Billus, Mia Carino, Marla Sussman and Jennifer Harper at Mosby's Philadelphia office. They could not have worked harder and they made doing this project a lot of fun. Thanks also to my colleagues at Kaiser Permanente including Mark Martinez MD, Janis Neuman MD, Vince Roger MD, Aaron Rubin, MD, and David Anderson MD, who have been most supportive of my sports medicine endeavors.

Robert Sallis, MD

CONTENTS

Sports Specific Problems

MEDICAL TOPICS

CHAPTER 1

Cardiac Rehabilitation

Mark D. Bracker, MD

I. Background Information
  A. History of cardiac rehabilitation.
    1. Epidemiology of work-related exercise and coronary heart disease (CHD): primary prevention.
      a. In 1953, Morris and associates published a landmark study of London transportation workers, postal employees, and British civil servants.[14,15,18,19]
        (1) When compared with bus drivers, bus conductors were found to be more physically active at work and had a lower incidence rate of first clinical episodes of coronary disease, a reduced case-fatality ratio, and a lower rate of early mortality.
        (2) Postal workers delivering mail on foot had lower rates of CHD than did sedentary supervisors.
        (3) Civil servants in jobs allowing for less exercise at work had rates of CHD that were influenced by their leisure time physical habits, such as vigorous sports play, yard work, and other activities.[1,4,16,17]
      b. Paffenbarger and his colleagues examined the records of San Francisco longshoremen as to their work activity and fatality rates as a result of CHD.[21]
        (1) Men who expended at least 8500 kilocalories (kcal) per week at work had significantly less risk of fatal CHD at any age than did men whose jobs required less exercise.
        (2) High energy workers had a lower risk of CHD than did low energy workers, independent of additional risk factors such as heavy cigarette smoking, obesity, blood pressure elevation, abnormal glucose metabolism, excessive blood cholesterol content, and prior incidence of CHD.
        (3) The risk of fatal CHD in high energy output cargo handlers with a history of myocardial infarction (MI) was half that in less active longshoremen with diagnosed heart disease.

2. Epidemiology of leisure time exercise and CHD.
   a. The Multiple Risk Factor Intervention Trial established an inverse relationship between leisure time physical activity and risk of coronary heart disease and total mortality among men engaged predominantly in light to moderate activities.[11]
   b. Leisure time exercise patterns and health status among college alumni have shown how past and present exercise relate to CHD risk.[22]
      (1) Alumni who reported engaging in light sports activity only had the same risk of CHD as those who played no sports at all.
      (2) Alumni who reported vigorous sports activity had a 27% less risk of CHD than those who did not.
      (3) Athletes who gave up their former energetic routines tended to have an even greater risk of CHD than did alumni who had never been active as student athletes.
      (4) In this study only a physically active adulthood was associated with lower CHD rates. Continued vigorous activity such as playing an endurance sport in adult life was independent of constitutional endowment or physical activity.
      (5) Five risk factors (adequate exercise, no cigarette smoking, weight control, no hypertension, no parental CHD) contribute independently to lowering the risk of CHD.
      (6) Hypertension is the most potent clinical risk factor but is least prevalent.
      (7) Sedentary life-style is highly prevalent and percentagewise represents the greatest contribution to risk of CHD in the population.
   c. More recent data from the Harvard Alumni Health Study demonstrates a graded inverse relationship between total physical activity and mortality. Vigorous activities (but not nonvigorous activities) were associated with longevity.[10]

B. Goal of cardiac rehabilitation: the role of exercise on secondary prevention of CHD.
   1. Cardiac rehabilitation may be defined as the process by which patients with cardiac diseases are returned to their optimal physical, psychological, social, emotional, vocational, and economic status.
      a. Short-term objectives include physical reconditioning, education about the disease process, and psychological support during the early recovery phase.
      b. Long-term objectives include identifying and treating risk factors, teaching and reinforcing health behaviors that improve prognosis, optimizing physical conditioning, and facilitating a return to occupational and avocational activities.
   2. Cardiac rehabilitation originated in the 1950s and was characterized by treating acute MI survivors with 3 to 6 weeks of bedrest followed by "armchair" care.[12]
      a. Early ambulation following MI was shown to be safe, and more formal programs of cardiac rehabilitation emphasize exercise training and vocational rehabilitation.[6]
      b. Exercise testing early after MI has become the standard of care in the past decade.[3]
      c. Risk stratification after coronary events allows for early treatment of high-risk patients with medication and revascularization by coronary angioplasty and surgery.

d. Low-risk cases are identified early, allowing comprehensive rehabilitative efforts to be started soon after a coronary event.[2,9]

II. Indications for Cardiac Rehabilitation
  A. Candidates for cardiac rehabilitation services.
    1. A health history that includes:
      a. Medical or surgical profile (or both).
      b. Pertinent medical records.
      c. Lipid/lipoprotein profile.
      d. Medications.
      e. Resting electrocardiography (ECG) and electrophysiological and signal-averaged ECG data.
      f. Cardiac angiographic data.
      g. Complications incurred during surgery or recovery.
      h. Noninvasive studies.
    2. Description of current symptoms.
    3. Coronary risk profile.
    4. Nutritional and body composition analysis (weight, height, body mass index, percent body fat).
    5. Cardiopulmonary assessment.
    6. Exercise stress test.
    7. Physical limitations and disabilities.
    8. Risk stratification.
  B. Absolute contraindications for entry into inpatient and outpatient exercise training.[5]
    1. Unstable angina.
    2. Resting systolic blood pressure >200 mmHg or resting diastolic blood pressure >100 mmHg.
    3. Significant drop (≥20 mmHg) in resting systolic blood pressure from patient's average level that is not a result of medications.
    4. Moderate to severe aortic stenosis.
    5. Acute systemic illness or fever.
    6. Uncontrolled atrial or ventricular arrhythmia.
    7. Uncontrolled tachycardia (>100 bpm).
    8. Symptomatic congestive heart failure.
    9. Third-degree heart block without pacemaker.
    10. Active pericarditis or myocarditis.
    11. Recent embolism.
    12. Thrombophlebitis.
    13. Resting ST segment displacement (>3 mm).
    14. Uncontrolled diabetes.
    15. Orthopedic problems that would prohibit exercise.
  C. Candidates for inpatient cardiac rehabilitation.
    1. Recent MI, coronary artery bypass surgery, or angioplasty.
    2. Residual ischemia, heart failure, and arrhythmias.
    3. Dilated cardiomyopathy, nonischemic heart disease.
    4. Concomitant pulmonary disease.
    5. Recent pacemaker or automatic implanted cardioverter-defibrillator.
    6. Recent heart valve surgery, aneurysm resection, or organ transplantation.
    7. Elderly patients.
    8. Other chronic diseases or complex medical problems.
  D. Candidates for outpatient cardiac rehabilitation.
    1. Completion of inpatient cardiac rehabilitation.

2. No disqualifying characteristics.
3. No concern that exercise will have a deleterious effect on the course of cardiac disease or other disorder and/or the patient's quality of life.

E. Risk stratification.[13]
1. Low risk.
a. No significant left ventricular dysfunction (i.e., ejection fraction ≥50%).
b. No resting or exercise-induced myocardial ischemia manifested as angina and/or ST segment displacement.
c. No resting or exercise-induced complex arrhythmias.
d. Uncomplicated MI, coronary artery bypass surgery, angioplasty, or anthrectomy.
e. Functional capacity ≥6 metabolic equivalents (METs) on graded exercise test 3 or more weeks after clinical event.
2. Intermediate risk.
a. Mild to moderately depressed left ventricular function (ejection fraction of 31%-49%).
b. Functional capacity >5-6 METs on graded exercise test 3 or more weeks after clinical event.
c. Failure to comply with exercise intensity prescription.
d. Exercise-induced myocardial ischemia (1-2 mm ST segment depression) or reversible ischemic defects (observed in nuclear radiography).
3. High risk.
a. Severely depressed left ventricular function (ejection fraction ≤30%).
b. Complex ventricular arrhythmias at rest or appearing/increasing with exercise.
c. Decrease in systolic blood pressure of >15 mmHg during exercise or failure to rise with increasing exercise workloads.
d. Survivor of sudden cardiac death.
e. MI complicated by congestive heart failure, cardiogenic shock, and/or complex ventricular arrhythmias.
f. Severe coronary artery disease and marked exercise-induced myocardial ischemia (>2 mm ST segment depression).

F. Monitoring.
1. The use of continuous or intermittent monitoring for a specific patient remains a matter of clinical judgment.
2. High-risk patients require the most extensive ECG monitoring, clinical supervision, and the most conservative exercise prescriptions.
3. All cardiac exercise programs should include the monitoring of blood pressure, heart rate, symptoms, and effort intolerance.

G. Length of program.
1. The appropriate length of time for patients to remain in each phase of cardiac rehabilitation takes into account the risk of disease progression and entry risk stratification.
a. Progression of new onset of coronary atherosclerosis.
b. Deterioration of quality of life.
c. Psychosocial dysfunction.
2. The length of time is determined by the following factors:
a. Evidence that the patient is clinically stable.
b. Achievement of the goals set at program entry.
c. Determination that the patient has received optimal or near optimal benefits.

III. Risk Factor Reduction
   A. Evaluation and treatment of hypercholesterolemia.
      1. The benefits of exercise, if any, may be due more to a decrease in risk factors than to actual improvement in cardiorespiratory fitness.
      2. The change in risk factors from exercise training programs may be small.
      3. Changes in body weight and skin fold thickness are negligible.
      4. Serum lipid values remain unchanged, and strenuous exercise may increase the protective plasma high-density lipoprotein (HDL) levels.[8]
   B. Smoking cessation.
      1. The percentage of cigarette smokers is lower in post-MI patients who exercise than in those who do not.
      2. More than a third of patients who exercise but continue to smoke make substantial reductions in their cigarette consumption.
      3. Exercise itself may contribute little to an improved risk factor profile in coronary patients; other components of the cardiac rehabilitation program may have a major impact on secondary prevention. All programs should include:
         a. Dietary modification.
         b. Stress management.
         c. Cessation of cigarette smoking.
         d. Control of hypertension.
         e. Control of hyperlipidemia.
   C. Vocational rehabilitation and psychosocial status.
      1. The psychological benefits of rehabilitation do not appear to be major.
         a. Psychological factors seem to play a relatively minor role in whether coronary patients return to work.
         b. 80% of coronary patients return to vocational function and preillness level of activity.
         c. Psychological problems after MI are responsible for 3% to 12% of patients not returning to work.[7]
   D. On the basis of several studies, expected improvements in psychosocial well-being cannot justify enrollment in cardiac exercise rehabilitation after MI.[20,23]

References

1. Chave SPW, Morris JN, Moss S, et al: Vigorous exercise in leisure time and the death rate: a study of male civil servants, *J Epidemiol Comm Health* 32:239-243, 1978.
2. DeBusk RF: Specialized testing after recent acute myocardial infarction—a review, *Ann Intern Med* 110:470-481, 1989.
3. DeBusk RF, Blomquist CG, Konchonkos NT, et al: Identification and treatment of low risk patients after acute myocardial infarction and coronary artery bypass graft surgery, *N Engl J Med* 314:161-166, 1986.
4. Epstein L, Miller GL, Stitt FW, et al: Vigorous exercise in leisure time, coronary risk factors, and resting electrocardiogram in middle-aged civil servants, *Br Heart J* 38:403-409, 1976.
5. Exercise prescription for cardiac patients. In *ACSM Guidelines for Exercise Testing and Prescription,* ed 4, Philadelphia, 1991, Lea & Febiger.
6. *The Exercise Standards Book,* Dallas, 1979, American Heart Association.
7. Gentry W: Psychosocial concerns and benefits in cardiac rehabilitation. In Pollack ML, Schmidt DH, editors: *Heart Disease and Rehabilitation,* ed 2, Boston, 1986, Wiley.
8. Goor R, Hosking JD, Dennis BH, et al: Nutrient intake among selected North American populations in the Lipid Research Clinics Prevention Study: comparison of fat intake, *Am J Clin Nutr* 41:299, 1985.
9. *Guidelines for Cardiac Rehabilitation Programs,* ed 2, 1995, Human Kinetics.
10. Lee IM, Hsieh C, Paffenbarger RS: Exercise intensity and longevity in men, *JAMA* 273:1179-1184, 1995.

11. Leon AS, Connett J, Jacobs DR, Ranramaa R: Leisure-time physical activity levels and risk of coronary heart disease and death: the Multiple Risk Factor Intervention Trial, *JAMA* 258:2388-2395, 1987.
12. Levine SA: 'Armchair' treatment of acute coronary thrombosis, *JAMA* 148:1365-1369, 1952.
13. McNeer JF, Margoho JR, Lee KL: Role of the exercise test in evaluating patients for ischemic heart disease, *Circulation* 57:64-70, 1978.
14. Morris JN: *Use of Epidemiology*, ed 3, New York, 1975, Churchill Livingstone.
15. Morris JN, Crawford MD: Coronary heart disease and physical activity of work: evidence of a necropsy survey, *Br Med J* 2:1485-1496, 1958.
16. Morris JN, Chave JPW, Adam C, et al: Vigorous exercise in leisure-time and the incidence of coronary heart-disease, *Lancet* 1:33-339, 1973.
17. Morris JN, Everitt MG, Pollard R, et al: Vigorous exercise in leisure-time: protection against coronary heart-disease, *Lancet* 2:1207-1210, 1980.
18. Morris JN, Heady JA, Raffle PA, et al: Coronary heart disease and activity of work, *Lancet* 2:1053-1057, 1111-1120, 1953.
19. Morris JN, Kagan A, Pattison DC, et al: Incidence and prediction of ischemic heart-disease in London busmen, *Lancet* 2:552-559, 1966.
20. O'Connor GT, Buring JE, Yusuf S, et al: An overview of randomized trials of rehabilitation with exercise after myocardial infarction, *Circulation* 80:234, 1989.
21. Paffenbarger RS, Gima AS, Laughlin ME, et al: Characteristics of longshoremen related to fatal coronary heart disease and stroke, *Am J Public Health* 61:1362-1370, 1971.
22. Paffenbarger RS, Wing AL, Hyde RT: Chronic disease in former college students. XVI. Physical activity as an index of heart attack risk in college alumni, *Am J Epidemiol* 108:161-175, 1978.
23. Roman O, Guitierez M, Lusic I, et al: Cardiac rehabilitation after myocardial infarction: 9 year controlled follow-up study, *Cardiology* 70:223, 1983.

CHAPTER 2

Hypertension

Jeffrey L. Tanji, MD

Mark E. Batt, MB, BChir

I. Overview
   A. Prevalence: 58 million Americans or about 15% to 20% of the U.S. adult population.
   B. Proven risk factor for myocardial infarction and stroke.
   C. Cardiovascular death is still the leading cause of mortality in the United States.
   D. Improvement in blood pressure control has resulted in a reduction in stroke and myocardial infarction (MI) in numerous epidemiological studies.
   E. Common in primary care practice.
      1. Hypertension is one of the leading causes for visits to physicians.
      2. Antihypertensive drugs comprise the leading prescription category in the United States.

II. Diagnosis
   A. New Joint National Committee on Detection, Evaluation and Treatment of High Blood Pressure guidelines were published in 1993.
      1. Systolic BP values:
         a. High normal—130-139 mmHg.
         b. Stage 1 (mild)—140-159 mmHg.
         c. Stage 2 (moderate)—160-179 mmHg.
         d. Stage 3 (severe)—180-209 mmHg.
         e. Stage 4 (very severe)—≥210 mmHg.
      2. Diastolic BP values:
         a. High normal—85-89 mmHg.
         b. Stage 1 (mild)—90-99 mmHg.
         c. Stage 2 (moderate)—100-109 mmHg.
         d. Stage 3 (severe)—110-119 mmHg.
         e. Stage 4 (very severe)—≥120 mmHg.
   B. Definitions.
      1. Primary, or essential hypertension (70% of all hypertensive individuals)—disease without a known underlying cause.

2. Secondary hypertension—disease as the result of an underlying condition:
   a. Cushing's disease.
   b. Pheochromocytoma.
   c. Hyperaldosteronism.
   d. Renal artery stenosis.
   e. Renal parenchymal disease.
   f. Coarctation of the aorta.

C. Diagnostic testing for hypertension.
   1. Three elevated blood pressure values at rest while seated are diagnostic of high blood pressure.
   2. 24-hour ambulatory blood pressure monitoring can be more accurate in determining the diagnosis but is not widely used.
   3. A markedly elevated blood pressure value during exercise or immediately postexercise in a normotensive individual has been associated with the subsequent development of hypertension. Exercise tests include:
      a. Bicycle ergometry testing.
      b. Step tests.
      c. Treadmill tests.
   4. Diagnostic exercise testing as a screening tool for hypertension remains in an investigative domain.

D. Laboratory testing for hypertensive subjects.
   1. Must weigh cost-benefit issues and understand that secondary hypertension (<5% of patients) is uncommon.
   2. Initial tests:
      a. Urinalysis.
      b. Electrocardiogram.
      c. Electrolytes.
      d. Renal function tests (creatinine, blood urea nitrogen).
   3. If secondary hypertension is suspected, further tests are necessary:
      a. 24-hour vanillylmandelic acid urine test.
      b. Chest x-ray.
      c. Renal scan.
      d. Renal arteriogram.

III. Exercise and Hypertension

A. Strong evidence exists that exercise (physical activity) results in enhanced blood pressure control.

B. Traditional paradigm—the greater the level of physical fitness, the better blood pressure control is for hypertensive patients.

C. This paradigm has been challenged by the American College of Sports Medicine (1993), and the Joint National Committee on Detection, Evaluation and Treatment of High Blood Pressure (1993) reported:
   1. Moderate intensity aerobic exercise (walking) may be optimal for blood pressure control.
   2. Exercise of high intensity (>80% of maximal heart rate) may increase resting blood pressure values.

D. Regular aerobic activity (55% to 70% of maximal heart rate) for 30 minutes on most days of the week may be optimal for blood pressure control.

E. Heavy resistance training is contraindicated in hypertensive individuals.

F. Light resistance training (20-30 repetitions per set) may enhance blood pressure control.

G. Mechanisms that explain the benefit of exercise on blood pressure:
   1. Decreased sympathetic tone.
   2. Decreased catecholamine levels.

3. Increased insulin sensitivity.
4. Relaxation response.
5. Endorphin-mediated postexercise blood pressure benefit.

IV. Therapy
- A. Nonpharmacologic therapy remains the initial step (3-6 month trial).
  1. Exercise.
  2. Salt restriction (30% of hypertensives are salt sensitive).
  3. Smoking cessation.
  4. Alcohol moderation.
  5. Caffeine moderation.
  6. Weight loss.
- B. Failure of nonpharmacologic therapy dictates the use of medications.
  1. Assess overall cardiovascular risk based on all factors and not just blood pressure values when deciding to institute medication therapy.
  2. Stage II (moderate) hypertension usually calls for pharmacologic therapy.
- C. Specific medications.
  1. Initial step calls for diuretics or beta-blockers.
     - a. Inexpensive
     - b. Major epidemiological studies use these agents to control blood pressure.
     - c. Hydrochlorothiazide.
       - (1) Maximum dose: 25 mg per day.
       - (2) Low rate of hypokalemia at this dose.
       - (3) Can be associated with dehydration in athletes.
     - d. Combined hydrochlorothiazide/triamterene
       - (1) Lower incidence of hypokalemia compared with hydrochlorothiazide
       - (2) Dehydration is still a risk, particularly among endurance athletes.
     - e. Cardioselective beta-blockers may be safe for athletes; nonselective beta-blockers are relatively contraindicated in athletes.
       - (1) Nonselective beta-blockers may limit maximal aerobic capacity (Vo_2 max) because of negative inotropic and chronotropic effects.
       - (2) Selective beta-blockers have fewer side effects but can limit Vo_2 max and increase perceived exertion in some athletes.
         - (a) Hyperthermia is a side effect of selective beta-blockers.
         - (b) Hyperkalemia can be a side effect, but the mechanism is unclear.
       - (3) Cardioselective beta-blockers.
         - (a) Metoprolol.
         - (b) Atenolol.
         - (c) Acebutolol.
         - (d) Betaxolol.
       - (4) Noncardioselective beta-blockers.
         - (a) Propranolol.
         - (b) Nadolol.
         - (c) Penbutolol.
         - (d) Timolol.
         - (e) Pindolol.
  2. Angiotensin-converting enzyme (ACE) inhibitors.
     - a. Reduce total peripheral resistance and enhance vasodilatation by blocking conversion of angiotensin I to angiotensin II.

b. Side effects profile is low in athletes, but these agents are costly.
   (1) Cough.
   (2) Concomitant use with nonsteroidal anti-inflammatory drugs can result in hyperkalemia.
c. Common ACE inhibitors.
   (1) Captopril.
   (2) Enalapril.
   (3) Benazepril.
   (4) Fosinopril.
   (5) Lisinopril.
   (6) Quinapril.
   (7) Ramipril.

3. Calcium channel blockers.
   a. Result in vasodilatation and decrease in total peripheral resistance by lowering calcium concentrations in vascular smooth muscle cells.
   b. Side effects profile is low in athletes, but cost is higher than diuretics or beta-blockers.
   c. Common agents.
      (1) Verapamil.
      (2) Nifedipine.
      (3) Diltiazem.
      (4) Felodipine.
      (5) Isradipine.
      (6) Nicardipine.
4. Alpha$_1$-adrenergic blockers.
   a. Mechanism of blood pressure lowering: block postsynaptic alpha$_1$-adrenergic smooth muscle receptors and lower total peripheral resistance.
   b. Particularly useful for patients with "syndrome X," hypertensive nephropathy, type II diabetes mellitus, obesity, and hyperlipidemia.
   c. Common agents.
      (1) Prazocin.
      (2) Doxazocin.
      (3) Terazocin.

Bibliography

American College of Sports Medicine: Physical activity, physical fitness and hypertension; position stand, *Med Sci Sports Exerc* 25:i-x, 1993.

American Heart Association: *Heart facts*, Dallas, 1988, AHA.

Boone JB, Levine M, Flynn MG, et al: Opioid receptor modulation of postexercise hypertension, *Med Sci Sports Exerc* 22:S106, 1990.

Davidoff R, Schamroth CL, Goldman AP, et al: Post-exercise blood pressure as a predictor of hypertension, *Aviat Space Environ Med* 53:591-594, 1982.

Dlin RA, Hanne N, Silverberg DS, et al: Follow-up of normotensive men with exaggerated blood pressure response to exercise, *Am Heart J* 106:316-320, 1983.

Gilders RM, Voner C, Dudley GA: Endurance training and blood pressure in normotensive and hypertensive adults, *Med Sci Sports Exerc* 21:629-636, 1989.

Gordon NF: Effect of selective and nonselective beta adrenoreceptor blockade on thermoregulation during prolonged exercise in heat, *Am J Cardiol* 55:74D-78D, 1985.

Harris KA, Holly RG: Physiological response to circuit weight training in borderline hypertensive subjects, *Med Sci Sports Exerc* 19:246-252, 1987.

Jette M, Landry F, Sidney K, et al: Exaggerated blood pressure response to exercise in the detection of hypertension, *J Cardiopulmonary Rehab* 8:171-177, 1988.

Joint National Committee on Detection, Evaluation and Treatment of High Blood Pressure, Coordinating Committee. Fifth report of the Joint National Committee on Detection, Evaluation and

Treatment of High Blood Pressure, Bethesda, MD, 1993, NHLBI, National High Blood Pressure Program.

Kaplan NM: The deadly quartet: upper body obesity, glucose intolerance, hypertriglyceridemia, and hypertension, *Arch Intern Med* 149:1514-1520, 1989.

Kiyonaga A, Arakawa K, Tanaka H, et al: Blood pressure and hormonal response to aerobic exercise, *Hypertension* 7:125-131, 1985.

MacDougall JD, Tuxen D, Sale DG, et al: Arterial blood pressure response to heavy resistance exercise, *J Appl Physiol* 58:785-790, 1985.

Tanji JL, Batt ME: Management of hypertension: adapting new guidelines for active patients, *Phys Sport Med* 23(2):47-55, 1995.

Tanji JL, Champlin JJ, Wong GY, et al: Blood pressure recovery curves after submaximal exercise: a predictor of hypertension at ten-year follow-up, *Am J Hypertens* 2:135-138, 1989.

Tipton CM: Exercise, training and hypertension: an update, *Exerc Sport Sci Rev* 19:447-505, 1991.

Tipton CM, Matthes RD, Marcus KD, et al: Influences of exercise intensity, age and medication on resting systolic blood pressure of SHR populations, *J Appl Physiol* 55:1304-1310, 1983.

Urata H, Tanabe Y, Kiyonaga A, et al: Antihypertensive and volume-depleting effects of mild exercise on essential hypertension, *Hypertension* 9:245-252, 1987.

CHAPTER 3

Exercise Testing and Prescription

Brent S. E. Rich, MD, ATC

I. General Overview
  A. Exercise testing and prescription are useful endeavors for the primary care sports medicine physician. In an office setting with the appropriate equipment the exercise test can be performed easily and with relative safety. Appropriate evaluation of results and recognition of serious conditions will alert the practitioner to early cardiac disease. An exercise prescription can be individualized with the information obtained from the exercise test.

II. Equipment
  A. Exercise devices.
    1. Treadmills.
      a. Most common device for exercise testing and prescription.
      b. Most people are familiar and comfortable with walking.
      c. Speed and slope can be adjusted for test variations.
      d. Side and front rails and emergency stop recommended.
    2. Bicycles.
      a. Most common method in Europe.
      b. Less expensive and takes up less space than treadmills.
      c. Less artifact on electrocardiography (ECG) because trunk is stationary.
      d. More difficult for novice bicycle rider.
    3. Arm ergometer.
      a. Useful for lower extremity–disabled persons.
      b. Often blood pressure readings are higher because of arm workload.
    4. ECG monitor.
      a. Recommended to print 12-lead ECG.
      b. Various brands on market to compile data.
      c. Do not rely on computer-generated ECG results. Clinicians should read all ECG and treadmill tests.

5. Ventilation equipment.
   a. Oxygen update information (Vo_2) can be assessed.
   b. Vo_2 max = the largest amount of oxygen used in the most strenuous exercise.
   c. Vo_2 max highly correlates with maximum cardiac output.
6. Advanced Cardiac Life Support equipment.
   a. Defibrillator and crash cart are strongly recommended.
   b. Establishment of an emergency plan is vital.
   c. It is recommended that personnel trained in cardiopulmonary resuscitation and ACLS conduct the test.
7. Cost.[4]
   a. Treadmill unit cost range = $18,000 to $24,000.
   b. Bicycle unit cost estimate = $13,000.
   c. Treadmill with ventilation system cost estimate = $40,000.
   d. Defibrillator unit cost range = $3000 to $5000.
   e. Average office charge for treadmill testing = $175 to $250.
   f. Medicare reimbursement = $125 to $200.

III. Indications and Contraindications
   A. Indications for exercise testing in a primary care sports medicine setting.
      1. Establishing an exercise prescription in patients who plan to enter a *vigorous* exercise program.
      2. Evaluating chest pain.
      3. Screening for coronary artery disease in asymptomatic men at risk.
      4. Evaluating dysrhythmias.
      5. Determining functional capacity.
      6. Determining the significance of exercise-induced asthma and the response to treatment.
   B. Indications for exercise testing done with or referred to a cardiologist.
      1. Evaluating high-risk patients with known ischemic heart disease.
      2. Evaluating response to antianginal or antihypertensive therapy in high-risk patients.
      3. Evaluation of post–myocardial infarction patients.
   C. Absolute contraindications to exercise testing.[1]
      1. Recent significant change in resting ECG suggestive of infarction or acute cardiac event.
      2. Recent complicated myocardial infarction.
      3. Unstable angina.
      4. Rapid ventricular or atrial dysrhythmia.
      5. Active or suspected myocarditis or pericarditis.
      6. Severe aortic stenosis.
      7. Severe left ventricular dysfunction.
      8. Pulmonary embolism or infarction within the past 3 months.
      9. Recent or active infection.
      10. Significant emotional distress (psychosis).
      11. Third-degree atrioventricular (AV) block.
      12. Thrombophlebitis.
      13. Acute infection.
   D. Relative contraindications to exercise testing.[1]
      1. Clinically significant hypertension (diastolic >120 mmHg or resting systolic >200 mmHg).
      2. Known electrolyte abnormalities (hypokalemia, hypomagnesemia).
      3. Moderate valvular or myocardial heart diseases.
      4. Frequent or complex ventricular ectopy.
      5. Fixed rate artificial pacemaker.

6. Chronic infectious disease (e.g., mononucleosis, hepatitis, acquired immunodeficiency syndrome).
7. Uncontrolled metabolic disease (e.g., diabetes, thyrotoxicosis, myxedema).
8. Neuromuscular, musculoskeletal, or rheumatoid disorders that are exacerbated by exercise.
9. Advanced or complicated pregnancy.

IV. Exercise Protocols
   A. Bruce protocol.
      1. Most common protocol.
      2. Appropriate for active patients because high workloads can be achieved.
      3. Changes occur both in speed and grade with each level.
      4. Rapid increases in workload.
      5. Stage 4 difficult because of speed (in between a walk and run for most patients).
   B. USAFSAM or modified Balke-Ware protocol.
      1. Use a single speed and vary slope between stages.
      2. Better in older/less active patients.
   C. Bicycle ergometry protocol.
      1. Most common is Astrand protocol.
      2. Constant pedaling rate as workload is increased.
      3. Difficult for some patients to maintain fixed pedaling rate.

V. Types of Exercise Tests
   A. Symptom-limited maximal test.
      1. Patient is in control as to when to terminate test.
      2. Maximal heart rate guide = 220 − age.
      3. Use of Borg scale of perceived exertion.
         a. In normal individuals, heart rate will approximate rating of perceived exertion (RPE) × 10 + 20 to 30 beats/min for RPEs of 11 to 16 and heart rates of 130 to 160 (using the original Borg scale).
         b. Numerous studies have demonstrated this scale to be a reproductive measure of exertion.

6		13	Somewhat hard
7	Very, very light	14	
8		15	Hard
9	Very light	16	
10		17	Very hard
11	Fairly light	18	
12		19	Very, very hard
		20	

      4. New rating scale

0	Nothing at all	6	
0.5	Very, very weak	7	Very strong
1	Very weak	8	
2	Weak	9	
3	Moderate	10	Very, very strong
4	Somewhat strong		
5	Strong	*	Maximal exertion

   B. Submaximal test.
      1. Used primarily for post–myocardial infarction patients to establish if they can perform activities of daily living.

2. Naughton protocol most commonly used.
3. Not recommended for exercise prescription or active patients.

VI. Exercise Test
   A. Patient preparation.
      1. Recommend limiting intake, except for usual medications, for 2 to 3 hours prior to the test.
      2. Wear loose-fitting, comfortable clothes.
      3. Shave abundant chest hair.
      4. No body oils or lotion.
      5. Cleanse skin with alcohol before electrode placement.
      6. Tape blood pressure cuff on the patient's arm.
      7. Obtain signed consent form after appropriate explanation of the benefits and risks before performing test.
   B. Baseline ECG.
      1. Preexercise ECG in supine and standing positions is recommended because the axis of the heart changes with position.
         a. Supine = the standard ECG position to use for comparison with past and future ECGs.
         b. Standing = the standard ECG position to use for comparison while the test is in progress.
   C. The exercise treadmill test.
      1. Demonstrate treadmill walking before starting test.
      2. Recommend light grip on bar for balance.
      3. Explain that blood pressure will be checked at every stage.
      4. Remind patient when stage (i.e., speed and slope) will change.
      5. Review the rating scale of perceived exertion.
      6. Review target/maximum heart rate.
      7. Recommend patient to stretch calf muscles before testing on Bruce protocol.
      8. Have patient inform examiner when nearing maximum effort.
      9. Encourage patient during the test.
      10. Monitor patient for 7-10 minutes posttest in supine position.
      11. Auscultate after peak exercise.
   D. Indications for terminating the test.
      1. General indications.
         a. Reaching target/maximum heart rate.
         b. Fatigue.
         c. Leg cramps.
      2. Absolute indications.[1]
         a. Patient's request.
         b. Acute or suspected myocardial infarction.
         c. Decrease in systolic blood pressure with increased workload.
         d. Serious dysrhythmias.
            (1) Second- or third-degree AV block.
            (2) Ventricular tachycardia or fibrillation.
            (3) Sequenced premature ventricular contractions.
            (4) Atrial fibrillation or flutter.
         e. Signs of poor perfusion.
            (1) Pallor.
            (2) Cyanosis.
            (3) Cold or clammy skin.
         f. Central nervous system symptoms.
            (1) Ataxia.
            (2) Vertigo.

(3) Visual or gait problems.
(4) Confusion.
g. Equipment malfunction.
3. Relative indications.[1]
a. Increasing chest pain/angina.
b. Marked (>2 mm) horizontal or downsloping ST segment or elevation.
c. Pronounced wheezing or shortness of breath, indicating exercise-induced asthma.
d. Hypertensive response to exercise (systolic blood pressure >260 mmHg, diastolic blood pressure >115 mmHg).
e. Acute onset of bundle branch block.
f. Supraventricular tachycardia.

VII. Interpretation of the Exercise Test
A. Components of the exercise test report.[5]
1. Reasons for ending test and symptoms.
a. Chest pain.
b. Fatigue.
c. Shortness of breath.
d. Leg cramps.
e. Exercise-induced wheezing/cough.
f. Achievement of maximum heart rate.
2. Heart rate and blood pressure response to exercise.
a. Heart rate should increase in linear fashion with exercise.
b. When heart rate does not rise appropriately, it may be an indicator of coronary artery disease.
c. Systolic blood pressure should increase linearly with exercise.
d. When systolic blood pressure does not rise appropriately, it may indicate ischemia.
e. Diastolic blood pressure should remain about the same throughout the test.
f. A greater than 10 mmHg rise in diastolic response may indicate a hypertensive response to exercise.
g. Double product (heart rate × systolic blood pressure) is an indicator of myocardial oxygen consumption.
3. Dysrhythmias.
a. Abnormal heart rhythm during exercise and in the recovery phase should be noted.
b. Unifocal premature ventricular contractions (PVCs) are not indicative of ischemia.
c. Couplets, multifocal PVCs, and ventricular tachycardia may be indicators of ischemia.
4. Functional aerobic response.
a. If maximal test is achieved, a metabolic equivalent (METS) (milliliters of oxygen per kg per minute) may be assigned and can be used in exercise prescription.
5. ECG response to exercise.
a. Normal response = J point depression and upsloping ST segment that returns to baseline by 80 msec beyond the J point.
(1) J point = area between the end of the QRS and ST segment.
b. Negative test.
(1) No chest pain.
(2) No ST changes.
(3) Exercise >12 minutes or 13 METS = good prognosis.[5]

(4) False-negative sensitivity rate = 75%.[3]

c. Positive test.

(1) Specificity = 80% to 90%.[5]

(2) False-positive rate = 10% to 20%.[5]

(3) Horizontal ST segment depression.

(4) Upsloping ST segment depression.

(5) Downsloping ST segment depression.

B. Exercise treadmill score.[6]

1. Definition: Exercise time (minutes) − (5 × ST deviation [mm]) − (4 × angina index).

2. Angina index.

a. 0 = no angina.

b. 1 = typical angina during exercise.

c. 2 = terminate test because of angina.

3. Four year survival based on score.

Risk	Score	Inpatients	Outpatients
Low	>5	.98	.99
Moderate	−10 to +4	.92	.95
High	<−10	.71	.79

VIII. Indication for Referral to a Cardiologist (i.e., Severe Ischemic Heart Disease)[5]

A. Early positive test.

1. Exercise duration <3 minutes.

2. Heart rate <120.

3. Double product (heart rate × systolic blood pressure) <15,000.

B. Downsloping ST depression.

C. ST depression >2.5 mm.

D. ST depression >8 minutes into recovery.

E. ST elevation in non–Q wave baseline.

F. Hypotensive response to exercise.

G. Significant dysrhythmia.

H. Any significant concern on the part of the patient or practitioner.

IX. Special Indications for Exercise Treadmill Testing of Athletes[10]

A. Sudden cardiac death (SCD) in athletes is rare.[9]

B. Coronary artery disease is the most common cause of SCD in athletes over the age of 30.

C. Screening tests for SCD are not indicated.[9]

D. There are variations in the heart's adaptation to exercise between different sports (e.g., the athletic heart syndrome).[9]

1. Isotonic exercise = cardiac dilatation.

2. Isometric exercise = cardiac wall thickening.

3. Pearls:

a. Blood pressure is usually normal.

b. Sinus bradycardia is common.

c. Sinus arrhythmia or ectopic beats that disappear with exercise are unremarkable.

d. 3rd and 4th heart sounds and systolic ejection murmurs are common.

e. First-degree and second-degree (Mobitz type I) AV blocks are often reported.

f. Ventricular enlargement occurs with exercise.

E. Bruce protocol indicated for testing.

X. Exercise Prescription
   A. Pearls:
      1. Physical activity: "any bodily movement produced by skeletal muscles that results in energy expenditure."[2]
      2. Exercise (a physical activity subset): "planned, structured, and repetitive bodily movement done to improve or maintain one or more components of physical fitness."[2]
      3. It has been estimated that 250,000 deaths per year in the United States may be due to lack of physical activity.[7]
      4. Most common reason for not exercising = lack of time.
      5. The physician's responsibility is to encourage regular physical activity as a life-style change for patients.
   B. 1995 recommendation from the Centers for Disease Control and Prevention and the American College of Sports Medicine.[8]
      1. Physical activity health benefits are proportionate to the total amount of minutes exercising or total calories expended.
      2. Every U.S. adult should engage in 30 minutes or more of moderate-intensity (i.e., 3-6 METS or 200 calories per day) physical activity on most days of the week.
      3. Intermittent bouts of activity (i.e., 8-10 minutes) to accumulate the 30 minute total are acceptable (i.e., a single bout of 30 minute continuous exercise is not required).
      4. A formal exercise program is not necessary (e.g., a 2 mile walk at 3-4 mile per hour pace is sufficient).
      5. Flexibility and muscle strengthening activities are additional components in a physical activity program.
      6. Benefits of physical activity.
         a. Lower cardiovascular disease incidence and mortality.
         b. Reduction of body fat.
         c. Improved psychological state.
         d. Resistance to disease, stress, and injury.
      7. It is not necessary for most adults to see a physician before starting a *moderate* physical activity program.
      8. Men >40 and women >50 years or individuals with chronic disease or risk factors for chronic disease who plan a *vigorous* exercise program (>60% of personal maximum oxygen consumption) should see their physician for evaluation and medical clearance.[1]

References

1. American College of Sports Medicine: *Guidelines for Exercise Testing and Prescription,* ed 4, Philadelphia, 1991, Lea & Febiger.
2. Caspersen CJ, Powell KE, Christenson GM: Physical activity, exercise, and physical fitness, *Public Health Rep* 100:125-131, 1985.
3. Detrano R, Froelicher VF: Exercise testing: uses and limitations considering recent studies, *Prog Cardiovasc Dis* 31:173-204, 1988.
4. Evans CH, Karunaratne HB: Exercise stress testing for the family physician: Part I. Performing the test, *Am Fam Physician* 45(1):121-132, 1992.
5. Evans CH, Karunaratne HB: Exercise stress testing for the family physician: Part II. Interpretation of the results, *Am Fam Physician* 45(2):679-688, 1992.
6. Mark DB et al: Exercise treadmill score for predicting prognosis in coronary artery disease, *N Engl J Med* 325:849-853, 1991.
7. McGinnis JM, Foege WH: Actual causes of death in the United States, *JAMA* 270:2207-2212, 1993.
8. Pate RR et al: Physical activity and public health. A recommendation from the Centers for Disease Control and Prevention and the American College of Sports Medicine, *JAMA* 273:402-407, 1995.
9. Rich BSE: Sudden death screening, *Med Clin North Am* 76:267-288, 1994.
10. Rink LD, Knowlan DM: Exercise treadmill testing in athletes. In Waller BF, Harvey WP, editors: *Cardiovascular Evaluation of Athletes. Toward Recognizing Young Athletes at Risk of Sudden Death,* Newton, NJ, 1993, Laennec Publishing.

CHAPTER 4

Cardiac Arrhythmias in the Athlete

Steven R. Neish, MD

Steven P. Van Camp, MD, FACSM, FACC

I. Overview
   A. Arrhythmias in athletes are common. Many findings that could be interpreted as abnormal using strict criteria can probably be considered normal in the trained athlete.
   B. Arrhythmias are not completely benign, however. Arrhythmias can be associated with syncope, sudden death, or limitations of exercise performance. This is especially true when the arrhythmias are associated with heart disease (e.g., coronary artery disease, postoperative congenital heart disease, myocarditis, cardiomyopathy).
   C. Arrhythmias likely to cause severe symptoms (e.g., syncope, sudden death) are those that cause extreme bradycardia or tachycardia. This includes complete atrioventricular (AV) block, ventricular tachycardia, and atrial flutter/fibrillation with a rapid ventricular response. Cardiac output (Q) is the product of heart rate (beats per minute) and stroke volume (milliliters of blood per beat). During extreme bradycardia the heart rate is insufficient regardless of the magnitude of the stroke volume. This is particularly true if the onset of bradycardia is acute. During excessive tachycardia the amount of time spent in diastole shortens so that ventricular filling is limited. This decreases stroke volume by sufficient magnitude that cardiac output drops irrespective of the increase in heart rate.

II. Effect of Exercise on Cardiac Rhythm
   A. Increase in heart rate is initially due to withdrawal of parasympathetic tone, followed by sympathetic predominance (circulating catecholamines and direct sympathetic stimulation).
   B. Changes in autonomic tone increase the rate of depolarization of the sinoatrial node, enhance AV conduction, and increase the rate of ventricular repolarization.
   C. Changes in the electrical properties of the heart play a prominent role in increasing myocardial oxygen consumption.

D. Effects in the abnormal heart.
  1. Ectopic focus may be suppressed as the depolarization of the sinus node increases, thereby suppressing the arrhythmia.
  2. Increased sympathetic tone may increase the depolarization rate of an ectopic atrial or ventricular focus, inducing a tachyarrhythmia.
  3. Catecholamines may increase delayed afterdepolarizations, leading to ventricular tachycardia.
  4. If there is cardiac hypertrophy or coronary artery disease, the increase in myocardial oxygen consumption/demand may not be matched by an increase in myocardial blood flow and myocardial oxygen delivery. This leads to ischemia and possible arrhythmia.

III. Normal Cardiac Rhythm in the Athlete
A. Effects of chronic exercise on cardiac rhythm.
  1. Lower resting heart rate and lower heart rate at submaximal exercise.
  2. Generally, peak heart rate is unchanged with training. (Workload at peak exercise usually increases with training, however.)
B. Arrhythmias associated with training. All of the following are normal effects of training on cardiac rhythm.
  1. Sinus bradycardia, wandering atrial pacemaker, and sinus pauses.
  2. Escape rhythms. Abnormal atrial focus, junctional rhythm, and idioventricular rhythm.
  3. AV conduction delay. First-degree and type I second-degree (Wenckebach) AV blocks are common. Type I second-degree AV block occurs in up to 40% of athletes evaluated with ambulatory electrocardiography.
  4. Premature ventricular complexes.
C. Athletes present special circumstances.
  1. Most competitive athletes are young and without heart disease, but they are involved in high intensity activities. High levels of mental stress typically accompany competition. If heart disease is present, it may not be apparent without investigation.
  2. We now see older athletes in their 70s, 80s, and even 90s in masters' competitions.
  3. Testing to provoke arrhythmias and to assess therapeutic efficacy should be tailored to the athlete's specific type of activity.
  4. Tests may need to be repeated, because training (or detraining) may affect cardiac rhythm.
  5. Compliance of athletes with therapeutic regimens is often less than ideal.
  6. The use of some drugs (e.g., beta-blockers) for treatment of arrhythmias may lead to disqualification by certain athletic governing authorities.

IV. 26th Bethesda Conference: Recommendations for Determining Eligibility for Competition in Athletes with Cardiovascular Abnormalities
A. The recommendations made by this conference serve as the framework for much of what follows. The conference was sponsored by the American College of Cardiology and the American College of Sports Medicine.
B. Recommendations for determining eligibility for athletes with cardiovascular abnormalities must be made considering the type of cardiovascular abnormality, its pathophysiologic severity, and the physiologic demands of the sport in which the athlete competes.
C. Address for reprints: American College of Cardiology, 9111 Old Georgetown Road, Bethesda, MD 20814. Attention: ACCEL Department.

V. Evaluation of the Athlete with Symptoms of Arrhythmia
   A. All arrhythmia symptoms.
      1. History regarding prodrome, presence of possible arrhythmia, medication usage, inciting events, family history of heart disease, syncope, or sudden death.
      2. Cardiovascular physical examination.
      3. Electrocardiography (ECG).
   B. Bradycardia.
      1. 24-hour ambulatory electrocardiogram.
   C. Tachycardia.
      1. 24-hour ambulatory electrocardiogram.
      2. Maximal, symptom-limited exercise test, especially if symptoms occur during exercise.
      3. Event monitor, if 24-hour ECG is normal or if symptoms are rare.
   D. Additional testing.
      1. If structural heart disease is suspected, evaluation should continue with echocardiography.
      2. In some cases, further testing beyond echocardiography will be necessary. This can include:
         a. Cardiac catheterization.
         b. Cardiac angiography.
         c. Coronary angiography.
         d. Endomyocardial biopsy.
         e. Electrophysiologic testing.

VI. Supraventricular Arrhythmias
   A. Bradycardia: resting bradycardia is extremely common in trained athletes. It is unusual for it to be of clinical significance.
      1. Sinus node dysfunction with sinus bradycardia. Without symptoms, resting sinus bradycardia with rates as low as 30 beats/minute can be thought of as normal.
      2. Indications for further investigation.
         1. Sinus pause >3 seconds.
         2. Sinoatrial exit block.
         3. Sick sinus syndrome (excessive bradycardia inducing atrial tachyarrhythmias).
      3. Further investigation. 24-hour ECG, exercise test, and echocardiography. If there is syncope, consider intracardiac electrophysiology testing.
      4. Recommendations.
         a. Isolated bradycardia may disappear with detraining.
         b. Symptomatic bradycardia may require placement of a permanent pacemaker.
         c. Asymptomatic bradycardia without evidence of underlying heart disease requires no treatment and no restrictions.
   B. Atrial flutter: usually associated with underlying heart disease. AV conduction typically improves during exercise so the ventricular rate may increase to dangerously high rates.
      1. Definition: regular sawtooth atrial flutter waves at a rate of 250–350 bpm. There is frequently decremental AV conduction where all atrial impulses do not penetrate through the AV node to reach the ventricle. The ventricular rate is typically ½ to ⅓ of the atrial rate. If there is 1:1 AV conduction, symptoms are often severe.
      2. Further investigation: athletes with atrial flutter should have a complete investigation to include echocardiography, 24-hour ECG, and exercise testing.

3. Recommendations.
   a. If the atrial flutter is controlled and there is underlying heart disease, low-intensity competition is allowed after 6 months without atrial flutter.
   b. If the heart is normal and the atrial flutter is no longer present whether or not treatment has been given, full competition can resume after 3 to 6 months.
   c. If the heart is normal and the ventricular rate is controlled by medication so that the heart rate is not above the appropriate normal sinus rate during exercise, patients can participate in low-intensity sports.
   d. Patients with uncontrolled atrial flutter should not exercise.

C. Atrial fibrillation: most common chronic arrhythmia in older adults. It also seems to be relatively common in adult athletes. Most often, it occurs in association with coronary artery disease or ventricular hypertrophy associated with systemic hypertension. It also occurs in patients with valvular disease, thyrotoxicosis, and metabolic derangements (e.g., hypokalemia). Substance abuse (e.g., alcohol, cocaine) may also be a cause.
   1. Definition: a disorganized rapid atrial arrhythmia. Classically, the ventricular rhythm is irregularly irregular.
   2. Further investigation: Investigation for underlying cardiac disease, including ECG and echocardiography, and evaluation for metabolic derangements. Also 24-hour ambulatory ECG may be done to evaluate the ventricular rate response.
   3. Recommendations.
      a. If there is no heart disease and the ventricular response to atrial fibrillation is controlled, all competition is permitted.
      b. If there is structural heart disease and the ventricular response is not excessive, the athlete should be limited according to recommendations based on the structural heart disease.
      c. If the patient is anticoagulated, sports with body collision should be avoided.

D. Paroxysmal supraventricular tachycardia. There are several different types. Patients with Wolff-Parkinson-White syndrome are treated differently than are patients without manifest preexcitation. Treatment may involve medications or radiofrequency ablation of the tachycardia circuit.
   1. Definitions.
      a. Supraventricular tachycardia: a rapid regular tachyarrhythmia resulting from an abnormal mechanism originating proximal to the bifurcation of the bundle of His, which does not have the morphology of atrial flutter.
      b. Wolff-Parkinson-White syndrome: criteria for diagnosis are (1) a PR interval that is shorter than normal for age and (2) a QRS complex with initial slurring (e.g., delta wave).
   2. Normal resting ECG (no preexcitation). The two most common mechanisms are AV node reentry and AV reentry over a concealed accessory connection.
      a. Further investigation: a 12-lead ECG. Demonstration of the tachycardia via 24-hour ambulatory ECG, exercise testing, and/or electrophysiology testing, either transesophageal or intracardiac. If intracardiac electrophysiology testing is performed, radiofrequency ablation of the tachycardia circuit should be considered.
      b. Recommendations.

(1) If supraventricular tachycardia does not develop during exercise, whether or not treatment is being given, competition can be unlimited.

(2) If there are severe symptoms, exercise should be restricted until treatment is commenced and there are no symptoms for 6 months.

3. Wolff-Parkinson-White syndrome: ventricular preexcitation associated with episodic supraventricular tachycardia. The typical tachycardia circuit involves conduction from the atria to the ventricles in the normal fashion through the atrioventricular node and the His-Purkinje system. This is followed by conduction from one of the ventricles to the atria through an accessory connection. Traversing the circuit in this direction causes narrow complex supraventricular tachycardia, known as orthodromic tachycardia. The pathway of the electricity can also be the opposite of that course. There is also a wide complex tachycardia known as antidromic tachycardia. Both of these tachycardias only rarely cause syncope or sudden death. An increased incidence of atrial flutter and atrial fibrillation is seen in Wolff-Parkinson-White syndrome. If the antegrade effective refractory period of the accessory pathway is sufficiently short, impulses can pass down the accessory pathway during atrial flutter/fibrillation frequently enough to induce ventricular tachycardia and ventricular fibrillation. This is associated with syncope and sudden death.

a. Further investigation.

(1) A 12-lead ECG and a 24-hour ambulatory ECG (preferably during athletic activity). Echocardiography can be used to look for associated structural cardiovascular abnormalities. An exercise test will show if exercise induces supraventricular tachycardia. Also, if the delta wave and the PR interval disappear during exercise, the antegrade effective refractory period of the accessory connection is probably long.

(2) If there are no symptoms and no structural heart disease, no further evaluation is necessary.

(3) If there are symptoms, the effective refractory period of the accessory connection should be measured. This can be done with a transesophageal pacing study in many patients. In others an intracardiac electrophysiology study is required.

(4) Some recommend intracardiac electrophysiology testing in all athletes with ventricular preexcitation. If this is performed, radiofrequency ablation of the accessory connection should also be considered at the same procedure.

b. Recommendations.

(1) Adult athletes with no symptoms and a normal heart can participate in all activities.

(2) Children and adolescents with ventricular preexcitation have less clearly defined risks, even in the absence of symptoms. Therefore, determination of their effective refractory period should be done, even in those without symptoms.

(3) If there is supraventricular tachycardia, the effective refractory period should be determined during exercise or isoproterenol infusion to accurately determine the pathway characteristics during exercise.

(4) In patients with a history of atrial flutter/fibrillation whose maximum ventricular rate during episodes is less than 240

bpm and who do not have a history of syncope or near syncope, the risk of sudden death appears to be low. They can participate in all sports.

(5) If the ventricular rate during atrial flutter/fibrillation is high or there is syncope or near syncope, athletes should be restricted to low-intensity sports. Additionally, radiofrequency ablation should be offered in most cases.

(6) If radiofrequency ablation (or surgical ablation) is successful and there is no tachycardia on followup electrophysiology testing or no tachycardia on long-term followup, the athlete can return to all competitive athletics.

E. Sinus node reentry tachycardia or atrial tachycardia. Evaluation is similar to patients with atrial flutter, although the likelihood of underlying heart disease is less, especially in younger athletes.

1. If the heart is normal and exercise does not induce an excessively high ventricular rate (over the normal maximum exercise heart rate for age), unlimited competition is allowed.
2. If the heart is normal, restrictions should be made based on the underlying heart disease.

VII. Abnormalities of AV Conduction

A. AV block describes a group of conditions that have in common delayed or absent AV conduction. In many athletes, this is simply due to cardiovascular fitness and high resting parasympathetic tone. Alternatively, it can be due to significant cardiac disease with damage to the AV node or His-Purkinje system. This is particularly true with certain more advanced types of AV block.

B. First-degree atrioventricular block. This is a common situation in endurance-trained athletes.

1. Definition: PR interval longer than the upper limit of normal for age.
2. Further investigation: if the 12-lead ECG is otherwise normal, no further evaluation is necessary. If the PR interval is markedly prolonged (≥300 msec) a 24-hour ambulatory ECG, exercise test, and echocardiogram should be performed. If there is further evidence of severe AV node pathology, electrophysiology testing should be performed to determine the site of conduction delay to allow prediction of future course and the possibility of progression to more severe degrees of AV block.
3. Recommendation: if there are no symptoms, no structural heart disease, and no worsening of AV block during exercise, all competition is permitted.

C. Mobitz Type I (Wenckebach) second-degree AV block. This is frequently present in trained athletes.

1. Definition: progressive prolongation of the PR interval before a non-conducted P wave.
2. Further investigation: 12-lead ECG, exercise test, and echocardiogram should be performed. A 24-hour ambulatory ECG during exercise may be useful.
3. Recommendations.
   a. If the above testing is normal except for the presence of Wenckebach, all competition is allowed.
   b. If the heart is abnormal but AV block disappears with exercise, all competition is allowed, depending on the severity of the underlying heart disease.
   c. If the AV block worsens with exercise or during the immediate postexercise recovery period, only low-intensity sports are al-

lowed. Intracardiac electrophysiology testing to determine the site of AV block should be performed. Affected athletes may benefit from permanent pacemaker implantation.

D. Congenital complete AV block. Rarely, an infant is born with AV block. This can be due to structural heart disease or to maternal collagen vascular disease. In some patients this is an asymptomatic situation.
   1. Definition of complete AV block: complete lack of transmission of atrial electrical impulses to the ventricles.
   2. Further investigation: An echocardiogram to look at heart size and to look for associated structural heart disease. A 12-lead ECG, 24-hour ambulatory ECG including a period during exercise, and an exercise test should be performed.
   3. Recommendations.
      a. If the heart is structurally and functionally normal, there is no syncope or near syncope, the QRS complex is narrow, the heart rate at rest is at least 40 bpm, the heart rate increases with exercise, and there are only rare or occasional premature ventricular complexes, all competition is allowed.
      b. If there is significant ventricular arrhythmia, symptoms, an excessively low heart rate at rest, or structural heart disease, a permanent pacemaker should be implanted.

E. Acquired complete AV block or Mobitz type II second-degree AV block. These conduction abnormalities occur in patients with coronary artery disease, myocarditis, and cardiomyopathy and those that have undergone cardiac surgery.
   1. Definition: type II second-degree AV block is a sudden failure of AV conduction without prolongation of the PR interval before the nonconducted P wave.
   2. Recommendation: These patients have an unacceptable rate of sudden death and should have a permanent pacemaker implanted, irrespective of competition. Type II second-degree AV block can advance to complete AV block without warning. Most experts recommend that all of these patients have permanent pacemaker implantation. Certainly a pacemaker should be in place before competition.

F. Pacemaker implantation. Patients with a permanent pacemaker should avoid sports with a danger of body collision to avoid damage to the pulse generator or pacemaker leads. Exercise ECG can help to assess pacemaker function during athletic activity. This can be useful to ensure that proper pacemaker settings and proper pacing mode are programmed in relation to the type of exercise performed.

VIII. Ventricular Arrhythmias

A. Premature ventricular complexes. Trained athletes often have a low resting sinus node rate. In this situation, ventricular escape beats frequently appear as premature ventricular complexes (PVCs). Typically, these disappear with exercise. PVCs can be a sign of underlying cardiac disease or a harbinger of more serious ventricular arrhythmia in the presence of underlying heart disease. Nevertheless, PVCs usually confer no added risk to athletes during competition. The frequency of PVCs may be increased by stress, sleep deprivation, caffeine, or alcohol. Only uniform single PVCs should be considered potentially normal.
   1. Definition: QRS complexes originating in the ventricular myocardium. They are not preceded by a P wave and tend to have a prolonged QRS duration.
   2. Further investigation.

a. Maximal exercise testing should be performed. The PVCs should disappear during exercise. Serious ventricular arrhythmias may manifest only at peak exercise, so a submaximal test that shows disappearance of PVCs is not completely reassuring. Return of PVCs during recovery is normal.
b. If structural heart disease is suggested by history, physical examination, 12-lead ECG, or exercise testing, further evaluation is necessary. Echocardiography, cardiac catheterization and angiography, and electrophysiologic testing should be considered.

3. Recommendations.
a. Athletes with a normal heart, no symptoms, and only single, uniform PVCs can compete without restriction.
b. Athletes with PVCs who have structural heart disease have an increased risk of sudden death and can only compete in low-intensity sports.

B. Ventricular tachycardia. Ventricular tachycardia is associated with a variety of conditions with ventricular muscle disease. These include coronary artery disease, dilated or hypertrophic cardiomyopathy, myocarditis, and postoperative congenital heart disease. In some cases the only sign of cardiac disease on noninvasive evaluation is the ventricular arrhythmia.

1. Definition: ventricular tachycardia is defined as three or more consecutive complexes that originate in the ventricular myocardium at a rate greater than the age-appropriate upper limit of the normal sinus rate. In adults this rate is 100 bpm. This should never be considered a variation of normal.
2. Further investigation.
a. Maximal exercise testing, 24-hour ambulatory ECG, and echocardiography.
b. Additionally, many experts recommend cardiac catheterization, endomyocardial biopsy, and intracardiac electrophysiologic testing.
3. Recommendations.
a. Athletes with ventricular tachycardia should avoid competition for 6 months following the last episode of ventricular tachycardia. This is true regardless of the etiology of the tachycardia and regardless of treatment. Before their reentry into competition, exercise testing and electrophysiologic study are recommended.
b. An exception to the above recommendation is the athlete with a normal heart; short (<10 beats), monomorphic, nonsustained episodes of ventricular tachycardia with a rate less than 150 beats per minute; and no symptoms. If exercise testing and ambulatory ECG during exercise do not show more serious ventricular arrhythmia, unlimited competition may be considered.

C. Ventricular fibrillation. This condition is almost uniformly associated with heart disease.

1. Definition: disorganized ventricular electrical activity without identifiable ventricular complexes on surface ECG.
2. Further investigation: similar to that for patients with ventricular tachycardia.
3. Recommendations: no competition is allowed for at least 6 months following the last episode of ventricular fibrillation. At that time only competition in low-intensity sports is allowed.

D. Long QT syndrome.
  1. Definition: corrected QT interval ≥460 msec suggests the presence of long QT syndrome. Nevertheless, some patients with the syndrome have a normal QT interval, and some without the syndrome have a statistically abnormal QT interval. The corrected QT interval is the QT duration divided by the square root of the RR interval.
  2. Recommendation: Patients with long QT syndrome, even those who are treated, have an increased risk of sudden death during athletic activity. These patients should avoid all competitive sports.

E. Automatic implantable cardioverter defibrillator (AICD). Patients with recurrent sudden death and ventricular arrhythmia may have an AICD implanted. Even if the AICD appears to successfully abort the arrhythmia, exercise may not be safe. There are little data regarding the ability of an AICD to terminate a potentially fatal arrhythmia during the stress of exercise.

IX. Syncope

A. Syncope and near syncope are common phenomena. There is a long list of causes of syncope. Syncope can be a clue to the presence of circulatory insufficiency due to cardiac disease. The most common type of syncope in athletes, particularly young athletes, is neurally mediated syncope. This entity exists in different forms and is known by many names. These include vasovagal syncope, cardioinhibitory syncope, autonomic dysfunction, and beta-adrenergic hypersensitivity.

B. Syncope that occurs during active exercise is more ominous. Investigation of patients affected frequently reveals a cardiac cause of syncope. On the other hand, syncope following exercise is most typically neurally mediated syncope.

C. Cardiac causes of syncope.
  1. Hypertrophic cardiomyopathy.
    a. Ventricular arrhythmia (probably the most common cause of syncope and sudden death in patients with hypertrophic cardiomyopathy).
    b. Left ventricular outflow tract obstruction (a rare cause of syncope).
    c. AV block.
    d. Atrial arrhythmias with rapid AV conduction.
  2. Coronary artery disease.
    a. Atherosclerosis.
    b. Anomalies of coronary artery origin or course.
  3. Long QT syndrome.
  4. Wolff-Parkinson-White syndrome. This implies a short antegrade effective refractory period of the accessory connection.
  5. Right ventricular dysplasia or right ventricular cardiomyopathy.
  6. Dilated cardiomyopathy.
  7. Myocarditis.
  8. Congenital heart disease.
    a. Postoperative congenital heart disease.
      (1) Tetralogy of Fallot.
      (2) Transposition of the great arteries.
      (3) Fontan procedure for single ventricle physiology.
    b. Severe unoperated congenital heart disease.
      (1) Aortic stenosis.

   (2) Tetralogy of Fallot.
   (3) Eisenmenger's syndrome.

D. Evaluation.
   1. History and physical examination. Usually these are the most helpful in making a diagnosis. Patients with neurally mediated syncope typically have a short prodrome, allowing them to sit or protect themselves from potential injury while fainting. They recover quickly once they are supine. They have recurrent episodes of lightheadedness, near syncope, and syncope. Physical examination is normal.
   2. ECG. Although the resting ECG is not sufficiently sensitive to detect all heart disease, careful examination will reveal abnormalities in the majority of patients who have a cardiac cause of syncope.
   3. 24-hour ambulatory ECG. The utility of the test in this setting is undefined. It should be used if there is abnormal tachycardia or bradycardia in association with altered consciousness.
   4. Echocardiography. If there is a family history of cardiomyopathy or signs of structural heart disease, this test is useful. Some physicians use it in all cases of syncope because the signs of cardiomyopathy can be cryptic. Physical examination may be normal, and no abnormalities or only subtle abnormalities may be apparent on the 12-lead ECG, even in the presence of hypertrophic or dilated cardiomyopathy.
   5. Tilt table testing. Although this test can elicit syncope and demonstrate abnormalities in heart rate and/or blood pressure in association with syncope, the reliability of this test as a useful diagnostic tool is uncertain. The positive and the negative predictive value of this test is sufficiently low so that this test cannot be used in isolation. Also, a positive test does not eliminate the possibility of life-threatening heart disease as a cause of syncope. Patients with life-threatening cardiac disease frequently have a "positive" tilt test. Before relying on the results of tilt table testing to help in diagnosis or management of a patient with syncope, cardiac causes of syncope should be excluded.
   6. Intracardiac electrophysiology testing. Without supportive evidence for arrhythmia this test rarely adds to the evaluation of a patient with syncope.

E. Recommendation: In a patient with syncope, exercise and competition should be restricted until a cause for the syncope has been identified. At that point recommendations should be made based on the underlying condition.

Bibliography

Biffi A et al: Usefulness of transesophageal pacing during exercise for evaluating palpitations in top-level athletes, *Am J Cardiol* 72:922-926, 1993.

Bjornstad H, Storstein L, Meen HD, Hals O: Ambulatory electrocardiographic findings in top athletes, athletic students, and control subjects, *Cardiology* 84:42-50, 1994.

Coumel P, Leenhardt A, Haddad G: Exercise ECG: prognostic implications of exercise induced arrhythmias, *PACE Pacing Clin Electrophysiol* 17:417-427, 1994.

Huston TP, Puffer JC, Rodney WM: The athletic heart syndrome, *N Engl J Med* 313:24-32, 1985.

Maron BJ, Mitchell JH: 26th Bethesda Conference: recommendations for determining eligibility for competition in athletes with cardiovascular abnormalities, *Med Sci Sports Exerc* 26:S223-S283, 1994.

Maurer MS, Shefrin EA, Fleg JL: Prevalence and prognostic significance of exercise-induced supraventricular tachycardia in apparently healthy volunteers, *Am J Cardiol* 75:788-792, 1995.

National Heart, Lung, and Blood Institute Working Group on Atrial Fibrillation: Atrial fibrillation: current understandings and research imperatives, *J Am Coll Cardiol* 22:1830-1834, 1993.

Neish SR, Freidman RA, Bricker JT: Exercise testing in patients with arrhythmias, *Pediatr Exerc Sci* 2:230-248, 1990.

Pelliccia A, Maron BJ: Preparticipation cardiovascular evaluation of the competitive athlete: perspectives from the 30-year Italian experience, *Am J Cardiol* 75:827-829, 1995.

Wisser WL et al: Cardiac dysrhythmias and sports, *Pediatrics* 95:786-788, 1995.

Zehender MT, Meinertz T, Keul J, Just H: ECG variants and cardiac arrhythmias in athletes: clinical relevance and prognostic importance, *Am Heart J* 119:1378-1391, 1990.

Zipes DP: Specific arrhythmias: diagnosis and treatment. In Braunwald E, editor: *Heart Diseases: A Textbook of Cardiovascular Medicine,* ed 4. Philadelphia, 1992, WB Saunders, pp 667-725.

CHAPTER 5

Sudden Death in Athletes

Steven P. Van Camp, MD, FACSM, FACC

I. Sudden Death
   A. Nontraumatic, unexpected death occurring instantaneously or within a few minutes of an abrupt change in a subject's clinical state.
   B. Generally excludes thermal injuries and drug-related deaths.

II. Sudden Death in Young Athletes (<30 years)
   A. Incidence: approximately 10–25 individuals per year in organized U.S. high school and college athletics.
   B. Predominantly males, unknown reasons.
   C. Structural, usually congenital, heart disease found on autopsy.
   D. Myocardial disorders.
      1. Hypertrophic cardiomyopathy (HCM).
         a. Most common cause of sudden death in young athletes.
         b. Genetic disorder.
         c. Hypertrophied, nondilated left ventricle in the absence of a cardiac or systemic disorder that produces left ventricular hypertrophy.
         d. Interventricular septum ≥15 mm with left ventricular free wall thickness normal or increased.
         e. Myocardial cellular disarray and abnormally thickened intramural coronary arteries with narrowed lumens may also be present.
         f. Diagnosis made by echocardiography.
         g. Symptoms may include syncope, chest discomfort, and dyspnea, although many individuals are asymptomatic.
         h. Murmur (if present): harsh, midsystolic, crescendo-decrescendo, heard best at left lower scapular border or apex. May be labile in intensity. Classically, though not invariably, it increases with increased contractility, decreased preload, and/or decreased afterload.
      2. Dilated cardiomyopathy.
      3. Myocarditis.
         a. Difficult to detect.
         b. Associated viral illness ± chest pain, electrocardiography (ECG) changes.

4. Right ventricular cardiomyopathy.
5. Nonspecific cardiomyopathy.

E. Coronary artery disorders.
   1. Congenital coronary artery anomalies.
      a. Any anomaly that may produce myocardial ischemia.
      b. Usually asymptomatic, may cause chest discomfort or syncope.
      c. Abnormal origins (including acute angulations) and/or courses (including passage between pulmonary artery and aorta).
      d. Anomalous origin of left coronary artery from right sinus of Valsalva; Most common coronary artery anomaly causing exertional SD.
      e. Anomalous origin of right coronary artery from left sinus of Valsalva.
      f. Coronary artery hypoplasia.
      g. Tunneled coronary arteries; precise role undefined.
   2. Atherosclerotic coronary artery disease (CAD). Rare, probably occurs only in presence of lipid abnormalities in young athletes.

F. Valvular disorders.
   1. Congenital aortic stenosis. Harsh, midsystolic murmur (usually grade 3 or louder).
   2. Mitral valve prolapse (MVP). Considered benign unless associated with:
      a. History of syncope.
      b. Family history of SD due to MVP.
      c. High grade premature ventricular complexes.
      d. Moderate or severe mitral regurgitation.
      e. Marfan's syndrome.

G. Aortic disorders.
   1. Aortic dissection and/or rupture due to Marfan's syndrome.
   2. Marfan's syndrome.
      a. Inherited disorder (typically autosomal dominant) of connective tissue due to mutations in fibrillin gene (chromosome 15q15-21).
      b. Aortic weakening, aortic aneurysm formation; subsequent dissection or rupture may be fatal.
      c. Musculoskeletal abnormalities.
         (1) Arm span > height.
         (2) Chest wall deformities.
         (3) Arachnodactyly.
      d. Cardiovascular abnormalities:
         (1) Aortic dilatation.
         (2) Aortic insufficiency.
         (3) Mitral valve prolapse.
      e. Contact or collision sports should be avoided.
      f. If aortic root normal, possibly selected sports (see section on Bethesda 26 Conference).

H. Electrophysiologic disorders.
   1. Wolff-Parkinson-White syndrome.
   2. Idiopathic long QT syndrome.
   3. Cardiac conduction system abnormalities.

I. Other congenital heart diseases (depends on the type and the pathophysiologic abnormalities).

J. Noncardiovascular conditions.
   1. Exertional hyperthermia.
   2. Exertional rhabdomyolysis and sickle cell trait.

3. Status asthmaticus and exercise-induced anaphylaxis.

III. Sudden Death in Mature and Older Athletes (>30 years)
  A. CAD
    1. Most common cause.
    2. Usually risk factors for CAD are present; may have prior history of CAD.
    3. May occur in asymptomatic individuals with high levels of fitness.
  B. Other causes in small minority of cases.

IV. Medical Screening
  A. Contraindications to vigorous exercise.
    1. Hypertrophic cardiomyopathy.
    2. Dilated cardiomyopathy.
    3. Right ventricular cardiomyopathy.
    4. Acute myocarditis.
    5. Significant coronary artery anomalies.
    6. CAD.
    7. Marfan's syndrome.
    8. Uncontrolled hypertension.
    9. Congestive heart failure.
    10. Coarctation of the aorta.
    11. Severe valvular heart disease (aortic stenosis [AS], pulmonic stenosis [PS]).
    12. Idiopathic long QT syndrome.
    13. Complex ventricular arrhythmias.
    14. Cyanotic congenital heart disease.
    15. Pulmonary hypertension.
  B. Relative contraindications.
    1. Uncontrolled atrial arrhythmias.
    2. Hemodynamically significant valvular heart disease (mitral stenosis [MS], mitral regurgitation [MR], aortic insufficiency [AI]).
  C. Screening for these abnormalities accomplished through the standard history and physical examination with special attention to:
    1. History—symptoms of exercise intolerance, exertional chest discomfort, syncope, near syncope, palpitations.
    2. Family history—sudden death, syncope, premature CAD.
    3. Physical examination—blood pressure, cardiac auscultation, body habitus suggestive of Marfan's syndrome.
    4. Additional tests if clinically indicated.
      a. Serum lipids.
      b. Resting ECG.
      c. Exercise stress test.
      d. Echocardiogram.
    5. Consider exercise stress test before starting a vigorous exercise program in individuals with multiple or severe risk factors for CAD or exertional symptoms.
  D. Athletic heart syndrome.
    1. Changes on physical examination, ECG, etc. that reflect adaptations to training rather than organic heart disease.
    2. Bradycardia, Gallop rhythms (S_3, S_4), innocent flow murmurs.
    3. Chest x-ray, echocardiogram: cardiac enlargement.
    4. ECG.
      a. Sinus bradycardia ± sinus arrhythmia (1st and 2nd degree) (Wenckebach type) atrioventricular block.
      b. P wave: right atrial enlargement (RAE), left atrial enlargement (LAE).

c. QRS: increased voltage ± interventricular conduction delay.
d. STT changes: early repolarization, juvenile T wave pattern, abnormal response to exercise.

V. Bethesda Conference 26: Recommendations for Determining Eligibility for Competition in Athletes with Cardiovascular Abnormalities
   A. Sponsored by the American College of Cardiology and American College of Sports Medicine.
   B. Published in the *Journal of the American College of Cardiology* (October 1994) and *Medicine and Science in Sports and Exercise* (October 1994).
   C. Recommendations for determining eligibility for athletes with cardiovascular abnormalities must be made considering the type of cardiovascular abnormality, its pathophysiologic severity, and the physiologic demands of the sport in which the athlete competes.
   D. Address for reprints: American College of Cardiology, 9111 Old Georgetown Road, Bethesda, MD 20814. Attention: ACCEL Department.

Bibliography

Huston TP, Puffer JC, Rodney WM: The athletic heart syndrome, *N Engl J Med* 313:24-32, 1985.

Maron BJ, Epstein SE, Roberts WC: Causes of sudden death in competitive athletes, *J Am Coll Cardiol* 7:204-214, 1986.

Maron BJ, Mitchell JH: Bethesda Conference 26. Recommendations for determining eligibility for competition in athletes with cardiovascular abnormalities, *Med Sci Sports Exerc* 26:S223-S283, 1994.

Thompson PD, Funk EJ, Carleton RA, et al: Incidence of death during jogging in Rhode Island from 1975 through 1980, *JAMA* 147:2535-2538, 1982.

Van Camp SP: Sudden death, *Clin Sports Med* 11(2):273-289, 1992.

Van Camp SP, Bloor C, Mueller FO, et al: Nontraumatic sports death in high school and college athletes, *Med Sci Sports Exerc* 27:641-647, 1995.

Waller BF, Roberts WC: Sudden death while running in conditioned runners aged 40 years or over, *Am J Cardiol* 45:1282-1300, 1980.

CHAPTER 6

Anemia and Blood Doping

E. Randy Eichner, MD, FACSM

I. Anemia
   A. Although any athlete can acquire any anemia, the primary care physician tends to encounter only three main anemias in athletes: (1) "sports anemia" (a dilutional pseudoanemia), (2) anemia secondary to "footstrike" or exertional hemolysis, and (3) iron deficiency anemia.
   B. Sports anemia. Athletes, especially endurance athletes, assuming they are training at sea level, tend to have lower hematocrit and hemoglobin concentrations than do sedentary counterparts. That is, athletes tend to be slightly "anemic" compared to norms in the general population. This has been called "sports anemia." Sports anemia, however, is a misnomer because the most common cause of a low hematocrit level in an athlete is a false anemia. This false anemia is due to regular aerobic exercise, which expands the baseline plasma volume, thus "diluting down" hematocrit and hemoglobin concentration. In other words, the lower hematocrit level of the endurance athlete is a dilutional pseudoanemia.
      1. Mechanism: Regular aerobic exercise expands baseline plasma volume as an adaptation or "overcompensation" to the acute loss of plasma volume, or hemoconcentration, that accompanies each workout. Strenuous exercise acutely reduces plasma volume by (a) increasing mean arterial blood pressure and thus capillary hydrostatic pressure, driving an ultrafiltrate of plasma into the tissues, (b) generating lactic acid in working muscle and other metabolites that increase tissue osmotic pressure, and (c) producing sweat, derived in part from blood plasma. To adapt, the body releases renin, aldosterone, and vasopressin to conserve water and salt and also adds albumin to the blood. As a result, baseline plasma volume expands.
      2. Degree: Degree of sports "anemia" (or expansion of baseline plasma volume) correlates with intensity of training regimen, ranging from a low of about 5% to a high of about 20%. It develops or increases within days of beginning or intensifying aerobic training. As a rule of

thumb, the general lower limit for hemoglobin concentration is 14 g/dl for men and 13 g/dl for women. The norm for moderate exercisers is 0.5 g/dl lower; that for elite aerobic athletes is 1.0 g/dl lower. So the lower limit of normal is 13 g/dl for an elite male distance runner (at sea level) and 12 g/dl for his female counterpart.

3. Benefit: Athletic pseudoanemia is integral to aerobic fitness. The expanded plasma volume—along with the adaptations of "athlete's heart"—increases the cardiac stroke volume, which overrides the fall in hemoglobin per unit of blood to deliver more oxygen to tissues. Athletes concerned about their "low" hemoglobin concentrations can be reassured that it is a sign of top aerobic fitness and therefore a benefit, not a detriment.

C. Footstrike hemolysis. Footstrike hemolysis is intravascular hemolysis, the bursting of red blood cells in the bloodstream as the foot strikes the ground. Initially attributed to impact, it is now called *exertional hemolysis* because it has been seen in distance swimmers, whose sport involves no impact. It has also been seen in rowers, aerobic dancers, and even weight lifters. In nonimpact sports, hemolysis may be a result of turbulence, acidosis, and elevated temperature in working muscles.

1. Diagnosis: The diagnostic triad is (a) elevated mean red cell volume (MCV), (b) elevated reticulocyte count, and (c) low haptoglobin level. These abnormalities are usually mild. The blood smear is usually normal; a rare crenated red cell may be seen. Exertional hemolysis elevates the MCV because older, smaller red cells are preferentially destroyed and replaced by younger, larger reticulocytes. Haptoglobin is consumed as it picks up free hemoglobin in the plasma and delivers it to the liver for salvage.

2. Treatment: For most recreational athletes, exertional hemolysis needs no treatment. It is usually so mild that it causes no anemia, because the bone marrow of the iron-replete athlete accelerates red cell production. In other words, reticulocytosis prevents anemia. For elite aerobic athletes, however, even mild hemolysis can cap the adaptive expansion of red cell mass that is key to top performance. Treatment involves mitigating impact. Among runners, for example, hemolysis can be lessened by "cushioning," namely through attention to weight, gait, shoes, and terrain. The runner free of hemolysis runs "light on the feet" in cushioned shoes on grass.

D. Iron deficiency anemia. The most common "true" anemia in athletes, as in the general population, is iron deficiency anemia.

1. Gender difference: Iron deficiency is common in female athletes, but rare in male athletes unless they have bleeding from the gastrointestinal (GI) tract.

2. Causes: Only tiny amounts of iron are lost in sweat, so the main cause of iron deficiency in athletic women (as in nonathletic women) is too little iron in their diet to meet physiological needs. Women who lose more than 60 ml of blood per menstrual period are more prone to iron deficiency. The recommended daily allowance for iron for women is at least 15 mg/day. Many elite female athletes, however, especially "low-weight" athletes (e.g., distance runners, gymnasts, ballet dancers), consume no more than 2000 kcal/day or only 12 mg of iron a day. Also, the iron in vegetarian diets is not highly bioavailable; studies suggest that female athletes who avoid red meat are prone to iron deficiency. Another cause is GI bleeding.

3. GI bleeding: GI bleeding—usually occult, minor, and brief and more common during racing than training—can occur in some distance runners, cyclists, and triathletes. On rare occasions athletes have had major bleeding episodes during races. The site is usually the stomach, apparently from superficial "stress ulcers," sometimes exacerbated by nonsteroidal antiinflammatory drugs. Occasionally, the site is the colon, from "ischemic colitis," as blood is diverted during racing from the gut to working muscles. These ulcers tend to heal quickly, but on rare occasions runners have had major ischemic colitis warranting subtotal colectomy.
4. Diagnosis: The diagnostic triad is (a) low MCV, (b) hypochromic, microcytic red cells in the blood smear, and (c) low serum ferritin level.
5. Management: Treatment involves ferrous sulfate given at 325 mg three times a day with meals. Advice for prevention: (a) eat more lean red meat and dark meat of chicken, (b) enhance iron absorption from bread and cereal by avoiding coffee or tea with meals and instead consuming a source of vitamin C, such as orange juice, (c) cook acid foods in cast iron pots to leach iron into food, and (d) eat poultry or seafood with dried beans or peas (the animal protein increases absorption of the iron in the legumes). An athlete that repeatedly develops iron deficiency anemia despite dietary advice should take ferrous sulfate at 325 mg three times a week for prevention.
6. Low ferritin: Contrary to myth, low ferritin without anemia does not sap athletic performance. But even mild anemia from iron deficiency saps performance, and it can be hard to separate mild iron deficiency anemia from athletic pseudoanemia. If in doubt, a 2-month trial of empiric iron therapy is wise. An increase in hemoglobin of at least 1 g/dl is the "gold standard" for iron deficiency anemia.

II. Blood Doping

Blood doping (blood boosting, blood packing, induced erythrocythemia) is the artificial raising of hematocrit by transfusing red cells or injecting recombinant human erythropoietin (rhEPO). In women, abusing anabolic steroids is a form of blood doping since they increase endogenous erythropoietin. Altitude training, although it raises hematocrit, is not blood doping.

A. Rationale. By boosting hematocrit without unduly raising blood viscosity, endurance performance is believed to be enhanced as a result of increased oxygen delivery to working muscles. From cross-sectional data mainly but also from sparse longitudinal data, it seems likely that elite aerobic athletes develop an increase in both red cell mass and plasma volume. Blood doping attempts to shortcut and mimic this athletic adaptation. Research on blood doping accelerated after the 1968 Olympic Games held at the high-altitude location of Mexico City. Nearly all the men's distance races were won by men born, bred, and trained in highlands. By 1972 research suggested that blood doping could enhance maximal oxygen uptake and brief, all-out running time to exhaustion. Beginning in 1972 and continuing today, dozens of elite endurance athletes—runners, skiers, triathletes, and others—have admitted or been accused of blood doping.

B. Methods. Historically, blood doping was via transfusion, most often autologous blood that had been withdrawn and stored for several weeks, enough time for the athlete to regenerate red cells (back to baseline hematocrit) and retrain. Recently, however, the preferred method has become rhEPO transfusion. In women, such as recent record-setting Chinese female swimmers and possibly also their female distance runners, abuse of anabolic steroids is a form of blood doping. This is because testosterone, for example, increases the action of endogenous erythropoietin. In fact, the normal gender difference in hematocrit (higher in men than women) stems from higher mean testosterone levels in men.

C. Effectiveness. In the 1980s, three controlled studies using freeze-preserved red cells found that blood doping could speed running time, from brief, all-out runs to 10-k races in the field. Only one study of rhEPO has appeared; it finds that boosting hematocrit from 45% to 50% (in male trained physical education students) can speed brief, all-out running time by 17%. Translated to world-class level, such studies suggest that, for example, a 10-k runner from sea level stands to gain a few seconds by blood doping. In the Olympic Games, of course, a few seconds separates winners from losers.

D. Side effects. Pilot data suggest that rhEPO can accentuate the exercise-induced rise in systolic blood pressure, but the main worry is that large or frequent doses of rhEPO will raise the hematocrit (and blood viscosity) to dangerous levels. It is known that some endurance athletes abuse rhEPO, sometimes along with testosterone and growth hormone. Many suspect that abuse of rhEPO or other drugs played a role in the spate of mysterious deaths in Dutch and Belgian cyclists between 1987 and 1990. It is plausible, for example, that a cyclist abusing rhEPO might start a race with a hematocrit of 55% to 60% and, with dehydration, end it with a hematocrit of 60% to 65%. Surely the combination of high hematocrit, elevated blood viscosity, dehydration, and long hours on the saddle increases the risk of venous or arterial thrombosis.

E. Conclusions. The use of rhEPO in sports is unethical and illegal, of course, but at present it cannot be detected with certainty. It is likely that a means of detection will soon become available. Until then, among possible solutions, these four are debated most often: (1) mark the drug, (2) control the drug, (3) sanction the drug but monitor the athletes, and (4) educate athletes and coaches to convince them that abusing rhEPO is not worth the risk. Unfortunately, some young athletes, believing they are immortal, will take huge risks to win. Probably, the solution depends on being able to detect abuse of rhEPO. The International Ski Federation now mandates regular blood sampling of athletes to detect doping, and a similar proposal is under study by the International Olympic Committee.

Bibliography

Cook JD: The effect of endurance training on iron metabolism, *Semin Hematol* 31:146-154, 1994.

Eichner ER: Anemia in female athletes, *Your Patient & Fitness* 3:3-11, 1989.

Eichner ER: Gastrointestinal bleeding in athletes, *Phys Sportsmed* 17:128-140, 1989.

Eichner ER: Runner's macrocytosis: a clue to footstrike hemolysis, *Am J Med* 78:321-325, 1985.

Eichner ER: Sports anemia, iron supplements, and blood doping, *Med Sci Sports Exerc* 24:S315-S318, 1992.

Eichner ER: Blood doping and performance. In Torg JS, Shephard RJ, editors: *Current Therapy in Sports Medicine,* ed 3, St Louis, 1995, Mosby–Year Book.

Ekblom B, Berglund B: Effect of erythropoietin administration on maximal aerobic power, *Scand J Med Sci Sports* 1:88-93, 1991.

Harris SS: Helping active women avoid anemia, *Phys Sportsmed* 23:35-48, 1995.

Selby GB, Eichner ER: Hematocrit and performance: the effect of endurance training on blood volume, *Semin Hematol* 31:122-127, 1994.

CHAPTER 7

Human Immunodeficiency Virus

E. Lee Rice, DO

I. General Overview
   A. The problem.[8–10,26]
      1. Acquired immunodeficiency syndrome (AIDS) is caused by the human immunodeficiency virus (HIV), which infects cells of the immune system and other tissues such as the brain.
      2. HIV is a member of the lentivirus subfamily of human retroviruses.
      3. HIV is transmitted through sexual contact or exposure to infected blood or blood products and from mother to neonate.
      4. Retroviruses produce the enzyme reverse transcriptase, which allows the virus's genetic information to be reproduced in host cells.
      5. HIV infects CD4+ T lymphocytes, a key component of the body's immune system, resulting in gradual deterioration of the body's immune function and susceptibility to life-threatening infection and malignancies.
      6. Since the time between HIV infection and getting sick (with AIDS) is sometimes longer than 10 years, there is a tremendous risk of disease spread by unknowingly infected persons.
      7. It appears that everyone who contracts HIV infection will eventually develop AIDS.
      8. To date there is no cure for AIDS, whose victims die prematurely due to AIDS-related diseases.
   B. Concerns regarding HIV and sports.[13,18]
      1. Medical evidence indicates that it is likely that there are HIV-infected players at the high school, college, and elite levels of American sports.
      2. Recent well-publicized accounts of HIV-positive athletes in competition have caused concern among athletes at all levels of competition that HIV infection may occur during sports participation.

3. Athletes, administrators, and the sports medicine community are faced with a number of concerns related to HIV and sports participation.
   a. What is the risk of an HIV-infected athlete transmitting the infection during sports participation?
   b. How does exercise affect the immune response and potential longevity of the HIV-infected athlete?
   c. What practical steps can be taken to prevent or minimize the risk of HIV transmission during sports participation?
   d. Should the HIV-infected athlete be excluded from sports participation?
   e. Should athletes be tested for HIV status?
   f. What are the significant medicolegal implications involved?

II. Epidemiology and Prevalence of HIV Infection[7-9,13,21,26]
   A. Approximately 1.25 million people in the United States presently infected with HIV.
   B. Over 250,000 patients diagnosed with AIDS worldwide.
   C. Over 150,000 AIDS deaths to date.
   D. Up to 50,000 new HIV infections recorded annually.
   E. 1% of males aged 20-49 HIV positive.
   F. One in 200 college students HIV positive.
   G. Leading cause of death in American men aged 25-44 and the fourth leading killer of women of the same ages.
   H. Infected population.[13,19,26]
      1. Gay or bisexual males: 52%.
      2. Intravenous (IV) drug abusers: 25%.
      3. Persons infected via heterosexual contact: 9%.
      4. Gay + IV drug abuse: 5%.
      5. Transfusion recipients: 2%.
      6. Uncertain: 7%.

III. Diagnosis
   A. Diagnosis based on presence of an illness characterized by one or more of the following "indicator" diseases, depending on the status of laboratory evidence of HIV infection (see box on p. 41).[23,26]
   B. Without laboratory evidence regarding HIV infection.
      1. Indicator diseases with definitive diagnosis.
         a. Candidiasis of the esophagus, trachea, bronchi, or lungs.
         b. Cryptococcosis, extrapulmonary.
         c. Cryptosporidiosis with diarrhea persisting >1 month.
         d. Cytomegalovirus disease of an organ other than liver, spleen, or lymph nodes in a patient >1 month of age.
         e. Herpes simplex virus infection causing a mucocutaneous ulcer that persists >1 month; or bronchitis, pneumonitis, or esophagitis of any duration affecting a patient >1 month of age.
         f. Kaposi's sarcoma affecting a patient <60 years of age.
         g. Lymphoma of the brain (primary) affecting a patient <60 years of age.
         h. Lymphoid interstitial pneumonia and/or pulmonary lymphoid hyperplasia (LIP/PLH complex) affecting a child <13 years of age.
         i. *Mycobacterium avium* complex or *Mycobacterium kansasii* disease, disseminated (at a site other than or in addition to lungs, skin, or cervical or hilar lymph nodes).
         j. *Pneumocystis carinii* pneumonia.
         k. Progressive multifocal leukoencephalopathy.
         l. Toxoplasmosis of the brain affecting a patient >1 month of age.

STATUS OF LABORATORY EVIDENCE

LABORATORY EVIDENCE FOR HIV INFECTION (ANY OF THE FOLLOWING CONDITIONS)

Serum reactivity for HIV antibody by a screening test (e.g., enzyme-linked immunosorbent assay [ELISA]) and subsequent HIV antibody tests positive (e.g., Western blot, immunofluorescence assay combined false-positive less than 0.001%[1]).

Positive test for HIV serum antigen.

Positive HIV culture confirmed by both reverse transcriptase detection and a specific HIV antigen test or in situ hybridization using a nucleic acid probe.

Positive result on any other highly specific test for HIV (e.g., nucleic acid probe of peripheral blood lymphocytes).

LABORATORY EVIDENCE AGAINST HIV INFECTION

A nonreactive screening test for serum antibody to HIV (e.g., ELISA) without a reactive or positive result on any other test for HIV (e.g., antibody, antigen, culture), if done.

LABORATORY EVIDENCE INCONCLUSIVE (NEITHER FOR NOR AGAINST INFECTION)

A repeatedly reactive screening test for serum antibody to HIV (e.g., ELISA) followed by a negative or inconclusive supplemental test (e.g., Western blot, immunofluorescence assay) without a positive HIV culture or serum antigen test.

C. With laboratory evidence of HIV infection.
   1. Any disease listed above in B.1., B.2., or B.3.
   2. Indicator diseases with definitive diagnosis.
      a. Bacterial infections, multiple or recurrent (any combination of at least two within a 2-year period), of the following types affecting a child <13 years of age:
         (1) Septicemia.
         (2) Pneumonia.
         (3) Meningitis.
         (4) Bone or joint infection.
         (5) Abscess of an internal organ or body cavity (excluding otitis media or superficial skin or mucosal abscesses), caused by *Haemophilus, Streptococcus* (including *Pneumococcus*), or other pyogenic bacteria.
      b. Coccidioidomycosis, disseminated (at a site other than or in addition to lungs or cervical or hilar lymph nodes).
      c. HIV encephalopathy (also called "HIV dementia," "AIDS dementia," or "subacute encephalitis due to HIV").
      d. Histoplasmosis, disseminated (at a site other than or in addition to lungs or cervical or hilar lymph nodes).
      e. Isosporiasis with diarrhea persisting >1 month.
      f. Kaposi's sarcoma at any age.
      g. Lymphoma of the brain (primary) at any age.
      h. Other non-Hodgkin's lymphoma of B cell or unknown immunological phenotype and the following histological types:
         (1) Small noncleaved lymphoma (either Burkitt or non-Burkitt type).
         (2) Immunoblastic sarcoma.

i. Any mycobacterial disease caused by mycobacteria other than *Mycobacterium tuberculosis,* disseminated (at a site other than or in addition to lungs, skin, or cervical or hilar lymph nodes).
j. Disease caused by *M. tuberculosis,* extrapulmonary (involving at least one site outside the lungs, regardless of whether there is concurrent pulmonary involvement).
k. *Salmonella* (nontyphoid) septicemia, recurrent.
l. HIV wasting syndrome (emaciation, "slim disease").

3. Indicator diseases diagnosed presumptively (in situations where patient's condition will not permit the performance of definitive tests or where accepted clinical practice is to diagnose presumptively based on the presence of characteristic clinical and laboratory abnormalities).
   a. Candidiasis of the esophagus.
   b. Cytomegalovirus retinitis with loss of vision.
   c. Kaposi's sarcoma.
   d. LIP/PLH complex affecting a child <13 years of age.
   e. Mycobacterial disease (acid-fast bacilli with species not identified by culture), disseminated (involving at least one site other than or in addition to lungs, skin, or cervical or hilar lymph nodes).
   f. *P. carinii* pneumonia.
   g. Toxoplasmosis of the brain affecting a patient >1 month of age.

D. With laboratory evidence against HIV infection.
   1. All other causes of immunodeficiency are excluded.
   2. In addition, the patient has had either:
      a. *P. carinii* pneumonia diagnosed by a definitive method.
      b. Any of the other diseases indicative of AIDS listed above in Section B.1. diagnosed by a definitive method.
   3. A T helper/inducer (CD4) lymphocyte count <400/mm^3.

IV. Laboratory Abnormalities
   A. General.[10]
      1. Anemia.
      2. Leukopenia.
      3. Thrombocytosis, thrombocytopenia.
      4. Elevated serum transaminase.
   B. Immunological studies.[9,10]
      1. Elevated IgG, IgM, IgA.
      2. Hypogammaglobulinemia.
      3. Reversed T helper/T suppressor cell ratio, due to progressive loss of CD4+ lymphocytes.
      4. Depressed lymphocyte response to mitogen, antigen.
      5. Decreased specific antibody responses.
      6. Decreased cytokine production (interferons, interleukins, tumor necrosis factor, lymphotoxin).
      7. Increased immune complexes.
      8. Delayed hypersensitivity skin test responses.
   C. Other.[10]
      1. Abnormal chest X-ray.
      2. Abnormal brain computed tomography scan.
      3. Evidence of multiple infections (bacterial, viral, fungal, protozoal).

V. Pathophysiology and Clinical Course of HIV Infection[7–9]
   A. After exposure, 2–12 weeks to develop antibodies.
   B. Helper T cells summon B cells, which make antibodies to HIV.

C. HIV invades T cells and replicates.
D. No symptoms during replication—HIV unrecognized.
E. Incubation period prior to symptom onset ranges from 6 months to >10 years.
F. Laboratory tests may take ≥6 months following infection to become positive.
G. Clinical course extremely variable (see box on p. 44).
H. Patients likely to die prematurely.
I. Cause of death commonly attributed to opportunistic infections, with HIV infection as the underlying cause.
J. With early diagnosis and health care, many patients live >10 years after diagnosis of HIV infection and AIDS, with no or very few symptoms.

VI. Treatment[5,10]
A. No cure presently available. Present drugs decrease the viral load and delay immunological decline.
B. Reverse transcriptase inhibitors.
1. Currently licensed medicines slow progress of the disease by inhibiting replication of the virus.
2. Zidovudine (AZT), dideoxyinosine, dideoxycytidine, stavudine (d4T), lamivudine (3TC).
C. Protease inhibitors.
1. Inhibit HIV protease activity and prevent HIV replication.
2. Indinavir, Saquinavir.
D. Research for vaccine continues.
E. New strains of the virus have been recently discovered, making total prevention by single vaccine unlikely. Multiple drug therapy often more efficacious than monotherapy.
F. Drugs, radiation, and surgery used to treat various illnesses of AIDS patients.

VII. Transmission of HIV
A. Dependent on degree and duration of exposure to infected blood or body fluids.[16]
B. HIV detected in many body secretions and fluids (blood, semen, bone marrow, saliva, tears, cervical secretions, cerebrospinal fluid, brain tissue, lymph node tissue, urine, feces, synovial fluids, amniotic fluids, and pleural fluid).[7,9,16,20]
C. HIV not transmitted via[2,7,15,20]
1. Saliva.
2. Tears.
3. Body contact.
4. Sweat.
5. Objects touched or used by HIV-infected individual.
D. Classification of body fluids based on quantity of HIV present.[8]
1. Very high: cerebrospinal fluid.
2. High: blood, semen, synovial fluid, amniotic fluid, pericardal fluid.
3. Moderate: vaginal and cervical secretions, breast milk.
4. Very low (not considered infectious): Tears, saliva, sputum, urine.
5. Probably none: sweat.
E. Methods of transmission.[6,7,9,20]
1. Sexual contact with infected individual (anal sex riskier than vaginal intercourse due to tendency of rectal mucosa to tear, allowing virus in semen to be directly transmitted to recipient's blood).
2. Intravenous drug use with contaminated needles.

MODIFIED CDC CLASSIFICATION OF HIV INFECTION

GROUP I: INITIAL INFECTION

Patients in this group may be designated as having symptomatic seroconversion or asymptomatic seroconversion.

Symptomatic infection may include a mononucleosis-like syndrome, aseptic meningitis, rash, musculoskeletal complaints, and hematological abnormalities, as well as other clinical and laboratory findings.

Asymptomatic infection may occur with or without hematological abnormalities.

GROUP II: CHRONIC ASYMPTOMATIC INFECTION

Patients in this group may be designated as having a normal laboratory evaluation, specified laboratory abnormalities or laboratory evaluation pending or incomplete.

Laboratory abnormalities associated with HIV infection include anemia, leukopenia, lymphopenia, decreased T helper lymphocyte count, thrombocytopenia, hypergammaglobulinemia, and cutaneous anergy.

GROUP III: PERSISTENT GENERALIZED LYMPHADENOPATHY

Patients in this group may be designated on the basis of laboratory evaluation in the same manner as those in Group II.

GROUP IV: OTHER DISEASES

Medical evaluation must exclude the presence of other concurrent illnesses that could explain the symptoms.

Subgroup IV-A: Constitutional Disease

Patients in this group may be designated as having fever >1 month, involuntary weight loss >10% of baseline body weight, diarrhea lasting >1 month, or any combination of these.

Subgroup IV-B: Neurological Disease

Category 1: Central nervous system disorders include (a) dementia, (b) acute atypical meningitis (occurring after initial infection), and (c) myelopathy.

Category 2: Peripheral nervous system disorders include (a) painful sensory neuropathy and (b) inflammatory demyelinating polyneuropathy.

Subgroup IV-C: Secondary Infectious Diseases

Category 1: Patients in this group may be designated as having one or more of the following: *P. carinii* pneumonia, chronic cryptosporidiosis, toxoplasmosis, extraintestinal strongyloidiasis, isosporiasis, candidiasis (esophageal, bronchial or pulmonary), cryptococcosis, disseminated histoplasmosis, mycobacterial infection with *M. avium* complex or *M. kansasii,* disseminated cytomegalovirus infection, chronic mucocutaneous or disseminated herpes simplex virus infection, and progressive multifocal leukoencephalopathy.

Category 2: Patients in this group may be designated as having one or more of the following: oral hairy leukoplakia, multidermatomal herpes zoster, recurrent *Salmonella* bacteremia, nocardiosis, tuberculosis, or oral candidiasis (thrush).

Subgroup IV-D: Secondary Cancers

Patients in this group may be designated as having one or more of the following: Kaposi's sarcoma, non-Hodgkin's lymphoma (small, noncleaved lymphoma or immunoblastic sarcoma), or primary lymphoma of the brain.

Subgroup IV-E: Other Conditions

Includes patients with clinical findings or diseases, not classifiable above, which may be attributed to HIV infection and/or which may be indicative of a deficit in cell-mediated immunity. Patients in this group may be designated on the basis of the types of clinical findings or diseases diagnosed (e.g., chronic lymphoid interstitial pneumonitis).

3. Transfusion of contaminated blood.
4. Infected mother to infant.
   a. Pregnancy.
   b. Childbirth.
   c. Nursing.
5. Improper medical or dental infection control procedures.

F. Relative risk of HIV transmission.[2,3,6,7,14]
   1. Transfusion with seropositive blood, 1 : 1.
   2. Seropositive mother to neonate, 1 : 4.
   3. Seropositive male to female during intercourse, 1 : 3 to 1 : 2500.
   4. Seropositive male to male (rectal receptive) intercourse, 1 : 19 to 1 : 50.
   5. Shared IV needle from seropositive drug abuser, 1 : 3 to 1 : 300.
   6. Seropositive female to male during intercourse, 1 : 32 to 1 : 2000.
   7. Health care worker with percutaneous needle stick with exposure to blood from HIV-infected patient, 1 : 300.
   8. Casual contact (hugging, kissing, sharing of eating utensils and glasses, sharing towels, combs, nail clippers, workers sharing use of inanimate objects, etc.), no reports of transmission.
   9. Cutaneous exposure to blood from HIV-infected patients, no reports of transmission.
   10. Day care workers who care for HIV-infected children and have frequent contact with body fluids, no reports of transmission.
   11. Transmission from infected food handlers, no reports of transmission.
   12. Transmission from biting insects, no report of transmission.

G. Additional factors that may affect risk of HIV transmission.[8,16]
   1. Hygienic practices.
   2. First aid procedures.
   3. Skin integrity (cuts and dermatitis).
   4. Immunological status.
   5. CD4-bearing cells at the exposure site.
   6. Severity of exposure (depth, extent, and tissue involved).
   7. Physical factors (temperature, pH, humidity).
   8. Age of the specimen (how long fluid has been outside the source).

H. Risk of transmission in sports.[2,6,7,14,20,21,27]
   1. No studies to evaluate risk of transmission in athletes during sports participation.
   2. No documented case of HIV transmission between athletes during sports participation.*
   3. Transmission theoretically possible through cutaneous and mucosal exposure.[15]
      a. Possibility considered sufficiently remote as to not be quantifiable.
      b. Risk of HIV transmission in football estimated conservatively at <1 per 85 million game contacts.[2]
      c. Theoretical requirements for transmission.[16]
         (1) Presence of infected athlete.
         (2) Occurrence of a bleeding wound or exudative skin lesion in the infected athlete.

*Single case report of Italian soccer player converting from HIV seronegative status to HIV seropositive 2 months following 1989 collision with HIV-positive player (questionable reliability and insufficient documentation).

(3) Presence in a susceptible athlete of a skin lesion or exposed mucous membrane that could serve as a portal of entry.
(4) Sustained contact between portal of entry and the infective material.
4. Sports involving greatest theoretical risk: boxing, wrestling, football, rugby, hockey, martial arts.[8]
5. Analogy with hepatitis.[6,13]
a. Hepatitis B 100 times easier to transmit from needle stick than HIV (3 in 10 for hepatitis B and 3 in 1000 for HIV).
b. No documented cases of hepatitis B transmission from sports contact in United States.

I. Risk to physicians and trainers.[13]
1. Probably similar to health care workers.
2. Approaches zero risk, assuming blood-borne pathogen precautions are heeded and utilized.

VIII. HIV-Infected Athletes

A. Exercise for HIV-positive persons.[6,13–15]
1. Aerobic exercise improves strength, fitness, mood, self-esteem, general well-being.
2. Exercisers experience a rise in CD4 counts in one study.
3. Reduced risk of some cancers due to exercise.
4. Exercise causes a reduction in stress and anxiety, which depress immune response.
5. Exercise stimulates an increase in endogenous opioids, which are immune system stimulators.
6. Studies have not proven clinically important improvement in immune status in HIV-positive persons due to exercise alone.
7. Individualization necessary regarding exercise and competition advice based on:
a. Athlete's current state of health.
b. Status of HIV infection.
c. Nature and intensity of training.
d. Stress factors involved.
e. Potential risk of HIV transmission.
8. No evidence that exercise of moderate intensity is deleterious to health of HIV-infected persons.
9. Severe psychological and/or physical stress may suppress immune system as well as overall state of mental and physical health in some persons.

B. Exclusion of HIV-infected athletes from competition.
1. No rationale for prohibition of HIV-infected athletes from athletic competition based on current medical and epidemiological information.
2. No present restrictions from competition for HIV-infected athletes from the International Olympic Committee or major sporting regulatory bodies in the United States.

IX. Precautions Against Risk of HIV Transmission in Sports[14,16,19–21]

A. Universal Precautions for health care workers developed by Centers for Disease Control and Prevention.
1. Use of appropriate barrier precautions when contact with blood or other bodily fluids is anticipated.
2. Contaminated skin surface and hands (even if gloves worn) washed immediately following exposure to body fluids.

3. Proper and safe use and disposal in appropriate containers of sharp instruments.
4. Utilization of "pocket masks" or similar resuscitation/ventilation devices during CPR.
5. Avoidance of direct patient contact by health care workers who have open, exudative, or weeping wounds or lesions.
6. Special vigilance regarding Universal Precautions by pregnant health care workers.

B. Specific precautions for sports.[13,14,17,19]
   1. Voluntary HIV testing made available for all at-risk athletes.
   2. Appropriate educational information regarding HIV, transmission, and risk behaviors made available for all involved.
   3. Pre-event preparation with proper care for existing wounds.
   4. Necessary equipment and supplies available for compliance with Universal Precautions.
   5. Latex or vinyl gloves worn by health care providers when contact with body fluids is anticipated and changed following each athlete exposure.
   6. Hands and other skin surfaces washed after gloves removed and/or body fluid contact. Athletes shower after competition.
   7. Contaminated surfaces cleaned with virus-inactivating solution following each match or exposure.
   8. "Pocket mask" or similar ventilation device used for cardiopulmonary resuscitation.
   9. Soiled laundry articles tagged and washed in hot water with HIV-inactivating detergent. Disposables used when possible with proper disposal procedures.
   10. Mouthpieces worn by athletes in at-risk sports.
   11. Receptacles containing HIV-inactivating solution provided for spitting.
   12. When significant amount of exposed blood present, remove athlete from contest, cleanse area, and apply barrier dressing to athlete.
   13. Athletes with open wounds covered with appropriate barrier dressing.
   14. Protective eye wear worn when appropriate.
   15. Vaccinations up to date for all athletes.
   16. Lack of protective equipment not a cause for delay of emergency care for life-threatening injuries.
   17. Postexposure prophylaxis.[9]
       a. Consideration for postexposure prophylaxis advised for individuals with direct HIV-infected blood contact to mucous membranes or to open cutaneous lesions.
       b. Zidovudine (AZT) may inhibit growth of HIV in infected patients.
       c. No definitive recommendation from U.S. Public Health Service due to limitations of current knowledge and concerns over toxicity, teratogenic effects, and possible carcinogenicity.
       d. Recommendations.
          (1) Develop system for evaluation, counseling, and follow-up after significant risk exposure.
          (2) Record circumstances in confidential medical record.
          (3) Inform source individual of incident and test for serological evidence of HIV, if consent is obtained.
          (4) Maintain confidentiality of source individual.

(5) If source has AIDS, is HIV-seropositive, or refuses testing, evaluate exposed person clinically and serologically for HIV infection. If seronegative, retest periodically for minimum of 6 months after exposure and advise individual to seek evaluation for any acute illness during followup period.
(6) Exposed individuals refrain from blood, semen, or organ donation and abstain from or use measures to prevent HIV transmission during intercourse during followup period.
(7) No further followup is necessary if source individual is HIV seronegative and has no clinical evidence of HIV infection, assuming no evidence of recent (last 6 months) exposure to HIV.

C. Disinfection of surfaces and equipment.[7,13]
1. Household bleach (5/15% sodium hypochlorite) at 1 : 10 dilution or "hospital disinfectants" recommended.
2. Acceptable alternative disinfectants include Lysol, hydrogen peroxide, Betadine, isopropyl alcohol.
3. Gloves should be worn and area scrubbed thoroughly.
4. Soiled waste stored in moisture-resistant bag and handled as biohazardous material and discarded appropriately.
5. Soiled laundry double bagged and washed with detergent for 25 minutes at 160°F.

X. HIV Testing
A. Mandatory testing.
1. Not justified based on medical reasons as a condition for athletic participation.
2. Problem areas include cost, legal implications, false positives, practicality, frequency, ethics, and justification.
3. Generally invalidated by courts due to invasion of privacy in face of lack of evidence regarding necessity of testing to protect other athletes.

B. Voluntary testing.[1,4,11]
1. Suggest to athletes with risk of exposure to blood-borne pathogens.
a. Multiple sexual partners.
b. Nonprescription drug injections (drugs of abuse and/or ergogenic aids).
c. Sexual contacts of at-risk persons.
d. Athletes with sexually transmitted diseases, including hepatitis B virus.
e. Blood transfusion before 1985.
2. Pretesting and posttesting counseling important; arranged by ordering physician.
3. State guidelines followed for informed consent and disclosure of results.
4. All athletes in at-risk sports may benefit from knowing HIV status.

XI. Legal Considerations[11,13,17,24]
A. Confidentiality.
1. Medical information belongs solely to the patient.
2. Patient only decides how and where medical information is disclosed (or parent/guardian in case of minor).
3. Exceptions involve reportable medical conditions governed by individual state laws. (AIDS currently reportable in all states while HIV infection is reportable in some states.)
4. Developing case law suggests physician, in sports medicine setting, may have duty to disclose or warn some individuals where there is a

risk of transmission, even though the possibility of virus transmission is remote.

5. No case has dealt with this particular issue (team physician's role in disclosing infected HIV status of one player to noninfected participants) to date.
6. Joint position statement by American Medical Society for Sports Medicine and American Academy of Sports Medicine declares that the "physician is not liable for failure to warn the uninfected opponent," and that the legal responsibility lies with the HIV-infected athlete.[14]
7. Physicians should keep up to date with state and federal statutes and regulations concerning confidentiality.

B. Exclusion of HIV-infected athletes from sports participation.
   1. No legal resolution in the United States regarding whether an HIV-infected athlete may be excluded from a contact sport because of potential risk of transmission to others.
   2. Legal exclusion generally possible where necessary to avoid exposing other participants to significant health and safety risks.
   3. Americans with Disabilities Act and the Rehabilitation Act of 1973.
      a. Prohibit unjustified discrimination against persons with contagious diseases who are otherwise qualified to participate in a sports event.
      b. Athletes creating "a significant risk of communicating an infectious disease to others" may be excluded from a sport unless "reasonable accommodations" will eliminate the risk, based on "reasonable medical judgments given the state of medical knowledge."
      c. Exclusion of HIV-infected athlete permissible if athlete unable to meet physical demands of the sport if supporting medical basis for that conclusion is established.

XII. Education[4,12,19]

A. Best method of prevention is education.
B. Sports medicine professionals should take lead.
C. Multiple issues need addressing with athletes, coaches, parents, administrators, trainers, families.
   1. Risk of HIV transmission through sexual contact.
   2. Effectiveness of condoms and spermicides in preventing HIV transmission.
   3. Possibility of HIV transmission through use of shared needles, including intravenous or intramuscular administration of ergogenic aids.
   4. Advisability of avoiding the sharing of articles of personal hygiene (razors, toothbrushes, etc.).
   5. The risk of HIV transmission during sports participation.
   6. Importance of timely reporting of significant injuries.
   7. Education and training regarding Universal Precautions.
   8. Elimination of unsupported fears and misconceptions regarding HIV and sports participation.
   9. Factual details concerning HIV testing.
D. Research still needed.
   1. Further elucidation concerning disease and sport-specific evaluation of the medical risks of athletic participation with blood-borne diseases is necessary.
   2. Sports medicine practitioners must lead the way.

References

1. Alden J: Screening and testing asymptomatic persons for HIV infection. In DeVita VT, Hellman S, Rosenberg SA, editors: *AIDS: etiology, diagnosis, treatment, and prevention,* Philadelphia, 1992 JB Lippincott, pp. 121-136, 421-429.
2. Brown LS et al: Bleeding injuries in professional football: estimating the risk for HIV transmission, *Ann Intern Med* 122(4):273-274, 1995.
3. Brown LS et al: HIV/AIDS policies and sports: the National Football League, *Med Sci Sport Exerc* April 26:4, 403-407, 1994.
4. Cohen MS: HIV and sexually transmitted diseases, The physician's role in prevention, Prevention of HIV and STDs, *Postgrad Med* 98:3, September 1995.
5. Drugs for AIDS and associated infections, *Med Lett* 33:52-58; 63-64;79-86, 1995.
6. Eichner ER: Immunity in athletes: are they at greater risk for infection? *Can J CME,* p. 904, Oct 1993.
7. Eichner ER: HIV threat for athletes, fear of contagion: mystique of blood, UCSD Sports Medicine, 1995.
8. Epstein FH: Mechanisms of disease; Pathogenesis of infection with human immunodeficiency virus, *N Engl J Med* 278-286, 1987.
9. Garl T, Hrisomalos ATC, Rink L: HIV virus & sports precautions against risk of contamination, US Olympic Committee, 1991.
10. Hecht M, Soloway B: *HIV infection—a primary care approach,* 1994, The Publishing Division of the Massachusetts Medical Society, Waltham, Massachusetts.
11. Herbert DL, editor: HIV/AIDS and Sports Participation, Medical-Legal Update, *Sports Med Dig* July 1992.
12. The Johns Hopkins School of Public Health and The National Basketball Players Association Fact Sheet on AIDS, 1992.
13. Johnson R: AIDS and Other Blood Borne Pathogens in Sports, Department of Family Practice, Hennepin County Medical Center, Minneapolis, MN.
14. Joint Position Statement by AASM and AMSSM, Human Immunodeficiency Virus (HIV) and Other Blood-Borne Pathogens in Sports.
15. Landry GL: HIV infection and athletes, *Sports Med Dig* 15(4), 1993.
16. Mast EE et al: Transmission of blood-borne pathogens during sports: risk and prevention, *Ann Intern Med* 122(4), 1995.
17. Mitten MF: Athletic participation with a contagious blood-borne disease, *Clin J Sports Med* 5:153-154, 1995.
18. National Football League AIDS Fact Sheet, Aug 1992.
19. National Football League's Policy on HIV/AIDS, adapted from materials developed by the John Hopkins School of Public Health in conjunction with the National Basketball Players Association.
20. NCAA Committee on Competitive Safeguards and Medical Aspects of Sports, Policy No 20: AIDS and Intercollegiate Athletics, April 1968, revised June 1991.
21. NCAA Guideline 2H, AIDS and Intercollegiate Athletics, April 1988.
22. Ostrow DG et al: Classification of the clinical spectrum of HIV infection in adults: information on AIDS for the practicing physician, July 1987.
23. Revision of the CDC Surveillance Case Definition for Acquired Immunodeficiency Syndrome, Centers for Disease Control, *MMWR* 36(Suppl 1), 1987.
24. The athlete's chances of contracting HIV, *Ann Intern Med* 122(4):271-274, 1995.
25. Torre D et al: Transmission of HIV-1 infection via sports injury, *Lancet* 335:1106, 1990 (letter).
26. US Public Health Service, County of San Diego, Department of Health Services: Facts about AIDS, Leaflet 4/86.
27. USOC Sports Medicine & Science Committee: A Report to all National Governing Bodies, Transmission of Infectious Agents During Athletic Competition, US Olympic Committee, 1991.

CHAPTER 8

Sexually Transmitted Disease

James L. Moeller, MD
David O. Hough, MD, FACSM

I. *Chlamydia trachomatis*
   A. More common than Neisseria gonorrhoeae (GC); 3-4 million cases per year.
   B. Obligate intracellular organism infects both females and males.
   C. Symptoms.
      1. Female (may be asymptomatic, 40% to 70%).
         a. Vaginal discharge.
         b. Dysuria.
         c. Lower abdominal pain.
         d. Low-grade fever.
      2. Male (may be asymptomatic).
         a. Penile discharge.
         b. Dysuria.
         c. Low-grade fever.
   D. Sequelae.
      1. Nongonococcal urethritis (NGU).
      2. Pelvic inflammatory disease (PID).
         a. Infertility.
         b. Ectopic pregnancy.
      3. Epididymitis.
   E. Transmission.
      1. Close sexual contact.
      2. Vertical transmission.
         a. Can lead to neonatal infection.
            (1) Ophthalmia neonatorum.
            (2) Pneumonia.
   F. Diagnostic tests.
      1. Culture: the "gold standard" but not an effective screening test.
      2. Direct antigen testing. Generally used when culture is negative but suspicion remains high.

a. Fluorescent antibody microscopy.
b. Enzyme-linked immunosorbent assay.

G. Treatment: antibiotics.
1. Doxycycline: 100 mg PO bid ×7 days. *Avoid in pregnant patient.*
2. Tetracycline: 500 mg PO qid ×7 days. *Avoid in pregnant patient.*
3. Erythromycin base: 500 mg PO qid ×7 days.
4. Erythromycin ethylsuccinate: 800 mg PO qid ×7 days.
5. Sulfisoxazole: 500 mg PO qid ×10 days.
6. Azithromycin: 1 g PO, single dose (compliance likely to be improved by single dose therapy).

H. Followup.
1. See patient 7-10 days after treatment; no repeat of culture is necessary.
2. Sexual partners should be treated.

II. *Neisseria gonorrhoeae*

A. Still a common sexually transmitted disease; 1-2 million cases per year.
B. Coinfection with *Chlamydia* is common: 40% to 50%.
C. Symptoms:
1. Female (up to 80% may be asymptomatic).
a. Yellow-green vaginal discharge.
b. Dysuria.
c. Dysfunctional uterine bleeding.
d. Dyspareunia.
2. Male (rarely asymptomatic).
a. Yellow-green penile discharge.
b. Dysuria.

D. Sequelae.
1. PID.
a. Infertility.
b. Ectopic pregnancy.
2. Septic arthritis.
3. Proctitis.

E. Transmission.
1. Close sexual contact.
2. Vertical transmission; may cause ophthalmia neonatorum.

F. Diagnostic tests.
1. Culture: the "gold standard." Sensitivities are important as penicillinase-producing and tetracycline-resistant strains exist.
2. GC antigen tests are available.
3. In males gram-negative diplococci seen on Gram stain of urethral smear is diagnostic.

G. Treatment: antibiotics. Because of the high rate of co-infection with *Chlamydia trachomatis,* treatment of *Chlamydia* in conjunction with treatment for the *N. gonorrhoeae* infection is recommended.
1. Ceftriaxone: 250 mg IM, single dose.
2. Cefixime: 400 mg PO, single dose.
3. Ofloxacin 400 mg PO, single dose. *Avoid if patient is pregnant or less than 18 years old.*
4. Ciprofloxacin: 500 mg PO, single dose. *Avoid if patient is pregnant or less than 18 years old.*
5. Ampicillin: 3.5 g PO with 1 g of probenecid.
6. Spectinomycin: 2 g IM, single dose. A good option when patient is allergic to penicillin or cephalosporins.

H. Followup
1. See patient in 7-10 days after therapy; no repeat culture necessary.
2. Sexual partners should be treated.

III. Syphilis
   A. Caused by the spirochete *Treponema pallidum.*
   B. Recent resurgence in disease incidence; annual incidence approximately 134,000.
   C. Four clinical stages.
      1. Primary syphilis—occurs 10-90 days after exposure.
         a. Characterized by a painless lesion (chancre) at the site of inoculation.
         b. Heals without treatment.
      2. Secondary syphilis—appears weeks to months later, characterized by:
         a. Maculopapular rash—includes palms and soles.
         b. Pink-gray papular rash on genital mucosa—condylomata lata.
         c. Lymphadenopathy.
         d. Spontaneous resolution.
      3. Latent syphilis—may last years.
      4. Tertiary syphilis—occurs in 33% of untreated patients.
         a. One third develop neurosyphilis.
            (1) Meningitis.
            (2) Peripheral neuropathy (i.e., tabes dorsalis).
            (3) Psychiatric illness.
         b. Two thirds develop cardiovascular syphilis.
            (1) Obliterative endarteritis.
            (2) Aortic insufficiency.
            (3) Aortic aneurysms.
   D. Transmission.
      1. Close sexual contact; transmission rate 33% after unprotected sex with an infected person.
      2. Vertical transmission.
         a. Incidence of congenital syphilis increasing.
         b. Congenital syphilis leads to fetal or perinatal death in 40% of cases.
   E. Diagnostic tests.
      1. Darkfield examination of a scraping from a primary or secondary lesion.
      2. Nontreponemal antibody tests.
         a. Rapid plasma reagin (RPR).
         b. Venereal Diseases Research Laboratory (VDRL).
         c. False-positive tests occur. A positive nontreponemal antibody test should be followed by a treponemal antibody test.
      3. Treponemal antibody test: fluorescent treponemal antibody-absorption test (FTA-ABS).
         a. Once positive, will remain positive for life.
         b. Cannot be used for followup.
   F. Treatment: antibiotics.
      1. Primary, secondary, or latent syphilis of <1 year.
         a. Benzathine penicillin G: 2.4 million units IM (drug of choice).
         b. Doxycycline: 100 mg PO bid × 14 days.
         c. Tetracycline: 500 mg PO qid × 14 days.
         d. Erythromycin: 500 mg PO qid × 14 days.
      2. Latent syphilis of >1 year or tertiary syphilis.
         a. Benzathine penicillin G: 2.4 million units IM weekly × 3 weeks.
         b. Doxycycline or tetracycline: as above for 4 weeks.
   G. Followup.
      1. Nontreponemal tests are followed at 3 and 6 months after treatment.
         a. Expect a 4× decrease within 3 months in cases of primary and secondary syphilis.

b. Expect a 4× decrease within 6 months in cases of early latent disease.
c. Failure to see a decrease; any increase indicates inadequate treatment or reinfection.
2. Treponemal tests remain positive for life and are not used for followup.

IV. Genital Herpes Simplex
A. Herpes simplex virus (HSV) is a DNA virus that infects mucous membranes through direct contact.
1. HSV type I: accounts for 85% to 90% of oral infections (cold sores).
2. HSV type II: accounts for 85% to 90% of genital infections.
B. Symptoms.
1. Primary infection: lasts 2-20 days.
a. Flu-like symptoms.
b. Blisters (may be painful).
c. Inguinal lymphadenopathy.
d. Lesions usually leave no scar upon resolution.
2. Latent phase. Virus lies dormant in nerve root ganglia. Virus may be reactivated; triggers include:
a. Stress.
b. Fatigue.
c. Skin irritation.
d. Poor diet.
e. Menstruation.
3. Recurrent infection.
a. Prodrome of pruritus and/or tingling may be present.
b. Symptoms usually less severe; duration usually shorter.
c. Constitutional symptoms usually absent.
C. Diagnostic tests.
1. Viral culture.
2. Tzanck smear.
D. Treatment.
1. Primary infection: treatment may decrease viral shedding and length of active infection.
a. Acyclovir: 200 mg PO 5× daily for 7-10 days.
b. Acyclovir: 5 mg/kg IV q8h for 5-7 days.
c. Acyclovir cream.
d. Valacyclovir: 500 mg PO bid × 10d.
e. Famciclovir: 125 mg PO bid × 10d.
2. Recurrent infection.
a. Acyclovir: 200 mg PO 5× daily for 5 days.
b. Acyclovir: 800 mg PO bid for 5 days.
c. Valacyclovir: 500 mg PO bid × 5d.
d. Famciclovir: 125 mg PO bid × 5d.
3. For patients who have >6 recurrences annually, daily acyclovir may decrease the number of recurrences.

V. Genital Warts
A. Caused by human papillomavirus (HPV). HPV infection associated with cervical dysplasia and carcinoma.
B. Condyloma acuminata (the typical lesion) are single or multiple papular growths with a reddish or white color. Usually asymptomatic.
1. May be pruritic.
2. May be painful.
C. Transmission by genital contact.

D. Diagnosed by appearance.
  1. 5% acetic acid will change these lesions to a white color.
E. Treatment (recurrence is high [80%]despite method used).
  1. Trichloroacetic acid 25% to 85%.
  2. Podophyllin 10% to 25%. *Avoid in pregnant patient.*
  3. Laser ablation.
  4. Electrodesiccation.
  5. Cryotherapy.

VI. Chancroid
  A. Caused by *Haemophilus ducreyi.*
  B. Symptoms and signs.
    1. One or more painful genital ulcers.
    2. Tender inguinal adenopathy.
      a. May worsen during therapy.
  C. Diagnosis.
    1. Culture is the gold standard yet is only 60% sensitive.
    2. Often confused with HSV and syphilis.
      a. 10% co-infection rate with HSV or *Treponema pallidum,* so tests for these organisms may be indicated.
  D. Treatment.
    1. Ceftriaxone: 250 mg IM, single dose.
    2. Azithromycin: 1 g PO, single dose.
    3. Alternatives.
      a. Erythromycin base: 500 mg PO qid × 7 days.
      b. Amoxicillin/clavulanic acid: 500 mg/125 mg PO tid × 7 days.
      c. Ciprofloxacin: 500 mg PO bid × 3 days. *Avoid if patient is pregnant or less than 18 years old.*
    4. Treat partners who had contact within 10 days of appearance of lesions.
  E. Followup.
    1. Reexamine the patient in 3-7 days after the initiation of therapy.
    2. No improvement at followup.
      a. Incorrect diagnosis?
      b. Co-infection?
        (1) HSV.
        (2) *Treponema pallidum.*
        (3) HIV.
      c. *H. ducreyi* is resistant to antibiotic?

VII. *Trichomonas vaginalis*
  A. The most common cause of sexually transmitted vaginitis.
  B. *Trichomonas vaginalis* is a flagellated protozoan.
  C. Symptoms and signs.
    1. Malodorous vaginal discharge (profuse, frothy).
    2. Vulvovaginal irritation.
    3. Punctate hemorrhages on the cervix ("strawberry cervix") may be present.
  D. Diagnosis.
    1. Wet mount preparation reveals motile trichomonads in about 80% of cases.
  E. Treatment.
    1. Metronidazole: 2 g PO, single dose.
    2. Metronidazole: 250 mg PO tid × 7 days.
    3. Metronidazole gel.
    4. Metronidazole is contraindicated in the first trimester of pregnancy; 20% saline douche may be used.

TABLE 8-1. Infectious organisms and treatments

Infectious Organism	Treatment
Chlamydia trachomatis	Doxycycline 100 mg po bid ×7d* Tetracycline 500 mg po qid ×7d* Erythromycin base 500 mg po qid ×7d Erythromycin ethylsuccinate 800 mg po qid ×7d Sulfisoxazole 500 mg po qid ×10d Azithromycin 1 gram po as a single dose
Neisseria gonorrhoeae	Ceftriaxone 250 mg IM single dose Ofloxacin 400 mg po as a single dose*^ Ciprofloxacin 500 mg po as a single dose*^ Ampicillin 3.5 grams po with probenecid 1 gram Spectinomycin 2 grams IM single dose
Treponema pallidum	Primary, secondary or early latent disease: Benzathine penicillin G 2.4 million units IM Doxycycline 100 mg po bid ×14d* Tetracycline 500 mg po qid ×14d* Erythromycin base 500 mg po qid ×14d Latent disease >1 year or tertiary disease: Benzathine penicillin G 2.4 million units IM weekly ×3wk Doxycycline 100 mg po bid ×4wk* Tetracycline 500 mg po qid ×4wk*
Herpes Simplex Virus	Primary infection: Acyclovir 200 mg po 5× daily for 7-10d Acyclovir 5 mg/kg IV q8h for 5-7d Acyclovir cream Valacyclovir 500 mg po bid × 10d Famciclovir 125 mg po bid × 10d Recurrent infection: Acyclovir 200 mg po 5× daily for 5d Acyclovir 800 mg po bid for 5d Valacyclovir 500 mg po bid × 5d Famciclovir 125 mg po bid × 5d
Human Papillomavirus	Trichloroacetic acid 25% to 85% Podophyllin 10% to 25%* Laser ablation Electrodesiccation Cryotherapy
Haemophilus ducreyi	Ceftriaxone 250 mg IM single dose Azithromycin 1 gram po as a single dose Erythromycin base 500 mg po qid ×7d Amoxicillin 500 mg/clavulanic acid 125 mg po tid ×7d Ciprofloxacin 500 mg po bid ×3d*^
Trichomonas vaginalis	Metronidazole 2 grams po as a single dose* Metronidazole 250 mg po tid ×7d* Metronidazole gel* 20% saline douche
Crab Lice	Kwell shampoo or lotion

*should be avoided in pregnant patient
^should be avoided in patients <18 years old

5. Partners should be treated simultaneously.

VIII. Crab Lice.
  A. Can infest any hairy area (scalp, axilla, genitals).
  B. Adult female crabs lay eggs, which are glued to hairs.
    1. Eggs (nits) may be visible on careful inspection.
    2. 7-10 days later the young lice emerge.
      a. 87°F is optimum temperature for survival.
      b. Most young lice feed on blood within 24 hours.
  C. Treatment.
    1. Kwell shampoo or lotion, followed by combing out the nits.
    2. Wash bed linens and clothes.

IX. Hepatitis (see Chapter 9)

X. Human Immunodeficiency Virus/Acquired Immunodeficiency Syndrome (see Chapter 7)

Bibliography

Braverman PK, Strasburger VC: Sexually transmitted diseases, *Clin Ped* 33(1):26-37, 1994.

Chambers CV: Sexually transmitted diseases, *Primary Care* 17(4):833-851, 1990.

Hook EW, Sondheimer S, Zenilman J: Today's treatment for STDs, *Patient Care* 29(4):40-56, 1995.

Majeroni BA: Chlamydial cervicitis: complications and new treatment options, *Am Fam Phys* 49(8):1825-1829, 1994.

Mogabgab WJ: Recent developments in the treatment of sexually transmitted diseases, *Am J Med* 91(6A):6A140S-6A144S, 1991.

Morgan RJ: Clinical aspects of pelvic inflammatory disease, *Am Fam Phys* 43(5):1725-1732, 1996.

Reed BD, Eyler A: Vaginal infections: diagnosis and management, *Am Fam Phys* 47(8):1805-1816, 1993.

US Preventive Services Task Force: Screening for sexually transmitted diseases, *Am Fam Phys* 42(3):691-702, 1990.

CHAPTER 9

Infectious Disease in Athletes

Herbert G. Parris, MD

I. Background
   A. There have been a number of epidemiological studies on the effects of exercise on the immune system.
      1. Some studies have revealed a protective advantage against respiratory illnesses in athletes. However, there have also been studies to show that athletes are more susceptible to illness because of their training.
      2. Further research in this area of sports medicine is needed before a consensus statement can be made.

II. Immune System and Exercise
   A. Laboratory studies.
      1. Lymphocytes.
         a. Overall increase in number with exercise.
         b. Increased ratio of T cells to B cells with enhanced function.
         c. Decreased concentration of IgA in saliva and nasal washings of high intensity swimmers.
         d. Clinical effect is uncertain because changes appear to be transient (<2 hours).
      2. Granulocytes.
         a. Transient increase, lasting 1-2 hours after exercise.
         b. Mechanism likely to involve extracellular fluid shifts and increases in catecholamine, interleukin-1, and cortisol levels.
      3. Complement.
         a. Limited studies reveal no effect with exercise.
      4. Interleukin-1.
         a. Increases acutely with exercise.
         b. An immunostimulant that may cause an increase in T cell/B cell activity.
      5. Interferon.
         a. Minimal increase with exercise (lasting <2 hours).
         b. Clinical significance is uncertain.

B. Summary.
   1. Varied clinical results when comparing effects of acute vs. chronic exercise.
   2. Uncertainty surrounding the clinical significance of the laboratory findings.
   3. Overtraining has been linked to an increased susceptibility for infections.

III. Physiological effects of fever (>100°F) and illness on exercise.
   A. Respiratory.
      1. Increased airway resistance.
      2. Decreased diffusion capacity.
      3. Decreased alveolar ventilation to pulmonary gas exchange ratio.
   B. Cardiovascular.
      1. Increased heart rate.
      2. Increased O_2 consumption.
      3. Decreased blood pressure.
      4. Decreased peripheral resistance.
      5. Decreased maximal workload.
   C. Musculoskeletal.
      1. Decreased muscle strength.
      2. Premature fatigue.
   D. Temperature regulation.
      1. Increased temperature set point in the hypothalamus.
      2. Increased risk of dehydration and heat-related illnesses.
   E. Athletic performance.
      1. Decreased endurance.
      2. Decreased strength.
      3. Decreased aerobic power.
      4. Decreased coordination.
      5. Decreased concentration.
      6. One or all of the above may lead to increased risk of injury.

IV. Illnesses.
   A. Upper respiratory tract infections.
      1. Etiology.
         a. Most common infections seen in athletes.
         b. Usually caused by adenoviruses or rhinoviruses.
      2. Signs and symptoms.
         a. Fever.
         b. Chills.
         c. Cough.
         d. Myalgias.
         e. Nasal congestion.
         f. Sore throat.
         g. Fatigue.
      3. Treatment.
         a. Supportive care.
            (1) Rest.
            (2) Fluids.
         b. Medication.
            (1) Antipyretics.
            (2) Decongestants.
            (3) Cough suppressants.
            (4) Throat lozenges.
      4. Return to play guidelines/recommendations.
         a. When afebrile or low-grade (<100°F).

b. Myalgias have resolved.
c. Gradual reconditioning.

B. Infectious mononucleosis.
1. Etiology
a. Caused by Epstein-Barr virus.
b. Incubation period, 30-50 days.
c. Excreted in saliva.
d. Low contagiousness.
e. Affects ages 15-24 years.
f. Males and females equally affected.
g. 90% of Americans have been infected by the age of 30.
2. Signs and symptoms.
a. Prodrome, day 3-5.
(1) Fatigue.
(2) Headache.
(3) Anorexia.
(4) Malaise.
(5) Myalgias.
b. Day 5-15.
(1) Sore throat (moderate to severe).
(2) Tonsillar enlargement.
(3) Fever.
(4) Tender lymphadenopathy (anterior and posterior cervical).
(5) By week two, 50% to 70% with palpable enlarged spleen.
(6) Jaundice in 10% to 15%.
(7) 5% to 15% with morbilliform rash.
3. Laboratory diagnosis.
a. Positive heterophil antibody absorption test.
b. Elevated white blood cell count with lymphocytosis (10% to 20% atypical lymphocytosis).
c. Mild elevation in liver function tests (LFTs), reflecting hepatitis.
4. Complications
a. Concurrent (Group A streptococcal pharyngitis 5% to 30% of cases).
(1) Treat with penicillin or erythromycin.
(2) Avoid ampicillin due to antibody-induced rash.
b. Airway obstruction, secondary to enlargement of tonsils and adenoids.
(1) Treat with high-dose parenteral corticosteroids.
(2) Emergency nasotracheal intubation may be needed.
c. Splenic rupture.
(1) Occurs in 0.1% to 0.2% of patients.
(2) Usually occurs between days 4-21 of symptomatic illness.
(3) May be spontaneous or traumatic.
(4) Clinically with pain in left upper quadrant with radiation to left shoulder.
(5) Pain worse with deep inspiration.
(6) Clinical signs and symptoms of hypovolemia later develop.
d. Neurological complications.
(1) Encephalitis and Guillain-Barré syndrome (rare).
e. Pneumonitis.
f. Hepatitis.
5. Treatment.
a. Supportive

(1) Acetaminophen for symptoms of myalgias, headache, and fever.
(2) Consider stool softener if enlarged spleen (straining may cause rupture).
(3) Monitor for any complications.

b. Corticosteroids
(1) Use for severe disease and complications (nonstreptococcal pharyngitis, hepatitis, hematological and neurological sequelae).
(2) Imminent airway compromise.

6. Return to play guidelines/recommendations.
a. 3 weeks after onset of illness, noncontact training if:
(1) Spleen is not enlarged or painful.
(2) Afebrile.
(3) Laboratory abnormalities have resolved.
(4) Other complications have resolved.
b. 4 weeks after onset of illness, contact and strenuous training if:
(1) No splenic enlargement (if clinically unsure, ultrasound for size [normal is <14 cm]).

C. Streptococcal pharyngitis.
1. Etiology
a. Group A beta-hemolytic streptococcus.
2. Signs and symptoms.
a. Sore throat.
b. Fever.
c. Enlarged exudative tonsils.
d. Tender anterior cervical lymphadenopathy.
3. Diagnosis.
a. History of streptococcal exposure.
b. Clinical signs and symptoms.
c. Rapid streptococcal testing (enzyme-linked immunosorbent assay or latex agglutination technique).
(1) 85% to 90% accurate.
d. Throat culture.
(1) 95% accurate.
(2) 24-48 hour delay for results.
4. Treatment
a. Penicillin.
b. Erythromycin or cephalosporins in penicillin-allergic patients.
c. Supportive care.
(1) Analgesics.
(2) Saline gargles.
(3) Antipyretics.
(4) Throat lozenges.
(5) Increased fluid intake.
(6) Rest.
5. Return to play guidelines/recommendations.
a. Treatment is initiated.
b. Afebrile.

D. Pneumonia.
1. Etiology.
a. Viral.
b. Streptococcus pneumonia.
c. Mycoplasma pneumonia.

2. Signs and symptoms.
   a. Fever.
   b. Rigors.
   c. Productive cough.
   d. Dyspnea.
   e. Abnormal auscultation.
3. Diagnosis.
   a. History and clinical examination.
   b. White blood cell count.
   c. Sputum smear and culture.
   d. Chest x-ray.
4. Treatment.
   a. Erythromycin or clarithromycin (empirical).
   b. Supportive care
5. Return to play recommendations/guidelines.
   a. Resolved symptoms of fever, cough, and dyspnea.

E. Gastroenteritis.
1. Etiology.
   a. Viral (most common).
      (1) Rotavirus.
      (2) Norwalk agent.
   b. Bacterial.
   c. Protozoal.
2. Signs and symptoms.
   a. Diarrhea.
   b. Abdominal cramping.
   c. Fever.
   d. Vomiting.
   e. Myalgias.
3. Diagnosis.
   a. History and clinical examination.
   b. Stool culture sometimes indicated.
4. Treatment.
   a. Antimotility drugs: Imodium or Lomotil.
   b. Supportive care: fluid replacement.
   c. Antibiotics if culture-positive bacterial infection. For "traveler's diarrhea," treat with trimethoprim/sulfamethoxazole or ciprofloxacin.
   d. *Giardia* (a protozoan), treat with metronidazole.
5. Return to play recommendations/guidelines.
   a. Well hydrated.
   b. Afebrile.
   c. Less frequent diarrhea.

F. Other illnesses (less common).
1. Hepatitis B
   a. Risk of spread from athlete to athlete via exposure to blood or body secretions.
   b. Monitor clinical signs/symptoms and laboratory abnormalities (LFTs and hepatitis B antigen/antibodies) before return to play.
2. Otitis media
   a. Return to play.
      (1) Afebrile.
      (2) Ear plugs if tympanic membrane is perforated.
3. Otitis externa

a. Return to play.
(1) No balance problems.
(2) Treatment is initiated.
(3) Protective ear plugs for water sport athletes.

4. Sinusitis
a. Return to play.
(1) Afebrile.
(2) Treatment initiated.

5. Dermatologic infectious diseases.
a. Herpes gladiatorum: no contact activities until lesions have resolved.
b. Impetigo: as above.
c. Molluscum contagiosum: may be transferred by close contact.
d. Tinea: as above.
e. Folliculitis: may compete once treatment is started.

G. Immunizations.
1. Tetanus booster every 10 years (5 years if wound is dirty).
2. Measles vaccine.
a. If born after 1957 and if first vaccination prior to 12 months of age should have booster.
b. Booster recommended prior to entering college.
3. Influenza vaccine should be encouraged for athletes competing in fall and winter sports.
4. Rubella vaccine.
a. Indicated for children over 12 months old.
b. Given as part of measles/mumps/rubella (MMR) vaccine: as above.

Bibliography

Brenner IKM, Shek PN, Shepard RJ: Infection in athletes, *J Sports Med Physical Fitness* 34(1):11-22, 1994.

Mellion MB, Sitorius MA, Butcher JD: Medical problems in athletes. In Birrer RB, editor: *Sports medicine for the primary care physician,* ed 2, Boca Raton, 1994, CRC Press, pp 123-134.

Nieman DC: Exercise, infection and immunity, *Int J Sports Med* 15:S131-S141, 1994.

Simon HB: Immune mechanisms and infectious disease in exercise and sports. In Strauss RH, editor: *Sports Medicine,* Philadelphia, 1991, WB Saunders, pp 95-116.

CHAPTER 10

Exercise-Induced Asthma

Robert J. Johnson, MD

I. Definition
   A. Exercise-induced asthma (EIA) is a transient increase in airway responsiveness following 5-8 minutes of strenuous exercise.
   B. It may also include moderate to severe airway obstruction within 5-8 minutes of cessation of exercise.
   C. The bronchospasm occurs in large and small airways.
   D. There may be a component of EIA that may occur 6-8 hours following the initial obstruction and recovery.

II. Historical Perspective
   A. 2 AD: Aretaeus, the Cappadocian—"If from running, gymnastic exercise, or any other work, the breathing becomes difficult, it is called Asthma."
   B. 1679: EIA was reported by Thomas Willis.
   C. 1698: Sir John Floyer wrote *A Treatise on Asthma*. "All Violent Exercise makes the Asthmatic to breathe short." He also determined dancing to be more asthmogenic than walking.
   D. 1864: Salter observed that the passage of cold, fresh air was a cause of EIA.
   E. 1946: Herxheimer reported the results of pulmonary function tests in six patients with EIA.
   F. 1962: Jones determined that strenuous exercise of 1-2 minutes duration resulted in bronchodilatation but strenuous exercise of 6-12 minutes duration resulted in obstruction with coughing and wheezing.

III. Performance Issues
   A. 9% of the 1976 and 1980 Australian Olympic teams had EIA.
   B. 67 of 597 athletes on the 1984 U.S. Olympic team had EIA. Of these 67 athletes, 32 had the diagnosis of EIA confirmed *after* they had qualified for the Olympic team.
   C. 41 of the 67 won medals (15 gold, 21 silver, and 5 bronze).

IV. Incidence
   A. Asthma: 7% of the general population have asthma. Of all asthmatics, 80% to 95% have EIA.
   B. Allergies: 15% to 20% of the population have allergies. About 40% of those with allergic rhinitis have EIA.
   C. 3% to 4% of the general population with neither asthma nor allergic rhinitis have EIA.
   D. Gender
      1. Childhood: male-to-female ratio = 2 : 1.
      2. Adulthood: male-to-female ratio = 1 : 1.

V. Pathophysiology (Theoretical)
   A. The first requirement is "twitchy" lungs.
   B. Hyperventilation.
      1. Loss of heat from the bronchi. At rest, inspired air is warmed and humidified in the nose, pharynx, and the first seven generations of bronchi. During strenuous exercise, minute ventilation may increase as much as 30 times ventilation at rest. The ventilation rate overwhelms the capacity of the respiratory tract to adequately warm inspired air. This cooling may be contributory.
      2. Water loss from the airway. Rapid ventilation in cold, dry air results in water loss from the bronchi, causing hyperosmolarity of the periciliary fluid. In response to the fluid loss, bronchoactive substances (histamine, leukotrienes, and prostaglandins) are released. These substances either act directly on smooth muscle or stimulate irritant or cold receptors, triggering neurogenic bronchoconstriction mediated by vagal influences. The release of neutrophil chemotactic factor (NCF), eosinophil chemotactic factor (ECF), and leukotrienes (LTC_4, LTD_4, and LTE_4) may initiate the delayed response (to be discussed later). The rapid ventilation associated with exercise usually necessitates switching from nasal breathing to oral breathing, which may increase the osmolality of the surface fluid by as much as 27%.
   C. Air pollution.
      1. Exercise increases pollutant delivery by bypassing the nose and increasing the ventilatory rate. The afferent irritant fibers trigger bronchoconstriction in response to the air-borne irritants. There may be a synergistic effect between SO_2 and cold air in triggering bronchospasm.
      2. Primary pollutants: SO_2, CO, NO_3, and particulate matter.
      3. Secondary pollutants: ozone, NO_2, etc.

VI. Clinical Presentation
   A. Common symptoms: dyspnea out of proportion to the task, postexercise cough, and/or poorer performance than training would suggest.
   B. Other associated symptoms: dyspnea, wheezing, chest tightness, and/or sputum production.
   C. Small children may complain of a "stomachache" or refuse to participate in strenuous play because of their inability to "keep up."

VII. Clinical Course
   A. Stimulus: exercise at intensities of 75% to 85% of the maximum heart rate will trigger bronchoconstriction in large and small airways. Wheezing plateaus at about 8 minutes after onset, with complete recovery in 30-90 minutes.
   B. Refractory period: occurs within 1-3 hours of the first exercise challenge. The refractoriness diminishes after 2 hours and is absent at 4

hours. The refractory period may be a response to increased sympathetic activity.

C. Late response: occurs 4-8 hours after original exercise challenge. Up to one half of children and 40% of adults with EIA will have this delayed bronchoconstrictive response. This may represent an inflammatory response. This occurs primarily in the small airways. Typically, the reduction in forced expiratory volume in one second (FEV_1) of the late response is *less than* the FEV_1 in the immediate response.

VIII. Diagnosis

A. Exercise challenge test: exercise for 6-8 minutes at an intensity of about 85% Vo_2 max (90% maximum heart rate). A 10% reduction (some sources suggest 15% reduction) in FEV_1 or peak expiratory flow rate suggests EIA.

1. Free-range running (may include too many variables).
2. Treadmill.
3. Bicycle ergometer.

B. Methacholine challenge test (provocative): the lower the concentration necessary to provoke a bronchospastic response, the more severe the problem. Seems to be of little practical application.

C. If history suggests EIA, may confirm with peak flow meter used by athlete. Have athlete undergo a trial of aerosolized therapy to evaluate for symptomatic improvement or improvement in peak flow.

IX. Exercise variables

A. Intensity of exercise: degree of bronchoconstriction postexercise is maximum when the activity is 65% to 75% Vo_2 max. Exercise at intensities >85% Vo_2 max results in little or no further change in bronchoconstriction.

B. Type of activity: "most" to "least" asthmogenic—outdoor run > treadmill run > cycling > swimming > walking.

C. Continuous activity > intermittent activity.

D. Environment: cold, dry > warm, moist.

X. Treatment.

A. Nonpharmacological.

1. Exercise in a high humidity environment. Inhaling water vapor maintained at 98.6°F is the most effective means of prevention but is also the most impractical.
2. Nose breathing (better warming, humidifying).
3. Slow, deep breathing.
4. Exercise at maximum work load >5 minutes to induce a refractory period.
5. Physical training (does not prevent asthma; rather, it improves endurance and alters the threshold of onset of symptoms).
6. Control or avoidance of environmental pollutants, when possible.
7. Control of associated problems such as allergic rhinitis or infections (sinusitis, bronchitis, pneumonia, etc.).

B. Pharmacological.*

1. $Beta_2$-agonists (sympathomimetic agents), aerosolized agents.
   a. Dose: two inhalations 10-15 minutes prior to activity.
   b. Onset of action occurs in 2-15 minutes, with a duration of action of several hours, perhaps as much as 4-6 hours.
   c. 90% effective.

***Note:** Treatments outlined in B.1.-B.3. are most effective in athletes with normal resting airway function.

2. Cromolyn sodium: Thought to be the most effective for prophylaxis. Inhibits both the immediate *and* late responses of EIA. Synergistic with $beta_2$-agonists.
   a. Dose: two inhalations about 15 minutes before activity.
   b. Acts by stabilizing the basement membrane of mast cells by blocking Ca^{++} reflux. May be effective up to 2 hours.
   c. 70% effective.
3. Corticosteroid aerosols.
   a. Must be taken on a regular basis using $beta_2$-agonists preexercise.
   b. Most effective in inhibiting late-phase asthma response.
4. Theophylline (rapid-release formulation).
   a. Dose: 5 mg/kg 1 hour before exercise.
   b. Side effects may limit effectiveness.
5. Sustained-release theophylline.
   a. Dose: 12-20 mg/kg/day to maintain a blood level of 7.5-20 g/ml.
   b. Effective in athletes with abnormal resting airway function who do not respond to therapies listed above in B.1. and B.2.
6. Ipratropium aerosol. Lessens symptoms, or may prevent symptoms as a bronchodilator.
7. Antihistamines. Minimally effective in reducing EIA.
8. Other possibilities. Prazosin (alpha-blockers). Ca^{++} channel blockers—act as either smooth muscle relaxant vs. mast cell stabilizer.
9. Combination therapy for the difficult patient. $Beta_2$-agonist → 15 minutes exercise → repeat $beta_2$ dose → cromolyn → ipratropium → exercise → $beta_2$-agonist

XI. Benefits of exercise for the patient with EIA.
   A. Increase tolerance and threshold levels which imply higher levels of provocation are necessary to induce bronchoconstriction.
   B. Decreased medication requirements.
   C. Improvement in aerobic capacity.
   D. Enhancement of self-image.

XII. Are there ergogenic effects of bronchodilators?
   A. No ergogenic effects—Aerosolized albuterol, cromolyn, H_1 antagonists, normal doses of aerosolized corticosteroids.
   B. Suspected ergogenic effects.
      1. Methyl xanthines—aminophylline has been shown to improve diaphragmatic contractility in normal individuals, which may render these individuals less susceptible to fatigue. Increased inotropy demonstrated but no consistent changes in stroke volume or ejection fraction have been shown. Caffeine—quantitative restriction because of reported ergogenic effects at 12 µg/ml.
      2. Glucocorticoids—Large doses during or prior to competition have shown 23% increase in cardiac output in 9 normals.
      3. Fenoterol and clenbuterol (banned by the International Olympic Committee).

XIII. Banned substances to avoid using in athletes.
   A. Oral $beta_2$ agonists, including clenbuterol.
   B. Sympathomimetic amines (Adrenaline, ephedrine, isoproterenol, etc).
   C. Oral glucocorticoids.
   D. A cast of thousands (see banned substance list).

COMMON ALLERGY/ASTHMA MEDICATIONS BANNED BY NCAA/USOC

DRUG	BANNED BY	KEY
Epinephrine HCL Solution	Both	ST
Metaproterenol Sulfate Tablets/Inhaler	USOC	ST
Albuterol Sulfate Tablets/Inhaler	Both	ST
Terbutaline Sulfate Tablets	Both	ST
Isoetharine Nebulizer	USOC	ST,AA
Isoproterenol Nebulizer	USOC	ST,AA
Ephedrine Sulfate Nebulizer	USOC	ST
Perbuterol Acetate Inhaler	USOC	ST,AA
Epinephrine Bitartrate Inhaler	Both	ST,AA,CC
Bitolterol Mesylate Inhaler	USOC	ST,AA
Theophylline	USOC	ST,SH
Diphylline	USOC	ST,SH
Bromodiphenhydramine HCL	Both	SH,AL,CC
Brompheneramine Maleate	USOC	SH
Azatadine Maleate	USOC	SH
Phenylephrine HCL	USOC	ST,SH
Chlorpheniramine Maleate	USOC	SH
Pseudoephedrine HCL	USOC	ST,SH
Phenylpropanolamine HCL	USOC	ST,SH
Phenindamine Tartrate	USOC	SH
Dextromethorphan HBR	Both	SH,AL,CC
Promethazine HCL	Both	SH,AL,CC
Oxymetazoline HCL	USOC	ST

KEY

BOTH = Banned by USOC and NCAA
USOC = Banned only by United States Olympic Committee
ST = Stimulants: most psychomotor and central nervous system stimulants
SH = Shooter: USOC bans most antihistamines for two sports involving riflery
AL = Contains alcohol, which is banned by NCAA for riflery competition
CC = Cough and cold decongestants permitted by NCAA, but remained banned by USOC

Adapted from Fuentes RJ, Rosenberg JM, Davis A: *Athletic Drug Reference* "95", Clean Data Inc., North Carolina, 1995, pp. 265-368 by Michael Moreno, MD.

Bibliography

Anderson SD: Exercise-induced asthma: new thinking and current management, *J Respir Dis* 7:48-61, 1986.

Anderson SD: Exercise-induced asthma: the state of the art, *Chest* 87:191S-197S, 1985.

Athletes and exercise-induced bronchospasm (symposium), *Med Sci Sports Exerc* 18(3):314-333, 1986.

Bierman CW: Exercise-induced asthma, *NER Allergy Proc* 9:193-197, 1988.

Fitch KD: The use of anti-asthmatic drugs: do they affect performance? *Sports Med* 3:136-150, 1986.

Grindel SH, McKeag DB: Management of the athlete with exercise-induced asthma, *Clin J Sports Med* 2:208-215, 1992.

Pierson WE: Exercise-induced bronchospasm in children and adolescents, *Ped Clin NA* 35:1031-1040, 1988.

Sly RM: Management of exercise-induced asthma, *Drug Ther* 95-100, 1982.

Speir WA et al: Exercise-induced asthma: meeting the challenge, *J Respir Dis* 4:10-13, 1983.

Voy RO: The U.S. Olympic committee experience with exercise-induced bronchospasm—1984, *Med Sci Sports Exerc* 18(3):328-333, 1986.

CHAPTER 11

The Diabetic Athlete

James M. Moriarity, MD

I. Introduction
   A. There are currently 14 million diabetic patients in the United States. Most are cared for by primary care physicians. The discovery of insulin liberated many juvenile onset diabetics from ketoacidosis and certain death. The arrival of the sulfonylurea agents provided a means of treatment for adult onset diabetes. With the advent of portable glucose scanners, diabetic patients have been able to achieve a greater degree of glucose control than was ever thought possible.
   B. The benefit of exercise in the treatment of diabetes has been advocated. Much research has been performed examining the use of exercise in the prevention and treatment of diabetes and its complications. Physicians will be challenged to provide information, encouragement, and in some cases permission for these athletes to compete.
II. Demographics
   A. Approximately 1 in 500 children under the age of 18 have insulin-dependent diabetes mellitus (IDDM).
   B. Between the ages of 30 and 50, 3% to 5% of the population have non–insulin-dependent diabetes mellitus (NIDDM).
   C. This percentage increases to nearly 20% of the population over the age of 65.
   D. Of the non–insulin-dependent group, 80% are obese.
   E. Diabetes is the leading cause of blindness in the United States.
   F. It is associated with a two- to four-fold rise in cardiovascular disease over controls.
   G. Diabetes is the most common etiology of end stage renal disease and a major contributor to peripheral and autonomic neuropathy.
III. Benefits of Exercise
   A. The Diabetes Control and Complications Trial Research Group study (published in the *New England Journal of Medicine* in 1993) clearly demonstrated in IDDM patients the beneficial effects of tight glucose control in the development and progression of diabetic complications.

1. One of the frequently asked questions is: "Will increased exercise improve glucose control?" In contrast to NIDDM patients, for whom exercise is unquestionably beneficial in the control of blood glucose, there are no convincing data to suggest a similar benefit for IDDM patients.
2. The increased insulin sensitivity bequeathed to regular exercisers with IDDM is in part counterbalanced by an increased need for additional calories and its risk of attendant hyperglycemia.

B. Exercise has been recommended in the treatment of diabetes since Hippocrates. The benefits of exercise in diabetes are many and include:
1. Reduced hyperinsulinemia.
2. Improvement in insulin sensitivity.
3. Reduced body fat.
4. Lower blood pressure.
5. Normalization of dyslipoproteinemias.

C. Insulin secretion and sensitivity.
1. Exercise has been shown to have a potentiating effect on the action of insulin in both insulin-dependent and non–insulin-dependent diabetics.
2. The precise reason for this glucose-lowering effect is unknown but is thought to involve activity of glucose receptors at the cell membrane.
3. Exercise can play a role in the prevention or delay of NIDDM. This was clearly demonstrated in a study of University of Pennsylvania alumni by Hemrich and associates, who found a 6% decrease in age-adjusted risk for every increment of 500 kcal energy expenditure per week.

D. Obesity induces a hyperinsulinemic state in normal individuals.
1. The etiology of this insulinemia stems from both increased beta cell production and reduced liver clearance of insulin as a consequence of increasing insulin resistance in peripheral tissues and the liver.
2. As long as insulin production matches insulin need, normoglycemia is maintained. A decrease in insulin production results in the onset of clinical diabetes.

E. Weight reduction, lipids, and diabetes.
1. Heath, Leonard, and Wilson studied the effects of exercise on diabetes in a Zuni Indian population. Diabetic patients who participated in a supervised exercise program reduced their weight and body fat, lowered their fasting blood sugars, and in most cases were able to discontinue hypoglycemic agents.
2. Exercise in diabetic patients has most of the same lipid-modifying effects as in nondiabetics.
3. High-density lipoprotein cholesterol does not seem to be similarly affected in IDDM but is lower than controls in NIDDM.

F. Hypertension.
1. The risk of hypertension is increased in diabetic populations.
2. It is not clear if increases in blood pressure are linked to hyperinsulinemia and its effect on renal tubular absorption of sodium or as a linked genetic cofactor of essential hypertension with dyslipoproteinemia and disordered carbohydrate metabolism (see article by Reaven and Hoffman).
3. Regular exercise is known to reduce both systolic and diastolic blood pressure.

G. Training benefit.
   1. Diabetic athletes demonstrate the same cellular increases in glycolytic and oxidative enzyme concentrations with training as controls.
   2. Glycogen storage in muscle is markedly decreased in diabetes, and training restores and enhances glycogen synthetase activity.
   3. Vo_2 max is reduced at baseline relative to controls but does demonstrate increases with training.
   4. Increases in capillarization in skeletal muscle seen with training are less apparent in diabetics with longer duration of disease.

IV. Risks of Exercise
   A. With the proper evaluation and care, some degree of exercise is possible in all patients with diabetes, regardless of attendant complications. There are, however, *contraindications* to *strenuous* exercise in diabetic patients with:
      1. Poor control.
      2. Proliferative retinopathy.
      3. Microangiopathy.
      4. Neuropathy.
      5. Nephropathy.
      6. Cardiovascular disease.
   B. Athletes with IDDM or NIDDM requesting permission to participate in strenuous exercise should be carefully screened for secondary complications. Table 11-1 outlines risks associated with exercise in athletes with diabetic complications.
   C. The most immediate and common problem associated with exercise and diabetes is the development of hypoglycemia.
      1. Hypoglycemia may occur during, shortly after, or 8-16 hours after conclusion of exercise.
      2. Sports such as long distance solo swimming, scuba diving, race car driving, and technically difficult rock climbing may pose difficulty in treatment of hypoglycemia.

V. Glucose Homeostasis in Normal and Diabetic Athletes
   A. Glucose is the principal source of energy for vigorous muscle usage and the only source of fuel for anaerobic activity.
      1. Glucose can be stored in muscle as glycogen, providing a ready but limited source of available fuel from the process of glycolysis.
      2. The major source of stored glycogen is the liver, from which it is released to the circulation for delivery to hungry muscle by the process of glycogenolysis.
      3. De novo synthesis of glucose occurs through the process of gluconeogenesis, whereby catabolized proteins and glycerol combine to form new molecules of glucose.
      4. Gluconeogenesis is the major contributor to increases in blood sugar in NIDDM.
   B. Free fatty acids are the primary source of fuel for prolonged aerobic exercise.
      1. Muscles have virtually unlimited supply of free fatty acids available from stores in the body's adipose tissue.
      2. The use of free fatty acids is limited by the availability of oxygen at the cellular level and the concentration of the cleaving enzyme lipoprotein lipase.
   C. The delivery of these fuels to the muscle metabolic machinery is a complex process, involving the interplay of the hormones insulin, glucagon, norepinephrine, cortisol, and growth hormone.

TABLE 11-1. Special precautions when recommending exercise for patients with insulin-dependent diabetes

Complication	Precaution
Retinopathy[1,2]	Avoid strenuous, high-intensity activities that involve breath holding (e.g., weight lifting and isometrics). Avoid activities that lower the head (e.g., yoga, gymnastics) or that risk jarring the head.
Hypertension	Avoid heavy weight lifting or breath holding. Perform primarily dynamic exercise using large muscle groups, such as walking and cycling at a moderate intensity.
Autonomic neuropathy[2]	Likelihood of hypoglycemia and hypertension. Elevated resting heart rate and reduced maximal heart rate. Use of RPE[3] recommended. Prone to dehydration and hypothermia.
Peripheral neuropathy	Avoid exercise that may cause trauma to the feet (e.g., prolonged hiking, jogging, or walking on uneven surfaces). Nonweight-bearing activities are most appropriate (e.g., cycling and swimming). Regular assessment of the feet recommended. The feet should be kept clean and dry. Careful choice of shoes for proper fit.
Nephropathy	Avoid exercise that raises blood pressure (e.g., weight lifting, high-intensity aerobic exercises, and breath holding).
All patients	Carry identification with diabetes information. Rehydrate carefully (drink fluids before, during, and after exercise). Avoid exercise in the heat of the day and in direct sunlight (wear hat and sunscreen when in sun).

From Campaigne BN, Lampman R: *Exercise in the clinical management of diabetes*, Springfield, IL, 1994, Human Kinetics.

D. The action of insulin in the body is anabolic.
   1. Insulin facilitates the passage of blood-borne glucose into the muscle cell for conversion to glycogen.
   2. In the liver insulin promotes glycogen synthesis while inhibiting its breakdown through its inhibition of glucagon.
   3. In fat cells insulin facilitates the uptake of glucose and stimulates its conversion to triglyceride, while likewise inhibiting the enzymes of lipolysis.
   4. Finally, insulin inhibits gluconeogenesis, thus exhibiting a protein-sparing effect.

E. The catecholamines, glucagon, growth hormone, and cortisol are all involved in the liberation of energy stores, with glucagon and epinephrine playing the most important roles.
   1. Glucagon directly stimulates glycogenolysis and gluconeogenesis.
   2. Epinephrine has similar action at the peripheral level and, in addition, stimulates lipolysis.

F. When exercise begins:
   1. Insulin levels decline.
   2. Catecholamine and glucagon levels rise.
G. As exercise progresses:
   1. All available glycogen stores are exhausted and glucose becomes available only through the process of gluconeogenesis or from ingested glucose.
   2. If glucose production fails to keep up with its removal from the circulation, hypoglycemia ensues.
H. Insulin resistance is a characteristic of diabetes, especially NIDDM.
   1. Insulin resistance is present peripherally at the muscle and adipocyte receptors and centrally in the liver.
   2. One of the consequences of hepatic insulin resistance is nonsuppression of glucagon activity, further contributing to the hyperglycemic state. As long as insulin output increases, normoglycemia is maintained. When insulin secretion declines, hyperglycemia ensues.

VI. Exercise and the Diabetic Athlete
   A. A diabetic athlete who begins exercise in a *well-controlled* state (blood sugar 100-200 mg/dl, no ketones) should experience little difficulty in completing activity lasting up to an hour. Muscle demands for glucose are met by stored muscle glycogen and available liver glycogen. If the athlete has timed activity to avoid peaking levels of injected insulin, there will be a steady or declining level of insulin and a rising level of glucagon ready to liberate glucose to hungry exercising muscle.
   B. An athlete who begins exercise in a *poorly controlled* state (sugar >250 mg/dl, plus ketones) risks worsening of hyperglycemia and eventual ketosis. Peripheral glucose uptake will be impaired by the relative or absolute lack of insulin, and unopposed glycogenolysis and gluconeogenesis from glucagon activity will add to the already high levels of circulating glucose.
   C. Finally, a diabetic athlete who begins exercise with a glucose level *<100* mg/dl and/or during a time of *peaking insulin activity* risks hypoglycemia. As the demands of exercise deplete muscle glycogen and blood sugar begins to fall, the liver is called on to release its supply. If the athlete's insulin levels are relatively high, glucagon is inhibited and glycogenolysis, gluconeogenesis, and release of glucose supplies cannot take place.
   D. *Therefore diabetic athletes should time exercise to coincide with steady or falling levels of insulin and rising levels of glucagon.*

VII. Preparticipation Evaluation
   A. There is no organized competitive sport in which diabetic athletes do not participate. The American Diabetes Association and the International Diabetic Athletes Association are two organizations that encourage and provide help to diabetic athletes in their pursuit of athletic excellence.
   B. The principal differences between competitive and therapeutic exercise are the risk of physical injury and impairment from the activity, the intensity and duration of training required to prepare for and sustain the activity, and the likelihood that the patient will be able to maintain the selected activity for many years.
   C. The preparticipation evaluation of a patient with diabetes should proceed in a logical and comprehensive manner.
      1. The first step in a preparticipation evaluation is to ensure that the minimal levels of care of the athlete are being met. The American

Diabetes Association has published standards of care for patients with diabetes (Table 11-2) and the preparticipation examination should not function as a substitute for ongoing medical care.

2. The second step is a history and physical examination that evaluates the specific requirements of the sport and the physical capabilities of the patient. This is no different than any other athlete seeking permission to compete.
3. Third is a diligent search for diabetic complications that may influence the type of exercise or sport permitted: specifically, retinopathy, nephropathy, cardiovascular disease, and neuropathy.
4. Fourth is a discussion with the patient and family about the anticipated changes in insulin dosage, dietary needs, strategies to avoid hypoglycemia, and necessity for increased glucose monitoring.

D. Treadmill testing is a useful adjunct in the evaluation of diabetic patients with complications of retinopathy or autonomic neuropathy and those at risk for cardiovascular disease.
   1. Exercise treadmill testing is recommended for all diabetic patients older than 35.
   2. Treadmill testing can also determine correlations between target heart rate, blood pressure, and perceived level of exertion and can give diabetic patients clues as to what self-determined set limits should be.

VIII. Strategies for Glucose Control During Exercise

A. Exercise, insulin, and meals should be timed with the following points kept in mind.
   1. Meals should be eaten 1 to 3 hours before exercise and should anticipate the intensity and duration of the exercise activity.
   2. Avoid exercising during times of peaking insulin activity.
   3. Do not begin exercise within 1 hour of insulin administration to prevent the possibility of a more rapid rate of insulin absorption from underlying exercising muscle.
   4. Check blood sugar before exercise; if >250 mg/dl, delay exercise; if <100 mg/dl, supplement with a snack.
   5. If exercise duration is >30 minutes, consider supplementing with glucose-containing fluids.
   6. Be prepared for hypoglycemia.
   7. After exercise, check blood sugar. If initiating a more intense training schedule, recheck sugar as needed to avoid delayed onset hypoglycemia.
   8. After exercise, replenish carbohydrate stores according to duration and intensity of activity in anticipation of next exercise session.

B. Portable glucose monitors have greatly aided the diabetic athlete in monitoring glucose levels. There can be no substitute for frequent glucose readings during the initiation of an exercise program, changes in training programs, or contests at times different from the customary training period.

C. Much has been written about the accelerated absorption rates of insulin injected subcutaneously over exercising muscles as opposed to a "neutral site" such as the abdomen.
   1. While there are differences in absorption rates, they are not consistently present nor is there strong evidence to say they are a cause of hypoglycemia.
   2. What do seem to be consistent are that insulin injected subcutaneously is absorbed more quickly over underlying exercising muscle

TABLE 11-2. American Diabetes Association (ADA) standards of care for patients with diabetes

Nature of Intervention	Recommended Frequency: Patients on Insulin	Recommended Frequency: Patients not on Insulin	Treatment Goal
HbA_{1c} evaluation	Quarterly	As often as needed to achieve and maintain near-normal blood glucose levels (usually quarterly)	Keep at or below 8%
Evaluation of FPG concentration	As often as needed	As often as needed (usually 4-6 times/year)	Keep at or below 140 mg/dl
Fasting lipid profile (total cholesterol, HDL, LDL, triglycerides)	Initially—subsequent frequency depends on results and treatment	Initially—subsequent frequency depends on results and treatment	LDL ≤130 mg/dl (no CHD) LDL ≤100 mg/dl (with CHD)
Urine protein evaluation	Yearly	Yearly	Negative
Determination for microalbuminuria	Yearly (if urine protein negative)	Yearly (if urine protein negative)	Negative
Office visit for diabetes (to include weight, blood pressure, foot examination)	Quarterly	Quarterly to semiannually	Education Management of diabetes and lipid disorders Early detection and treatment of complications
Telephone follow-up	As needed—sometimes weekly	As needed—sometimes weekly	Adjustment of insulin doses and encouragement to comply with regimen
Self-monitoring of blood glucose	Daily—preprandially and before bedtime (snack) ideal (regimen based on patient's needs)	As needed, based on patient preference	As close to normal as possible, based on patient circumstances
Ophthalmology referral	Yearly	Yearly	Early treatment and detection of diabetic retinopathy

HbA_{1c} = glycosolated hemoglobin; FPG = fasting plasma glucose; LDL = low-density lipoprotein; CHD = coronary heart disease.
From Peters AL, McCullough DK, Hayward RA, et al: Delayed diagnoses of NIDDM, Journal of Clinical Outcomes 1(2):13, 1994

and that massage or heat applied to the injection site increases absorption rates.

3. The athlete should understand that injection site absorption may be influenced by exercise and that alterations in glucose levels may be affected.

D. Inadvertent injection of insulin intramuscularly rather than subcutaneously definitely is associated with a more rapid onset of action and should be avoided preexercise. This circumstance can be prevented by grasping the injection site with a pinch technique and injecting at an oblique angle rather than perpendicular to the skin and by using shorter needles (<8 mm).

E. Differences in absorption rates of porcine versus genetically engineered human insulin have been observed.
   1. Human insulin is absorbed faster than porcine insulin at rest.
   2. Both are absorbed faster with exercise but porcine slightly more.
   3. The net effect is that there are few differences overall between human and porcine insulin and they are not very significant to the exercising athlete.

F. A comparison of peak action and duration of activity of the commonly used insulins is included in Table 11-3.

G. As stated previously, the strategy of a well-controlled, normoglycemic athlete planning an exercise activity is to time the onset of activity so as to coincide with decreasing insulin activity and increasing levels of blood sugar. Table 11-4 provides a general strategy to achieve this goal.

H. The *duration and intensity* of the exercise determine the *amount* of additional food intake the athlete requires for exercise. The *preexercise* blood sugar determines the *timing* of food intake. These amounts vary

TABLE 11-3. Activity characteristics of insulins*

	Onset (hr)	Peak (hr)	Duration (hr)
Rapid acting			
Insulin injection (regular)	½-1	2-4	5-7
Prompt insulin zinc suspension (Semilente)	1-3	2-8	12-16
Intermediate acting			
Insulin zinc susp. (Lente)	1-3	6-12	24-28
Isophane insulin susp. (NPH)	1-3	6-12	24-28
Long acting			
Extended insulin zinc susp. (Ultralente)	4-6	18-24	36+
Protamine zinc insulin susp. (PZI)	4-6	14-24	36+

*Onset, peak, and duration of action vary considerably and are dependent upon the individual patient, injection site, vascularity, and temperature.
From Campaigne BN, Lampman R: *Exercise in the clinical management of diabetes*, Springfield, IL, 1994, Human Kinetics.

TABLE 11-4. General guidelines for avoiding hypoglycemia during and after exercise

Blood glucose monitoring
1. Monitor blood glucose immediately before, during (every 30 min), and 15 min after exercise.
2. Delay exercise if blood glucose is 250 mg/dl or higher or if ketones are present.
3. Consume carbohydrates if blood glucose is ≤80-100 mg/dl.
4. Learn individual glucose response to different types of exercise.
5. Avoid exercising late at night.

Insulin
1. Decrease insulin dose:
   a. Intermediate-acting insulin: Decrease by 30% to 35% on the day of exercise.
   b. Intermediate- and short-acting insulin: Omit dose of short-acting insulin that precedes exercise.
   c. Multiple doses of short-acting insulin: Reduce the dose prior to exercise by 30% to 35% and supplement carbohydrates.
   d. Continuous subcutaneous infusion: Eliminate mealtime bolus or increment that precedes or immediately follows exercise.
2. Avoid exercising muscle underlying injections of short-acting insulin for 1 hr after injection.
3. Do not exercise at the time of peak insulin action.

Adapted from Vitung JA, Schneider SH, Ruderman NB. In Pandolf K, editor: *Exercise and sport sciences reviews*, vol 16, New York, 1988, McGraw-Hill, pp 285-304. In Campaigne BN, Lampman R: *Exercise in the clinical management of diabetes*, Springfield, IL, 1994, Human Kinetics.

per individual. A general guideline for food intake adjustments is in Table 11-5.

I. Exercise of prolonged duration requires that the athlete replenish depleted glycogen stores in liver and muscle. This is best accomplished within 4 hours after conclusion of the exercise or competition. Carbohydrates moderately high in glycemic index are recommended.
J. Delayed hypoglycemia occurring 1 to 12 hours postexercise can afflict diabetic athletes who have failed to ingest adequate carbohydrates necessary for muscle and liver glycogen replenishment. It is important for patients beginning exercise programs or those altering training schedules to test blood sugar frequently in the hours following exercise. For this reason also, it may be prudent to avoid late evening training regimens or, in the case where there is late competition, to provide box lunches for the bus ride home.

TABLE 11-5. General guidelines for making food adjustments for exercise

Type of Exercise and Examples	If Blood Glucose is:	Increase Food Intake By:	Suggestions of Food to Use
Exercise of short duration and of low to moderate intensity (walking a half mile or leisurely bicycling for less than 30 minutes)	less than 100 mg/dl	10 to 15 gms of carbohydrate per hour	1 fruit or 1 starch/bread exchange
	100 mg/dl or above	not necessary to increase food	
Exercise of moderate intensity (one hour of tennis, swimming, jogging, leisurely bicycling, golfing, etc.)	less than 100 mg/dl	25 to 50 gms of carbohydrate before exercise, then 10 to 15 gms per hr of exercise	½ meat sandwich with a milk or fruit exchange
	100 to 180 mg/dl	10 to 15 gms of carbohydrate	1 fruit or 1 starch/bread exchange
	180 to 300 mg/dl	not necessary to increase food	
	300 mg/dl or above	don't begin exercise until blood glucose is under better control	
Strenuous activity or exercise (about one to two hours of football, hockey, racquetball, or basketball games; strenuous bicycling or swimming; shoveling heavy snow)	less than 100 mg/dl	50 gms of carbohydrate, monitor blood glucose carefully	1 meat sandwich (2 slices of bread) with a milk and fruit exchange
	100 to 180 mg/dl	25 to 50 gms of carbohydrate, depending on intensity and duration	½ meat sandwich with a milk or fruit exchange
	180 to 300 mg/dl	10 to 15 gms of carbohydrate	1 fruit or 1 starch/bread exchange
	300 mg/dl or above	don't begin exercise until blood glucose is under better control	

From Etzwiler DD et al: *Learning to live well with diabetes,* Minnetonka, MN, 1987, Chronimed Publishing, p 157. Copyright 1991 by International Diabetes Center, Park Nicollet Medical Center. Adapted by permission.

Bibliography

Campaigne BN, Lampman R: *Exercise in the clinical management of diabetes,* Springfield, IL. 1994, Human Kinetics.

The Diabetes Control and Complications Trial Research Group: The effect of intensive treatment of diabetes on the development and progression of long-term complications in Insulin Dependent Diabetes Mellitus, *N Eng J Med,* 329:977-986, 1993.

Gordon NF: *Diabetes, your complete exercise guide,* The Cooper Clinic and Research Institute Fitness Series. Champaign, IL. 1993, Kinetics.

Heath GW, Wilson RH, Smith J, Leonard BE: Community-based exercise and weight control: Diabetes risk reduction and glycemic control in Zuni Indians, *Clin Nutr* 53(suppl 6):16425-16465.

Helmrich SP, Raglund DR, Leung RW, et al: Physical activity and reduced occurrence of non-insulin-dependent diabetes mellitus, *N Eng J Med,* 325(3):147-152.

Landry G, Allen D: Diabetes mellitus and exercise, *Clin Sports Med,* p 403, April 1992.

Polansky K, Given B, Hirsch L, et al: The basal hyperinsulinemia of obesity is due to enhanced insulin secretion, *Clin Res* 34:552a.

Reaven GM, Hoffman BB: A role for insulin in the etiology and course of hypertension? *Lancet* 2(8556):435-437.

Robbins DC, Carleton S: Managing the diabetic athlete, *Physician Sports Med,* p 45, Dec 1989.

Sherman W, Albright A: Exercise and type I diabetes, Gatorade Sports Science Exchange, No 25.

Sherman W, Albright A: Exercise and type II diabetes, Gatorade Sports Science Exchange, No 37.

Stater MA: Managing diabetes in older adults, *Physician Sports Med,* p 66, March 1991.

Suton JR: Metabolic response to exercise in normal and diabetic individuals. In Strauss R, editor: *Sports Medicine,* Philadelphia, 1984, WB Saunders.

CHAPTER 12

Gastrointestinal Problems in Athletes

Jeffrey A. Housner, MD

Gary A. Green, MD

I. Introduction
   A. Exercise has been found to have several positive effects on the gastrointestinal (GI) tract.
      1. Decrease in constipation.
      2. Possible decrease in incidence of colon cancer.[100,101]
   B. Exercise has been associated with several gastrointestinal (GI) symptoms, and being physically active does not preclude the development of GI pathology.
   C. Studies on the association between the GI tract and exercise are difficult to interpret due to several factors.
      1. Problems tend to be multifactorial and there is difficulty in controlling for all variables (i.e., diet, exercise intensity, etc.).
      2. Many studies lack an adequate denominator, making a true incidence of symptoms difficult to determine.
      3. Studies sometimes use artificial means to measure parameters (e.g., exercising with an esophageal manometer), and this may influence outcomes.
      4. Many studies have not controlled for common underlying diseases, such as irritable bowel syndrome, which may have similar symptoms.
      5. Many studies rely on low response rate surveys, which introduces selection bias.
      6. Reliance on a subject's dietary recall as an assessment of diet may result in inaccuracies.
   D. This chapter summarizes the existing literature and makes consensus recommendations for the clinician.
   E. Further research is needed to answer many of the clinical questions regarding the relationship between the GI tract and exercise.

II. Incidence
   A. First case reports of exercise-related diarrhea appeared in the late 1970s and early 1980s,[13,30,97] and the first survey of running-related GI symptoms was published in 1981.[109]

B. Incidence of GI complaints (see Table 12-1).

C. An *increase* in all GI complaints is associated with the following conditions.[8,9,39,45]

1. Dehydration.
2. Greater exercise intensity.
3. Training status.
    a. Untrained > trained.
    b. Improvement in preexisting GI problems with regular training.
4. Younger > older.
5. Female > male, especially during the menstrual cycle.
6. Type of exercise (i.e., running > cycling, swimming, speed skating, and cross-country skiing).
7. Large precompetition meal, rich in fat, protein and dietary fiber, and taken shortly before exercise.
8. Highly concentrated drinks (e.g., containing glucose, honey, maple syrup) or food substances such as caffeine, protein, herb extracts, or salt tablets.

D. Most common cause to stop during a run is *urge to defecate.*

E. Sullivan and associates[107] published the first case-controlled survey (see Table 12-1).

1. Running is not likely to be sole precipitant of upper GI symptoms; other factors may include eating, drinking, belching, and maximal exertion.
2. Lower GI symptoms may be caused by running, or the "running lifestyle" (i.e., increased fiber and fruit in the diet).

III. Etiology of Upper GI Problems

A. Esophageal function.

1. Esophageal sphincter pressure (ESP)—conflicting results.
    a. Mean *decrease* in lower ESP in athletes with heartburn[94] and during 30-minute bicycle ergometer test.[23]
    b. Mean *increase* in lower ESP measured immediately postexercise compared to preexercise values in asymptomatic athletes.[117]
    c. No change detected in lower ESP[71] or in upper ESP[23] during exercise
2. Gastroesophageal reflux.
    a. Exercise induces gastroesophageal reflux.[51,102,103,119]
    b. Effect of exercise on gastroesophageal reflux is more potent in subjects who also experience reflux at rest.[8]
    c. Running induces highest frequency of gastroesophageal reflux,[51] more so than bicycling and weight lifting.[15]
    d. Exercise in fed state leads to more reflux than in fasted state.
    e. Esophageal reflux can aggravate myocardial ischemia and produce abnormalities in persons with both normal and stenotic coronary arteries.[58,94]
    f. Pretreatment with H_2 blockers is effective in reducing esophageal acid exposure and running-associated reflux.[51]
3. Esophageal motility—amplitude, duration, and frequency of esophageal contractions—decreased steadily with increasing exercise intensity in both trained[103] and untrained subjects.[102]

B. Gastric secretion.

1. Gastric acid secretion has been found to be unaffected[28] or decreased[54,82] by exercise.
2. Seven-fold increase in concentration of intragastric bile acids found in military recruits subjected to physical stress.[78]

TABLE 12-1. Incidence of gastrointestinal symptoms associated with exercise

Reference	No. of Subjects (% response)	% Male	Event	Upper GI Tract (%)				Lower GI Tract (%)			
				Loss of Appetite	Heartburn	Nausea	Vomiting	Abdominal Cramps	Urge to Defecate	Bowel Movement with Exercise	Diarrhea
Sullivan et al.[107]	57	70	Running Club	50	10	6	6		30		
Keeffe et al.[45]	707 (41.6)	86	Marathon								
Easy run					8.8	1.8	0.3	10.9	38.6	18.4	8.2
Hard run					9.5	11.6	1.8	19.3	36.4	16	10
After run					3.5	12.7	1.8	13.9	38.2	34.9	14.2
Worobetz and Gerrard[118]	70 (59)	87	Enduro*	41	11	21	0.6		54	44	26
Riddoch and Trinick[87]	471 (27)	92	Marathon								
Easy run				3	6	2	0.2	10	20		14
Hard run				28	13	20	4	31	42		28
After run				30	9	21	5	20	43		32
Worme et al.[116]	67 (44)	73	Triathlon	13	9	6	2	4			18
Sullivan et al.[105]			Running Club								
Runners	93 (93)	65			19†	4‡	—	20	60¶		60‡
Controls	95 (95)	63			22	8	2	21	30		40

*800-m swim, 25-km cycle, 5-km canoe, 12-km run.
†$p < .05$.
‡$p < .01$.
¶$p < .001$.

C. Gastric emptying—affected by multiple variables.
   1. Exercise intensity.
      a. Up to about 70% $Vo_{2\,max}$, gastric emptying is accelerated* or unchanged.[28]
      b. When $Vo_{2\,max}$ is greater than 70%, gastric emptying is delayed.[21,27,82]
   2. Training status/type of exercise—at exercise intensities up to about 70% $Vo_{2\,max}$, training status or type of exercise did not influence rate of gastric emptying.[43,85]
   3. Dehydration reduces gastric emptying rate.[86]
   4. Hormonal.
      a. Gastrin[28] and motilin[108] *increase* gastric emptying.
      b. Catecholamines[44,83] and endorphins[14] *decrease* gastric emptying.
      c. The overall effect of hormones on gastric emptying during exercise remains obscure because of interindividual variability, wide fluctuations in hormonal blood levels, and large interactions among the multiple hormones produced during exercise.
   5. Composition of the ingested solution.
      a. Fluid osmolality does not affect gastric emptying rate.[75]
      b. The following factors *decrease* gastric emptying rate.[10]
         i. Higher caloric density.†
         ii. ↑ temperature.
         iii. ↑ amino acid content.
         iv. ↑ fatty acid content.
         v. ↑ acidity.
         vi. Solid meal
      c. The body will vary gastric emptying in response to changes of the caloric content of the ingested fluid to maintain isocaloric and isoosmotic jejunal contents.[72]

IV. Recommendations to the Athlete for Prophylaxis and Treatment of Upper GI Symptoms[9,38]
   A. Reduce the level of exertion of the exercise, followed by a gradual increase in intensity.
   B. Adequate fluid intake during exercise should be part of every training session and competitive event.
   C. Liquid foods can be taken as a precompetition meal and also during exercise; however, fat and protein should be minimized.
   D. Whenever fluid intake is the first priority, drinks should be cold and low in carbohydrate.
   E. Whenever carbohydrate intake is of first priority, drinks may contain up to 10% glucose.
   F. When maximal intake rates of both carbohydrate and water are desired, the optimal concentration should be in the range of isotonicity.
   G. Solid foods should be avoided during the last 3 hours prior to competition.
   H. Pretreatment with H_2 blockers is effective in reducing nausea[2] and running-associated reflux[51] without impairment in psychomotor performance or cardiovascular response.[60]
   I. Omeprazole may be considered for short-term and maintenance therapy for athletes with upper GI symptoms.

*References 12, 21, 29, 31, 62, 74.

†All factors considered, the caloric content of the ingested fluid appears to be the primary determinant of gastric emptying.

V. Etiology of Lower GI Problems
  A. Intestinal motility and transit.
    1. Gastroduodenal.
      a. Duodenal contents signal gastric emptying.[3]
      b. Fatty acids in the duodenum result in an increase in duodenal contractions and a subsequent decrease in gastric emptying rate.[8]
      c. No change of duodenal function during exercise.[8]
    2. Small intestine.
      a. Exercise induces *delay* in small bowel transit time.[12,26,69,70]
      b. During the luteal phase of the menstrual cycle, transit is delayed.[113]
    3. Colonic transit.
      a. Segmental colonic transit times evaluated by Robertson and associates[90] failed to reach statistical significance.
      b. Colonic transit time probably increases secondary to greater colonic secretion during exercise, which dilutes luminal contents.[8]
    4. Whole gut mean transit time (WGMTT).
      a. Primarily a colonic event that is subject to wide variation.
      b. Moderate aerobic exercise (aerobic jogging,[5] bicycling,[104] jogging,[19] treadmill[90]) has no effect on bowel transit time when diet is held constant.
      c. Conflicting results in the past[47,48,59] secondary to long duration of colonic transit, making detection of possible exercise-induced changes difficult.
      d. Harrison and coworkers[42] suggest that running may tend to normalize gut transit time, thereby *"speeding the slow and slowing the fast."*
      e. Total body strength training programs decrease WGMTT.[49]
      f. Upright movements certainly increase colonic motility compared with complete inactivity.[5]
      g. Hyperthermia does not alter WGMTT.[41]
  B. Mesenteric blood flow.
    1. Exercise causes a quantitative redistribution of tissue blood flow.
    2. Splanchnic and gastric blood flow may be reduced by as much as 70% to 80% at $VO_{2\,max}$[16,32,50,91,112] and reduced to 30% to 40% of resting values at 70% $VO_{2\,max}$.[93]
      a. This may induce local O_2 and energy deficits, resulting in changes in absorption and secretion that lead to GI symptoms observed in endurance athletes.
      b. Carbohydrate absorption decreased when blood flow is decreased.[111,115]
    3. Training at a given exercise intensity lessens the exercise-induced reduction in splanchnic circulation.[17,92,93]
      a. Possibly secondary to enhanced O_2 extraction in trained muscle tissue and improved metabolic capacity, resulting in reduced metabolite accumulation and less blood shift from the GI tract to the muscle.[18,25,106]
      b. May explain decrease in reported GI symptoms after adequate training or when relative exercise intensity is reduced.
    4. Both splanchnic[35] and gastric[37] blood flow increases with eating.
      a. It is possible that small feedings during athletic endurance events may prevent GI blood flow from falling to critical levels.
      b. It has been postulated that liquid feedings during exercise may prevent gut ischemia.[8]

C. Mechanical.
  1. Abdominal vibrations/movements greater in:
    a. Running vs. cycling.[84]
    b. Running vs. walking.[61]
    c. Faster running vs. slower running.[4,57]
  2. Compression of the colon by psoas muscle hypertrophy.[22]

D. Neuroendocrine.
  1. Significant hormonal changes during exercise include an increase in plasma levels of prostaglandins, endorphins, gastrin, secretin, motilin, glucagon, somatostatin, pancreatic polypeptide, peptide histidine methionine (PHM), and vasoactive intestinal peptide.[73,88,99,108]
    a. Increased pancreatic polypeptide levels and a fall in plasma insulin stimulate colonic relaxation.[33,110]
    b. PHM and vasoactive intestinal peptide decrease anal sphincter pressure.[76]
  2. Green[36] theorized increased parasympathetic tone in athletes at rest with subsequent release of catecholamines during exertion may cause decreased transit time.

E. Absorption and permeability.
  1. Impaired intestinal absorption from decreased mesenteric blood flow may cause an osmotic load, resulting in GI distress and diarrhea.
  2. Exercise-induced increases in intestinal permeability have been demonstrated,[67,77] which may lead to the passage of macromolecules and bacteria through the intestinal wall and cause inflammation.

VI. Recommendations to the Athlete
  A. Avoid any foods or drugs (e.g., caffeine) that exacerbate lower GI tract symptoms.
  B. Athletes suffering frequently from diarrhea or the urge to defecate may benefit from complete nutritional liquid (low in fiber content) during the last day preceding the competition so that GI contents will be minimized.
  C. The athlete suffering from lactose intolerance should obviously avoid dairy products, as well as high-protein drinks and sports supplements that contain lactose.[11]
  D. Loperamide may be helpful in the athlete with exercise-induced fecal urgency or diarrhea.[46]
  E. Cathartics should be avoided owing to their dehydrating effect.
  F. All athletes should consult with the specific governing body that regulates their respective sport in regards to banned substances.

VII. Nonexercise Causes of Abdominal Problems in Athletes
  A. Irritable bowel syndrome—this disease affects 10% of the population and may mimic exercise-related symptoms.
  B. Inflammatory bowel disease—especially in the presence of rectal bleeding.
  C. Colon cancer—especially in older individuals with symptoms of weight loss, change in color/caliber of stool, rectal bleeding, etc.
  D. Superior mesenteric and portal vein thrombosis—case report has been published of an amateur cyclist who became ill with fever and abdominal pain during a backpacking trip.[63]
  E. "Spontaneous" abdominal adhesions—case report has been published of an endurance athlete with recurrent abdominal pain without prior abdominal surgery treated by laparoscopic adhesiolysis.[52]

VIII. Gastrointestinal Bleeding
  A. Incidence.
    1. Recurrent hematochezia initially reported in 1980 in a medical student.[30]
    2. Various surveys of GI bleeding and exercise have been conducted (see Table 12-2).
    3. GI bleeding was more pronounced with strenuous training or after competitive events than during practice runs and subsided when physical effort was reduced.[1,24,98]
    4. Selby and colleagues[98] followed college runners and found that 55% had guaiac-positive stools more than once during a full season.
  B. Source.
    1. Usually not identified.
    2. The stomach has been reported to be a frequent site of running-associated GI hemorrhage.[68]
    3. Gaudin[34] showed two types of pathological changes in the gastric antrum associated with decreased splanchnic blood flow.
      a. Submucosal hemorrhage and edema.
      b. Disorder of epithelial function with decreased mucosal secretion.
    4. Schwartz and associates[95] performed panendoscopy in seven marathon runners with occult fecal blood loss and found oozing gastric antral erosions in two runners and patchy areas of hyperemia and eroded mucosa in the splenic flexure of a third runner.
    5. No instances of esophageal or small intestinal bleeding have been reported.[64]
    6. A thorough history and physical evaluation is necessary in all instances of frank GI bleeding, regardless of its relation to exercise.
  C. Etiology.
    1. Ischemia—most likely etiology.
      a. During maximal exercise, blood flow to the gut is reduced by as much as 80%, regardless of the state of physical training.[9]
      b. Fluid losses and hyperthermia contribute to decreased perfusion of the GI tract.
      c. Restoration of blood flow to the gastric and intestinal microcirculation allows the injury to heal quickly, thus explaining the absence of endoscopic findings in runners who have endoscopy more than 3 days after a competitive race.[95]
    2. Trauma.
      a. Running (and, to a lesser extent, bicycling and swimming) causes pressure changes in the abdomen.[84]
      b. The "cecal slap syndrome" has been postulated to cause bleeding as the cecum slaps against the pelvis,[80] but this has never been proven.
      c. Injury by psoas muscle hypertrophy.[22]
      d. Cecal volvulus may develop.[81]
    3. Medication.
      a. Large quantities of nonsteroidal antiinflammatory drugs (NSAIDS) or aspirin may contribute to gastric, small intestinal, or colonic inflammation or ulcers.[6,105]
      b. The use of NSAIDS or aspirin has not, however, correlated with Hemoccult-positive conversion in most series.[64]
  D. Treatment.
    1. Depends on location and severity of bleeding.
    2. Acutely, the athlete is treated the same as any patient who presents with GI bleeding.

TABLE 12-2. Survey of gastrointestinal bleeding

Reference	No. of Subjects (% response)	% Male	Event	Method	Result (%) Preevent	Postevent
Porter[79]	39 (9.4)		Marathon	Post-race Hemoccult	0	7.40
Keeffe et al.[45]	707 (41.6)	86	Marathon	Survey bright red blood per rectum		1.2-2.4
Halvorsen et al.[40]	63 (3)	89	Marathon	Pre- and post-race Hemoccult	7.90	12.70
McCabe et al.[55]	125 (21)	54	Marathon	Pre- and post-race Hemoccult	–	– (66)
					+	+ (6)
					+	– (5)
					–	+ (23)
McMahon et al.[56]	32 (59)	?	Marathon	Pre- and post-race Hemoccult	3	22
Baska et al.[1]	35 (36)	97	Ultramarathon	Pre- and post-race Hemoccult	3	85
Halvorsen et al.[39]	279 (10)	81	Marathon	Overt blood in stool		3

3. Most cases are self-limited and resolve spontaneously.
4. Hemorrhagic gastritis can be treated with H_2 blockers or by reducing exercise intensity below symptomatic levels, then gradually increasing intensity to "train the gut."[64]
5. An elemental, semihydrolyzed diet has been recommended for the treatment of hemorrhagic colitis,[7] but its efficacy has not been thoroughly tested.

E. Prevention.
1. Misoprostol is effective in peptic ulcer disease and in preventing mucosal damage from NSAIDS.[114]
2. H_2 blockers help heal gastritis and prevent its recurrence.[20]
3. Cimetidine reduced the percentage of Hemoccult-positive conversion in an ultramarathon,[2] and subsequent double-blind trials using cimetidine suggest a reduction in exercise-associated bleeding; however, these studies failed to reach statistical significance.[65,66]
4. Acid suppression with H_2 blockers can be used prophylactically before exercise in selected patients with a negative workup for a source of GI bleeding.

IX. Exercise and Hepatobiliary Function

A. Liver.
1. Elevated levels of aminotransferases are often found in athletes but are usually thought to be of muscular origin.[89]
2. Blood flow to the liver during exercise decreases to 80% of preexercise levels.[93,120]
3. Liver damage can occur as a result of shock or exertional heatstroke, but this is a rare occurrence.[68]

B. Gallbladder.
1. Exercise may reduce lithogenicity of bile, possibly leading to reduced frequency of gallstones.
2. Conversely, it has been hypothesized that running-associated intravascular hemolysis may lead to increased excretion of bilirubin in bile, thereby resulting in the formation of pigment gallstones.[53]
3. No firm studies to confirm these suppositions.

X. Conclusions

A. GI symptoms are a frequent complaint in athletes, especially endurance athletes.
B. The initial workup of the athlete with GI symptoms needs to include evaluation for nonexercise-related causes before assuming exercise is the cause.
C. Once other causes have been excluded, treatment can focus on prevention; inadequate hydration is the most frequent culprit.
D. Further research is needed to better establish both the positive and negative effects of exercise on the GI tract.
E. Despite the frequency of reported symptoms, it is rare that GI complaints cause an athlete to discontinue participation in sports.

References

1. Baska RS et al: Gastrointestinal bleeding during an ultramarathon, *Dig Dis Sci* 35(2):276-279, 1990.
2. Baska RS, Moses FM, Duester PA: Cimetidine reduces running-associated gastrointestinal bleeding, *Dig Dis Sci* 35:956-960, 1990.
3. Bass P, Russell J: Electric and motor relations of the stomach and small intestine in gastric emptying. In Dubois and Castell, editors: *Esophageal and gastric emptying*, Boca Raton, 1984, CRC Press, pp 57-64.
4. Bhattacharya A et al: Body acceleration distribution and oxygen uptake in humans during running and jumping, *J Appl Physiol* 49:881-887, 1980.

5. Bingham SJ, Cummings JH: Effect of exercise and physical fitness on large intestinal function, *Gastroenterology* 97:1389-1399, 1989.
6. Bjarnson I et al: Nonsteroidal antiinflammatory drug-induced intestinal inflammation in humans, *Gastroenterology* 93:480-489, 1987.
7. Bounous G, McArdle AH: Marathon runners: the intestinal handicap, *Med Hypotheses* 33:261-264, 1990.
8. Brouns F, Beckers E: Is the gut an athletic organ? Digestion, absorption and exercise, *Sports Med* 15(4):242-257, 1993.
9. Brouns F: Etiology of gastrointestinal disturbances during endurance events, *Scand J Med Sci Sports* 1:66-77, 1991.
10. Brouns F, Saris WHM, Rehrer NJ: Abdominal complaints and gastrointestinal function during long-lasting exercise, *Int J Sports Med* 8:175-189, 1987.
11. Brukner P, Khan K, editors: Gastrointestinal symptoms during exercise. In *Clinical Sports Medicine*, Sydney, Australia, 1993, McGraw-Hill, p 600.
12. Cammack J, Read NW, Cann PA: Effect of prolonged exercise on the passage of a solid meal through the stomach and small intestine, *Gut* 23:957-961, 1982.
13. Cantwell JD: Gastrointestinal disorders in runners, *JAMA* 246:1494-1495, 1981.
14. Chapman WP, Rowlands EN, Jones CM: Multiple balloon kymographic recording of the comparative action of demerol, morphine, and placebos on the motility of the upper small intestine in man, *N Engl J Med* 243:171-177, 1950.
15. Clark CS et al: Gastroesophageal reflux induced by exercise in healthy volunteers, *JAMA* 261:3599-3601, 1989.
16. Clausen JP: Effect of physical training on cardiovascular adjustments to exercise in man, *Physiol Rev* 57:779-815, 1977.
17. Clausen JP et al: Central and peripheral circulatory changes after training of the arms or legs, *Am J Physiol* 225:675-682, 1973.
18. Clausen JP, Trap-Jensen J: Effects of training on the distribution of cardiac output in patients with coronary artery disease, *Circulation* 42:611-624, 1970.
19. Coenen C et al: Does physical exercise influence bowel transit time in healthy young men? *Am J Gastroenterol* 87(3):292-295, 1992.
20. Cooper DT et al: Erosive gastritis and gastrointestinal bleeding in a female runner. Prevention of bleeding and healing of the gastritis with H_2-receptor antagonist, *Gastroenterology* 92:2019-2023, 1987.
21. Costill DL, Saltin B: Factors limiting gastric emptying during rest and exercise, *J Appl Physiol* 37:679-683, 1974.
22. Dawson D, Khan A, Shreeve D: Psoas muscle hypertrophy: mechanical cause for "Jogger's Trots," *Br Med J* 291:787-788, 1985.
23. DeMeirleir K et al: Esophageal function during dynamic exercise, *Med Sci Sports Exerc* 22:2, 1990 (abstract 595).
24. Dobbs TW et al: Gastrointestinal bleeding in competitive cyclists, *Am Coll Sports Med* 20:S78, 1988.
25. Elsner RW, Carlson LD: Post-exercise hyperemia in trained and untrained subjects, *J Appl Physiol* 17:436-440, 1962.
26. Evans DF, Foster GE, Hardcastle JD: Does exercise affect small bowel motility in man? *Gut* A1012, 1989.
27. Evans DF, Foster GE, Hardcastle JD: Does exercise affect the migrating motor complex in man? In Roman C, editor: *Gastrointestinal motility*, Boston, 1984, MTP Press, pp 277-284.
28. Feldman M, Nixon JV: Effect of exercise on post-prandial gastric secretion and emptying in humans, *J Appl Physiol* 53:851-854, 1982.
29. Fordtran JS, Saltin B: Gastric emptying and intestinal absorption during prolonged severe exercise, *J Appl Physiol* 23(3):331-335, 1967.
30. Forgoros RN: Runner's trots: Gastrointestinal disturbances in runners, *JAMA* 243(17):1743-1744, 1980.
31. Foster C, Costill DL, Fink WJ: Gastric emptying characteristics of glucose and glucose polymer solutions, *Res Q Exerc Sport* 51:299-305, 1980.
32. Fronek K: Combined effect of exercise and digestion on hemodynamics in conscious dogs, *Am J Physiol* 218:555-559, 1970.
33. Galbo H, editor: Gastro-entero-pancreatic hormones. In *Hormonal and metabolic adaption to exercise*, New York, 1983, Thieme Press, pp 59-61.
34. Gaudin C, Zerath E, Guezennel CY: Gastric lesions secondary to long distance running, *Dig Dis Sci* 35(10):1239-1243, 1990.
35. Granger DN et al: Intestinal blood flow, *Gastroenterology* 78:837-863, 1980.
36. Green GA: Gastrointestinal disorders of the athlete, *Clin Sports Med* 11(2):453-469, 1992.
37. Guth PH, Leung FW: Physiology of the gastric circulation. In Johnson LR, editor: *Physiology of the gastrointestinal tract*, New York, 1987, Raven Press, pp 1031-1053.

38. Halvorsen FA, Ritland S: Gastrointestinal problems related to endurance event training, *Sports Med* 14(3):157-163, 1992.
39. Halvorsen FA et al: Gastrointestinal disturbances in marathon runners, *Br J Sports Med* 24(4):266-268, 1990.
40. Halvorsen FA, Lyng J, Ritland S: Gastrointestinal bleeding in marathon runners, *Scand J Gastroenterol* 21:493-497, 1986.
41. Harris A, Keeling WF, Martin J: Identical orocecal transit time and serum motilin in hyperthermia and normothermia, *Dig Dis Sci* 35(10):1281-1284, 1990.
42. Harrison RJ et al: Exercise and wheat bran: effect on whole-gut transit, *Proc Nutr Soc* 39:22A, 1980.
43. Houmard JA et al: Gastric emptying during one hour of cycling and running at 75% $VO_{2\,max}$, *Med Sci Sports Exerc* 23(3):320-325, 1991.
44. Jenkinson DH, Morton IKM: The role of alpha- and beta-adrenergic receptors in some actions of catecholamines on intestinal smooth muscle, *J Physiol* 188:387-402, 1967.
45. Keeffe EB et al: Gastrointestinal symptoms of marathon runners, *West J Med* 141:481-484, 1984.
46. Keeling WF, Harris A, Martin BJ: Loperamide abolishes exercise-induced orocecal liquid transit acceleration, *Dig Dis Sci* 38(10):1783-1787, 1993.
47. Keeling WF, Harris A, Martin BJ: Orocecal transit during mild exercise in women, *J Appl Physiol* 68:1350-1353, 1990.
48. Keeling WF, Martin BJ: Gastrointestinal transit during mild exercise, *J Appl Physiol* 63:978-981, 1987.
49. Koffler KH et al: Strength training accelerates gastrointestinal transit in middle-aged and older men, *Med Sci Sports Exerc* 24(4):415-419, 1992.
50. Konturek S, Falser J, Obtulowicz W: Effect of exercise on gastrointestinal secretions, *J Appl Physiol* 34:324-328, 1973.
51. Kraus BB, Sinclair JW, Castell DO: Gastroesophageal reflux in runners: characteristics and treatment, *Ann Intern Med* 112:429-433, 1990.
52. Lauder TD, Moses FM: Recurrent abdominal pain from abdominal adhesions in an endurance athlete, *Med Sci Sports Exerc,* in press.
53. Leslie BR, Sander RNW, Gerwin LE: Runner's hemolysis and pigment gallstones, *N Engl J Med* 313:1230, 1985.
54. Markiewicz K et al: Furosemide effect on gastric basal secretion during exercise and post exercise restitution in healthy subjects, *Acta Pol Pharm* 33:296-304, 1982.
55. McCabe ME et al: Gastrointestinal blood loss associated with running a marathon, *Dig Dis Sci* 31:1229-1232, 1986.
56. McMahon LF et al: Occult gastrointestinal blood loss in marathon runners, *Ann Intern Med* 100(6):846-847, 1984.
57. Meijer GA, Westerterp KR: Assessment of daily physical activity using synchronous recording of heart rate and body acceleration, *Proc Nutr Soc* 47:25A, 1988.
58. Mellow MH et al: Esophageal acid perfusion in coronary artery disease, *Gastroenterology* 85:306-312, 1983.
59. Meshkinpour H, Kemp C, Fairshter R: Effect of aerobic exercise on mouth-to-cecum transit time, *Gastroenterology* 96:941-983, 1989.
60. Montgomery LC, Deuster PA: Effects of antihistamine medication on exercise performance: implications for sports people, *Sports Med* 15(3):179-185, 1993.
61. Montoye HJ et al: Estimation of energy expenditure by a portable accelerometer, *Med Sci Sports Exerc* 15:403-407, 1983.
62. Moore JG, Datz FL, Christian PE: Exercise increases solid meal gastric emptying rates in men, *Dig Dis Sci* 35:428-432, 1990.
63. Moriarity JM: Abdominal pain and fever, *Med Sci Sports Exerc* 23(4):S81, 1991.
64. Moses FM: Gastrointestinal bleeding and the athlete, *Am J Gastroenterol* 88(8):1157-1159, 1993.
65. Moses FM et al: The effect of cimetidine on ultramarathon-associated gastrointestinal bleeding, *Am J Gastroenterol* 86:A336, 1991.
66. Moses FM et al: Effect of cimetidine on marathon-associated gastrointestinal symptoms and bleeding, *Dig Dis Sci* 36:1390-1394, 1991.
67. Moses FM et al: Alterations in intestinal permeability during prolonged high intensity running, *Gastroenterology* 100:A472, 1991.
68. Moses FM: The effect of exercise on the gastrointestinal tract, *Sports Med* 9(3):159-172, 1990.
69. Moses FM et al: Lactose absorption and transit during prolonged high intensity running, *Am J Gastroenterol* 84:1192, 1989.
70. Moses FM et al: Oral cecal transit time during a two hour run with ingestion of water or glucose polymer, *Am J Gastroenterol* 83:1055, 1988.
71. Motil JJ et al: Case report: exercise induced gastroesophageal reflux in an athletic child, *J Pediatr Gastroenterol Nutr* 6:989-991, 1987.

72. Murray R: The effects of consuming carbohydrate-electrolyte beverages on gastric emptying and fluid absorption during and following exercise, *Sports Med* 4:322-351, 1987.
73. Naveri H, Kuoppasalmi K, Harkonen M: Metabolic and hormonal changes in moderate and intense long-term running exercises, *Int J Sports Med* 6:276-281, 1985.
74. Neufer PD, Young AJ, Sawka MN: Gastric emptying during walking and running: effects of varied exercise intensity, *Eur J Appl Physiol* 58:440-445, 1989.
75. Noakes TD, Rehrer NJ, Maughan RJ: The importance of volume in regulating gastric emptying, *Med Sci Sports Exerc* 23:307-313, 1991.
76. Nurko S, Dunn BM, Rattan S: Peptide histidine isoleucine and vasoactive intestinal polypeptide cause relaxation of opossum anal sphincter via two distinct receptors, *Gastroenterology* 19:619-624, 1982.
77. Oektedalen O et al: Changes in the gastrointestinal mucosa after long distance running, *Scand J Gastroenterol* 27:270-274, 1992.
78. Oektedalen O et al: The influence of prolonged physical stress on gastric juice components in healthy man, *Scand J Gastroenterol* 23:1132-1136, 1988.
79. Porter AMW: Do some marathon runners bleed into the gut? *Br Med J* 287:1427, 1983.
80. Porter AMW: Marathon running and the cecal slap syndrome, *Br J Sports Med* 16:178, 1982.
81. Pruett TL, Wilkins ME, Gamble WG: Cecal volvulus: a different twist for the serious runner, *N Engl J Med* 312:1262-1263, 1985.
82. Ramsbottom N, Hunt JN: Effect of exercise on gastric emptying and gastric secretions, *Digestion* 10:1-8, 1974.
83. Reese MR et al: The effect of beta-adrenoreceptor agonists and antagonists on gastric emptying in man, *Br J Clin Pharmacol* 10(6):551-554, 1980.
84. Rehrer NJ, Meijer GA: Biomechanical vibration of the abdominal region during running and bicycling, *J Sports Med Phys Fitness* 31(2):231-234, 1991.
85. Rehrer NJ et al: Gastric emptying with repeated drinking during running and bicycling, *Int J Sports Med* 11(3):238-243, 1990.
86. Rehrer NJ et al: Effects of dehydration on gastric emptying and gastrointestinal distress while running, *Med Sci Sports Exerc* 22(6):790-795, 1990.
87. Riddoch C, Trinick T: Gastrointestinal disturbances in marathon runners, *Br J Sports Med* 22(2):71-74, 1988.
88. Riddoch C et al: Gut hormones and exercise, *Regul Pept* 18:343, 1987.
89. Ritland S, Foss NE, Gjone E: Physical activity in liver disease and liver function in sportsmen, *Scand J Soc Med Suppl* 29:221-226, 1982.
90. Robertson G et al: Effects of exercise on total and segmental colon transit, *J Clin Gastroenterol* 16(4):300-303, 1993.
91. Rowell LB et al: Splanchnic vasomotor and metabolic adjustments to hypoxia and exercise in humans, *Am J Physiol* 247(2 Pt 2):H251-H258, 1984.
92. Rowell LB: Human cardiovascular adjustments to exercise and thermal stress, *Physiol Rev* 54:75-159, 1974.
93. Rowell LB, Blackmon JR, Bruce RA: Indocyanine green clearance and estimated blood flow during mild to maximal exercise in upright man, *J Clin Invest* 43:1677-1690, 1964.
94. Schofield PM et al: Exertional gastroesophageal reflux: a mechanism for symptoms in patients with angina pectoris and normal coronary angiograms, *Br Med J* 294:1459-1461, 1987.
95. Schwartz A, Vanagunas A, Kamel P: The etiology of gastrointestinal bleeding in runners: A prospective endoscopic appraisal, *Ann Intern Med* 113:632-633, 1990.
96. Scobie BA: Correspondence, *N Z Federat Sports Med* 6:31, 1978.
97. Selby G, Fram D, Eichner ER: Effort-related gastrointestinal blood loss in distance runners during a competitive season, *Am Coll Sports Med* 20:S79, 1988.
98. Semple CG, Thompson JA, Beastall GH: Endocrine response to marathon running, *Br J Sports Med* 19:148-151, 1985.
99. Severson SK et al: A prospective analysis of physical activity and cancer, *Am J Epidemiol* 130:522-529, 1989.
100. Slattery ML et al: Physical activity, diet, and risk of colon cancer in Utah, *Am J Epidemiol* 128:989-999, 1988.
101. Soffer EE et al: Effect of graded exercise on esophageal motility and gastroesophageal reflux in nontrained subjects, *Dig Dis Sci* 39(1):193-198, 1994.
102. Soffer EE et al: Effect of graded exercise on esophageal motility and gastroesophageal reflux in trained athletes, *Dig Dis Sci* 38(2):220-224, 1993.
103. Soffer EE, Summers RW, Gisolfi C: Effect of exercise on intestinal motility and transit in trained athletes, *Am J Physiol* 260:G698-G702, 1991.
104. Stamm CP et al: Colonic ulcerations associated with nonsteroidal anti-inflammatory drug ingestion, *Gastrointest Endosc* 37:260, 1991.
105. Stenberg J: Muscle blood flow during exercise: effects of training. In Larsen OA, Malmborg RO, editors: *Coronary heart disease and physical fitness,* Copenhagen, 1971, Munksgaard, pp 80-83.

106. Sullivan SN, Wong C, Heidenheim P: Does running cause gastrointestinal symptoms? A survey of 93 randomly selected runners compared with controls, *N Z Med J* 107(984):328-331, 1994.
107. Sullivan SN et al: Gastrointestinal regulatory peptide responses in long-distance runners, *Physician Sports Med* 12:77-82, 1984.
108. Sullivan SN: The gastrointestinal symptoms of running, *N Engl J Med* 304(15):915, 1981.
109. Tache Y: Nature and biological actions of gastrointestinal peptides, *Clin Biochem* 17:77-81, 1984.
110. Varro GE, Garris JA, Geenen JE: Effect of decreased local circulation on absorptive capacity of a small intestine loop in the dog, *Am J Dig Dis* 10:170-177, 1965.
111. Wade OL et al: The effect of exercise on the splanchnic blood flow and splanchnic blood volume in normal men, *Clin Sci* 15:457-463, 1956.
112. Wald A et al: Gastrointestinal transit: the effect of the menstrual cycle, *Gastroenterology* 80: 1497-1500, 1981.
113. Watkinson G, Hopkins A, Akbar FA: The therapeutic efficacy of misoprostol in peptic ulcer disease, *Postgrad Med J* 649(Suppl 1):60-73, 1988.
114. Williams JH, Mager M, Jacobsen ED: Relationship of mesenteric blood flow to intestinal absorption of carbohydrates, *J Lab Clin Med* 63:853-862, 1964.
115. Worme JD et al: Dietary patterns, gastrointestinal complaints, and nutrition knowledge of recreational triathletes, *Am J Clin Nutr* 51(4):690-697, 1990.
116. Worobetz LJ, Gerrard DF: Effect of moderate exercise on esophageal function in asymptomatic athletes, *Am J Gastroenterol* 81:1048-1051, 1986.
117. Worobetz LJ, Gerrard DF: Gastrointestinal symptoms during exercise in Enduro athletes: prevalence and speculations on aetiology, *N Z Med J* 98:644-646, 1985.
118. Yazaki E, Evans DF: Long distance running increases post-prandial gastroesophageal reflux, *Gastroenterology* 100:A189, 1991.
119. Zeeh J et al: Steady-state extrarenal sorbitol clearance as a measure of hepatic plasma flow, *Gastroenterology* 95:749-759, 1988.

CHAPTER 13

Genitourinary Problems

Aaron L. Rubin, MD

I. Trauma
  A. Kidney
    1. Minor renal trauma (accounts for 85% of cases).
      a. Includes contusion, subcapsular hematoma, superficial cortical laceration.
    2. Major renal trauma (accounts for 15% of cases).
      a. Deep lacerations extending into collecting system, large retroperitoneal and perinephric hematomas, fractured kidneys.
      b. Worse injuries with lower degree of trauma occur with renal abnormality such as horseshoe kidney, megaureter, malignancy, ureteropelvic junction obstruction.
    3. Vascular injury (accounts for <1% of cases).
    4. Evaluation.
      a. History, physical examination, and urinalysis.
        (1) Mechanism and force of injury are important.
        (2) May be associated with intraabdominal trauma and rib fracture.
      b. Sonography.
      c. Computed tomography.
      d. Intravenous pyelography.
      e. Surgical exploration.
    5. Treatment.
      a. Immediate resuscitation of the athlete is the initial concern when the injury is sufficient to cause renal damage. Hemorrhage is the most important early complication.
      b. Always consider referral for urology consultation if kidney is damaged.
      c. Most minor trauma can be treated nonsurgically.
        (1) Prescribe bedrest, hydration, analgesic agent.
        (2) Advise athlete to avoid strenuous activity for 2 to 3 weeks.

(3) Rebleeding typically occurs 15-20 days after injury when clot resolves.

d. Major trauma often requires invasive management.
   (1) 15% of all patients have delayed bleeding.
   (2) Postinjury hypertension occurs in 1% to 33% of cases.
   (3) Pedicle injuries and shattered kidneys usually need surgery.

B. Collecting system.
   1. Ureters: injury uncommon.
   2. Bladder.
      a. Low incidence of injury.
      b. Associated with pelvic fracture.
   3. Urethra.
      a. Associated with straddle injuries.
      b. Injury more commonly occurs in male patients.
      c. Pain, inability to void, and blood at meatus.
      d. Requires urgent urological referral.
      e. Traumatic urethritis may occur in cyclists from chronic irritation and may be confused with prostatic hypertrophy because of dysuria, outflow obstruction, pyuria, or hematuria. Treatment includes ensuring a proper saddle position (horizontal or only slightly elevated) and increased padding in seat or shorts. Trauma may be increased by use and positioning of "aero" bars.

C. Scrotum
   1. Contusion: look for associated testicular injury.
   2. Laceration.
   3. Mass.
      a. Testicular cancer is one of the most common forms of solid malignancy in the 16- to 35-year-old male patient.
      b. Varicocele: varicosity of internal spermatic veins without symptoms is present in 9% to 19% of men.
      c. Hydrocele: fluid-filled tunica vaginalis. Hydrocele that develops acutely without evidence of trauma or infection may be due to malignancy.
      d. Hematocele: due to blood accumulation in the tunica vaginalis secondary to trauma.

D. Testis.
   1. Contusion: most frequent injury.
   2. Rupture, dislocation: if suspected, urologist should be consulted.
   3. Torsion of spermatic cord.
      a. Genetic predisposition probably exists. Often associated with trauma.
      b. Should be suspected if pain and swelling in a single testicle occur, especially after minor trauma.
      c. Pain often increases when testicle is lifted above the symphysis, whereas pain from epididymitis is usually decreased by this maneuver.
   4. Evaluation.
      a. Physical examination.
      b. Sonography: may be helpful for diagnosing rupture and torsion. Is highly operator dependent and varies between medical centers. Has a high false-negative rate.
      c. Testicular scan: ^{99m}Tc-pertechnetate scan results are 90% to 100% accurate for diagnosing torsion.
      d. Surgical exploration: early exploration and treatment (within 4 hours) improves outcome.

5. Treatment.
   a. Prevent injury by using proper safety equipment: most often worn by baseball catchers, hockey and lacrosse goalies, and persons with previous injury.
   b. Contusion: use ice, elevation, support.
   c. Rupture, dislocation, torsion: surgical exploration is advised, although some have had success with manual derotation of torsion. Generally during torsion the left testicle rotates counterclockwise, and the right rotates clockwise (as observed from foot of bed).

E. Penis.
1. Contusion: most common injury.
2. Fracture: from direct trauma in erect state. Should be considered another urological emergency for evacuation of clot and repair of tunica albuginea.
3. Laceration.
4. Pudendal neuropathy: numbness, tingling in scrotum and penile shaft, which may be noted in a cyclist. Treatment is the same as that for traumatic urethritis.

F. Female genitalia: injuries either of lower incidence or reported less.
1. Vulval trauma can occur in cycling.
2. Vaginal trauma is associated with waterskiing falls.

II. Exercise-Induced Injury

A. Hematuria: most common upper limit of normal is three erythrocytes per high-powered field.
1. Incidence reported to be 55% in football and rowing, 80% in swimming, lacrosse, and track, 20% in marathon runners, and 50% in ultramarathon runners. Also found in 5% of Israeli Air Force recruits and 15% of students in one study and 49% in another.
2. Mechanisms include increased permeability of glomerulus, trauma from direct blows or jarring of kidneys, and bladder irritation.
3. Amount of hematuria increases with intensity and duration of activity.
4. Consider other sources of hematuria, such as infection, interstitial nephritis, renal papillary necrosis, hemorrhagic cystitis, and nephrolithiasis.
5. Not all that is red is blood. Pharmaceutical agents (phenazopyridine, rifampin, nitrofurantoin, quinine, phenytoin), vegetable dyes, myoglobin, and hemoglobin in urine may mimic hematuria.
6. Initial symptom of genitourinary tract cancer is often painless hematuria.
7. Evaluation.
   a. History: note onset, trauma, flank pain, renal colic, discharge, frequency and urgency of voiding, dysuria, clots passed, edema, pharyngitis, viral illness, impetigo, sickle cell anemia, or drug use.
   b. Physical examination.
   c. Urinalysis.
   d. Repeat urinalysis in 24-48 hours (without exercise).
   e. Urine culture.
   f. Intravenous pyelography.
   g. Cystoscopy.

B. Proteinuria.
1. Occurs in 70% to 80% of athletes.
2. Related to duration and intensity of exercise.
3. Related to decreased renal blood flow, decreased glomerulofiltration rate during exercise. May also be related to increased plasma renin activity, which enhances glomerular permeability.

4. Generally clears in 1-2 days.
5. Evaluation.
   a. History: assess recent infections (especially streptococcal), history of renal disease, collagen vascular disease, edema, drug use, and family medical history.
   b. Dipstick urinalysis for protein determination is good for screening, but many false-positive tests result from such factors as concentrated urine, hematuria, alkaline urine, or contamination by an antiseptic agent or medication.
   c. Common protein values for dipstick urinalysis:

Trace	15-29 mg/dl
1+	30-99 mg/dl
2+	100-299 mg/dl
3+	300-999 mg/dl
4+	≥1000 mg/dl

   2+ or greater usually represents clinically important proteinuria.
   d. Repeat urinalysis after 24-48 hours without exercise. Consider further evaluation of patients with values ≥2+, even if urine clears.
   e. Use serum blood urea nitrogen and creatinine determinations, 24-hour urine collection for determination of protein and creatinine clearance, urine protein electrophoresis, and intravenous pyelography.
   f. No evidence exists that routine screening for proteinuria is an important part of evaluating an athlete before participation in sports. Proteinuria is benign in all but 0.1% of cases.

III. Infections
   A. Discuss safer sex and investigate potential problems and questions.
   B. Urethritis.
      1. Nongonococcal urethritis.
         a. Infection with *Chlamydia trachomatis, Ureaplasma urealyticum, Trichomonas,* or *Candida.*
         b. Diagnosis.
            (1) Mucopurulent discharge is the main symptom in male patients. Female patients are often asymptomatic.
            (2) Culture and Gram's staining are indicated.
         c. Treatment.
            (1) *Chlamydia, Ureaplasma:* Nonpregnant and nonallergic patients—tetracycline, 500 mg four times daily for 7 days, doxycycline, 100 mg twice daily for 7 days. Pregnant patients—erythromycin, 500 mg four times daily for 7 days.
            (2) *Trichomonas* in the nonpregnant patient—metronidazole, 2 g as a single dose or 500 mg twice daily or 250 mg three times daily for 7 days.
      2. Gonorrhea.
         a. *Neisseria gonorrhoeae* infection.
         b. Diagnosis.
            (1) Discharge is the main symptom, but the disease may be asymptomatic.
            (2) Culture recommended. Gram's staining shows gram-negative intracellular diplococci.
         c. Treatment.

(1) Ceftriaxone, 250 mg intramuscularly or cefixime, 400 mg orally plus oral doxycycline, 100 mg twice daily for 10 days if the patient is not allergic or pregnant.

(2) Many other regimens are available for use with doxycycline, 100 mg twice daily for postgonococcal urethritis: spectinomycin, 2 g intramuscularly, given once; oral ciprofloxacin, 500 mg given once; oral norfloxacin, 800 mg given once; oral amoxicillin, 3 g with probenecid.

C. Epididymitis.
   1. *Chlamydia*, gonococcal, or *Escherichia coli* infection.
   2. Diagnosis: symptoms are testicular pain, tender epididymis.
   3. Treatment
      a. Gonococcal or *Chlamydia* infection (more common in patients <35 years old): treatment is as indicated above
      b. *Escherichia coli* infection (more common in patients ≥35 years old): treat with trimethoprim-sulfamethoxazole, ciprofloxacin.

D. Prostatitis.
   1. Same organisms and age ranges as for epididymitis.
   2. Diagnosis: do rectal examination.
   3. Treatment: as described above.

E. Cystitis.
   1. Multiple organisms responsible.
   2. Diagnosis: for symptoms of frequency and urgency of voiding and dysuria, do urinalysis and urine culture.
   3. Treat with trimethoprim-sulfamethoxazole, cephalosporins, tetracyclines. Obtain culture results to aid in treatment.

F. Herpes simplex.
   1. Diagnosis: painful vesicular lesions.
   2. Treatment: oral acyclovir, 200 mg five times daily for 10 days.

G. Tinea cruris
   1. Diagnosis: pruritus; microscopic evaluation with potassium hydroxide reveals hyphae.
   2. Treatment: keep area clean and dry, treat with miconazole, clotrimazole, econazole creams. Hydrocortisone 1% cream may be added if the area is irritated. Treatment-resistant cases may benefit from griseofulvin, 500 mg twice daily or ketoconazole, 200 mg daily for 4-6 weeks.

Acknowledgment

The Medical Editing Department, Kaiser Foundation Research Institute, provided editorial assistance. C. Mark Page, MD, reviewed the manuscript.

Bibliography

Bragg LE: Athletic injuries of the thorax and abdomen. In Mellion MB, Walsh WM, Shelton GL, editors: *The team physician's handbook*, Philadelphia, 1990, Hanley & Belfus, pp 371-373.

Briner WW, Howe WB, Jain RK: Scrotal injury in a high school football player, *Physician Sportsmed* 18(11):64-68, 1990.

Cass AS, Luxerberg M: Testicular injuries, *Urology* 37:528-530, 1991.

Cianflocco AJ: Renal complications of exercise, *Clin Sports Med* 11:437-451, 1992.

Diamond DL: Sports-related abdominal trauma, *Clin Sports Med* 8:91-99, 1989.

Eichner ER: Hematuria: a diagnostic challenge, *Physician Sportsmed* 18(11):53-63, 1990.

Elliot DL, Goldberg L, Eichner ER: Hematuria in a young recreational runner, *Med Sci Sports Exerc* 23:892-894, 1991.

Fournier GR Jr, Laing FC, McAninch JW: Scrotal ultrasonography and the management of testicular trauma, *Urol Clin North Am* 16:377-385, 1989.

Mueller EJ, Thompson IM: Bladder carcinoma presenting as exercise-induced hematuria, *Postgrad Med* 84:173-176, 1988.

Noujaim SE, Nagle CE: Acute scrotal injuries in athletes: evaluation by diagnostic imaging, *Physician Sportsmed* 17(10):125-130, 1989.

Schneider RE: Genitourinary trauma, *Emerg Med Clin North Am* 11:137-145, 1993.

Sitorius MA, Mellion MB: General medical problems in athletes. In Mellion MB, Walsh WM, Shelton GL, editors: *The team physician's handbook,* Philadelphia, 1990, Hanley & Belfus, pp 173-174.

Tanagho EA, McAninch JW, editors: *Smith's general urology,* San Mateo, CA, 1992, Appleton & Lange.

York JP: Sports and the male genitourinary system: kidneys and bladder, *Physician Sportsmed* 18(9):116-129, 1990.

York JP: Sports and the male genitourinary system: genital injuries and sexually transmitted diseases, *Physician Sportsmed* 18(10):92-100, 1990.

CHAPTER **14**

The Geriatric Athlete

Edward D. Snell, MD

Robert J. Dimeff, MD

I. Epidemiology
   A. People >65 years of age comprise 12.5% of the population.[3,6,13]
      1. Persons over 85 comprise the fastest growing part of the population.
      2. The over 65 part of the population is estimated to comprise ~25% of the population by the year 2050.
   B. Americans have an increasing life expectancy.*
      1. Women live 18.6 years past 65.
      2. Men live 14.7 years past 65.
   C. Increased sedentary life-style demonstrates need to reinforce exercise in the elderly.[10]
      1. Healthy life-style leads to a *healthier* life.
      2. With exercise people lead a more carefree life-style.
      3. Exercise leads to less time spent in hospital/medical office.[1,10]
      4. The greatest threat to the aging athlete is inactivity!
   D. Injury patterns in the elderly are less traumatic and more due to chronic overuse degenerative processes.

II. Physiology of Aging
   A. General.
      1. Disuse changes are similar to those seen with aging.
      2. Disuse changes are potentially reversible.
         a. Start exercises early.
         b. Enjoyable routines to ensure compliance.
   B. Cardiovascular changes.
      1. Decreased maximum heart rate (loss of 1 beat/year).
      2. Elevated systolic and diastolic blood pressure (10-40 mmHg).[2]
      3. Decreased cardiac output ~8%/decade starting at age 25 (20% to 30% decline by 65 years).[2,13]
      4. Decreased stroke volume ~30% by 85.

*References 2, 8, 12, 13, 17, 18, 25, 27, 28, 31.

5. Little change in ejection fraction.
6. Sedentary individuals have a progressive decrease in maximal oxygen uptake ($Vo_{2\ max}$) at an average rate of 10%/decade starting at age 25.

C. Respiratory: increase in work of breathing by 20%.
1. Increased residual volume (30% to 50% by age 70).
2. Decreased vital capacity (40% to 50% by age 70).[2]
3. Increased forced residual capacity (30% to 50% by age 70).[2]
4. Decreased thoracic mobility.
5. Increased lung compliance.

D. Renal changes.
1. Decreased absolute number of glomeruli.
2. Decreased plasma volume and renal blood flow secondary to cardiovascular changes.
3. Decreased glomerular filtration rate (GFR) with decreased blood flow.
4. Decreased concentrating ability.

E. Metabolic changes.
1. Decreased intracellular and total body water.
2. Increased body fat.
3. Decreased glucose tolerance.
4. Decreased thyroid function.
5. Increased lipids and total and low-density lipoprotein cholesterol.
6. Decreased muscle mass.
7. The metabolic *potential* for aerobic and anaerobic activity on the cellular level changes minimally with age.
8. Decline in resting metabolic rate.[21]
   a. Men: 3% to 4%/year after age 40.
   b. Women: 3% to 4%/year after age 50.
9. Decline in energy and macronutrient intake.[21]
10. Glycolytic enzyme and high energy phosphates are not affected by aging.[26]

F. Neuropsychiatric changes.
1. Decreased cognitive function.[4]
   a. Minimal decline in the autonomic processes (actions that are done without conscious attention).
   b. Decline in processing resources or behavioral slowing.
   c. Increased decline in patients with Parkinson's disease, depression, manic-depressive psychosis, schizophrenia, and cardiovascular disease.
2. Spinal cord axons decline by ~40% by age 60.[2,4]
3. Nerve conduction velocity of remaining axons slows by ~10% by the age of 60.[4]
4. Decreased sensory, cerebellar, and motor function.
5. Decreased brain mass.
6. Increase in resting sympathetic nervous system.

G. Musculoskeletal changes.[2,4]
1. Bone mass plateaus at 30 years.
   a. Rate of loss of trabecular bone (50% over life).
      (1) Men: loss starts at age 25-30 and progresses at a rate of 1.2%/year.
      (2) Women: loss starts at 25-30 and progresses at a rate of 1.2%/year.
   b. Rate of loss of cortical bone starts at 30-40 years.
      (1) Men: 0.3% to 0.5%/year starting at age 40 and increasing to 0.5% to 1%/year at ~70.

(2) Women: 0.3% to 0.5%/year starting at age 30, increasing 2% to 3%/year for the first 8-10 years postmenopause, and then slowing again to 0.5% to 1%/year. If estrogen replacement is given, this change is not seen.

2. Cartilage/tendon/ligament.
   a. Collagen fibers have an increased cross-linking.
   b. Decreased water and glycosaminoglycan content.
   c. Decreased cross-sectional area.
   d. Increased stiffness and possible injury.
   e. Decreased fiber bundle, thickness, and capillarization.
3. Muscle has a peak power at 20-30 years, with power athletes reaching a greater peak than their sedentary counterparts.[7]
   a. Muscle undergoes a reduction in size and mass of 3% to 5%/decade with a loss of ~20% to 30% between 30 and 80 years.[21,25,28]
   b. Decreased number of muscle fibers.[25]
      (1) Type II fiber (fast twitch) loss is probably greater than the type I fibers (slow twitch) loss.
      (2) Loss of fibers may be secondary to age-related damage to muscle cell without regeneration.
      (3) Loss of fibers may be secondary to the loss of neuromuscular units (axons).
   c. Decreased size of fibers.
      (1) Type I fibers remain intact.
      (2) Type II and IIa undergo reductions in size.[25]
   d. Decreased contractility properties of muscle.
   e. Muscle atrophy of disuse shows similar changes compared to aging, but the loss of fiber size is mainly seen in type 1 fibers.

III. Preexercise Evaluation
   A. History.
      1. Medical illnesses.
         a. Chronic lung diseases.
         b. Coronary heart disease.
         c. Peripheral arterial disease.
         d. Diabetes.
         e. Hypertension.
         f. Renal insufficiency.
         g. Thyroid/malignancies.
         h. Osteoarthritis.
      2. Surgery/hospitalizations with any resulting deficits.
      3. Medications.
         a. Diuretics, angiotensin-converting enzyme inhibitors.
         b. Insulin/oral hypoglycemics.
         c. Alpha-, beta-, and calcium channel blockers.
         d. Major tranquilizers.
      4. Immunizations.
         a. Tetanus.
         b. Influenza.
         c. Pneumococcus.
         d. Other.
      5. Allergies.
         a. Environmental.
         b. Medication induced.
      6. Social history.
         a. Smoking.
         b. Alcohol.

c. Occupation.
d. Income.
e. Living situation.
f. Social support systems (families, friends, acquaintances).

5. Family history.
   a. Sudden death.
   b. Coronary heart disease.
   c. Stroke.
   d. Hypertension.
   e. Diabetes.
   f. Thyroid disease.
   g. Psychiatric diseases.
6. Review of systems.
   a. Pulmonary/cardiothoracic.
      (1) Dyspnea on exertion (DOE).
      (2) Orthopnea.
      (3) Snoring/sleep apnea.
      (4) Chronic cough/hemoptysis.
      (5) Chest pain/pressure, especially with exertion.
      (6) Palpitations.
      (7) Diaphoresis.
      (8) Syncope and near syncope.
      (9) Previous myocardial infarction.
   b. Orthopedic.
      (1) Joints.
         (a) Previous strains (residual deficiency).
         (b) Swelling.
         (c) Pain or night pain.
         (d) Loss of motion.
         (e) Mechanical (locking or instability).
      (2) Bone.
         (a) Fractures/total joints.
         (b) Treatment.
         (c) Residual deformity.
      (3) Muscle.
         (a) Previous strains (residual deficiency).
         (b) Pain.
         (c) Weakness.
      (4) Chronic pain syndromes.
   c. Peripheral vasculature: claudicatory symptoms (burning, paresthesia and weakness with activity).
   d. Neurological/psychiatric.
      (1) Syncope/presyncope.
      (2) Cerebrovascular accidents.
      (3) Concussions.
      (4) Dizziness/vertigo.
      (5) Gait disturbances (weakness, history of falls).
      (6) Incontinence.
      (7) Neuropathies.
      (8) Seizures.
      (9) Depression.

B. Physical Examination.
   1. Vital signs.
      a. Blood pressure with orthostatic measurements.
      b. Heart rate.

c. Height.
d. Weight.
e. Body composition.
(1) Lean muscle mass.
(2) Fat content.

2. Cardiopulmonary.
a. Murmurs or rubs: supine and standing, S_1, S_2, S_3, or S_4.
b. Breath sounds.
c. Peripheral vascular examination (palpation of pulses).

3. Abdominal.
a. Previous surgical scars.
b. Hernia.
c. Masses.
d. Bruits.

4. Orthopedic.
a. Neck.
b. Shoulders.
c. Elbow/hand/wrist.
d. Back.
e. Hips.
f. Knees.
g. Ankles/feet.

5. Neurological.
a. Mental status.
b. Cranial nerves.
c. Sensory.
d. Strength.
e. Reflexes.
f. Cerebellar.
g. Gait.

C. Investigations.

1. Routine blood work/laboratory tests.
a. Complete blood count with differential.
b. Electrolytes.
c. Renal function.
d. Cholesterol/lipid profile.
e. Hemoccult.
f. Thyroid panel and reactive plasma reagin (RPR).
g. Further blood work, depending on medications and history.
(1) Liver function tests if on medications metabolized by the liver for >1 month.
(2) Iron studies if abnormalities in complete blood count or if symptoms of ulcers, lower gastrointestinal bleeding, or decreased exercise tolerance.

2. Radiographs as needed based on the patient's medical history and examination.

3. Electrocardiography (ECG) and rhythm strip should be ordered on all geriatric patients; there is debate over further age-related testing.[29]

4. Graded exercise testing.
a. Cycle ergometry: advantages.
(1) Inexpensive equipment.
(2) Easy, accurate blood pressure (BP) and ECG readings.
(3) Less chance of accidents.
(4) Can be used in patients with joint instability, gait abnormality, visual impairment, or peripheral ischemia.

b. Cycle ergometry: disadvantages.
   (1) Unfamiliar activity.
   (2) Uncomfortable seat.
   (3) Leg fatigue may occur before completion of test.
c. Treadmill testing: advantages.
   (1) Easy to master.
   (2) Uses major muscle groups.
d. Treadmill testing: disadvantages.
   (1) Difficult to record BP measurements and ECG measurements.
   (2) Increased risk of falls and accidents.
   (3) Unable to express work and power in measurable terms.
e. Reasons to discontinue stress testing.
   (1) Second- or third-degree heart block or sustained arrhythmias (supraventricular tachycardia or any ventricular tachycardia).
   (2) >1 mm of ST elevation that is new.
   (3) Systolic BP decrease of 10 mmHg or reading of >250 mmHg.
   (4) Diastolic BP increase of 20 mmHg or reading of >120 mmHg.
   (5) Angina.
   (6) Orthostatic symptoms.
   (7) Volitional fatigue.

5. Body composition.
   a. Weight and height charts are often inaccurate due to vertebral collapse and accentuated kyphosis in the elderly.
   b. Underwater weighing is still the most accurate but presents obvious practical difficulties.
   c. Skin fold thickness affords a relatively good way to monitor progress throughout training.

IV. Physiologic Changes with Exercise and Training
   A. Cardiovascular.
      1. Decreased heart rate, diastolic and systolic BP, and lactate levels.
      2. Improve cardiovascular recovery after exercise.
      3. Increase duration of submaximal exercise.
      4. Increased $\dot{V}O_{2\,max}$.
      5. Uncertain change in stroke volume and cardiac output.[20,28]
   B. Respiratory.
      1. Increased vital capacity.
      2. Increased minute ventilation.
      3. Increased lung compliance.
      4. Decreased work of breathing.
   C. Metabolic.
      1. Increased resting metabolic rate.
      2. Increased hormone levels such as insulin-like growth factor, growth hormone, epinephrine, and norepinephrine.[21,23]
      3. Decrease in total cholesterol with increase in high-density lipoproteins.
      4. Decreased total body fat and increased muscle mass.
   D. Neuropsychiatric.[26]
      1. Increased motor unit recruitment and synchronization.
      2. Augmented neural drive to the skeletal muscle.
      3. Increased coordination.
      4. Enhancement of cognitive processing speed, performance, and learning.
      5. Decreased anxiety, depression, and chronic pain.
      6. Elevated mood and increased self-esteem.

E. Renal.[5]
   1. Exercise at 65% $Vo_{2\ max}$ may decrease renal blood flow by up to 75% and decrease GRF up to 50%.
   2. Greater chance of dehydration and renal damage.
   3. Prehydrate with water to decrease risk.

F. Musculoskeletal.
   1. Bone.
      a. Increase in bone mass and density with weight-bearing exercise.
      b. Decrease in rate of cortical bone mass and density loss.[14,16]
   2. Cartilage/ligament/tendon.[9]
      a. Increase in prolyl hydroxylase.
      b. Increase in tensile strength, tangent modulus, and elastic efficiency of collagen.
      c. Increase in joint mobility and flexibility.
      d. Be aware that age-related changes in collagen may increase risk of injury.
   3. Muscle.[11,22,25]
      a. Increase in aerobic mitochondrial oxidative capacity.
      b. Transformation of type IIb to IIa fibers.[25]
      c. Increase in capillarization.
      d. Muscle fiber hypertrophy.
      e. Increase in strength.
      f. Rhabdomyolysis damage to T tubules, sarcoplasmic reticulum, and mitochondria.
      g. Decreased reparative capabilities increase recovery time after exercise.

V. Changes in Disease States with Exercise
   A. Artherosclerotic heart disease.
      1. Exercise may initially increase cardiovascular symptoms: need to use graded exercise test before progressing.
      2. Increased efficiency of oxygen utilization and consumption.
      3. Enhanced left ventricular performance.
      4. Slower progression of cardiovascular disease.
   B. Chronic obstructive pulmonary disease.
      1. Exercise may initially increase bronchospasm and pulmonary symptoms.
         a. May have to increase medications (O_2, beta-agonists, steroids).
         b. Close followup is important: can monitor progress with pulmonary function tests (PFTs) or flowmeter.
      2. Increased aerobic exercise tolerance with time.
   C. Diabetes mellitus.
      1. Exercise increases glucose utilization, causing a decrease in blood sugars.
      2. Monitor blood sugar frequently and make necessary medication adjustments, especially initially.
         a. Type I: decrease insulin dosage.
         b. Type II: may decrease or discontinue medications.
   D. Peripheral vascular disease.
      1. Exercise may initially increase claudicatory symptoms.
      2. Increased efficiency of oxygen utilization and consumption.
      3. Slows progression of disease.
   E. Hypertension.
      1. Exercise may initially increase BP.
      2. Over time can decrease diastolic and systolic BP up to 10-20 mmHg.[2]

F. Osteoporosis.
   1. Increased risk of stress fracture.
   2. Begin at low-impact and low-intensity exercise to minimize risk.
   3. Weight-bearing exercise may increase bone mineral density and mass.[13]
G. Osteoarthritis.
   1. Age is greatest risk factor.[15]
   2. Increased symptoms of pain, swelling, and stiffness.
   3. Adjust exercise program by minimizing impact loading to increase comfort and decrease symptoms.
   4. Treat acute exacerbations.
   5. Individualize exercise of joint replacement patients to minimize risk of trauma (discourage high-impact loading exercises and activity).
   6. Increased maximal oxygen capacity and muscle strength will improve functional status.

VI. Exercise Prescription[19]
A. Individualize according to:
   1. Age.
   2. Fitness level.
   3. General health status.
   4. Status and control of chronic diseases.
B. Goals of exercise.
   1. Increased cardiovascular endurance.
   2. Increased muscle strength and endurance.
   3. Increased joint flexibility.
   4. Increased lean body mass.
   5. Decreased body fat.
   6. Decreased sedentary life-style habits.
   7. Increased ability to perform activities of daily living.
   8. Improved social contacts.
   9. Increased life span with decreased morbidity.[27]
C. Motivation and cooperation.
   1. Define and set realistic goals.
   2. Exercises should be interesting and accessible.
   3. Exercise equipment must take into account patient abilities and disabilities.
   4. Ensure proper supervision, especially with weight equipment and complex tasks.
   5. Match exercise with patient's skill and fitness levels.
   6. Exercise should be performed with friends and social contacts to improve adherence and compliance.
   7. Incorporate practical activities such as walking instead of driving and use of hand tools instead of power tools.
   8. Psychological improvements occur along with physiological benefits.
   9. Begin at a relatively "young" old age.
D. Adverse effects and injuries are more prevalent in the geriatric athlete.
   1. Dehydration and heat illness.
      a. Increased heat production due to biomechanical insufficiency.
      b. Decreased heat dissipation due to decreased sweat production, increased subcutaneous fat, and poor vasomotor regulation.
      c. Blunted thirst response.
      d. Impaired thermoregulation.

2. Hypothermia.
   a. Decreased heat production due to poor vasomotor regulation, peripheral vascular disease, decreased metabolic rate, and decreased shivering response.
   b. Cold environment can also increase the risk of bronchospasm and angina.
3. Overuse injuries.
   a. 85% of geriatric sports injuries.[2]
   b. Increased risk due to physiological changes of aging.
   c. Evaluate and treat promptly.
   d. Can be a major pitfall in the exercise program.
4. Traumatic injuries.
   a. Increased risk of falls due to poor balance and coordination, decreased visual acuity, and orthostatic hypotension.
   b. Increased risk of fractures due to decreased bone density and mass.

E. Aerobic training.
1. Mode.
   a. Target large major muscle groups.
   b. A proper warmup period of 10-15 minutes followed by stretching exercises is important.
   c. Emphasize walking, swimming, bicycling, and other low-impact loading exercises.
   d. Program should be easy to follow with continuous dynamic repetitive exercises.
   e. A gradual cooldown period of 10-15 minutes followed by a stretching program is essential.
2. Intensity.
   a. Most important factor in determining improvement in cardiovascular fitness.
   b. Map out a training heart zone (exercise performed at 25% to 50% $Vo_{2\,max}$ will result in a training effect).[2]
   c. Begin with lower-intensity exercise.
      (1) Tailor to baseline fitness level.
      (2) Safer.
      (3) Adjust intensity as fitness level improves.
3. Duration.
   a. Goal is 30-60 minutes activity.
   b. Begin at 5-10 minutes and gradually increase duration as fitness improves (5% to 10% increments).
   c. Increased duration improves weight loss.
4. Frequency.
   a. Begin with frequency of two times per week.
   b. Gradually increase frequency of exercise over 3- to 4-week period.
   c. Cardiovascular fitness: two to three sessions per week.
   d. Weight control: five to seven sessions per week but at a decreased intensity level.

F. Strength training.
1. Mode.
   a. Use major large muscle groups.
   b. Gradual warmup period of 5-10 minutes utilizing general stretching.
   c. 8-10 exercises with the major muscle groups.
   d. Lift at moderate to slow speeds through the full range of motion.

   e. Avoid Valsalva maneuver while weight lifting.
   f. No 1 RM lifts (the maximum amount of weight an individual can lift one time but not two times).
2. Intensity: voluntary contraction against a fixed weight.
   a. Amount of weight being lifted.
   b. Most important factor in determining strength improvement.
   c. Recommend weight that can be lifted 10-15 times (10-15 RM).
3. Repetitions.
   a. Number of lifts per set.
   b. Recommend 10-15 RM per set.
4. Set.
   a. Group of repetitions.
   b. Recommend two to three sets per session.
5. Duration.
   a. Amount of time spent lifting.
   b. Recommend less than 60 minutes per session.
6. Frequency
   a. Number of days of weight lifting per week.
   b. Recommend 2 days per week.
   c. Allow 2 days of recovery time.

References

1. Astrand PO: Why exercise? *Med Sci Sports Exerc* 24:153-162, 1992.
2. Barry HC, Eathorne SW: Exercise and aging, *Med Clin North Am* 78(2):357-376, 1994.
3. Bouchard C et al: *Exercise, fitness, and health: a consensus of current knowledge,* Champaign, IL, 1990, Human Kinetics Books, pp 127-131.
4. Chodzko-Zajko W, Moore KA: Physical fitness and cognitive functioning in aging, *Exerc Sports Sci Rev* 22:195-220, 1994.
5. Cianflocco AJ: Renal complications of exercise, *Clin Sports Med* 11(2):437-451, 1992.
6. Cohen RA, Van Nostrand JF: *Health data on older Americans, United States,* Washington, DC, 1992, US Government Printing Office.
7. Ferretti G et al: Determinants of peak muscle power: effects of age and physical conditioning, *Eur J Appl Physiol* 68:111-115, 1994.
8. Fogelholm M, Kaprio J, Sarna S: Healthy lifestyles of former Finnish world class athletes, *Med Sci Sports Exerc* 26(2):224-229, 1994.
9. Gartee GD: Aging skeletal muscle: response to exercise, *Exerc Sports Rev* 22:91-120, 1994.
10. Heath GW et al: Physical activity patterns among adults in Georgia: results from the 1990 behavioral risk factor surveillance system, *Southern Med J* 87(4):435-439, 1994.
11. Judge JO, Whipple RH, Wolfson LI: Effects of resistive and balance exercises on isokinetic strength in the older person, *J Am Geriatr Soc* 42:937-946, 1994.
12. Karvonen MJ et al: Longevity of endurance skiers, *Med Sci Sports Exerc* 6:49-51, 1974.
13. Kerlan RK editor: Sports medicine and the older athlete, *Clin Sports Med* 10(2), 1991.
14. Krall EA, Dawson-Hughes B: Walking is related to bone density and rates of bone loss, *Am J Med* 96:20-26, 1994.
15. Lane NE et al: The risk of osteoarthritis with running and aging: a 5-year longitudinal study, *J Rheumatol* 20(3):461-468, 1993.
16. Menkes A et al: Strength training increases regional bone mineral density and bone remodeling in middle-aged and older men, *J Appl Physiol* 74(5):2478-2484, 1993.
17. Paffenberger RS et al: The association of changes in physical activity level and other lifestyle characteristics with mortality among men, *N Engl J Med* 328:538-545, 1993.
18. Paffenberger RS et al: A natural history of athleticism and cardiovascular health, *JAMA* 252: 491-495, 1984.
19. Pate RR et al: *ACSM guidelines for exercise testing and prescription,* ed. 4, Philadelphia, 1991, Lea & Febiger.
20. Pelliccia A et al: The upper limit of physiologic cardiac hypertrophy in highly trained elite athletes, *N Engl J Med* 324:295-301, 1991.
21. Poehlman ET, Arciero PJ, Goran MI: Endurance exercise in aging humans: effects on energy metabolism, *Exerc Sports Sci Rev* 22:251-284, 1994.
22. Pyka G et al: Muscle strength and fiber adaptations to a year-long resistance training program in elderly men and women, *J Gerontol* 49(1):M22-M27, 1994.

23. Pyka G, Taaffe DR, Marcus R: Effect of a sustained program of resistance training on the acute growth hormone response in older adults, *Hormone Metab Res* 26:330-333, March 1994.
24. Paffenbarger RS, Jr. et al: Physical activity, all-cause mortality, and longevity of college alumni, *N Engl J Med* 314:605-613, 1986.
25. Rogers MA, Evans WJ: Changes in skeletal muscle with aging: effects of exercise training, *Exerc Sports Sci Rev* 21:65-102, 1993.
26. Sandvick L et al: Physical fitness as a predictor of mortality among middle-aged Norwegian men, *N Engl J Med* 328:533-537, 1993.
27. Sarna ST et al: Increased life expectancy of world class athletes, *Med Sci Sports Exerc* 25:237-244, 1993.
28. Seals DR et al: Enhanced left ventricular performance in endurance trained older men, *Circulation* 89:198-205, 1994.
29. 17th Bethesda Conference, *J Am Coll Cardiol* 24(4):845-899, 1994.
30. Van Saase JL et al: Longevity of men capable of vigorous physical activity exercise: a 32 year follow-up of 2259 participants in the Dutch 11 cities ice skating tour, *Int Med J* 301:1409-1411, 1990.

CHAPTER 15

Dermatology

William D. Knopp, MD

I. Introduction

The athlete develops many dermatological problems that are not unique to participation in sports, but there are particular problems that occur in direct relation to equipment use, direct contact with other athletes, or environmental exposure. This chapter will focus on these specific problems.

II. Viral Infections

A. Herpes simplex (herpes labialis, cutaneous herpes, herpes gladiatorum, herpetic whitlow).

1. Etiology. Nongenital herpes skin infections are caused by herpes simplex virus (HSV) 1 or, less commonly, HSV 2. Ninety percent of adults have been infected with HSV 1. Infection is transmitted by direct contact with open lesions or, less often, through a fomite (wrestling mat, equipment). In wrestling, epidemic spread of infection is called "herpes gladiatorum." Stress, sun exposure, illness, or weight loss may stimulate a recurrence.

2. Signs and symptoms.

a. Incubation is a few days to a few weeks.

b. Grouped, clear vesicles (1-3 mm) on an erythematous base on the lips (herpes labialis), skin (cutaneous herpes), and the fingertips (herpetic whitlow).

c. Primary infection may cause constitutional symptoms of fever, malaise, headache, sore throat, and regional lymphadenopathy. Recurrent infections usually do not cause systemic symptoms.

d. Infection can be confirmed with Tzanck test or culture.

e. Wrestlers often have facial lesions in the trigeminal nerve distribution, with the most serious complication being herpes keratitis (VI distribution).

f. Recurrence may be preceded by burning or itching hours to days before lesions are visible.

3. Treatment.
    a. Acyclovir 200 mg PO five times a day for 7-10 days. This is most effective if given when prelesion symptoms are present but is of questionable benefit when lesions are already present.
    b. Topical acyclovir is of questionable benefit.
    c. Drying agents such as 5% to 10% benzoyl peroxide, astringents, or tretinoin gel or cream may enhance healing of existing lesions.
    d. Prophylaxis with acyclovir should be considered if recurrences are frequent or 24-48 hours before exposure to known causes of recurrence.
    e. Sunscreens may prevent reactivation.
    f. Consider human immunodeficiency virus (HIV) infection if frequency of recurrences increases without explanation.
4. Participation/prevention.
    a. Due to the high infectivity of HSV infections, participation is permitted only when the crusting or eschar has cleared.
    b. Prevention would be improved if infected athletes are detected early and excluded from participation until healing occurs.

B. Herpes zoster.
1. Etiology.
    a. Recurrence of varicella virus in unilateral, dermatomal distribution.
    b. Stress, illness, sun exposure, or weight loss may initiate recurrence.
2. Signs and symptoms: grouped, clear vesicles with erythematous base in a dermatomal distribution most commonly on the trunk; appearance is similar to HSV lesions.
3. Treatment: acyclovir 800 mg five times per day for 7-10 days.
4. Participation/prevention: same as for HSV infections.

C. Molluscum contagiosum.
1. History/etiology.
    a. A pox virus.
    b. Transmitted by direct contact with lesion or through sexual contact.
2. Signs and symptoms: flesh-colored papules (1-2 mm) without underlying erythema on face, trunk, extremities, or genitalia.
3. Treatment: Cryocautery, curettage, retinoic acid, trichloroacetic acid, electrodesiccation, salicylic acid.
4. Participation/prevention: may participate if adequately covered with dressing.

D. Common warts.
1. History/etiology.
    a. Human papillomavirus; multiple types.
    b. Transmitted via fomite or direct contact.
2. Signs and symptoms.
    a. Single or multiple verrucous papules primarily on the hands and feet.
    b. Thrombotic speckling at base of lesion if pared down.
    c. Skin markings absent on lesion.
3. Treatment.
    a. Cryocautery, podophyllin, 5-fluorouracil, electrodesiccation; intralesional bleomycin and interferon have been used.
    b. Potentially scarring therapies should be particularly avoided on the hands and feet.

4. Participation/prevention: no restrictions for participation, although coverage recommended.

III. Bacterial Infections

A. Impetigo/ecthyma.

1. History/etiology.
   a. *Streptococcus* (beta-hemolytic) or *Staphylococcus* infection.
   b. *Streptococcus* may cause glomerulonephritis.
   c. Skin to skin contact or fomite (particularly wrestling mats).
2. Signs and symptoms.
   a. Honey-colored crusted macules, papules, or bullae with erythematous base; single or clustered.
   b. Begins on face, extremities, or trunk and spreads rapidly over a period of days.
   c. Ecthyma involves the superficial dermis and causes shallow ulcers.
   d. Favors skin folds, areas subject to friction, or areas of occlusion.
   e. If atopic or contact dermatitis present, patient is at risk for secondary impetiginization.
3. Treatment.
   a. Mupirocin is the most effective topical agent.
   b. Multiple lesions often require oral agents such as cefadroxil, cephalexin, dicloxacillin, amoxicillin/clavulanate, erythromycin.
   c. Streptococcal species are showing increased resistance to erythromycin.
   d. Lesions should be cleaned with soap and water or peroxide before applying ointment and dry dressing.
4. Participation/prevention.
   a. Due to infectious nature of impetigo and possibility of systemic infection or glomerulonephritis, the lesions should be clear of crusting before participation is allowed.
   b. In 15% to 20% of patients, colonization of nasal mucosa may occur. This can be eradicated with thrice daily application of mupirocin for 1 week. Consider treatment of teammates and family members in recurrent cases.
   c. Prevention is paramount and includes meticulous cleaning of wrestling mats (antiseptic cleaners are available) and other equipment as well as good personal hygiene.

B. Folliculitis and furunculosis.

1. History/etiology.
   a. Infection with *Staphylococcus aureus* and beta-hemolytic streptococci.
   b. Same risk factors as impetigo.
   c. Hot tub folliculitis caused by *Pseudomonas*.
   d. Individuals treated with oral or topical antibiotics for acne can develop gram-negative folliculitis.
   e. Carbuncles may form if individual furuncles coalesce.
2. Signs/symptoms.
   a. Papular, pustular, or nodular lesions usually about a hair follicle.
   b. Tender, fluctuant abscesses may occur.
3. Treatment.
   a. Early lesions may respond to cefadroxil, cephalexin, or dicloxacillin.
   b. If pustules or abscesses present, amoxicillin/clavulanate or clindamycin may be required as well as incision and drainage.
   c. Topical agents are usually not sufficient.

   d. Hot tub folliculitis may respond to oral ciprofloxacin or may require intravenous therapy for *Pseudomonas* species.
4. Participation/prevention: may not participate in contact sports or swimming until furuncles are healed. May participate if folliculitis can be adequately covered.

C. Erythrasma.
1. History/etiology: *Corynebacterium minutissimum* are the causative bacteria.
2. Signs/symptoms.
   a. Dull red-brown plaques that occur in the groin, axilla, or webs of feet.
   b. Exacerbated by hot, moist conditions.
   c. May mimic tinea cruris or intertrigo.
   d. Appears as coral red fluorescence on Wood's light.
3. Treatment.
   a. Topical erythromycin or clindamycin.
   b. May require oral tetracycline or erythromycin for 10-21 days.
4. Participation/prevention.
   a. No restrictions.
   b. Cotton underclothes.
   c. Dry environment.

D. Pitted keratolysis.
1. History/etiology.
   a. *Corynebacterium* or multibacterial infection.
   b. Caused by profuse sweating and warm environment.
   c. Asymptomatic.
2. Signs/symptoms.
   a. Soles of feet show multiple pits (1-15 mm) in the stratum corneum.
   b. Skin malodorous.
3. Treatment.
   a. Drying agents such as 20% aluminum chloride (Drysol).
   b. Erythromycin 2% solution, benzoyl peroxide, 5% formaldehyde soaks, or acetic acid soaks.
   c. Resistant cases require oral erythromycin.
4. Participation/prevention.
   a. Frequent change of dry cotton socks.
   b. Well-ventilated shoes.

IV. Fungal and yeast infections.

A. Tinea corporis/tinea cruris/tinea pedis/tinea capitis.
1. History/etiology.
   a. Tinea corporis/pedis/capitis caused by dermatophytes.
   b. *Candida albicans* is the most common cause of yeast infections.
   c. Moist locations such as feet, intertriginous areas are the most common sites, but in athletes who sweat profusely, nonintertriginous sites are vulnerable to infection.
2. Signs/symptoms.
   a. Tinea pedis presents as a dry, erythematous scaling of the soles, sometimes with fissuring of soles. In severe cases macerated, erosive, or bullous lesions develop in the web spaces. Bacterial superinfection is common. Blistering (vesicular) tinea may be confused with contact dermatitis or dyshidrotic eczema.
   b. Tinea cruris causes pruritic, scaling, coalescent patches or plaques in the inguinal folds, sparing the scrotum and penis, whereas in-

fections caused by *Candida* spp. cause pruritic, red plaques with satellite lesions involving the penis and scrotum.
   c. Tinea corporis presents as erythematous, scaling plaques with central clearing on the trunk, face, and extremities.
   d. Tinea capitis appears as raised plaques with hair loss on the scalp.
3. Treatment.
   a. Topical imidazoles are first-line therapy, followed by the allylamines (dermatophytes).
   b. 1 : 10 acetic acid soaks may enhance healing of tinea pedis.
   c. 3 days of topical steroid may reduce pruritus and erythema.
   d. Oral griseofulvin (dermatophytes), ketoconazole, fluconazole, and itraconazole are useful in resistant or widespread cases.
4. Participation/prevention.
   a. Frequent change of clothing.
   b. Drying powders.
   c. Rarely, may need daily application of antifungal.
   d. Cotton clothing, breathable shoes.
   e. May participate if area covered.

B. Tinea versicolor.
1. History/etiology.
   a. Infection with *Pityrosporum orbiculare,* a normal inhabitant of hair follicles and sebaceous glands.
   b. More frequent in individuals with diabetes, immunosuppression, or genetic predisposition.
2. Signs/symptoms.
   a. Fine scaling macules, which may coalesce on upper chest, back, arms, and neck and are either hyperpigmented or hypopigmented.
   b. The yeast produces decarboxylic acid, which acts as a sun screen.
   c. KOH preparation reveals a spaghetti (hyphae) and meatballs (yeast) appearance.
   d. Generally asymptomatic, but may be pruritic.
   e. May occasionally cause folliculitis.
3. Treatment.
   a. Topical treatment includes 2.5% selenium sulfide lotion or shampoo, either one application overnight or 15 minutes each night for 7 nights.
   b. Topical imidazoles bid for 2-3 weeks.
   c. Oral ketoconazole 200 mg daily 1 hour prior to exercise for 3 days.
   d. Repigmentation may take weeks to months.
4. Participation/prevention.
   a. No contraindication to participation.
   b. May be recurrent, impossible to eradicate organism.
   c. Selenium sulfide, salicylic acid, or sulfur shampoo 1-2 times per month may help prevent recurrences.

V. Mechanical Disorders

A. Blisters.
1. History/etiology.
   a. Shearing force at friction points cause cleavage at the spinous layer of the epidermis.
   b. Occurs more frequently in the untrained athlete who has not undergone epidermal hyperplasia.
   c. Abrupt shearing forces may cause immediate blister and can occur under a callus.

d. Predisposition in hyperhydrotic individuals.
2. Signs/symptoms.
 a. Clear or blood-filled vesicle or bulla with or without an erythematous base.
3. Treatment.
 a. Needle drainage to maintain epidermal roof as dressing.
 b. Apply adhesive tape and moleskin.
 c. Occlusive dressings (Duoderm, etc.) can speed healing and reduce pain. The blister must be deroofed and the dressing applied every 3 days until healed.
 d. Antibiotic ointments prevent infection and speed healing.
4. Participation/prevention.
 a. 1% tannic acid soaks can promote hyperplasia and increase blister threshold.
 b. Vaseline and adhesive tape decrease friction; talc prevents excessive moisture accumulation.
 c. Chalk for gymnasts.
 d. Gloves, proper footwear, sport specific socks.
 e. Toe glides.

B. Calluses (tyloma)/corns (clavi).
1. History/etiology.
 a. Epidermal hyperplasia at the basal layer of epidermis caused by friction and shearing forces.
 b. External forces (shoes, equipment) and internal forces (enlarged condyle, bony prominences).
2. Signs/symptoms.
 a. Calluses are conical areas of hyperkeratosis with the apex directed externally, usually at bony prominences or areas of excessive pressure.
 b. Hard corns are similar to calluses with the apex directed subcutaneously.
 c. Soft corns occur interdigitally and appear as white, macerated epidermis. This is most common between the fourth and fifth toes.
3. Treatment.
 a. Soak to soften epidermis, then pare down with scalpel or sand down with pumice stone.
 b. A corn requires removal or thinning of core.
 c. Salicylic acid (Duofilm) application will cause gradual thinning of epidermis.
 d. Surgery may be required to eliminate bony abnormalities.
 e. Orthotics can reduce pressure.
 f. Toe separators or lamb's wool reduce friction and discomfort.
4. Prevention/participation.
 a. Proper footwear.
 b. Orthotics, toe separators, lamb's wool.

C. Black heel (talon noir).
1. History/etiology.
 a. Same pathogenesis as friction blisters but more common in sports that require quick stops and starts.
 b. Rupture of superficial epidermal capillaries.
2. Signs/symptoms.
 a. Black macule usually at heel.
 b. Can be differentiated from a nevus or melanoma by easy removal with shaving of superficial stratum corneum.

3. Treatment: none.
4. Participation/prevention.
   a. Proper footwear.
   b. Vaseline, moleskin, adhesive tape.

D. Intertrigo.
1. History/etiology.
   a. Erythema and maceration in groin, axilla, and inframammary folds secondary to friction and excessive moisture.
   b. Superinfection with yeast or bacteria is common.
   c. Obesity or large breasts a strong contributor.
2. Signs/symptoms: Moist, erythematous, sometimes macerated skin in intertriginous areas.
3. Treatment.
   a. Burow's compresses.
   b. Hydrocortisone cream.
   c. Topical antibacterial or antifungal.
4. Participation/prevention.
   a. Keep area dry.
   b. Cotton clothing with frequent changes.
   c. Proper bras.
   d. Weight loss.

VI. Allergic and Irritant Contact Dermatitis

A. History/etiology.
1. Irritant contact dermatitis is nonallergic and secondary to an irritating substance or physical agent.
2. Allergic contact dermatitis is secondary to acquired hypersensitivity to specific allergen.
3. Allergic reactions are due to five major allergens.
   a. *Rhus* (poison ivy, oak, and sumac).
   b. Paraphenylenediamines (blue/black dyes).
   c. Nickel compounds.
   d. Rubber compounds.
   e. Chromates (tanned leather, metal parts).
4. Other allergens include diethylthiourea compounds (e.g., neoprene, shoe glues) and topical medications (e.g., salicylates, menthol, antibiotics).
5. Rubber compounds in face masks, mouthpieces, support hose, athletic shoes, wet suits, and orthopedic equipment are common sources of allergic contact dermatitis. Specific manufacturers can suggest alternatives and the likely allergen.

B. Signs/symptoms.
1. Erythematous, pruritic papules, plaques to vesicular or bullous lesions that appear 1-7 days after exposure.
2. Patch testing may be useful in identifying inciting agent.

C. Treatment.
1. Topical steroids for 7-14 days is usually sufficient.
2. Oral antihistamines (diphenhydramine, hydroxyzine) and aspirin reduce pruritus.
3. Oral steroids in severe or extensive cases.

D. Participation/prevention.
1. Create barrier between skin and agent (e.g., two pairs of socks).
2. Nonsensitizing substitutes are the most effective form of prevention. Companies often offer alternatives that they or other manufacturers produce.

VII. Environmental Exposures
   A. Sunburn: very common in athletes secondary to outdoor exposure. Treatment and prevention are similar to those for nonathletes and will not be discussed. Waterproof sunscreens should be frequently applied to prevent sunburn and, more importantly, to prevent photoaging and skin neoplasms later in life.
   B. Frostbite (see Chapter 17B).

VIII. Insect Bites
   A. Insect bites are common in athletes.
   B. Team physicians should be aware of athletes with a history of severe reactions such as urticaria, angioedema, or anaphylaxis and should have oral antihistamines and injectable epinephrine (Epipen) available at sporting events.

IX. Pilosebaceous Disorders: Acne Mechanica
   A. History/etiology.
      1. Superficial folliculitis caused by occlusion, heat, friction, moisture, or pressure from athletic clothing and equipment.
      2. Chin straps, sweatbands, helmets, shoulderpads, spandex clothing, and other equipment are common causes.
      3. Often seen in prepubescent athletes without acne vulgaris.
   B. Signs/symptoms: multiple erythematous papules and pustules at area of contact and friction.
   C. Treatment.
      1. Reduce friction.
      2. Natural fibers such as cotton prevent occlusion and excessive moisture and reduce maceration.
      3. Immediate cleansing after exercise.
      4. Occasionally, topical tretinoin is helpful.
      5. Topical or oral antibiotics seldom required.
   D. Participation/prevention: same as treatment.

X. Striae Distensae
   A. History/etiology: tears in the dermis secondary to mechanical stress, muscle hypertrophy, breast development, pregnancy, or anabolic or prolonged corticosteroid use both oral and topical.
   B. Signs/symptoms: linear areas of fine wrinkling that are skin colored or slightly erythematous.
   C. Treatment: none.
   D. Participation/prevention: prevention only by avoidance of steroid use. Natural causes such as pregnancy and growth are not preventable.

Bibliography

Amundson LH: Managing skin problems in athletes. *The team physician's handbook,* Philadelphia, 1990, Hanley and Belfus, Mosby–Year Book, pp 236-250.

Bergfeld WF, Helm TN: *The skin:* Sports medicine, Philadelphia, 1991, WB Saunders, pp 117-131.

Elston DM, Bergfeld WF: Skin diseases of the hands and feet, *Phys Sportsmed* 22(3):40-50, 1994.

Fisher AA: Allergic contact dermatitis, *Phys Sportsmed* 21(3):65-72, 1993.

Katchis SD, Hershman EB: Broken nails to blistered heels, *Phys Sportsmed* 21(5):95-104, 1993.

Nelson M: Stopping the spread of herpes simplex, *Phys Sportsmed* 20(10):117-127, 1992.

Reichel M, Laub D: From acne to black heel: common skin injuries in sports, *Phys Sportsmed* 20(2):111-118, 1992.

Rustad OJ: Outdoors and active: relieving summer's siege on skin, *Phys Sportsmed* 20(5):163-176, 1992.

Scheinberg RS: Stopping skin assailants: fungi, yeasts, and viruses, *Phys Sportsmed* 22(7):33-39, 1994.

Scheinberg RS: Exercise-related skin infection: managing bacterial disease, *Phys Sportsmed* 22(6):47-58, 1994.

CHAPTER 16

Ear, Nose, and Throat Problems

Allen C. Felix, MD

I. Otological Problems
   A. Otitis media.
      1. Etiology.
         a. Most common bacterial agents: *Streptococcus pneumoniae, Haemophilus influenzae,* and *Moraxella catarrhalis.*[21]
         b. History of recent upper respiratory tract infection and fever.
         c. Characterized by severe pain, a sense of fullness, or decreased hearing.
      2. Signs/symptoms.
         a. Diagnosis made by otoscopy.
         b. Bulging, immobile, erythematous tympanic membrane with effusion typically seen.
         c. Vesicles suggest a viral or *Mycoplasma* infection (bullous myringitis).
         d. Flat (type B) tracing on tympanogram.[12]
         e. Conductive hearing loss (during Weber's test, vibration heard best in affected ear).
      3. Treatment.
         a. Preferred antibiotic is amoxicillin; if no response in 48 hours, change medication.
         b. Penicillin-allergic patients require erythromycin or trimethoprim/sulfamethoxazole.
         c. For associated tympanic membrane rupture, add antibiotic-containing eardrops.
         d. Followup examination recommended in 2-4 weeks to confirm resolution of effusion.
         e. If infection fails to clear or if effusion persists beyond 10 weeks, refer patient to otolaryngologist.[12]
         f. Do not prescribe decongestant or any other medication that may disqualify the athlete from competition at which drug testing is done.[24]

4. Complications.
   a. Mastoiditis, labyrinthitis, meningitis.
   b. Suspected when patient fails to respond within 10 days or is worse after a few days.
5. Miscellaneous.
   a. Air travel not recommended until normal appearance and function of ear return.[3]
   b. May return to play if patient is afebrile and, in swimmers or divers, if tympanic membrane is intact and nondraining.[31]

B. Otitis externa.
1. Etiology/epidemiology.
   a. Swimming, waterskiing, scuba diving, surfing, or prolonged water exposure.
   b. Infection of external canal usually due to *Pseudomonas, Proteus,* or fungus.
   c. Chronic itching may result from recurrent manipulation of ear canal with cotton swab or bobby pin.
   d. Higher incidence in poorly chlorinated pools and fresh water.[22]
   e. Greater risk in surfers with exostosis in ear canal.[17]
2. Signs/symptoms.
   a. Pathognomonic sign is pain on manipulation of auricle.
   b. External canal is edematous and erythematous; tympanic membrane is usually normal.
   c. Symptoms also include occasional hearing loss and/or watery discharge.
   d. In fungal infections, canal lining appears fuzzy and is dotted with black specks, and exudate may have musty odor.[32]
3. Treatment.
   a. The foundation of proper initial treatment involves cleansing of the ear canal.[24]
   b. Referral to otolaryngologist for suction under magnification may be required.
   c. Prescribe antibiotic eardrops with or without steroids and/or drying agent four times daily.
   d. Acidifying drops such as acetic acid otic solution are useful for mild inflammation.
   e. If canal is swollen and drops cannot penetrate it, place a cotton ear wick in the ear canal for 24-48 hours.
   f. Use analgesic agents as needed (substantial narcotic medication may be needed).[27]
   g. Keep canal dry during treatment, and recheck and repeat process every 24-72 hours.
   h. Use systemic antibiotic agents if nodes are enlarged and/or fever occurs; then culture.[27]
   i. May return to water sports within 2-3 days after onset of treatment, although abstaining for 7-10 days is recommended[22]; others recommend no return to swimming until resolution of infection.[12]
4. Complications.
   a. Malignant otitis externa (*Pseudomonas* osteomyelitis of the temporal bone).
   b. More common in diabetic patients.
5. Prevention.
   a. Maintaining normal earwax and bacterial flora constitutes the best protection.[6]

b. A few drops of baby oil in the ears before swimming can help protect them.[16]
c. Acidifying, drying eardrops applied prophylactically after swimming also are effective.
d. An effective home remedy is one or two drops of equal parts white vinegar, 70% isopropyl alcohol, and water.[3]
e. Thoroughly drying ear canal by using a handheld hairdryer also is helpful.[22]

C. Auricular hematoma.
1. Etiology/epidemiology.
a. Common in contact sports such as boxing, rugby scrum, wrestling, judo.
b. Caused by trauma or friction. Most often occurs anteriorly at junction of perichondrium and elastic cartilage of ear.[26]
2. Signs/symptoms.
a. Gross edema, usually on anterior aspect of ear.
b. Acutely tender to palpation.
3. Complications.
a. Failure to evacuate hematoma may lead to necrosis and fibrosis, resulting in deformation (cauliflower ear, scrum ear, boxer's ear; Fig. 16-1).
b. Infection may lead to perichondritis or chondritis requiring intravenous antibiotic agents.
4. Treatment.
a. Aseptic needle aspiration (25- or 27-gauge needle) within 24 hours after injury.
(1) Incision and drainage may be required.
(2) Incision is made in helical fold or under antihelical curl.

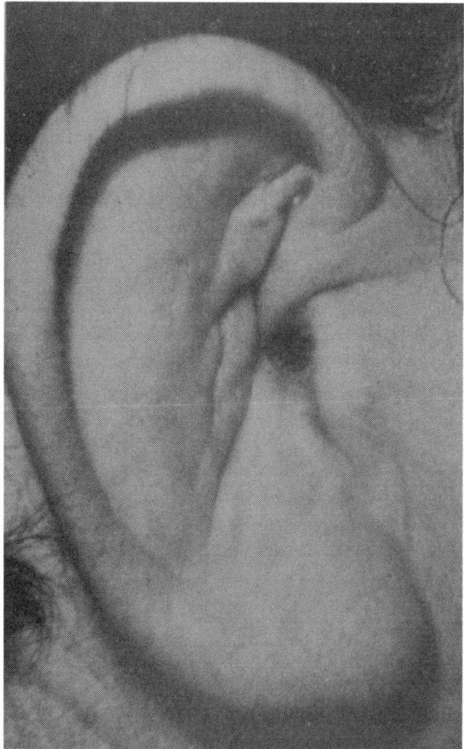

FIGURE 16-1
Cauliflower ear after hematoma. (Reproduced by permission of author and publisher from Schuller DE, Schleuning AJ, editors: *DeWeese and Saunders' Otolaryngology: head and neck surgery*, ed 8, St Louis, 1994, Mosby–Year Book, p 436.)

(3) Debridement by specialist if patient is seen >7-10 days after injury.

b. Anesthesia for evacuation of hematoma (using large-bore, 18-gauge needle) or for incision and drainage is applied anteriorly and posteriorly at base of pinna.[16]

c. No dressing is required if hematoma does not recur within 1 hour of successful aspiration[2]; otherwise, pressure dressing is indicated for 2-3 days.

d. Several pressure dressing options are available.[7,12,16]

(1) Compression suture dressing.

(2) Collodion-cotton cast.

(3) Plaster of Paris cast or silicone mold.

(4) Mastoid dressing.

e. Antibiotic agent is warranted if suturing or incision and drainage are done.

f. Nonsteroidal antiinflammatory agents and aspirin should be avoided.

g. After dressing is applied, daily followup is recommended to avoid pressure necrosis, infection, or allergic reaction.

h. Recommendations for return to activity after drainage and application of dressing.

(1) Some allow full activity,[5,26] although ear protector should be worn.[5]

(2) Others recommend no competition while wearing mastoid dressing.[2]

(3) Still others suggest avoiding potential head trauma during healing.[27]

5. Prevention.

a. Ear protectors, headgear, lubricant such as Vaseline (not allowed in matches).[19]

b. 50% decrease in incidence of auricular hematomas reported in wrestlers who consistently wore protective headgear during training and competition.[25]

c. Ice and pressure applied at end of practice or game or whenever apparent problems exist also help.[16]

D. Barotrauma.

1. Etiology/epidemiology.

a. Tissue injury from inability to equilibrate pressure difference across tympanic membrane.[19]

b. May affect any structure from external auditory canal to inner ear.

c. Vessel rupture within tympanic membrane[8] and rupture of tympanic membrane are the most common.

d. Primarily seen in scuba divers.

2. Signs/symptoms.

a. Otalgia, blood-tinged sputum, tinnitus, muffled hearing, ear fullness.

b. Erythematous, depressed tympanic membrane (ear squeeze) or bulging tympanic membrane (reverse ear squeeze).[19]

3. Treatment.

a. Decongestant may be helpful.

b. Avoid diving until symptoms resolve and ear heals.

4. Prevention.

a. Treat underlying problem (cerumen impaction, sinus polyp, osteoma, exostosis).[19]

b. Avoid diving if suffering from sinusitis, allergic rhinitis, or severe upper respiratory tract infection.[16]
c. Use antihistamine agents cautiously to avoid rebound edema.
d. Equalize pressure during descent by using Valsalva maneuver.[8]

E. Tympanic membrane perforation.
1. Etiology/epidemiology.
a. Most commonly seen in scuba divers.
b. May also be due to a blow to the unprotected ear, as in water polo, diving, surfing, skiing, or, more rarely, boxing, football,[16] or martial arts.[17]
c. Less frequently associated with blasts to the ear, as in riflery.[2]
2. Symptoms.
a. Otalgia, otorrhea, vertigo.
b. Conductive hearing loss and tinnitus.[1]
3. Complications.
a. Acute: hemotympanum, dislocation of ossicles, vomiting, vertigo, and disorientation (hazardous for scuba divers).
b. Chronic: fistula, cholesteatoma, infection.
4. Treatment.
a. Conservative; in most cases healing occurs spontaneously, but observation is necessary until perforation heals.
b. 90% heal within 8 weeks.[1,9]
c. Topical or oral antibiotic agents indicated in contaminated perforation (e.g., with sea water).
d. Referral to otolaryngologist is appropriate.
e. Precautions during later participation in water sports required to prevent infection.[2]
f. If symptoms are mild, athlete may return to play.[10]
g. No scuba diving until perforation heals.[2]

F. Ear laceration.
1. Usually occurs when an earring is pulled through earlobe.
2. Anesthesia and suturing for acute injuries.
3. In complex lacerations affecting cartilage, athlete should be referred to an otolaryngologist.

G. Ear avulsion.
1. Rare in sports.
2. Compression dressing is placed over wound.
3. Severed auricle should be placed on ice or in cold saline.[2]
4. Immediate surgical evaluation required.

II. Nasal problems.
A. Nasal fracture.
1. Etiology/epidemiology.
a. Usually results from contact with elbow or knee, ball, or, occasionally, projectile.
b. More common in rugby, football, boxing,[31] hockey, basketball, and wrestling.
c. Most common facial fracture.
d. Usually associated with fracture of ascending process of maxilla or nasal process of frontal bone.[27]
2. Examination.
a. Essentially a clinical diagnosis.
b. Most common signs include deformity, epistaxis, tenderness, crepitation, and periorbital and subconjunctival ecchymosis.[20]

c. Inspect nasal septum for septal hematoma, exposed cartilage, or displacement.
d. Radiographic examination generally provides little practical information for management.

3. Treatment.
a. Control bleeding, close wounds, and drain septal hematoma.[18]
b. Advise athlete to keep head elevated and place icepacks on nose for first 24-48 hours.
c. The patient should be prescribed oral antibiotic agents[13] and receive adequate analgesia.
d. Reduction should be done under general or local anesthesia, usually managed by a specialist.
(1) Best to reduce before swelling occurs, but if immediate reduction is not possible, when edema subsides.
(2) Definitive treatment within 4 days for children and within 10-12 days for adults.[23]
e. Protective equipment recommended for contact or collision sports to prevent further injury or redisplacement.

4. Complications.
a. Septal hematoma or permanent saddle-nose deformity or both (Fig. 16-2).[28]
b. With more severe injury, damage may extend to cribriform plate, resulting in cerebrospinal fluid leakage, continued epistaxis, and infection.[20]
c. Presence of bull's-eye or halo upon testing drainage fluid by using filter paper indicates cerebrospinal fluid leakage.[13]

B. Epistaxis.
1. Etiology.

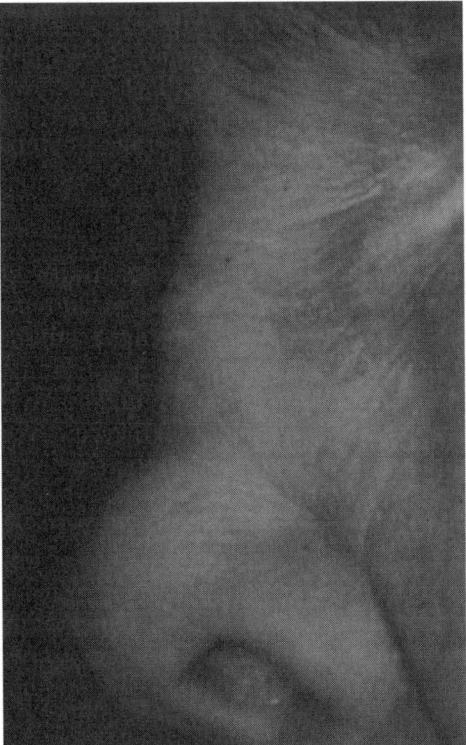

FIGURE 16-2
Saddle-nose deformity. (Reproduced by permission of author and publisher from Sessions RB, Troost T: The nasal septum. In Cummings CW et al, editors: *Otolaryngology: head and neck surgery*, ed 2, St Louis, 1993, Mosby–Year Book, p 801.)

a. Trauma secondary to contact or collision sports.
b. Spontaneous type.
    (1) Desiccation of the nasal mucosa in dry climates or at higher altitudes (e.g., as occurs in snow skiers).[11]
    (2) Usually occurs on either side of anterior inferior nasal septum (Little's area) which contains confluence of vessels (Fig. 16-3).[11]
c. Anterior epistaxis accounts for 9% of nasal bleeding episodes.
d. Epistaxis from nasal fracture often emanates from nasal roof or nasal conchae[30] with resultant anterior and posterior bleeding.
e. Persistent bleeding may be caused by undiagnosed nasal fracture.
f. Bleeding that becomes more dilute suggests basal skull fracture.[19,20]
g. Consider preexisting nasal conditions in recurrent epistaxis (e.g., hypertension or nasopharyngeal angiofibroma).

2. Examination.
    a. Exact site of bleeding must be determined when not controlled by nasal pressure.
    b. Blood clots should be removed by suction, or instruct patient to blow nose.
3. Treatment.
    a. Anterior epistaxis is usually controlled with nasal pressure applied by thumb and index finger placed on either side of ala for 2 to 5 minutes.
    b. Athlete should be sitting upright with head elevated and slightly forward.
    c. Additional pressure may be applied over midline of upper lip.
    d. Posttraumatic epistaxis usually resolves spontaneously within several minutes.
        (1) Without obvious impairment or deformity, no immediate treatment is indicated.
        (2) Examine in 1-2 days to confirm airway patency and rule out delayed septal hematoma.[21]

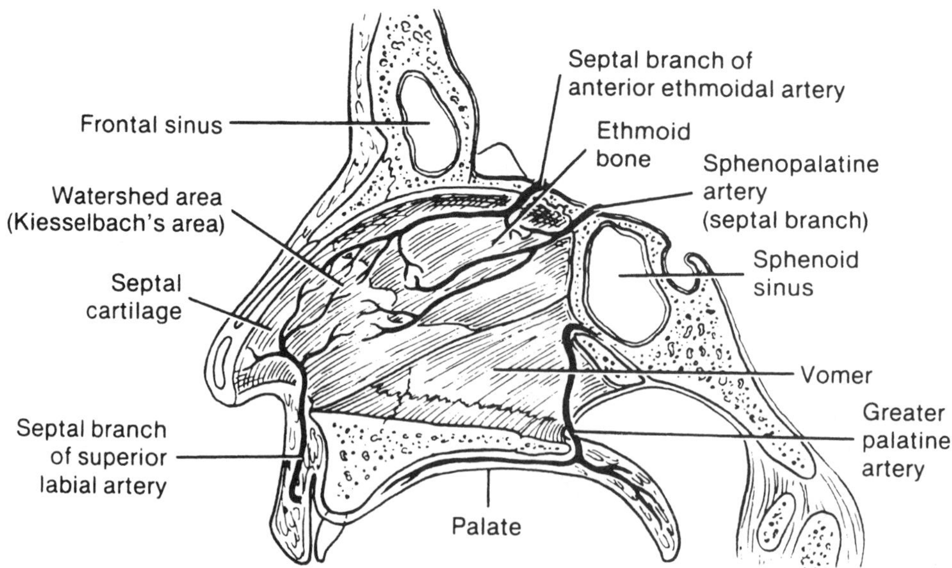

FIGURE 16-3
Blood supply to nasal septum. Little's area is site of most anterior nose bleeds. (Reproduced by permission of author and publisher from Maceri DR: Epistaxis and nasal trauma. In Cummings CW et al, editors: *Otolaryngology: head and neck surgery,* ed 2, St Louis, Mosby–Year Book, p 728.)

e. If bleeding continues after 10-15 minutes of direct pressure, a cotton pledget soaked in epinephrine 1 : 1000 or an over-the-counter vasoconstrictor such as phenylephrine or oxymetazoline placed in the anterior nose helps to promote vasoconstriction.[30]
f. If treatment is unsuccessful, transport athlete to emergency care facility for further evaluation.
g. In clinic, clinician may apply pledget soaked in solution of topical anesthetic and vasoconstrictor.
    (1) Cocaine solution 4% or 10%.
    (2) Phenylephrine 1%, followed by topical lidocaine spray 10%.[30]
h. If bleeding decreases and discrete site is identified, cauterize with silver nitrate.
    (1) Electrocautery also is an option; use with caution to avoid septal perforation.
    (2) Microscopic cautery may be used in hospital.[15]
    (3) After cautery, apply topical antibiotic ointment 2-3 times daily, and instruct athlete not to blow or pick at nose for 24 hours.
i. For persistent bleeding, anterior nasal packing is indicated when:
    (1) No specific bleeding site is identified.
    (2) Bleeding does not respond to cautery.
    (3) Posterior bleeding site is inaccessible to cautery.[30]
j. Anterior nasal packing should be left in place for 72 hours.
    (1) Physical activity, hot showers, and hot beverages should be avoided.
    (2) Sports activity should be avoided for 2 weeks after packing removal.[30]
k. Posterior epistaxis requires placement of anterior and posterior packs.
    (1) Insert 16 or 18 French Foley catheter; then insert balloon and inflate with 10-15 ml of saline.
    (2) Kits with anterior and posterior hemostatic balloons also are available.[20]
l. Referral is indicated for posterior or simultaneous anterior and posterior bleeding.

4. Prevention.
    a. Petrolatum applied to nasal mucosa twice daily and/or before athletic events.
    b. Vaporizer or humidifier should be used while sleeping.

C. Septal hematoma.
1. Etiology.
    a. Occurs from trauma, which produces a shear injury.
    b. Perichondrium separates from underlying cartilage.[14]
2. Examination.
    a. Enlarged, bluish, discolored septum obstructing nasal passage.
    b. Palpation confirms boggy, fluctuant swelling.
3. Treatment.
    a. Needle aspiration or small incision in dependent portion of hematoma.[2]
    b. Anterior nasal packs applied for 7 days so perichondrium adheres to cartilage.
4. Complications.
    a. May lead to septal necrosis if left untreated.
    b. If sufficiently widespread, may lead to collapse of nasal septum, producing saddle-nose deformity.[16]

    c. If abscess forms in hematoma, cartilage destruction is accelerated, and intracranial sepsis may follow.[14]

III. Throat and Maxillofacial Problems
  A. Trauma.
    1. Patients with maxillofacial or throat trauma must always be evaluated for airway obstruction.
    2. Injuries prone to cause obstruction.[13]
      a. "Flail" mandible.
      b. Maxillary fracture.
      c. Tongue laceration.
      d. Hematoma of sublingual, nasopharyngeal, lateral pharyngeal, or retropharyngeal area.
      e. Fractured larynx.
    3. Facial or neck trauma is common in hockey, field hockey, lacrosse, basketball, or baseball.
    4. Facial fractures are usually seen only in high-velocity sports, such as skiing and equestrian events.[16]
    5. Most facial fractures are nondisplaced; however, accurate diagnosis is essential.
    6. Signs of facial fracture include (Table 16-1):
      a. Malocclusion.
      b. Facial asymmetry of cheek, nose, jaw.
      c. Periorbital ecchymosis.
      d. Diplopia.
    7. Maintain a suspicious attitude for possible fractures.
    8. A specialist is necessary for definitive treatment.
    9. Establish airway patency, control bleeding, and transport athlete promptly in semiprone position after protecting spine.[13,16]
  B. Laryngeal trauma.
    1. Usually due to direct blow to neck.
    2. Signs include throat pain, pain on swallowing, swelling, crepitus over anterior neck, and respiratory distress.
    3. Stridor, hoarseness, and hemoptysis are serious signs.[4]

TABLE 16-1. Facial Fractures: Signs, Symptoms, and Examination Findings

Maxillary Fracture	Mandibular Fracture	Zygomatic Fracture
Signs include bilateral edema, periorbital ecchymosis, diplopia, malocclusion, missing or avulsed teeth, and facial lengthening, which is pathognomonic.[13] Classified by fracture line location (Le Fort I, II, III) Diagnosed by attempting to move upper jaw while stabilizing head with other hand.[16]	Signs include gingival hematoma, instability, deformity, and malocclusion.[4] Ecchymosis in floor of mouth is pathognomonic for mandibular fracture.[13] Mandibular deviation to the side of injury occurs when mouth is opened. A step defect is often palpable along the inferior border.	Signs include periorbital ecchymosis, diplopia, numbness over cheek, and associated epistaxis. Cheek is usually flattened but may be enlarged from edema. Associated eye injury or additional facial bone fracture is typical.

4. Obliteration of normal cartilaginous landmarks is diagnostic of fracture.
5. Athletes who have no symptoms or signs of laryngeal fracture after neck trauma may return to play but must be monitored for airway compromise.[10]

C. Dentoalveolar trauma.
1. Partial avulsion.
   a. If tooth is slightly depressed in bone or is loose or if numbness or pain is felt upon pressure, athlete should see dentist as soon as possible.[16]
   b. May anesthetize with lidocaine 2% (if available).
   c. Reposition tooth into socket and stabilize with mouthguard or wire ligatures.
   d. Start treatment with oral antibiotic[29] and analgesic agents.[13]
   e. If asymptomatic, athlete may resume play.[16]
   f. Mouthguard strongly recommended for prevention.
2. Complete avulsion.
   a. Clean root of tooth with milk, saline, or saliva; do not brush.[13]
   b. Handle tooth by crown,[29] and reimplant tooth as soon as possible.
   c. If unable to reimplant, transport in milk, in buccal vestibule of athlete, or under athlete's tongue.
   d. If reimplanted within 30 minutes, 90% chance of tooth being retained.
   e. Start antibiotic agents, and refer athlete to endodontist as soon as possible.
3. Tooth fracture.
   a. Small fracture not sensitive to air is compatible with continuing play, but evaluation within 24 hours is recommended.
   b. Larger fracture exposing pulp should receive dental treatment, preferably within 2-3 hours of injury.[16]

Acknowledgment

The Medical Editing Department, Kaiser Foundation Research Institute, provided editorial assistance.

References

1. Berger G, Finkelstein Y, Harell M: Non-explosive blast injury of the ear, *J Laryngol Otol* 108:395-398, 1994.
2. Davidson TM, Neuman TR: Managing ear trauma, *Phys Sportsmed* 22(7):27-32, 1994.
3. Davidson TM, Neuman TR: Managing inflammatory ear conditions, *Phys Sportsmed* 22(8):56-60, 1994.
4. Davis TS, Carlton JM: Injuries of the face. In Grana WA, Kalenak A, editors: *Clinical sports medicine,* Philadelphia, 1991, WB Saunders, pp 125-129.
5. Dimeff RJ, Hough DO: Preventing cauliflower ear with modified tie-through technique, *Phys Sportsmed* 17(3):169-173, 1989.
6. Eichel BS: How I manage external otitis in competitive swimmers, *Phys Sportsmed* 14(8):108-113, 1986.
7. Grosse SJ, Lynch JM: Treating auricular hematoma: success with a swimmer's nose clip, *Phys Sportsmed* 19(10):99-102, 1991.
8. Kindwall EP, Strauss RH: Medical aspects of scuba and breath-hold diving. In Strauss RH, editor: *Sports medicine,* ed 2, Philadelphia, 1991, WB Saunders, pp 409-430.
9. Kristensen S et al: Traumatic tympanic membrane perforations: complications and management, *Ear Nose Throat J* 68:503-516, 1989.
10. Lowery DW: Soft tissue trauma of the head and neck, *Phys Sportsmed* 19(10):21-24, 1991.
11. Maceri DR: Epistaxis and nasal trauma. In Cummings CW et al, editors: *Otolaryngology: head and neck surgery,* ed 2, St Louis, 1993, Mosby–Year Book, pp 723-736.
12. Miser WF: Acute minor illnesses and exercise. In Lillegard WA, Rucker KS, editors: *Handbook of sports medicine: a symptom-oriented approach,* Boston, 1993, Andover Medical Publishers, pp 237-248.

13. Mulrean JC, Davis SM: Maxillofacial injuries. In Lillegard WA, Rucker KS, editors: *Handbook of sports medicine: a symptom-oriented approach,* Boston, 1993, Andover Medical Publishers, pp 33-41.
14. O'Donoghue GM, Bates GJ, Narula AA: *Clinical ENT: an illustrated textbook,* New York, 1992, Oxford University Press.
15. Quine SM et al: Microscope and hot wire cautery management of 100 consecutive patients with acute epistaxis: a superior method to traditional packing, *J Laryngol Otol* 108:845-848, 1994.
16. Reid DC: *Sports injury assessment and rehabilitation,* New York, 1992, Churchill Livingstone.
17. Renneker M: Medical aspects of surfing, *Phys Sportsmed* 15(12):96-105, 1987.
18. Renner GJ: Management of nasal fractures, *Otolaryngol Clin North Am* 24:195-213, 1991.
19. Robinson T, Birrer RB: Ear injuries. In Birrer RB, editor: *Sports medicine for the primary care physician,* ed 2, Boca Raton, FL, 1994, CRC Press, pp 365-366.
20. Robinson T, Greenberg MD: Nasal injuries. In Birrer RB, editor: *Sports medicine for the primary care physician,* ed 2, Boca Raton, FL, 1994, CRC Press, pp 367-369.
21. Sanford JP: *The Sanford guide to antimicrobial therapy.* Dallas, 1994, Antimicrobial Therapy Inc.
22. Schelkun PH: Swimmer's ear: getting patients back in the water, *Phys Sportsmed* 19(7):85-90, 1991.
23. Schendel SA: Sports-related nasal injuries, *Phys Sportsmed* 18(10):59-74, 1990.
24. Schuller DE, Bruce RA: Ear, nose, throat, and eye. In Strauss RH, editor: *Sports medicine,* ed 2, Philadelphia, 1991, WB Saunders, pp 189-203.
25. Schuller DE et al: Auricular injury and the use of headgear in wrestlers, *Arch Otolaryngol Head Neck Surg* 115:714-717, 1989.
26. Schuller DE, Dankle SD, Strauss RH: A technique to treat wrestlers' auricular hematoma without interrupting training or competition, *Arch Otolaryngol Head Neck Surg* 115:202-206, 1989.
27. Schuller DE, Schleuning AJ, editors: *DeWeese and Saunders' Otolaryngology: head and neck surgery,* ed 8, St Louis, 1994, Mosby–Year Book.
28. Sessions RB, Troost T: The nasal septum. In Cummings CW et al, editors: *Otolaryngology: head and neck surgery,* ed 2, St Louis, 1993, Mosby–Year Book, pp 786-806.
29. Sitorius MA, Mellion MB: General medical problems in athletes. In Mellion MB, Walsh WM, Shelton GL, editors: *The team physician's handbook,* Philadelphia, 1990, Hanley & Belfus, pp 161-178.
30. Stevens H: Epistaxis in the athlete, *Phys Sportsmed* 16(12):31-40, 1988.
31. Tu HK, Davis LF, Nique TA: Maxillofacial injuries. In Mellion MB, Walsh WM, Shelton GL, editors: *The team physician's handbook,* Philadelphia, 1990, Hanley & Belfus, pp 302-312.
32. Yanagisawa E, Kmucha S: Diseases of the external and middle ear. In Lee KJ, editor: *Textbook of otolaryngology and head and neck surgery,* New York, 1989, Elsevier, pp 63-102.

CHAPTER 17A

Environmental Concerns: Heat

Brent S.E. Rich, MD, ATC

I. Significance of Heat Illness
   A. Actual incidence of heat illness is unknown because of underreporting.
   B. Prevalence of heat illness is based on field experience and believed to be in the thousands per year.
   C. 84 deaths secondary to heatstroke in football from 1955 to 1990.[1]
   D. Heat illness continuum: heat stress → heat cramps → heat exhaustion → heatstroke → death.

II. Pathophysiology of Heat Accumulation and Loss
   A. Definitions.
      1. Heat load = internal (metabolic) heat + external (environmental) heat.
      2. Heat dissipation = removal of heat by one of four methods.
         a. Radiation = heat transfer by electromagnetic waves (may be source of heat gain in warmer climates).
         b. Conduction = transfer of heat from warmer to cooler objects (only 2% of body heat is normally lost by conduction).[6]
         c. Convection = movement of heat away from the body by the movement of the ambient air.
         d. Evaporation = conversion of liquid to gas.
      3. Pearls.
         a. Environmental temperature >35°C (95°F) = all heat loss through evaporation.
         b. Humidity >75% = evaporation slows and sweating becomes inefficient.[4]
         c. Humidity >90% and temperature >95% = body loses no heat![4]
   B. Thermoregulation.
      1. Anterior hypothalamus: afferent skin receptors and body core send impulses to the hypothalamus, which controls the autonomic nervous system affecting the following.

a. Sympathetic nervous system.
   (1) Decreased vasoconstriction.
   (2) Increased skin blood flow.
b. Parasympathetic nervous system: controls sweating mechanism.

2. Sweating mechanism.
   a. Sweating rate in heavy exercise.[4]
      (1) 0-30 seconds = no sweat.
      (2) 30 seconds to 3 minutes = sweating begins.
      (3) 3-10 minutes = linear increase in sweating.
      (4) >10-15 minutes = sweat rate levels off.
   b. Composition of sweat: Na^+ and Cl^- > K^+ and Mg^+.[3]
   c. Acclimation of the sweating mechanism.
      (1) Earlier initiation of sweating.
      (2) Increased rate of sweating.
   d. Pearls.
      (1) Loss of Na^+ (not K^+) leads to heat cramps.
      (2) There is a cumulative loss of Na^+ with continued sweating.
3. Risks for heat emergencies.
   a. Vigorous physical activity leads to cumulative fluid loss.
   b. Diuretic beverages (coffee, tea, and caffeinated beverages).
   c. Vapor-impermeable clothing.
   d. Effects of drugs.

Drugs	Effects
1. Amphetamines, cocaine	Increase muscle activity
2. Anticholinergics	Block parasympathetic activity
3. Beta-blockers	Decrease cardiac output, limit skin blood flow
4. Alpha-adrenergics (decongestants)	Vasoconstriction, limit skin blood flow
5. Diuretics (including alcohol)	Decrease intravascular volume
6. Haloperidol	Decrease thirst

   e. Poor muscle conditioning.
   f. Lack of acclimation.
   g. Obesity.
   h. Extremes of ages.
      (1) Elderly:
         (a) Myocardial dysfunction/valvular heart disease = limited cardiac output.
         (b) Decreased muscle mass (replaced by fat) = decreased total body water.
         (c) Decreased cutaneous blood supply.
         (d) Renal deterioration = impaired ability to regulate electrolytes and water.
         (e) Elderly illness (arthritis, cerebrovascular disease, cataracts, dementia) = impaired mobility and decreased fluid intake.
      (2) Children: greater ratio of surface area to body mass, leading to increased surface area for radiant, convective, and conductive heat gain.[2]

III. Exertional Heat Syndromes
   A. Heat stress.
      1. Pathophysiology: increased temperature.
      2. Symptoms.
         a. Increased heart rate.

b. Increased blood pressure.
c. Dizziness.
d. Restlessness.
e. Fatigue.
f. Emotional lability.
g. Mild changes in mentation.

3. Treatment.
   a. Mild cooling.
   b. Oral rehydration with water.

B. Heat cramps.
   1. Pathophysiology: total body salt deficiency (i.e., Na^+ not K^+). Core temperature = normal.
   2. Symptoms.
      a. Muscle spasms/cramps.
      b. Weakness.
      c. Fatigue.
      d. Nausea and vomiting.
      e. Tachycardia.
   3. Treatment.
      a. Mild cooling.
      b. Oral rehydration with electrolyte solution.
      c. Gentle stretching.
      d. Ice affected muscles.
      e. Prehydration.
      f. Add extra table salt to food.
      g. Salt tablets are not indicated secondary to irritation of gastrointestinal tract.

C. Heat exhaustion.
   1. Pathophysiology hallmark: hypovolvemia.
      a. Dehydration.
      b. Electrolyte loss.
      c. Core temperature = normal/slightly elevated but <40°C (104°F).
   2. Symptoms.
      a. Orthostatic vital signs.
      b. Syncope.
      c. Dyspnea.
      d. Weakness.
      e. Piloerection.
      f. Profuse sweating.
      g. Cutaneous flushing.
      h. Decreased urine output.
      i. Nausea and vomiting.
      j. Irritability, headache.
      k. Absence of serious central nervous system dysfunction.
   3. Treatment.
      a. Moderate cooling.
      b. Remove to cool environment.
      c. Remove excess clothing.
      d. Spray lukewarm water and cool with fans.
      e. Oral hydration = cool water 1 L/hour for several hours.
      f. Intravenous (IV) fluid replacement, if necessary.

D. Heatstroke.
   1. Pathophysiology hallmark = hyperthermia.
      a. Result = thermoregulatory failure.
      b. Core temperature >40°C (104°F).

c. "Classic": hot, dry skin.[5]
d. "Exertional": profuse sweating.
e. Volume depletion → peripheral vasoconstriction → decreased heat transfer to periphery.

2. Symptoms.
   a. Hypotension.
   b. Vomiting.
   c. Diarrhea.
   d. Coma.
   e. Seizures.
   f. Change in mental status.
3. Serious effects.
   a. Abnormal lab values.
      (1) Elevated liver enzymes.
      (2) Elevated creatine phosphokinase.
      (3) Proteinurea.
      (4) Granular casts.
      (5) Hematuria.
      (6) Myoglobinuria.
   b. Neurological injury.
   c. Disseminated intravascular coagulation.
   d. Organ failure.
   e. Rhabdomyolysis.
   f. Adult respiratory distress syndrome.
4. Mortality = function of duration and intensity of hyperthermia.
5. Poor prognosis.
   a. Temperature >42°C.
   b. Liver function enzymes (aspartate transaminase) >1000 in first 24 hours.
   c. Coma >2 hours.
6. Treatment.
   a. Goal = rapid cooling to a core temperature of 39°C (102°F).
   b. Remove to cool environment.
   c. Remove excess clothing.
   d. Spray lukewarm water and cool with fans.
   e. IV fluid challenge (D5 1/2 NS or D5 NS). (Watch closely; avoid cerebral and pulmonary edema.)
   f. Oxygen and respiratory assistance.
   g. Monitor urine output.
   h. Monitor core body temperature every 5-10 minutes.
   i. Ice water baths.
   j. Monitor serum liver enzymes and coagulation time.
   k. Avoid alcohol baths (in children alcohol intoxication through absorption and flash burns from friction rub).

IV. Prevention
   A. Heat illness is preventable.
      1. Recognize high-risk conditions.
      2. Education.
      3. Wear light, vapor-permeable clothing.
      4. Prehydration.
         a. 8 oz before and 4 oz every 15-20 minutes.
         b. Runners = 100 to 200 ml of water every 2-3 km.
         c. 625-1250 ml of fluid intake per hour of exertion.
      5. Heat acclimation.
         a. Gradually over 10-14 days.

b. Daily exposure to work and heat.
c. Train 1-2 hours in same heat.

Effects.

a. Earlier initiation of sweating.
b. Increased rate of sweating.
c. Earlier vasodilatation.
d. Lower core body temperature.
e. Increased plasma volume at rest.
f. Decreased heart rate for work stress.
g. Decreased sweat Na^+ concentration.
h. Increased thermal comfort.
i. More hypotonic sweat.

6. Monitor weight before and after practice.
   a. Dehydration = 3% of body weight.
   b. If >5% loss = stop activity, rest, and reevaluate in 24 hours.
   c. If >7% loss = medical evaluation.
7. Gradual physical conditioning: new/transfer athletes = be aware of early practices!
8. Avoid heat after history of previous episode of heatstroke: Consider exercise trial.
9. Schedule water breaks.
10. Wet bulb globe temperature (WBGT) = (0.7 Twb) + (0.2 Tg) + (0.1 Tdb) or (0.567 Tdb) + (0.393 Pa) + 3.94 (Twb = temperature of a wet bulb thermometer; Tg = temperature of a black globe thermometer; Tdb = temperature of a dry bulb thermometer; Pa = environmental water vapor pressure.)
    a. At WBGT >19.0°C, increased risk.

V. Pearls.
   A. Muscle tissue stores more water than fat tissue.
      1. Muscle = 75% to 80% water.
      2. Fat = 10% water.
   B. Thirst is *not* an indicator of decreased body water: can lose 1.5 L of body water before perceiving thirst.
   C. Ability to do work decreases with dehydration.
      1. Fluid loss of 2% of body weight = decreased work ability.[4]
      2. Fluid loss of 4% to 5% of body weight = decreased endurance.
   D. 1 lb of weight loss = 450 ml of fluid.
   E. Fluid replacement.
      1. If event lasts <1 hour = water replacement is adequate.
      2. If event lasts >1-3 hours = carbohydrate solution should be added to water.

References

1. Allman FL: The effects of heat on the athlete, *J Med Assoc Georgia* 81:307-310, 1992.
2. Bar-Or O: Temperature regulation during exercise in children and adolescents. In Gisolfi CV, Lamb DR, editors: *Youth, exercise, and sport. Perspectives in exercise science and sports medicine,* vol 2, Indianapolis, 1989, Benchmark, pp 335-367.
3. Bergeron MF et al: Fluid and electrolyte losses during tennis in the heat, *Clin Sports Med* 14(1):23-32, 1995.
4. Halpern B: Fluid and electrolyte replacement in athletes, *Sports Med Digest* 16(7):1-5, 1994.
5. Sterner S: Summer heat illnesses, *Postgrad Med* 87(8):67-73, 1990.
6. Yarbrough BE: Heat-related disorders, *Hosp Med,* pp 81-91, June 1991.

CHAPTER 17B

Environmental Concerns: Hypothermia and Frostbite

Murray E. Allen, MD

HYPOTHERMIA

I. Objectives
   A. Understand the epidemiology, physiology, and pathophysiology of accidental hypothermia.
   B. Understand the initial evaluation and management of adverse cold exposure.
   C. Be aware of some advanced issues in hypothermia management.

II. Definition
   A. Core body temperature <35°C (95°F).
   B. In the clinical setting this is usually unintentional or accidental.

III. Epidemiology
   A. True incidence: unknown due to a large underreporting of this condition. Since it probably occurs quite regularly and is treated often very successfully with simple rewarming at home, it is often not reported to doctors or hospitals.
   B. Commonest setting for reporting: urban areas, usually in the northern climates. This could reflect the presence of large populations exposed to cold temperatures, with an abundance of doctors and hospitals. Individuals in rural areas are equally exposed, but there could be a slightly greater awareness of the dangers of cold exposure in rural areas and therefore the deleterious results of cold exposure do not appear as often. Lack of understanding of the concerns for hypothermia have led to occurrences of fatal hypothermia, even in Florida.
   C. Primary hypothermia: occurs in previously healthy persons following cold exposure. This grouping can be broken down into:
      1. Accidental, homicidal, or suicidal causes.
      2. Immersion or nonimmersion causes.
   D. Secondary hypothermia: occurs in persons with other significant debilitating disease that compromises their ability to maintain normother-

mia (e.g., cancer, systemic disease, trauma, sepsis, etc.). Underreporting of this type of hypothermia is common. Subtle factors such as fatigue, overwork, physical and/or psychological stress, lack of sleep, and lack of adequate nourishment can also be factors in otherwise healthy persons. Persons on drugs or alcohol or with other metabolic diseases such as diabetes, hypothyroidism, or central nervous system disorders may respond poorly to cold stress.

IV. Physiology of Cold Exposure
   A. Basal heat production: about 40-60 kcal/m^2 BSA/hour. (BSA = body surface area.) The thermostat is set at about 37°C. Thermogenesis of shivering is due to muscle action, and therefore heat production, between 35° and 32°C. Below this point, shivering often stops, a point of maladaption. Vigorous muscle contraction can produce 20 to 25 times more heat than during rest.
      2. Peripheral control: reflex vasoconstriction and autonomic shunting of blood helps pool blood around the central organs and brain and allows the periphery to cool. Upon rewarming, this cold peripheral blood can add more coolant to the central core, causing an afterdrop.
      3. Endocrinological thermogenesis: facilitated through release of adrenocorticotropic hormone, thyroid hormone, insulin, and catecholamines.
      4. Adaptive response: simply means seeking a warm place, adding more clothes. Some persons who become confused during hypothermia will actually undress, a paradoxical or maladaptive response, which leads to progressive hypothermia.

V. Mechanisms of Heat Exchange
   A. Radiation: all objects are continually emitting electromagnetic heat waves. The sun emits the most. Reflected radiation can come from other objects, even snow. Radiant heat can be absorbed by the body from other warmer surrounding objects but can also be emitted to other objects. Usually, loss of heat due to radiant exchange is not great. Being adequately dressed will allow for radiant heat from the body to be absorbed by the clothing. With proper clothing, only some of this heat will then be radiated to the surroundings.
   B. Conduction: this process involves the direct transfer of heat through a liquid, solid, or gas from one molecule to another. This method trans-

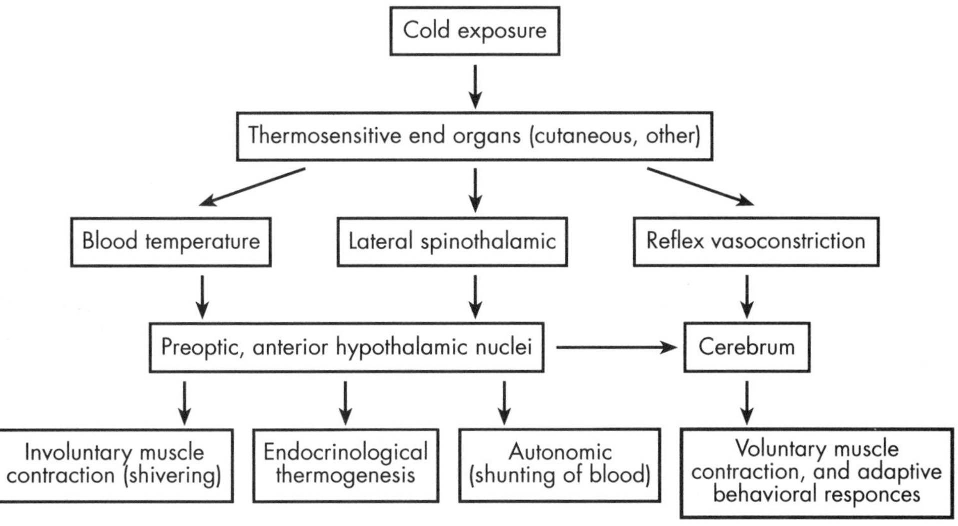

fers heat from deep in the shell to the surface without actual circulation. Conductive heat loss is through heating of molecules at the surface of the skin. If the surface is air, the loss is minor; if the surface is water, the loss is greater. Water can absorb several thousand times the heat of air, and water can conduct the heat away from the surface much easier. Keep dry is the adage in cold weather. Wet clothing will allow for serious heat loss.

C. Convection: if air movement at the skin is slow, then the air can be warmed and will act as a zone of insulation. If convection is high, the heat is carried away from the body surface. Air currents of 4 mph are about twice as effective in removing heat than 1 mph; this is the "windchill factor." In water, lying still will build up a layer of warm water, while swimming will cause more convection of warm water away from the body. Again, proper clothing with a wind barrier at the surface is important to prevent the wind from convecting away the heat. Among swimmers, there is little help from preventing convection loss.

D. Evaporation: this provides the greatest physiological defense against overheating but is the greatest hazard for heat loss. As water at the surface vaporizes, it loses heat during the change from fluid to gas. For each liter of water that vaporizes, 580 kcal are extracted from the body and transferred to the environment. The 3 million or so sweat glands secrete hypotonic saline solution, which evaporates at the surface. The cooled skin in turn cools the surface blood, which returns to the core. For the average inactive adult, about 500 ml fluid are lost through normal sweating during a routine day but only a small amount of sumped heat is actually lost from this fluid per se. The most heat loss is not due to fluid loss but rather from the evaporation. Clinically, persons who work hard in cold weather will sweat, which in turn moistens their clothing to the surface, which in turn acts as a wick to facilitate evaporative loss.

E. Respiration: this loss is from actual fluid loss from the moist lung air. It is similar to sweat loss and only accounts for a small amount of the total heat loss. The average inactive adult will lose about 300 ml fluid from respiration during a routine day. Although cold dry air will increase this loss, it is not a major contributor to heat loss.

VI. Clothing for Cold Weather

A. Clothing for cold weather is all important, especially in sports where heat is produced in abundance. The body is attempting to lose the excess heat from the core but in turn is trying to preserve heat at the surface. What starts out as overheating during exercise, if not controlled, can lead to excess heat loss and hypothermia. Here are some key features of clothing that can reduce this possible dilemma.

1. One or two layers at the surface can wick the moisture away from the skin. Cotton is the worst; it will actually retain lots of moisture and facilitate loss due to convection. Wool is a good wick; it moves moisture to the surface but keeps it away from the skin surface. However, it also retains lots of moisture. The current favorite for the first layer is synthetic material such as polypropylene or its variants. This type of material will wick the moisture away from the body surface, causing it to bead at the outer surface.
2. The next layer can be more of the same, a synthetic or wool that acts as an insulator to retain heat and allows movement of moisture to the surface.
3. The outer layer should be a windproof layer, preferably with some waterproofing capability to shed rain or snow. If this layer is too effi-

cient at shedding rain, it may also prevent moisture beading of underlying moisture to the surface and can build up lots of sweat on the inside. Gore-Tex materials can allow moisture to move in one direction, out.

B. All of this layering is designed to prevent the buildup of a continuous uninterrupted layer of moisture between the skin surface and the environmental surface of the clothing. Although this prevents conductive loss, it also reduces radiant and evaporative loss as well.

VII. Hypothermic Zones

A. Mild zone: zone of adaptive responses.

C°	F°	Features
37.6	99.6	Normal rectal temperature.
37	98.6	Normal oral temperature.
36	96.8	Initial adaptive response, increase in metabolic rate (noted as increased calorie needs in cold weather).
35	95.0	Maximum shivering-induced thermogenesis.
34	93.2	Maximum respiratory drive, apathy, dysarthria, amnesia, poor judgment.
33	91.4	Ataxia, sometimes profound apathy, defenselessness.

B. Moderate zone: zone of loss of adaptation.

C°	F°	Features
32	89.6	Stupor, drop in oxygen consumption.
31	87.8	No more shivering.
30	86.0	Bradycardia, drop of cardiac output, arrhythmia, poikilothermia (temperature same as environment).
29	85.2	Coma develops, reduced pulse and respiration, pupils dilate.
28	82.4	Oxygen consumption and pulse reduced 50%, pending ventricular fibrillation.
27	80.6	Loss of reflexes.

C. Severe zone: nonrecoverable, except with extraordinary measures.

C°	F°	Features
26	78.8	No response to pain, major acid-base disturbances.
25	77.0	Pulmonary edema.
24	75.2	Profound hypotension.
23	73.4	Lack of corneal reflexes.
22	71.6	Maximum risk of ventricular fibrillation.
20	68.0	Lowest resumption of cardiac electromechanical activity.
19	66.2	Flat electroencephalogram.
18	64.4	Asystole.
16	60.8	Lowest adult accidental hypothermia survival.
9	48.2	Lowest therapeutic hypothermia survival.

VIII. First Aid in the Field

A. Prevention: key issue. It is important to be aware of weather conditions and dress appropriately. Layered clothing or sometimes a simple umbrella helps. Proper headgear is important; lots of heat can be lost from the exposed scalp. Always be aware that hypothermia is a possible event in any climate zone where wind and moisture can penetrate to the body. If sporting out of doors for prolonged duration, many athletes pace themselves to the level of sufficient heat production to achieve goals, yet not so hard as to oversweat, which leads to moist clothing and heat loss. If working in very cold weather, this pacing is very important, as is having extra clothing kept safe in a dry compartment. Knowing the out of doors and shelter building is key to reducing cold exposure. Knowledge of the early signs of hypothermia and taking the appropriate steps early are perhaps the most important steps in preventing serious hypothermia. The listless, slow, somewhat apathetic athlete may not be lazy or unmotivated but instead may be hypothermic.

B. The first step in the field: stop and recognize the problem. Retreat from whatever intended goals were planned to deal with the now important issue of preserving heat. Find shelter, or make a shelter. Remove wet clothing, replace with dry clothes, even if you have to trade between persons. In a group the warm bodies should hold close to the cold person, even to being near naked in a sleeping bag together (regardless of sex), you can always sort out the embarrassment later (a dead person is not embarrassed!). Hot fluids are helpful. Arrange evacuation. Handle the cold person gently. In the field, taking rectal temperature readings is awkward, partly due to lack of an adequate hypothermic thermometer and due to the need to expose the victim to the elements to insert the thermometer.

C. The second step in hospital: warm blankets and heaters such as lights and hot fans will help. Warm, moist oxygen is very helpful; some hospitals have special heated devices that warm up the core quite quickly. Be careful of accepting core temperature readings from regular thermometers or the tympanic thermometers, which have a limited range.

D. Serious hypothermia: requires a full team of experts. Necessitates the careful evaluation of core temperatures, acid base balance, electrolytes, electrocardiography, with the inclusion of major intervention. Patients must be handled with great care; physical jarring can set off ventricular fibrillation. Rewarming might have to be delayed until full cardiorespiratory resuscitation is available. During the rewarming phase, a person may go from asystole to ventricular fibrillation quite easily and not respond to defibrillation until core temperature rises to greater than 30°C. Also required are fluid balance measures, IV warming, hyperglycemia/hypoglycemia watch, coagulation considerations, possible peritoneal lavage with warmed fluids, and in rare cases full cardiopulmonary circulatory bypass. Persons who are hypothermic due to immersion and drowning present serious challenges due to electrolyte imbalances, which can be difficult to manage whether they were immersed in salt or fresh water.

E. Remember, *"a person is not dead, until they are both warm and dead."*

FROSTBITE

I. Objectives
   A. Understand the basic causes of frostbite.
   B. Understand its early recognition, prevention, and treatment.

II. Definition: localized cold injury with or without hypothermia, due to freezing of tissue, usually starting with the skin.

III. Pathological Phases

A. Prefreeze phase: secondary to surface chilling; tissue temperatures range between 3° and 10°C. Usually cutaneous sensation is abolished at about 10°C. At this level there are some cellular membrane changes with plasma leakage and edema due to damage to the vascular endothelium.

B. Freeze-thaw phase: tissue temperatures below freezing, at −6° to −15°C, with early crystalline formation both intracellularly and extracellularly. The most vulnerable tissues are endothelium, nerve, and bone marrow. Lesser vulnerable tissues are muscle, cartilage, and bone. Bone marrow is vulnerable tissue but is farthest from the cold. Cellular dehydration and shrinkage occurs. Microembolic showers clog the vasculature. Repeated freeze-thaw events can be very damaging to tissue, similar to burns.

C. Vascular stasis phase: vessels first develop vasospasm and then may dilate before coagulation. With crystalline development, there is superimposition of plasma leakage.

D. Late ischemic phase: associated with thrombosis, arterio-venous shunting, and gangrene. Tissues denature.

IV. Clinical Presentation (Classic Categories):

A. First degree: seen with white patches on the skin surface, often painless and numb. There is no tissue loss, but sometimes edema occurs if not treated immediately. The skier with the swollen nose probably suffered a first-degree frostbite during the day and may not have noticed it. In cold weather it is important to keep an eye open for white patches on companions. This usually occurs on nose, ears, cheeks, and fingertips, and even penis tips in some runners in cold weather. Involved fingers usually feel numb and clumsy before they turn white. During the rewarming phase of fingers or toes there can be extreme pain. It is best to rewarm these tissues as fast as possible. Simple remedies are facing away from the wind, put hands on nose or ears, place hands inside jacket or armpits. Change mitts with a warm-handed friend. Swinging arms around like a helicopter will sometimes force blood into the fingers and help speed up warming. Rewarming in warm to hot water is helpful, but be careful to have a normal sensate person test the water first to prevent hot water burns. The same principle applies to using an oven to warm up hands or feet, which is normally not recommended due to the dangers of overheating. Folklore methods such as rubbing the offended part with snow or ice should be discouraged. Once recovered, there is seldom any serious problem after. Almost all persons living in the far north have experienced this type of frostbite.

B. Second degree: white patch not caught in time or the fingers left frosted too long. Persistent cold, pale skin that does not blanch with pressure is a poor sign. Vesiculation or blistering with surrounding edema and erythema may be seen. The blisters are usually clear. After rewarming (see above), popping or debriding the blisters is sometimes helpful, but sepsis is a concern; antibiotics may be necessary. Aloe skin cream is often used here. Splint and pad the damaged sites carefully. Tetanus toxoid is recommended. If tissue loss is minor, then recovery from these blisters is the same as if they occurred from friction or burning, essentially over the next few weeks with reepithelialization. These same tissues may be more vulnerable to refrosting for the next few months. If any numbness occurred that did not clear in a few hours or that lasted up to a week, then deeper tissue damage occurred and these tissues might be more vulnerable to cold injury for the next several years.

C. Third degree: the blisters are larger, deeper, and purplish with blood. The swelling and redness of the surrounding tissues can be quite dramatic. There is quite probably deep tissue injury and maybe some permanent loss. Gentle hydrotherapy may help to clean the wounds. If there is little tissue loss, there will still most likely be prolonged numbness of the area and vulnerability to cold injury for years to life. Sometimes the swelling and blistering can be very dramatic, yet there is no tissue loss and recovery is full. Early appearances can sometimes be deceiving. In some cases of deep frostbite, especially of hands or feet, when there will be several days before a person can reach help, the frozen limb should not be rewarmed until it can stay warm. Repeated freeze-thaws are very damaging to tissues and may invoke sepsis as well.

D. Fourth degree: complete tissue freeze with loss of dermas and exposure of deeper tissues, with mummification including muscle and bone. The demarcation zone is sometimes difficult to predict, and time should be given for the tissues to decide for themselves which parts will fall off and which will stay. Mummification looks horrible but is painless, and the natural healing at the deep demarcation site is usually better than resorting to amputation.

Bibliography

Auerback PS, Geater ED: *Management of wilderness and environmental emergencies,* St Louis, 1989, Mosby.

Donzl DF: *Accidental hypothermia,* The Wilderness Medical Society. Philadelphia, 1972.

McArdle WD, Katch FI, Katch VL: *Exercise physiology,* Philadelphia, 1981, Lea & Febiger.

McCauley RL et al: Frostbite injuries: a rational approach based on the pathophysiology, *J Trauma* 23:143-147, 1983.

Mills WF: Summary of treatment of the cold-injured patient, *Alaska Med* 15:56, 1973.

CHAPTER **17C**

Environmental Concerns: Altitude Illness

Ferdy Massimino, MD, MPH

I. Definition of Altitude
  A. High altitude: 1500-3500 m (5,000-11,500 feet).
    1. Physiological effects.
      a. Decreased inspired oxygen
      b. Decreased exercise performance
      c. Increased ventilation at rest
    2. Mountain sickness common with rapid ascent above 2500 m (8000 feet).
  B. Very high altitude: 3500-5500 m (11,500-18,000 feet).
    1. Physiological effects.
      a. SaO_2 <90%
      b. Arterial PO_2 (PaO_2) <60 torr.
      c. Extreme hypoxemia may occur during exercise, sleep, and altitude illness.
    2. Most common range of altitude for serious altitude illness.
  C. Extreme altitude: >5500 m (18,000 feet).
    1. Physiological effects: marked hypoxemia and hypocapnia.
    2. Progressive deterioration of physiological function outstrips acclimation.

II. Physiology of Acclimation
  A. Definition of acclimation: process by which individuals gradually adjust to hypoxia to enhance survival and performance.
  B. Overview of physiological factors that *increase* with acclimation.
    1. *Acute* (days to weeks).
      a. Ventilation: increases immediately and stays high.
      b. Heart rate: eventually returns to normal.
      c. Cerebral blood flow: depends on the balance between hypoxic vasodilatation and hypocapnia-induced vasoconstriction.
      d. Hematocrit: increases immediately due to decreased plasma volume, which correlates with increased diuresis.
      e. Diuresis

A GLOSSARY OF HIGH-ALTITUDE TERMS

P_B	Barometric pressure (torr)
PO_2	Partial pressure of oxygen
P_IO_2	Inspired PO_2 {0.21 × [P_B − 47 torr (water vapor pressure at 37°C)]}
P_AO_2	PO_2 in alveolus
P_ACO_2	PCO_2 in alveolus
PaO_2	PO_2 in arterial blood
$PaCO_2$	PCO_2 in arterial blood
SaO_2%	Arterial oxygen saturation (%HbO_2/total Hb)
R	Respiratory quotient (CO_2 produced/O_2 consumed)

Alveolar Gas Equation: $P_AO_2 = P_IO_2 - P_ACO_2/R$

Reproduced from Hackett PH, Roach RC, High Altitude Medicine. In: Auerbach PS, editor: Wilderness Medicine ed. 3, St. Louis, Mosby–Year Book.

2. Chronic (weeks to months).
   a. Ventilation: remains high.
   b. Heart rate: returns to normal.
   c. ↑ red blood cell mass: due to increased erythropoiesis.
   d. Tissue becomes more efficient at extracting oxygen by mechanisms not yet understood.
3. Hyperventilation: hallmark of acclimation to altitude.
   a. Attempt to maintain alveolar PO_2.
   b. Mediated by the carotid body function that is called the hypoxic ventilatory response (HVR).
   c. Produces hypocapnic alkalosis, which results in secondary bicarbonate diuresis.
4. HVR.
   a. Mediated by carotid bodies.
   b. Probably genetically determined.
   c. Athletes with low HVR tend to do poorly at altitude.
5. Factors affecting HVR.
   a. Decrease HVR.
      (1) Long residence at altitude.
      (2) Sedative, hypnotic drugs, alcohol.
      (3) Fragmented sleep.
   b. Increase HVR.
      (1) Acute sudden exposure to altitude.
      (2) General stimulants (caffeine).
      (3) Respiratory stimulants (progesterone).
   c. No effect on HVR.
      (1) Physical conditioning.
      (2) Age.
      (3) Gender.
6. Circulatory effects.
   a. Increased catecholamine activity causes:
      (1) ↑ blood pressure.
      (2) ↑ heart rate.
      (3) ↑ cardiac output.
      (4) ↑ venous tone.
   b. Decreased plasma volume causes ↓ stroke volume.
   c. Hypoxic pulmonary vasoconstriction causes:
      (1) ↑ pulmonary vascular resistance.
      (2) ↑ pulmonary artery pressure/pulmonary hypertension.

d. Cerebral blood flow (CBF) depends on a balance of hypoxic vasodilation and hypocapnic vasoconstriction: CBF appears to increase at altitude.

7. The blood and tissue oxygen transfer
   a. ↑ hematocrit at altitude due to diuresis.
   b. Erythropoiesis begins within hours of arriving at altitude, but increased red cell mass requires several weeks.
   c. At altitude, tendency of hemoglobin to bind oxygen (left shift) due to alkalosis (Bohr effect) is offset by the right shift due to 2,3, DPG.
   d. In skeletal muscle, increased capillary density and mitochondrial density occurs.
8. Sleep at high altitude.
   a. Fragmented sleep stages with frequent awakenings.
   b. Periodic breathing, similar to Cheyne-Stokes breathing normal above 3000 m (≈10,000 feet).
9. Acetazolamide decreases periodic breathing. Improves quality of sleep at altitude.
10. Exercise.
    a. $Vo_{2\ max}$ decreases by 10% for each 1000 m (3200 feet) of altitude gain above 1500 m (≈5000 feet).
    b. Submaximal endurance increases with acclimation.
    c. Increased ventilation causes breathlessness.
11. Training at high altitude.
    a. Optimal training for increased performance at high altitude depends upon:
       (1) Altitude of residence.
       (2) Athletic event.
    b. For aerobic events (lasting more than 3-4 minutes) at altitudes above 2000 m (7000 feet), 10-20 days necessary to maximize performance.
    c. For events above 4000 m (13,000 feet), acclimation at an intermediate altitude is recommended.
    d. Highly anaerobic events of intermediate altitudes only require arrival at the time of the event, although altitude illness may become a problem.
    e. Benefits of training at high altitude for subsequent performance enhancement at or near sea level are dependent on choosing the training altitude that:
       (1) Maximizes the benefits.
       (2) Minimizes the "detraining" inevitable when $Vo_{2\ max}$ is limited altitude >1500-2000 m (5000-7000 feet).

III. High-Altitude Syndromes
   A. High-altitude syndromes as a continuum: distinctions between the various high-altitude syndromes are not sharp, nor do they occur in isolation.
      1. Acute mountain sickness (AMS).
      2. High-altitude pulmonary edema (HAPE).
      3. High-altitude cerebral edema (HACE).
      4. High-altitude deterioration.
      5. Chronic mountain sickness.
      6. Neurological syndromes.
   B. AMS.
      1. Incidence (see Table 17C-1).

TABLE 17C-1. Incidence of Altitude Illness in Various Groups

Study Group	Number at Risk per Year	Sleeping Altitude (m)	Maximum Altitude Reached (m)	Average Rate of Ascent*	Percent with AMS	Percent with HAPE and/or HACE
Western State visitors	30 million	–2000 –2500 –≥3000	3500	1-2	18-20 22 27-42	0.01
Mt. Everest trekkers	6000	3000-5200	5500	1-2 (fly in) 10-13 (walk in)	47 23	1.6 0.05
Mt. McKinley climbers	800	3000-5300	6194	3-7	30	2-3
Mt. Rainier climbers	6000	3000	4392	1-2	67	—
Indian soldiers	Unknown	3000-5500	5500	1-2	†	2.3-15.5

AMS, Acute mountain sickness; *HAPE,* high-altitude pulmonary edema; *HACE,* high-altitude cerebral edema.
*Days to sleeping altitude from low altitude.
†Reliable estimate unavailable.

2. Symptoms.
   a. Headache: usually throbbing, bitemporal or occipital, worse at night and on awakening.
   b. Malaise: may induce disabling lassitude.
   c. Anorexia: with or without nausea.
   d. Dizziness.
   e. Insomnia.
   f. Mimics symptoms of hangover (*beware*).
3. Physical findings.
   a. Early stage: lack of physical findings.
   b. Advanced stage: might include findings associated with pulmonary or cerebral edema.
   c. Ataxia is useful sign of severe AMS.
   d. Nailbed cyanosis, papilledema, and altered level of consciousness may be present with severe AMS.
   e. Severe AMS is often associated with HAPE, HACE.
4. Differential diagnosis.
   a. Viral illness.
   b. Hangover.
   c. Exhaustion.
   d. Dehydration.
   e. Hypothermia.
   f. Sedative/hypnotic medications.
   g. Carbon monoxide poisoning.
5. Ataxia: single most useful sign for recognizing the progression of AMS from mild to severe.
6. Proposed pathophysiology of AMS (see Fig. 17C-1).
7. Natural history.
   a. Usually self-limited.
   b. If untreated, may persist for several weeks.
   c. May progress to HAPE, HACE, death.
   d. Responds well to treatment.
   e. Severity correlates with altitude and rate of ascent.
8. Management.
   a. Stop ascent and allow for acclimation at same altitude. *Never leave sick person alone* (buddy system).
   b. Descend if not improving despite treatment.
   c. Descend immediately for ataxia, decreased consciousness, or pulmonary edema.
9. Treatment options for mild AMS.
   a. Descend until symptoms improve; 500-1000 m may be sufficient.
   b. Acclimation: 12 hours to 4 days.
   c. Acetazolamide 125-250 mg PO tid.
   d. Symptomatic treatment.
   e. Hyperbaric chamber.
10. Additional treatment of severe AMS.
    a. Oxygen.
    b. Dexamethasone 4 mg PO or IM q6h.
11. Portable hyperbaric chambers.
    a. First inflatable model developed by Igor Gamow (Gamow bag).
    b. Inflated by foot pump and maintains air exchange through popoff valves.
    c. Interior pressure is 2 psi (0.14 atmosphere, 103 torr)
12. Prevention of AMS by graded ascent.
    a. Gradual ascent to sleeping altitude of 3000 m (9800 feet).

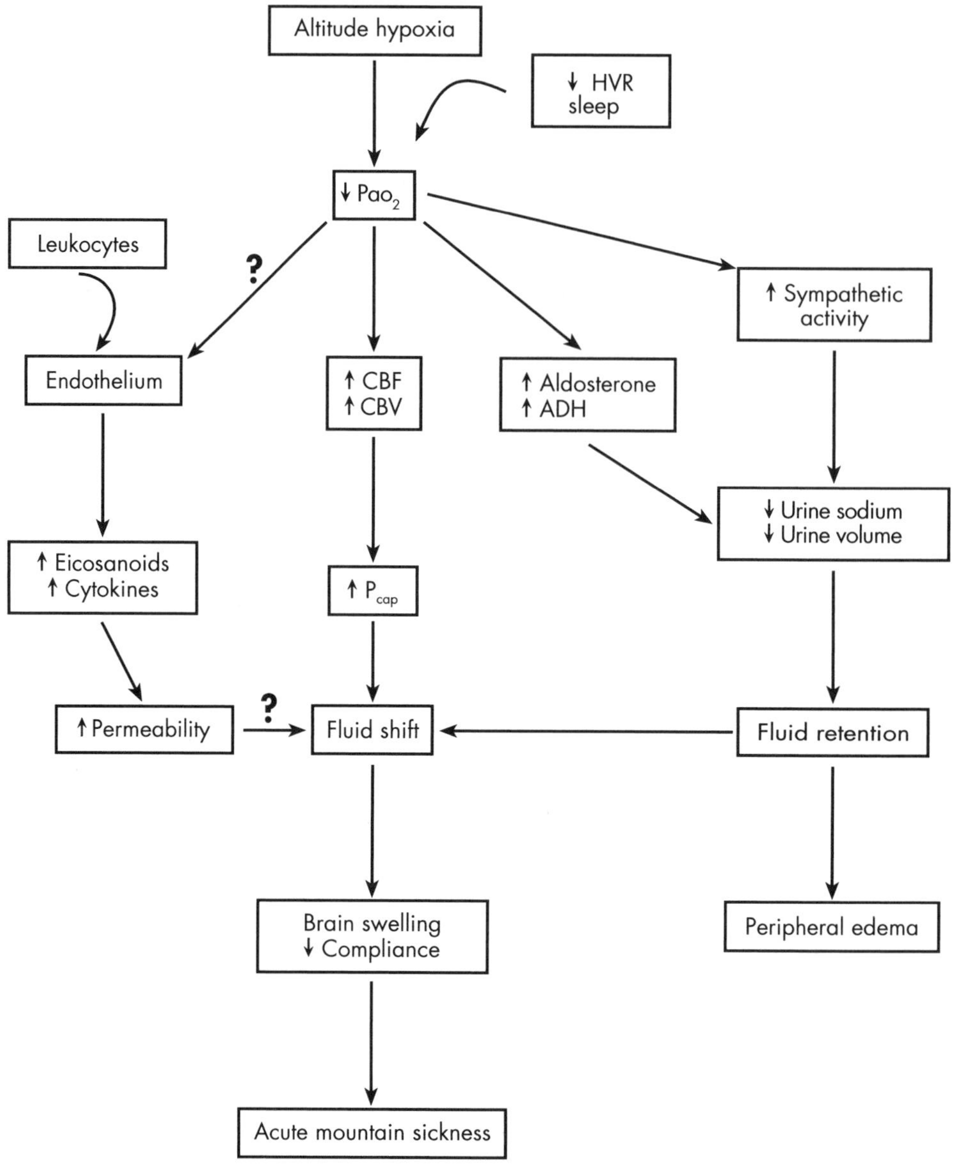

FIGURE 17C-1

Proposed pathophysiology of acute mountain sickness. *HVR*, Hypoxic ventilatory response; *CBF*, cerebral blood flow; *CBV*, cerebral bood volume; P_{cap}, capillary pressure; *ADH*, antidiuretic hormone. Reproduced from Hackett PH, Roach RC: High-altitude medicine. In Auerbach PS, editor: Wilderness Medicine, ed. 3, St. Louis, Mosby–Year Book.

    b. Two to three nights at 2800 or 3000 m.
    c. Extra night for every 600-900 m (1000 feet).
    d. Above 2800 m, limit nightly altitude gain to 800 m (3000 ft).
13. Other aids to acclimation.
    a. Climb high, sleep slow.
    b. High-carbohydrate diet.
    c. Mild exercise; avoid overexertion.
    d. Avoid alcohol and sedative/hypnotic medications.
14. Acetazolamide speeds natural acclimation.
    a. Inhibits carbonic anhydrase, which catalyzes both steps in the bicarbonate equation.
    b. CO_2 accumulates in tissues, including respiratory centers.

15. Physiological effects of acetazolamide.
    a. Diuresis with bicarbonate ion excretion causes decreased pH (metabolic acidosis).
    b. Increased ventilation.
    c. Improves arterial oxygen saturation.
16. Indications for acetazolamide.
    a. Rapid forced ascent to altitude over 3000 m (9800 feet).
    b. Past medical history (PMH) of recurrent AMS or HAPE.
    c. Treatment of AMS.
    d. Periodic breathing or fragmented, disturbed sleep.
17. Dosage of acetazolamide.
    a. 5 mg/kg/day in two or three divided doses.
    b. Prevention: 125-250 mg bid to begin 24 hr before ascent to altitude and continue to end of first day.
    c. Treatment: 250 mg bid until improved.
    d. Sleep: 250 mg at dinnertime.
18. Adverse effects of acetazolamide.
    a. Peripheral paresthesias, polyuria.
    b. Less commonly, nausea, drowsiness.
    c. Ruins taste of carbonated beverages; inhibits taste buds.
    d. Sulfa drug (hypersensitivity, marrow suppression, crystalluria).

C. HACE
1. May be conceptualized as a severe form of AMS.
2. Primarily global in nature, focal signs may be present.
3. Progression of cerebral signs and symptoms in the setting of AMS.
4. If untreated, HACE is fatal.
    a. Proposed pathophysiology-progression of same mechanism as AMS.
    b. Treatment should begin at first suspicion of HACE.
        (1) Descent is critical.
        (2) Temporizing measures include
            (a) Oxygen (2-4 L/min).
            (b) Dexamethasone 4-8 mg initially, then 4 mg q6h (IM, IV, or PO).
            (c) Hyperbaric chamber while arranging descent.

D. HAPE
    a. Most common cause of death from high-altitude illnesses.
    b. Most often occurs after second night at new altitude.
    c. Abrupt onset.
    d. Noncardiogenic type of pulmonary edema.
1. Signs/symptoms.
    a. Early symptoms may be indistinguishable from AMS.
    b. Progression to shortness of breath at rest and with exertion.
    c. Right middle lobe best heard in right axilla is affected first.
    d. Pink or blood-tinged productive sputum.
    e. Crackles in bases bilaterally on auscultation.
2. Radiographic findings.
    a. Patchy infiltrates.
    b. Normal heart size.
3. Proposed pathophysiology (see Fig. 17C-2).
4. Treatment.
    a. Descent, minimize exertion.
    b. Mild cases: bedrest, oxygen.
    c. Severe cases: high flow oxygen (4-6 L/min) and descent.
    d. Various maneuvers to improve gas exchange: positive end expiratory pressure (EPAP), pulmonary toilet, hyperbaric chamber.

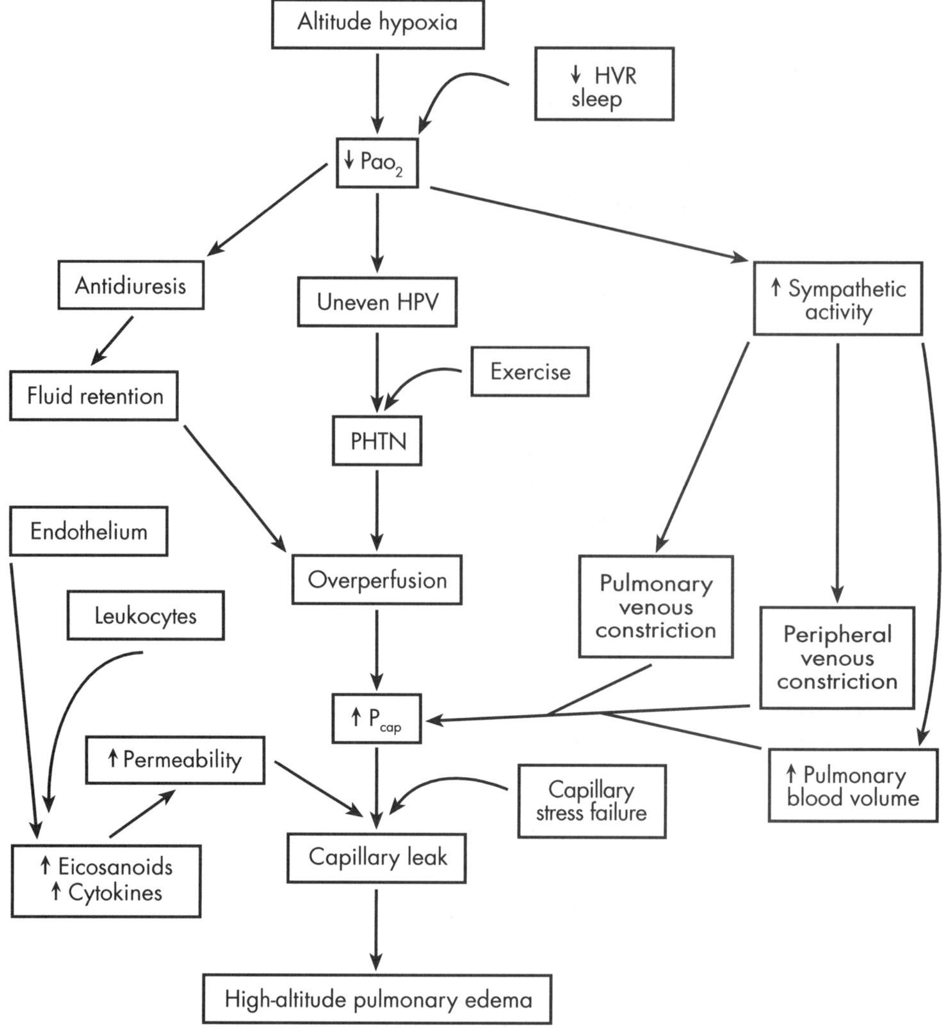

FIGURE 17C-2
Proposed pathophysiology of high-altitude pulmonary edema. *HVR*, Hypoxic ventilatory response; *HPV*, hypoxic pulmonary vasoconstriction; *PHTN*, pulmonary hypertension; P_{cap}, capillary pressure.

5. Pharmacological therapy.
   a. Drugs are not treatment of choice.
   b. Drugs that may be useful include:
      (1) Diuretics (furosemide 20-40 mg IV).
      (2) Vasodilators (nifedipine, morphine).
   c. Steroids not helpful.
6. Predisposing factors.
   a. Heavy exertion at altitude.
   b. Male, children (both sexes).
   c. Reentry of high-altitude residents.
   d. Pulmonary hypertension.
   e. Cold?

E. Thrombosis: coagulation and platelet disorders.
   1. Coagulation abnormalities at altitude may lead to platelet microemboli as well as a variety of thromboembolic phenomena (DVT, cerebral and pulmonary emboli, thrombosis).

2. More recent data show that these coagulation abnormalities appear after HAPE is established.
3. Dehydration plays an important role as do postulated abnormalities of clotting and fibrinolysis.

F. Peripheral edema.
1. Fascial edema, peripheral swelling common.
2. Not serious; resolves with descent, diuretic.
3. May be associated with AMS, HACE, HAPE.
4. Mandates a careful examination.

G. High-altitude retinopathy.
1. Tortuous and dilated retinal veins; disc hyperemia.
2. Retinal hemorrhages common above 5200 m (17,000 feet).
   a. Usually asymptomatic.
   b. Resolve spontaneously without descent.
3. Retinal hemorrhages are symptomatic only if over macula, which may cause blindness.
4. Cotton-wool exudates are rare.
5. Most physicians would view the appearance of this syndrome as a contraindication to further visits to high altitude due to the disturbing suggestion that a look at the fundi may be a mirror of similar vascular changes in the brain itself.

H. High-altitude flatus expulsion (HAFE).
1. Unwelcome spontaneous passage of colonic gas.
2. Potential mechanisms include
   a. Expansion of bowel gas with ascent.
   b. Intestinal hypermotility.
   c. High-fiber diet.
3. Palliative measures include:
   a. Digestive enzymes.
   b. Simethicone.
   c. High-complex carbohydrate diet.

I. High-altitude pharyngitis and bronchitis.
1. High-altitude sore throat and cough nearly universal after 2 weeks above 5500 m (18,000 feet).
2. Respond poorly to antibiotics.
3. Due to respiratory heat loss, membrane drying.
4. Treatment: hard candy, lozenges, steam, fluids, face mask.
5. Resolve amazingly after descent.

J. Immune suppression
1. Infections common; difficult to treat.
2. T lymphocyte function mildly impaired; therefore resistance to bacterial infections is impaired. Antibiotics may not be effective until descent.
3. B lymphocyte function not affected; therefore resistance to viral infection is not reduced.
4. Active immunization is maintained.

K. Preexisting medical conditions.
1. Contraindications to high altitude.

Contraindications	Cautions
Uncompensated congestive heart failure (CHF)	CHF
Pulmonary hypertension	Arrhythmias
Sickle cell anemia	Cerebrovascular disease
Moderate-severe chronic obstructive pulmonary disease (COPD)	Sleep apnea
	Seizure disorders

2. Medical conditions OK at high altitude.
   a. Young and old; fit and unfit.
   b. Obesity, diabetes.
   c. Following coronary artery bypass graft, stable angina, compensated CHF
   d. Asthma, mild COPD.
   e. Controlled hypertension.
   f. Pregnancy.
3. Chronic lung disease
   a. Hypoxemia and pulmonary hypertension worsen at altitude.
   b. Maximize pulmonary function prior to ascent.
   c. Individuals with mild to moderate COPD may do well.
   d. Arterial oxygen saturation at altitude can be predicted based on sea level values. Patients with a predicted saturation below 75% should receive supplemental oxygen.
4. Atherosclerotic heart disease.
   a. Little hard data.
   b. No data for increased coronary events.
   c. Increased catecholamines might increase arrhythmias.
   d. Angina threshold may be decreased.
5. Hypertension.
   a. Blood pressure increases mildly in healthy persons.
   b. Patients should continue usual medications.
   c. Hypertension in visitors to altitude is transient: not treated.
6. Sickle cell disease.
   a. Altitude can cause sickle cell crisis, even in aircraft.
   b. Consider supplemental oxygen for hemoglobin SC.
   c. Usual treatment plus descent.
7. Pregnancy: recommendations.
   a. Commercial air travel is safe.
   b. Complicated pregnancy: avoid altitude exposure.
   c. Pregnant lowland women should avoid:
      (1) Staying above 4000 m (13,000 feet).
      (2) Going above 6,000 m (19,000 feet).

Bibliography

Auerbach PS, Goehr EC: *Management of wilderness and environmental emergencies,* ed 2, St Louis, 1989, CV Mosby.

Hackett PH: *Mountain sickness: prevention, recognition and treatment,* New York, 1980, American Alpine Club.

Hackett PH, Rennie D: Acute mountain sickness, *Semin Resp Med* 5(2):132-140, 1983.

Hackett PH, Roach RC: Medical therapy of high altitude illness, *Ann Emerg Med* 16(9):980-986, 1987.

Houston CS: *Going higher,* Houston, 1983, Burlington.

Hultgren HN: High altitude medical problems, *West J Med* 131:8-23, 1979.

Rennie D: See Nuptse and die, *Lancet* 2:1177-1179, 1976.

Singh I et al: Acute mountain sickness, *N Engl J Med* 280:175-184, 1969.

Sutton JR, editor: *Man at altitude, Semin Resp Med* 5(2), 1983 (whole issue devoted to altitude pathophysiology).

Sutton JR, Jones NC, Houston CS, editors: *Hypoxia: man at altitude,* New York, 1982, Thieme-Stratton (Proceedings of the Banff Symposium).

CHAPTER 18

The Preparticipation Examination

Robert E. Sallis, MD

I. Overview
   A. Estimates are that >1 million physician hours are consumed annually in examining >6 million young athletes.
   B. Cost effectiveness questioned: Risser et al. looked at 763 adolescent athletes screened. They found only 16 athletes with clinically significant problems. Two were disqualified, and one was treated before participation. Cost of identifying these three problems was $4537 per problem.
   C. Studies show preparticipation evaluation disqualified only 0.3% to 1.3% of athletes, and only 3.2% to 13.5% required consultation.

II. Goals
   A. Detect any condition that may limit participation.
   B. Detect any condition that may predispose an athlete to injury during competition.
   C. Meet legal or insurance requirements. (At least 35 states require yearly examination.)
   D. Determine general health of athlete.
      1. Answer health-related questions.
      2. Counsel on life-style issues and high-risk behavior.
      3. Assess physical maturity (Tanner stage, Table 18-1).

III. Format
   A. Private office with primary care physician.
      1. Advantages: better continuity of care, easier to do counseling there.
      2. Disadvantages: higher cost, less communication with school or athletic staff.
   B. Group examination (usually done as a station-by-station examination).
      1. Advantages: more cost effective, usually done at school with athletic staff present.
      2. Disadvantages: lack of privacy, poor followup.

TABLE 18-1. Maturity Staging Guidelines

Boys

Stage	Pubic Hair	Penis	Testis
1	None	Preadolescent	Preadolescent
2	Slight, long, slight pigmentation	Slight enlargement	Enlarged scrotum, pink, slight ruga
3	Darker, starts to curl, small amount	Longer	Larger
4	Coarse, curly, adult type, but less quantity	Increase in glans size and breadth of penis	Larger, scrotum darker
5	Adult, spreads to inner thighs	Adult	Adult

Girls

Stage	Pubic Hair	Breasts
1	Preadolescent (none)	Preadolescent (no germinal button)
2	Sparse, lightly pigmented, straight, spread to medial border of labia	Breast and papilla elevated as small mound: areola diameter increased
3	Darker, beginning to curl, increased	Breast and areola enlarged; no contour separation
4	Coarse, curly, abundant, but less than adult	Areola and papilla form secondary mound
5	Adult female triangle, spreads to medial surface	Mature, nipple projects, areola part of general breast contour

Adapted and reproduced by permission of the author and publisher from Tanner JM: *Growth at adolescence; with a general consideration of the effects of hereditary and environmental factors upon growth and maturation from birth to maturity,* ed 2, Oxford, 1962, Blackwell Scientific Publications, pp 28-39.

IV. Frequency and Timing
   A. Most states require yearly examination. However, every 3-4 years with yearly update as needed is probably adequate.
   B. Best time is 4-6 weeks before season starts to allow sufficient time for further evaluation and treatment of any problems found.

V. Content
   A. Many schools provide a specific form. If not, the American Academy of Family Physicians Athletic Competition Health Screening Form is recommended (Fig. 18-1).
   B. Medical history.
      1. Has been shown to identify 63% to 74% of problems affecting athletes.
      2. Is best completed by parents of adolescent athletes.
   C. Cardiovascular assessment.
      1. Critical history question: "Have you ever felt dizzy, fainted, or actually passed out while exercising?" May be a sign of outflow tract obstruction.
      2. Benign systolic murmurs are common in athletes. If a murmur is grade III or higher and/or diastolic, further evaluation is recom-

Preparticipation Sports Evaluation

School ______________________
Age______ Grade______ Sex ______
Sports ______________________

Health History

Athlete/Parent or Guardian

Provide the following Information

	YES	NO
Chronic/recent illness? Hospitalization?		
Surgery?		
Injury		
Bone/joint injuries?		
Missing organs		
Dizziness, fainting convultions?		
Frequent headaches?		
Knocked out/concussion?		
Wear glasses/contacts?		
Hearing problems?		
Asthma/chronic cough?		
Hernia?		
Recurrent skin disease?		
Current medications List		
Family history of heart disease or unexpected death at young age?		
Other family history of disease?		
Allergy to medication? List		
Immunizations current?		
Date of last tetnus		
Date of last measles		
Other		
For women only Has menses started?		
Age at first menses		
Are periods regular?		

The above is correct and current to the best of my knowledge

______________________ __________
Athlete/parent or guardian* Date

*Parent or guardian if less than 18 years old

Family Physician ______________ Phone ________
Address ______________________

	Satisfactory			Comments
	Yes	No	NE	
Ht				
Wt				
BP				
General				
Head				
Eyes				
ENT				
Dental				
Chest				
Heart				
Abdomen				
Genitalia				
Skin				
Ortho				
Flex/ Strength				

Follow-up recommendations:

Sports participation approved: Yes_____ No_____ Restricted _____
Limitations:

____
Physician Date

WHITE COPY—CHART YELLOW COPY—PATIENT COPY

FIGURE 18-1

Preparticipation Sports Evaluation Health History form. (By permission of the author and publisher: Southern California Permanente Medical Group, Inc., Los Angeles, Calif: 1991; Adapted from American Academy of Family Physicians, Commission on Public Health and Scientific Affairs: Athletic Competition Health form, Kansas City, MO; 1984, American Academy of Family Physicians.

mended. Accentuation with Valsalva maneuver should alert the physician to possible outflow tract obstruction such as in hypertrophic cardiomyopathy or aortic stenosis.

3. Ventricular ectopy may suggest cocaine abuse.
4. Upper limits of blood pressure *not* requiring evaluation.
   a. 130/75 mmHg for children <10 years of age.
   b. 140/85 mmHg for children age >10 years of age.
   c. Systolic hypertension in young athletes is frequently related to anxiety or inappropriate cuff size in husky adolescents (ages 13 through 17).
5. Simultaneous palpation of radial and femoral pulses for asymmetry is a good screening test for coarctation of the aorta.

D. Musculoskeletal assessment.
   1. Look for preexisting injury because it is likely to recur. The knees, shoulders, and ankles are at greatest risk.
   2. Two-minute orthopedic examination is a useful screening tool (Table 18-2).

E. Other organ systems (see box on p. 155).
   1. Lungs (asthma).
   2. Abdomen (hepatosplenomegaly, masses).
   3. Genitourinary tract (single testicle, hernia, Tanner stage).
   4. Skin (infectious disease, acne).

TABLE 18-2. The Two-Minute Orthopedic Examination

Instructions	Observation
Stand facing examiner	Acromioclavicular joints, general habitus
Look at ceiling, floor, over both shoulders; touch ears to shoulders	Cervical spine motion
Shrug shoulders (examiner resists)	Trapezius strength
Abduct shoulders 90 degrees (examiner resists at 90 degrees)	Deltoid strength
Fully rotate arms externally	Shoulder motion
Flex and extend elbows	Elbow motion
Arms at sides, flex elbows 90 degrees; pronate and supinate wrists	Elbow and wrist motion
Spread fingers; make fist	Hand or finger motion and deformity
Tighten (contract) quadriceps; relax quadriceps	Symmetry and knee effusion; ankle effusion
"Duck walk" 4 steps (away from examiner with buttocks on heels)	Hip, knee, and ankle motion
Walk back to examiner	Shoulder symmetry, scoliosis
Knees straight, touch toes	Scoliosis, hip motion, hamstring tightness
Raise up on toes, raise heels	Calf symmetry, leg strength

Reproduced by permission of the author and publisher from American Academy of Pediatrics, Committee on Sports Medicine: *Sports medicine: health care for young athletes,* Elk Grove Village, IL, 1991:54, American Academy of Pediatrics.

AREAS TO EMPHASIZE IN THE PREPARTICIPATION PHYSICAL EXAMINATION

GENERAL
- Height
- Weight
- Body habitus (especially for weight-determined sports)

SKIN
- Jaundice
- Herpetic lesions
- Impetigo
- Severe acne

VISUAL ACUITY
- Severe myopia
- Amblyopia
- Single eye

FUNDUSCOPIC SIGNS
- Detached retina
- Early atherosclerotic change
- Diabetic retinopathy

LUNGS
- Asthma
- Bronchitis

CARDIOVASCULAR SYSTEM
- Murmurs
- Uncontrolled hypertension
- Cyanosis

ABDOMEN
- Hepatosplenomegaly
- Masses

BACK
- Scoliosis
- Kyphosis
- Lordosis

GENITOURINARY SYSTEM
- Single testicle
- Hernia
- Sexual maturity by Tanner staging

MUSCULOSKELETAL SYSTEM
- Unstable knee and ankle ligaments
- Recurrent shoulder dislocation
- Assessment of elbow stability
- Painful Osgood-Schlatter disease
- Assessment of muscular development
- Marfan syndrome

NEUROLOGIC SYSTEM
- Gross coordination
- Gait abnormality

Reproduced by permission of the author and publisher from Tanji JL: The preparticipation physical examination for sports, *Am Fam Physician* 42(2):399, 1990.

VI. Diagnostic Tests
- A. The most commonly recommended laboratory tests are complete blood count and urinalysis. Consensus is that they should *not* be done routinely.
  1. Consider obtaining routine hematocrit in women athletes.
  2. Do cholesterol testing as indicated.
- B. Routine electrocardiogram and/or echocardiogram are not cost effective when used as screening tests.
- C. Exercise stress testing may be indicated in an adult athlete before starting an exercise program.

VII. Clearance
- A. After a problem is found, consider the following in deciding whether to clear an athlete to participate.
  1. Does problem place the athlete at increased risk of injury?
  2. Is any other participant at risk of injury because of the problem?
  3. Can the athlete safely participate with treatment (medication, rehabilitation, bracing, or padding)?
  4. Can limited participation be allowed while treatment is initiated?
  5. If clearance is denied only for certain activities, in what activities can the athlete safely participate?
- B. The American Academy of Pediatrics recommendation for participation in competitive sports is a useful guide in deciding about clearance (Tables 18-3 and 18-4).

TABLE 18-3. Recommendations for Participation in Competitive Sports: Classification of Sport*

		Noncontact		
Contact/ Collision	**Limited Contact/ Impact**	**Strenuous**	**Moderately Strenuous**	**Nonstrenuous**
Boxing	Baseball	Aerobic dancing	Badminton	Archery
Field hockey	Basketball	Crew	Curling	Golf
Football	Bicycling	Fencing	Table tennis	Riflery
Ice hockey	Diving	Field		
Lacrosse	Field	Discus		
Martial arts	High jump	Javelin		
Rodeo	Pole vault	Shotput		
Soccer	Gymnastics	Running		
Wrestling	Horseback riding	Swimming		
	Skating	Tennis		
	Ice	Track		
	Roller	Weight lifting		
	Skiing			
	Cross-country			
	Downhill			
	Water			
	Softball			
	Squash, handball			
	Volleyball			

Adapted and reproduced by permission of the author and publisher from American Academy of Pediatrics, Committee on Sports Medicine: Recommendations for participation in competitive sports, *Pediatrics* 81:737, 1988.

*First, sports events may be divided into groups depending on degree of strenuousness and probability of collision. Each medical condition for which classification of sports may be allowed can then be assessed.

C. The "26th Bethesda Conference: Recommendations for Determining Eligibility for Competition in Athletes with Cardiovascular Abnormalities" covers guidelines for clearance in athletes who have congenital heart disease and other cardiovascular abnormalities.

VIII. Exercise-Related Sudden Death

A. Preparticipation screening is the primary preventive tool. However, the incidence of exercise-related sudden death is rare: 0.2-0.5 deaths per 100,000 adolescents per year.

B. Cause is usually cardiac: if athlete is <30 years of age, a structural heart problem is usually implicated; if >30 years of age, usually coronary artery disease.

C. Cause.

1. Hypertrophic cardiomyopathy.

a. Symptoms: palpitations, syncope, chest pain, dyspnea on exertion.

TABLE 18-4. Recommendations for Participation in Competitive Sports by Medical Condition

	Contact/ Collision	Limited Contact/Impact	Noncontact		
			Strenuous	Moderately Strenuous	Nonstrenuous
Atlantoaxial instability	No	No	Yes[a]	Yes	Yes
Acute illness	[b]	[b]	[b]	[b]	[b]
Cardiovascular					
Carditis	No	No	No	No	No
Congenital heart disease	[d]	[d]	[d]	[d]	[d]
Eyes					
Absence or loss of function of one eye	[e]	[e]	[e]	[e]	[e]
Detached retina	[f]	[f]	[f]	[f]	[f]
Hypertension					
Mild	Yes	Yes	Yes	Yes	Yes
Moderate	[c]	[c]	[c]	[c]	[c]
Severe	[c]	[c]	[c]	[c]	[c]
Inguinal hernia	Yes	Yes	Yes	Yes	Yes
Kidney: Absence of one	No	Yes	Yes	Yes	Yes
Liver: Enlarged	No	No	Yes	Yes	Yes
Musculoskeletal disorders	[c]	[c]	[c]	[c]	[c]
Neurological disorders					
History of serious head or spine trauma, repeated concussions, or craniotomy	[c]	[c]	Yes	Yes	Yes
Convulsive disorder					
Well controlled	Yes	Yes	Yes	Yes	Yes
Poorly controlled	No	No	Yes[g]	Yes	Yes[h]

(Table continued on following page.)

TABLE 18-4. Recommendations for Participation in Competitive Sports by Medical Condition (cont'd)

	Contact/ Collision	Limited Contact/Impact	Noncontact		
			Strenuous	Moderately Strenuous	Nonstrenuous
Ovary: Absence of one	Yes	Yes	Yes	Yes	Yes
Respiratory					
Pulmonary insufficiency	[i]	[i]	[i]	[i]	Yes
Asthma	Yes	Yes	Yes	Yes	Yes
Sickle cell trait	Yes	Yes	Yes	Yes	Yes
Skin: boils, herpes, impetigo, scabies	[j]	[j]	Yes	Yes	Yes
Spleen: Enlarged	No	No	No	Yes	Yes
Testicle: Absent or undescended	Yes[k]	Yes[k]	Yes	Yes	Yes

[a]Swimming: no butterfly, breast stroke, or diving starts.
[b]Needs individual assessment (e.g., contagiousness to others, risk of worsening illness).
[c]Needs individual assessment.
[d]Patients with mild forms can be allowed a full range of physical activities: patients with moderate or severe forms or who have undergone surgery should be evaluated by a cardiologist before athletic participation.
[e]Availability of American Society for Testing and Materials (ASTM)-approved eye guards may allow competitor to participate in most sports, but this must be decided for each athlete.
[f]Consult ophthalmologist.
[g]No swimming or weight lifting.
[h]No archery or riflery.
[i]May be allowed to compete if oxygenation remains satisfactory during a graded stress test.
[j]No gymnastics with mats, martial arts, wrestling, or contact sports until not contagious.
[k]Certain sports may require protective cup.
Reproduced by permission of the author and publisher from: American Academy of Pediatrics. Committee on Sports Medicine. Recommendations for Participation in Competitive Sports. *Pediatrics* 1988; 81:738.

b. Examination: high-frequency systolic ejection murmur at left lower sternal border; increases with Valsalva maneuver, decreases with squatting.
c. Diagnosis: do echocardiogram.

2. Congenital coronary artery anomalies.
   a. Types.
      (1) Origin of left coronary artery from right sinus of Valsalva.
      (2) Single coronary artery.
      (3) Origin of coronary artery from pulmonary artery.
      (4) Coronary artery hypoplasia.
   b. Symptoms: exertional chest pain or syncope.
   c. Diagnosis: do angiogram.
3. Marfan syndrome.
   a. Diagnosis: need two of four major features.
      (1) Family history.
      (2) Cardiovascular abnormality (aortic aneurysm, mitral valve prolapse, congestive heart failure symptoms).
      (3) Musculoskeletal abnormality (arm span greater than height, kyphoscoliosis, anterior thoracic deformity).
      (4) Ocular abnormality (ectopic lens, myopia).
   b. If syndrome is suspected, obtain genetic and cardiology consultation (including echocardiogram). (See suggested screening format for Marfan syndrome in the box below)
4. Coronary artery disease.
   a. Consider exercise stress testing for:
      (1) Men >45 years of age, women >55 years of age.
      (2) Those with risk factors: diabetes, smoking, family history of heart disease, total cholesterol level >250 mg/dl, high-density lipoprotein cholesterol <30 mg/dl.
      (3) Anyone with exertional chest pain, syncope, or palpitations.
5. Valvular disorders.
   a. Mitral valve prolapse: relation to sudden death is questionable.

SUGGESTED SCREENING FORMAT FOR MARFAN SYNDROME

Screen all men >6 feet and all women >5 feet, 10 inches in height with echocardiogram and slit-lamp examination when any two of the following are found:

- Family history of Marfan syndrome*
- Cardiac murmur or midsystolic click
- Kyphoscoliosis
- Anterior thoracic deformity
- Arm span greater than height
- Upper to lower body ratio >1 standard deviation below the mean
- Myopia
- Ectopic lens

Reproduced by permission of the author, editor, and publisher from Hara JH, Puffer JC: The preparticipation physical examination. In Mellion MB, editor: *Office management of sports injuries & athletic problems*, Philadelphia, 1988, Hanley & Belfus, p 8.

*This finding *alone* should prompt further investigation.

b. Aortic stenosis: often results in sudden death with or without exercise.
6. Cardiac conduction system abnormalities.
   a. Idiopathic long QT syndrome.
      (1) QT interval >440 ms.
      (2) Frequently suspected in cases of sudden death in athletes without structural heart problems.
      (3) May produce syncope or near syncope.

D. Screening.
1. History: family history; syncope, exertional chest pain, or dyspnea on exertion.
2. Examination: Marfan habitus; murmur.
3. Electrocardiogram/chest x-ray film: reassuring if both are normal.
4. Exercise stress test, Holter monitoring, and angiogram should be done as indicated by history and examination findings.

Acknowledgment

The Medical Editing Department, Kaiser Foundation Research Institute, provided editorial assistance.

Bibliography

American Academy of Family Physicians, American Academy of Pediatrics, American Medical Society for Sports Medicine, American Orthopaedic Society for Sports Medicine, and American Osteopathic Academy of Sports Medicine: Pre-participation physical evaluation (PPE), 1992. Joint Publication. (8800 Ward Parkway, Kansas City, MO 64114).

American Academy of Pediatrics, Committee on Sports Medicine: Recommendations for participation in competitive sports, *Pediatrics* 81:737-739, 1988.

American Academy of Pediatrics, Committee on Sports Medicine: *Sports medicine: health care for young athletes,* Elk Grove Village, IL, 1991:54, American Academy of Pediatrics.

Feinstein RA, Soileu EJ, Daniel WA: National survey of preparticipation physical examination requirements, *Physician Sports Med* 16(5):51-59, 1988.

Fields FB, Delaney M: Focusing the preparticipation sports examination, *J Fam Pract* 30:304-312, 1990.

Hara JH, Puffer JC: The preparticipation physical examination. In Mellion MB, editor: *Office management of sports injuries & athletic problems,* Philadelphia, 1988, Hanley & Belfus, pp 1-10.

Risser WL et al: A cost-benefit analysis of preparticipation examinations of adolescent athletes, *J Sch Health* 55:270-273, 1985.

Preparticipation Sports Evaluation Health History form. Southern California Permanente Medical Group, Inc., Los Angeles, CA: 1991.

Tanji JL: The preparticipation physical examination for sports, *Am Fam Physician* 42(2):397-402, 1990. [published erratum appears in *Am Fam Physician* 42(4):930, 1990.]

Tanner JM: *Growth at adolescence; with a general consideration of the effects of hereditary and environmental factors upon growth and maturation from birth to maturity,* ed 2. Oxford, 1962, Blackwell Scientific Publications.

26th Bethesda Conference: recommendations for determining eligibility for competition in athletes with cardiovascular abnormalities, January 6-7, 1994, *Med Sci Sports Exerc* 26(10 Suppl):5223-83, 1994. [published erratum appears in *Med Sci Sports Exerc* 26(12), 1994.]

Van Camp SP: Exercise-related sudden death: risks and causes, *Physician Sports Med* 16(5):97-112, 1988.

CHAPTER 19

Exercise Physiology

Peter B. Raven, PhD, FACSM

I. Definition: exercise physiology is a branch of the discipline of physiology that focuses on the integration of all the physiological functions that enable the human to exercise (i.e., perform work).

II. Muscle Action
   A. To do work, muscles:
      1. Contract or shorten (concentric).
      2. Lengthen or extend (eccentric).
      3. Remain the same length (isometric—static).
   B. All of these actions require the integration of neural signals from the motor cortex to the muscle(s) that produce a chain of biochemical reactions, resulting in the transformation of the potential chemical energy to the mechanical energy of muscle action.

III. Energy Metabolism: there are three main energy sources for the muscles to draw on.
   A. Creatine phosphate (CP) and adenosine triphosphate (ATP).

$$\left.\begin{array}{r} ATP \rightarrow P_1 + ADP \\ + \\ ATP + C \leftarrow CP \end{array}\right\}$$ These reactions occur rapidly and the amount of CP available to regenerate energy stores as ATP is very small.

   B. Nonoxidative metabolism (sometimes known as anaerobic metabolism) has two forms.
      1. Glycogenolysis: the degradation of glycogen (the body's store of carbohydrate)
      2. Glycolysis: the dissolution of sugars (i.e., glucose).
         a. These processes convert glycogen or glucose to lactic acid and regenerate energy stores of ATP. However, if lactic acid is allowed to build up, muscle contraction is compromised.
         b. This buildup of lactic acid is thought to be a component of muscle fatigue.

c. For continuous recovery of the immediate energy stores, CP and the nonoxidative metabolism require oxygen. These reactions are the main factor in the continuous reestablishment of the energy stored in ATP and are known as the *oxidative energy system.*

C. Oxidative energy system (or aerobic) metabolism can be maintained at a submaximal level as long as substrates are available to provide fuel to the oxidative process. Oxidation of fuels occurs in the tricarboxylic acid (Krebs) cycle. These chemical reactions occur in the mitochondria of the muscle and are linked to oxygen use via the respiratory chain. As the intensity of exercise increases, the speed at which the reactions occur in the respiratory chain and the Krebs cycle increases.

1. The fuels or substrates used during exercise are primarily carbohydrates and fats.
2. Oxygen consumption (Vo_2) is tightly coupled with the intensity of the exercise performed. Because carbohydrates are the main energy substrate and their supply is limited, the body uses alternative fuels, such as lipids, to retard the use of the carbohydrate. This transfer from carbohydrate to fat utilization is known as carbohydrate sparing. In long-endurance events the main part of the performance occurs with the intensity of exercise below the lactate threshold (i.e., when lactate begins to appear within the bloodstream) and is primarily fueled by lipids.

IV. Cardiovascular and Ventilatory Responses to Exercise

A. A measure of the circulatory capacity to delivery oxygen is obtained by performing a maximal oxygen uptake test ($Vo_{2\,max}$). $Vo_{2\,max}$ is defined as the greatest rate of oxygen utilization during exercise. It is determined by measuring oxygen uptake (Vo_2) at rest and at increasing workloads until a plateau of oxygen uptake is achieved ($Vo_{2\,max}$) with an increase in workload. Exercise can be performed above the plateau but requires a greater contribution of energy from the nonoxidative metabolism, with a consequent marked increase in lactic acid production. The measurement of maximal aerobic power is an assessment of the organism's cardiorespiratory reserves. A review of some basic expressions of cardiopulmonary physiology identifies the interrelationships among some key parameters and variables.

B. Like height and weight, $Vo_{2\,max}$ is a reproducible characteristic of the individual showing insignificant day-to-day variation. $Vo_{2\,max}$ is used as a means of scaling cardiovascular responses in % $Vo_{2\,max}$ in different individuals.

Maximal Aerobic Power ($VO_{2\,max}$) = Cardiac Output$_{max}$(Q_{max}) × Arteriovenous Oxygen Difference$_{max}$ ($A\text{-}Vo_2DIFF_{max}$)

Cardiac Output$_{max}$ (Q_{max}) = Heart Rate$_{max}$ (HR_{max}) × Stroke Volume$_{max}$ (SV_{max})

V. Cardiovascular Responses to Exercise

A. At the onset of exercise responses to the command signals include:

1. A reduction in the vascular resistance of the working muscle.
2. An increased pumping action by the heart with an increased cardiac contractility and an increase in heart rate.
3. An increase in pulmonary ventilation.

B. The remarkable aspect of this regulation is the strong relationship between exercise-induced demand for oxygen and the cardiovascular and ventilatory responses required to deliver the oxygen to the working tissues.

C. Cardiac output (Q).
   1. Cardiac output increases linearly with oxygen uptake (Vo_2), with a slope of 5 L/min of Vo_2.
   2. Maximal recorded and believable cardiac output = 42 L/min.

D. Stroke volume (SV).
   1. This parameter decreases approximately 40% when an individual stands upright from supine rest.
   2. The heart (stimulated at the onset of exercise) in conjunction with the muscle pump returns the upright exercising stroke volume to a level equivalent to supine rest values rapidly.
   3. SV remains constant up to the level of $Vo_{2\ max}$ in moderately active individuals.
   4. Endurance-trained athletes, however, seem to increase stroke volume throughout the progressive increase in workload. Athletes have very high resting and exercise stroke volumes.
   5. In general, cardiac disease reduces pump function and therefore stroke volume.
   6. Stroke Volume. Changes in stroke volume are regulated by factors that are both extrinsic and intrinsic to the heart.
      a. Changes related to venous return or preload, which elicit the classic Frank-Starling mechanism (i.e., for an increase in end diastolic volume there is an increase in stroke volume).
      b. Changes in afterload (i.e., systolic blood pressure). The intrinsic factors that affect stroke volume are those that alter contractility or inotropy.
         (1) Increases in heart rate increase calcium ion release, which increases contractility (treppe effect).
         (2) Increases in sympathetic drive via central command or feedback from the muscle or peripheral baroreceptors, thereby increasing contractility.
         (3) General sympathetic activation resulting in release of epinephrine from the adrenal gland, which also increases contractility via β_1-receptor stimulation.

E. Heart rate (HR).
   1. The heart rate rises linearly with increasing rate of oxygen uptake.
   2. The slope of the rise in HR is inversely related to the individual's $Vo_{2\ max}$.
   3. Maximal heart rates range from 190-196 bpm and depend on age ($220 - Age = HR_{max}$).
   4. The range of HR change during exercise is related to the resting heart rate.
   5. Some athletes have resting heart rates lower than 40 bpm and therefore have a greater range than the unfit sedentary individual, who has a HR at rest of 70-80 bpm.

F. Arteriovenous oxygen difference ($A\text{-}Vo_2DIFF_{max}$).
   1. This measures maximal oxygen extraction of the working tissues; it widens with increasing overall rate of oxygen uptake.
   2. At rest $A\text{-}Vo_2DIFF$ = 4-5 ml O_2/100 ml or 25% extraction; at $Vo_{2\ max}$ it increases to 15-17 ml/100 ml or 80% to 85% extraction.

G. Regulation of the cardiovascular response to exercise
   1. The initial increase in heart rate with exercise from rest to 100-110 bpm is primarily a result of vagal withdrawal.

2. Cardiac acceleration above 100-110 bpm is predominantly due to increases in sympathetic activity with a continuation of vagal withdrawal.

H. Arterial blood pressure (BP) and total vascular conductance. Arterial pulse pressure (systolic BP–diastolic BP) increases with maximal exercise, primarily due to increasing systolic pressure.
   1. Mean BP rises only moderately (approximately 25 mmHg).
   2. Conductance or blood flow through the working muscles rises directly with cardiac output.
   3. The increase in blood flow is brought about by increased cardiac output and preferential redistribution of blood flow to the working muscles and away from nonexercising areas (e.g., the splanchnic bed).
   4. This increase in blood flow is pulsated in phase with the muscle contraction through a dilated working muscle vascular bed.
   5. Locally released metabolites, particularly adenosine, result in vasodilatation of the vessels of the muscle.

I. Systemic arteriovenous oxygen difference. Arterial O_2 depends on hemoglobin concentration, O_2 binding capacity, alveolar Po_2, pulmonary diffusion capacity, and alveolar ventilation.
   1. Arterial O_2 content is well maintained during exercise, although saturation may drop from 96% to 93% because of the Bohr effect (rightward shift of O_2/desaturation curve) due to a decrease in pH and an increased temperature.
   2. Hemoglobin concentration (and hence its effective O_2 carrying capacity) rises 10% because of fluid shifts out of the vascular compartment.
   3. Venous O_2 content decreases to approximately 2 ml/100 ml in venous blood draining from the active musculature, whereas mixed venous blood may decrease to 3-4 ml/100 ml. This is due to increased O_2 extraction by the working muscle and regional vasoconstriction of resting organs.

J. Ventilatory responses to exercise.
   1. Ventilation volume (V) is the amount of air passing in and out of the lungs in 1 minute. Physiologically, the inspired minute volumes (V_I) equal expired minute volume (V_E). Because of gas exchange at the alveolar surfaces, measured V_I does not equal V_E, yet corrections can be made to account for these differences. V_E is expressed in liters of air (L/min). Ventilation volume per minute (V_E) increases linearly with increasing rate of oxygen uptake (1 L O_2/min uptake = 25 L/min V_E) until approximately 50% to 70% $Vo_{2\ max}$. At this point, the ventilation threshold, the ventilation increases exponentially and 1 L O_2/min uptake = 35 L/min V_E.
   2. Tidal volume (V_T) increases linearly with increasing workload up to two thirds of the vital capacity and then levels off as the workload increases to maximum.
   3. Respiratory rate (RR) increases linearly with increasing workload up to a maximum rate of 35-50 breaths/min at maximal work at sea level.
   4. The ventilatory response is the primary determinant of arterial blood gas and acid base status during exercise.
   5. Maximal ventilatory capacity is measured as the maximal voluntary ventilation (MVV) in 15 seconds ($MVV_{.25}$) expressed as L/min.
   6. Individual $MVV_{.25}$ ranges from 160-260 L/min depending on the size of the individual and respiratory muscle fitness.

7. Maximal exercise expired ventilation volumes ($V_{E\ max}$) range from 100-170 L/min standardized at body temperature and pressure saturated with water at body temperature (BTPS). In normal, healthy individuals exercise exhaustion usually occurs at a V_E of approximately 70% of $MVV_{.25}$ (or $V_{E\ max}/MVV_{.25}$ = 70%). In some highly fit individuals, however, exhaustion may occur at $V_{E\ max}$ of approximately 90%.

K. Ventilatory threshold. As noted previously, ventilation at higher intensities of exercise increases exponentially with increasing power output. The workload (or rate of oxygen consumption) at which the ventilatory response to graded exercise first departs from linear is the ventilatory threshold (VT), sometimes referred to as the anaerobic threshold. Although the physiological mechanism that underlies VT remains a matter of debate, VT occurs at a work rate that corresponds closely to the intensity at which lactic acid begins to accumulate in the blood.
  1. The rapid increase in ventilation that occurs at exercise intensities at VT may be a result of the bicarbonate buffer system, which helps to maintain blood pH by buffering metabolically produced acid to carbon dioxide and then transporting excess carbon dioxide to the lung for excretion.
  2. Most individuals who exercise regularly are able to perceive VT as the exercise intensity at which breathing becomes somewhat labored and talking becomes difficult.
  3. Because VT and blood lactic acid accumulation occur at similar exercise intensities in most persons, VT provides a convenient marker for the upper end of the exercise intensity range usually applied in "aerobic" training programs.
  4. At exercise intensities above VT, rapid accumulation of lactic acid in the muscle and blood results in cessation of exercise.
  5. Thus prescribed aerobic exercise programs often employ an exercise intensity below VT.

VI. Adaptations to Exercise Training
  A. Aerobic training significantly improves the oxygen transport system and increases $Vo_{2\ max}$ by increasing both the maximal cardiac output and the maximal arteriovenous oxygen difference.
  B. This change occurs primarily by improvements in central circulation and cardiac function, peripheral circulation, and skeletal muscle metabolism.

VII. Skeletal Muscle
  A. The specific adaptations that occur within the skeletal muscle depend on the frequency, duration, and intensity of the contractions or on the amount of overload imparted for the specific actions. Skeletal muscle adaptations to endurance, sprint, and weight training represent adaptive responses to the specific training mode involved.
  B. Endurance training. The general effects of endurance training are enhanced skeletal muscle oxidative capacity (resulting in improvement in endurance performance), increased fatty acid utilization, and decreased glycogen utilization during prolonged exercise. Presumably, with an increased oxidative potential, less of a disturbance in homeostasis occurs for a given level of work, minimizing the accumulation of adenosine diphosphate (ADP) and activation of glycolysis, thereby sparing glycogen and enhancing fat utilization. Furthermore, the enhanced oxidative capacity of type I and type IIa fibers allows more work to be done before nonoxidative glycolysis or glycogenolysis and

type IIb fiber recruitment are required, minimizing or delaying the onset of lactic acid accumulation.

C. Sprint training. Spring training induces changes in enzymatic activities in skeletal muscle similar to those observed with endurance training. However, a change in fiber type contractile properties can occur with sprint training. Repeated bouts of exercise at 90% to 100% of $Vo_{2\ max}$ can produce a decrease in the proportion of type I fibers and an increase in the proportion of type IIc fibers. Similar results were reported when endurance athletes were placed on an "anaerobic" training program, and a decrease in type I myofiber twitch time was observed after high-intensity training.

D. Strength training. The primary adaptation of skeletal muscle to strength training is an increase in muscle bulk that results from hypertrophy of existing fibers. The cross-sectional area of the trained fibers, primarily the type IIa fibers, increases to accommodate additional sarcomeres formed parallel to the existing myofibrils. Fiber type conversion does not appear to occur. The contractility of the fibers (i.e., the maximal tension produced per square millimeter of muscle tissue and per crossbridge interaction) is not altered by strength training.

   1. In general, the overall gain in strength is proportional to the increase in cross-sectional area of the muscle. In the early stages of training, however, strength may increase more rapidly than muscle bulk because of increased motor unit recruitment and coordination.
   2. Muscle bulk may increase more than strength if hypertrophy alters the attachment angle to bone and reduces the mechanical advantage of the lever arm. The cross-sectional areas and strength of connective tissue also increase in response to muscle overload and strength training.
   3. Little or no change in muscle enzyme activities occur with strength training.
   4. Traditional high-resistance isotonic training regimens do not appear to enhance oxidative or glycolytic enzyme activities.

VIII. Ligaments and Bone

A. More and more information is being obtained on the effects of endurance, sprint, and strength training on mineralized tissues (ligaments, bones, and cartilage). In all cases weight-bearing activities increase tensile strength and thickness of the special tissues. Obviously, training of these tissues occurs in concert with skeletal muscle training.

B. Cardiac function and central circulation.

   1. Resting cardiac output is not altered, but maximal cardiac output can be twice as large in a well-trained endurance athlete as in an untrained subject of the same body size.
   2. The ability of an individual to achieve a high maximal cardiac output is probably related to genetic factors and to a prolonged period of endurance training.
   3. Maximal heart rate is not affected by endurance training and is usually the same in highly trained athletes as in untrained subjects.
   4. The higher maximal cardiac outputs are exclusively a result of the heart's ability to eject a larger maximal stroke volume.
   5. The increased maximal stroke volume is a result of:
      a. Increased cardiac dimensions.
      b. A significantly greater absolute left ventricular mass (eccentric hypertrophy) normalized to lean body mass in endurance-trained athletes as compared to that in sedentary subjects.

6. In addition, endurance training increases preload. An augmented preload independently produces an increase in stroke volume by the Frank-Starling mechanism. Evidence suggests that preload is increased after endurance training by an increase in total blood volume consequent to an increase in plasma volume.
7. The effective left ventricular diastolic compliance is increased after endurance training, which also enhances submaximal or maximal preload.
8. Endurance-trained individuals have a reduced heart rate at rest and at any given level of submaximal exercise.
9. The presence of sinus bradycardia and sinus arrhythmia at rest in endurance-trained individuals is attributable to a shift of autonomic balance in favor of the parasympathetic nervous system and a decrease in intrinsic heart rate.
10. Intrinsic heart rate is the heart rate obtained with complete cardiac blockade (using atropine and metoprolol) of the autonomic nervous system.
11. Cardiac output is not significantly changed at submaximal workloads by endurance training; therefore stroke volume is elevated at all levels of submaximal work.
12. The changes in heart rate and stroke volume improve "efficiency" of the heart at submaximal workloads.
13. The enhanced preload, decreased afterload, and unaltered or slightly augmented contractility result in a dramatically increased maximal stroke volume.

C. Peripheral vascular resistance and tissue oxygen extraction. Endurance training is associated with a reduction in total peripheral resistance, or afterload, during exercise. This reduction in peripheral resistance is a result of an increase in vascularity and enables the endurance athlete to achieve levels of cardiac output double those of a sedentary subject at similar arterial pressures during maximal exercise.
   1. The maximal tissue oxygen extraction (arteriovenous oxygen difference) increases after endurance training. This effect is brought about by an increase in the diffusion gradient for oxygen between the capillaries and the active skeletal muscle cells and the total myoglobin content of trained muscle. These changes within the skeletal muscle tissue enhance the diffusion capacity of oxygen at the tissue level.
   2. In addition, tissue oxygen extraction within the active muscle is enhanced by the increased capillary density that occurs with endurance training. The total number and the density (total number per gram of tissue) of capillaries increase. The increased capillary density results in an increased capillary diffusion surface area and is advantageous for nutrient and metabolic byproduct exchange.
   3. The size of the arterial tree also increases as a result of endurance training because of the opening of dormant collateral vessels.
   4. Endurance training also increases the degree of shunting of blood away from the splanchnic and renal circulations at maximal exercise.
   5. These changes improve redistribution of blood flow during exercise and act in concert with the increased tissue extraction to augment total body arteriovenous oxygen difference.

D. Pulmonary system. In the untrained individual, arterial oxygen tension is maintained at maximal workloads, demonstrating that pulmonary factors do not limit oxygen transport in normal individuals.

1. Maximal oxygen transport through the lungs is not significantly improved by endurance training.
2. Furthermore, in the untrained individual, the capacity for oxygen transport by respiration is greater than that of the circulation. This mismatch is dramatically reduced, however, as the level of exercise training improves the cardiovascular capacity for oxygen transport.
3. Oxygen saturation and content may begin to decrease near maximal work in elite endurance athletes. Therefore it appears that in some elite athletes the pulmonary system may contribute to the limitation of $Vo_{2\,max}$ by reducing the amount of oxygen carried by the blood.

CHAPTER 20

Sports Psychology

Aurelia Nattiv, MD

William D. Parham, PhD

I. Introduction
  A. What is sports psychology?
    1. Definition: broadly speaking, sports psychology is the application of psychology and the study of human behavior to the field of athletics.
    2. Applied vs. academic settings.
      a. Sports psychologists work in applied settings (with high school, collegiate, professional, and elite teams) as well as academic settings.
      b. In applied settings, performance enhancement and traditional clinical services (individual and group counseling) are offered.
      c. In academic settings, sports psychology courses are taught and research on the myriad areas related to athletic performance is conducted.
  B. Historical roots.
    1. Developmental history.
      a. Coleman Griffith, a psychologist at the University of Illinois, is considered by many to be the father of sports psychology. His books, *Psychology of Coaching* (1926) and *Psychology of Athletics* (1928), are considered milestone contributions.
      b. Little applied or research activity occurred from the 1920s through the 1950s. There was some activity in the 1960s in the form of professional associations being started as well as sports psychology professional journals.
      c. The field of sports psychology received a tremendous boost in interest during the 1970s and especially during the 1980s, spawned largely by the Olympics.
    2. Current state.
      a. Sports psychologists are recognized as an integral and essential component of the multidisciplinary approach to the care of athletes, working closely with the primary care physicians and other

members of the health care team to optimize the health care of the athlete.

b. Controversy exists regarding basic issues such as professional identity (e.g., who is a sports psychologist), training, and boundaries of the sports psychology field.

II. Selected Topics in Sports Psychology*

A. Psychopathology in the athlete.

1. Psychological profile of the athlete.

a. The "Iceberg Profile": Morgan and others have shown repeatedly that athletes tend to score higher on vigor and extroversion and lower on tension, depression, anger, fatigue, neuroticism, and confusion (profile of mood states [POMS]).

b. Psychopathology: athlete vs. nonathlete.

(1) According to Morgan, success in sports is inversely correlated with psychopathology.

2. Developmental issues.

a. Psychological impact of increasing organization of youth sports.

b. Pressures placed on youth in sports from parents, coaches, others during vulnerable periods of development.

c. Dealing with winning and losing in a healthy way.

d. Psychopathology in youth: conversion reactions, reflex sympathetic dystrophy, etc.

3. Psychodynamic factors.

a. Sudden performance failures (choking).

b. Prolonged performance failures (slump).

c. Emotional factors leading to injury.

d. Interpersonal problems.

e. Training associated problems.

f. Others.

4. The elite athlete.

a. Less psychopathology overall, according to Morgan.

b. External pressures: society, coaches, parents, peers, media, etc.

c. Internal pressures: perfectionistism, high achievers, goal oriented.

5. Athletes and personality traits: Are specific personalities attracted to certain sports or is personality a consequence of sports participation?

a. Obsessive-compulsive behaviors.

(1) Exercise "addiction" and compulsive behavior.

(2) Eating disorders.

(3) Relationship of compulsive running to anorexia nervosa?

b. Risk-taking behavior.

(1) Higher risk-taking behavior seen in collegiate (less in high school) athletes compared to their nonathletic peers in areas of motor vehicle safety (less use of seatbelts and helmets), quantity of alcohol consumption per sitting (e.g., greater quantity per sitting), and sexual behaviors (less safe sex, greater frequency of sexual partners and less contraceptive use).

(2) Male athletes seem to have higher risk-taking behaviors overall.

(3) Sport-specific patterns are seen.

c. Thrill seeking behavior: type "T" personality (thrill seeking)?

*Topics have been selected for their clinical relevance to the field of sport psychology. Although not all-encompassing, the topics discussed will give the healthcare professional a framework of some of the important areas of psychological concern in the athletic setting.

d. Extroverts vs. introverts.
   (1) Most athletes are extroverts.
   (2) Distance runners tend to be more introverted.
e. Gender differences.
   (1) Few studies.
   (2) Disordered eating patterns more common in women athletes.
f. Sport-specific differences.
   (1) Few studies.
   (2) Risk-taking behaviors have sport-specific patterns.

6. Athletes and mental illness: in general, athletes have less psychopathology.
   a. Depression.
      (1) Less endogenous depression in athletes.
      (2) Often related to burnout, overtraining, injury.
   b. Burnout/overtraining.
      (1) Very common in athletes.
      (2) Probably underdiagnosed.
      (3) Depression.
   c. Eating disorders.
      (1) Prevalence of 15% to 62% in female athletes (based on limited studies).
      (2) More common in sports with subjective judging and emphasis on appearance and leanness (gymnastics, figure skating, ballet dance) and endurance sports (distance running) where leanness is often associated with enhanced performance by the athlete and coach.
   d. Substance abuse: alcohol and drug use (frequency) among high school and college athletes is same or less than nonathletes with exception of steroids and smokeless tobacco.
   e. Anxiety disorders: less common in athletes.
   f. Neuroticism: less common in athletes.
   g. Conversion reactions: few reported cases in pediatric population, felt to be secondary to stress of sports participation.
   h. Reflex sympathetic dystrophy: reportedly higher in certain groups of young athletes (Micheli) — highly competitive gymnasts, figure skaters, upper-middle class, Caucasian (lack of studies).
7. Treatment issues.
   a. Prevention is key.
   b. Psychotherapy: primary treatment modality in most cases.
   c. Behavioral therapy: often used in conjunction with psychotherapy.
   d. Pharmacotherapy.
      (1) Potential adverse effect on coordination, vision, and subsequent performance.
      (2) Effect on hydration, electrolyte balance.
      (3) Monitoring the athlete/working closely with psychiatrist.
      (4) Drug testing: National Collegiate Athletic Association/United States Olympic Committee (NCAA/USOC)-banned substances.
8. Related areas.
   a. Postinjury and postoperative psychological adjustment.
   b. Life stress and athletic injury.
   c. Exercise as therapy for anxiety and mood disorders.
9. Summary.
   a. Athletes in general have a more favorable psychological profile compared to their nonathlete counterparts.

b. The physician caring for the athlete needs to be familiar with the psychological problems that may occur in the athletic context.
c. Referral mechanisms need to be in place for psychological and psychiatric care with a professional familiar with sports medicine who works closely with the primary care/team physician.

B. Psychological effects of intensive childhood training.
1. Are youth sports too stressful?
a. Psychological arousal and self-report measures of stress in youth.
(1) Physiological monitoring used in earlier studies: was this measuring stress vs. positive emotion?
(2) Self-reported anxiety slightly higher during athletic season.
(3) Anxiety levels in individual sports greater than in team sports.
b. Winning and losing in youth sports.
(1) Inverse relationship between fun and anxiety in youth sports, independent of victory or defeat.
(2) Fear of failure is a main source of anxiety.
(3) Competitive stress contributes significantly to drop-out rates in youth sports.
(4) Competitive stress can cause impaired performance, increased risk of athletic injury, sleep disturbances.
c. Youth sports: developing a balance is the key.
2. Potential maladaptive psychological effects of intensive childhood training.
a. Promotion of asocial behavior?
b. Promotion of aggressive behavior?
c. Anxiety/stress provoking?
d. Compromising academic performance?
e. Development of pathogenic eating behaviors.
f. Development of burnout.
g. Lower self-esteem.
3. Potential maladaptive psychophysiological effects.
a. Stress-related gastrointestinal distress.
b. Other physiological manifestations.
c. Reflex sympathetic dystrophy.
4. Potential adaptive effects of intensive childhood training.
a. Increased self-esteem.
b. Development of coping skills.
c. Development of social skills.
d. "Mental toughness."
e. Development of a sense of mastery.
5. The physician's role in prevention/treatment of psychological problems related to youth sports participation.
a. Decrease situational demands associated with:
(1) Winning and losing.
(2) Coaching roles and relationships.
(3) Parents' roles and responsibilities.
(4) Organization and administration of sports programs.
b. Implementation of stress management programs for youth.
c. Assist in the development of coping skills.
d. Team approach.

C. Psychological burnout in athletes.
1. Concept of burnout.
a. Stress-based model.
b. Social-based model.

2. Symptoms.
   a. Early: growing state of fatigue, irritability, loss of enthusiasm, frustration.
   b. Intermediate: increasing fatigue, withdrawn, physical distress (stomach upset, headaches, shortness of breath, body aches, overeating or undereating), loss of motivation, etc.
   c. Advanced: total lack of energy, convinced not good enough, low self-esteem, cynicism, feelings of alienation.
3. The "at risk" athlete.
   a. Adolescent.
   b. Elite/highly competitive.
   c. Perfectionist.
   d. "Type A."
   e. "Other oriented."
   f. Lack of assertiveness skills.
4. Factors leading to burnout ("demotivators").
   a. Lack of positive feedback from coaches.
   b. Lack of perceived control.
   c. Lack of social connectedness.
   d. Recurrent physical injury.
   e. Competitiveness of sport.
   f. Social consequences of sport participation.
   g. Identifying self as athlete vs. individual.
   h. Pressures placed on athlete by society to excel.
5. Differential diagnosis of burnout.
   a. Anemia.
   b. Exercise-induced bronchospasm.
   c. Medication.
   d. Overtraining.
   e. Depression.
   f. Endocrine or metabolic disease.
   g. Cardiac disease.
   h. Neuromuscular disease.
   i. Infection.
   j. Decreased motivation.
   k. Decreased ability to focus.
6. Treatment of burnout.
   a. Early diagnosis.
   b. Identifying susceptible individuals/prevention.
   c. Rest from sport.
   d. Psychotherapy.
   e. Supportive team.
   f. Empowering athlete as individual.
   g. Burnout as a positive experience/opportunity for change and growth.

D. Anxiety and sport performance.
   1. Anxiety.
      a. Definition: emotional reaction that consists of a unique combination of feelings of tension, apprehension, nervousness, unpleasant thoughts, and physiological changes (Spielberger 1989)
      b. General measures: Spielberger's State-Trait Anxiety Scale (STAI).
         (1) Measures state anxiety (the transitory aspect of anxiety that can vary in intensity and change across time) and trait anxiety (the more constant and unchanging aspect of anxiety); the predisposition to perceive situations as threatening.

(2) Most widely used measure of state and trait anxiety.
(3) Has established construct validity and demonstrated sensitivity in athletes.

c. Sport-specific measures: Cognitive-Somatic Anxiety Questionnaire (CSAI-2).
(1) Assesses cognitive and somatic sport state anxiety, as well as self-confidence.
(2) Felt to be more specific to athletes.

d. Multidimensional measures.
(1) Measures several different dimensions of anxiety.
(2) Complex.
(3) Experimental in athletes at this time.

e. Common sources of anxiety in the athlete.
(1) Fear of failure and of making a mistake.
(2) Expectations of others.
(3) Poor preparatory training and physical state.
(4) Fear of injury.
(5) Media.
(6) Unforeseen events.
(7) Personal issues/concerns unrelated to athletics.

2. Assessment of athletic performance.
a. Coach/subjective rating.
b. Personal best or season average.
c. Criterion-referenced method: dividing athlete's attained performance by a standardized reference.

3. Theories of anxiety-performance relationship.
a. Inverted U Hypothesis (Yerkes and Dodson).
(1) Optimal performance associated with moderate levels of arousal or anxiety.
(2) Very low levels of arousal/anxiety (apathy) and very high levels of arousal/anxiety (nervousness) associated with a decreased level of performance (relationship between arousal and performance takes on an inverted U shape).
(3) Not as well accepted in the sports psychology literature as it once was.

b. Zone of Optimal Function Theory (Hanin).
(1) Optimal performance is best when the athlete's precompetition anxiety level is within a relatively narrow range or zone.
(2) Most widely accepted theory of anxiety and performance relationship, especially with individual sports (less research with team sports).
(3) Many elite athletes found to perform best under high levels of anxiety—supporting theory.

c. Drive Theory.
(1) States that performance is a function of drive and habit strength.
(2) Theory is not well accepted.

4. Mechanisms underlying anxiety-performance relationship.
a. Perceptual or attentional narrowing.
(1) As anxiety increases, there is a narrowing of visual field from peripheral to foveal.
(2) Elimination of task-irrelevant cues.
(3) High-level athletes score high on visual information processing.

5. Interventions.
   a. Not all interventions need to focus on decreasing anxiety, as anxiety may help performance in some athletes.
      (1) Successful athletes tend to perceive anxiety as desirable.
      (2) The athlete's control over the anxiety is an important concept (vs. anxiety controlling the athlete).
      (3) The absolute level of precompetition anxiety may not be as important as the consistency in the anxiety level.
   b. Interventions or coping strategies proposed to improve performance.
      (1) Well-established preperformance routines: helps with attention focus.
      (2) Simulation training (i.e., listening to a tape of a screaming crowd before a big game—elimination of external distractions).
      (3) Goal-setting skills.
      (4) Imagery.
      (5) Positive self-talk.
      (6) Relaxation strategies.
      (7) Importance of a social support system.
   c. No one intervention has proven more successful for all athletes for performance enhancement; need to individualize interventions.
6. Summary.
   a. Anxiety is not an enemy and may be productive if controlled.
   b. Considerable variability exists in optimal precompetition anxiety responses.
   c. Interventions must be individualized.
   d. Coping strategies may be helpful.
   e. More research is needed in the anxiety-performance relationship.

E. Coping with athletic injury.
   1. Psychological factors predisposing to injury in the athlete.
      a. Tension.
      b. Depression.
      c. Academic stress.
      d. Social problems.
      e. Family dysfunction.
      f. Intrapersonal struggles.
      g. Life stress events.
   2. Emotional responses of athletes to injury.
      a. Loss-of-Health Model (Kubler-Ross).
         (1) Denial.
         (2) Anger.
         (3) Bargaining.
         (4) Depression.
         (5) Acceptance.
      b. Athlete's vs. nonAthlete's Responses (POMS tests).
         (1) Frustration.
         (2) Depression.
         (3) Anger.
      c. More seriously injured athletes.
         (1) Increased emotional response to tension, depression, anger.
         (2) Less vigor.
         (3) Increased emotional responses for 1 month after injury (?).
   3. Psychological strategies/coping techniques for the injured athlete.
      a. Strategies for intervention.
         (1) Problem focused.

(2) Behaviorally oriented.
(3) Achievable goals.
(4) Minimize uncertainty.

b. Specific techniques.
(1) Relaxation methods.
(2) Visualization.
(3) Cognitive restructuring.

F. Performance enhancement.
A set of cognitive, affective, and behavioral tools and procedures designed to assist athletes in executing their athletic tasks with maximum precision and consistency by tapping the wellspring of talent and inner strength that each possesses.

1. Arousal.
   a. An energizing function that contributes to the level at which athletic activity is produced and maintained.
   b. Arousal is influenced by the cortex, reticular formation, the hypothalamus, and the limbic system, all of which interact with the adrenal medulla and the somatic autonomic systems.
   c. Arousal can be measured physiologically (i.e., electroencephalography, heart rate and blood pressure measurement), biochemically (i.e., epinephrine and norepinephrine levels) and via questionnaire (i.e., STAI, CSAI-2).
2. Goal setting.
   a. Deciding on a desired outcome and designing a strategy to achieve that outcome within a specified period of time.
   b. Goals can be short term (e.g., daily, weekly, monthly) or longer term (i.e., quarterly, every year, every 5 years, etc.).
   c. Goal effectiveness research suggests that goal setting clearly and consistently facilitates performance.
3. Relaxation techniques.
   a. Bringing about a state of physiological calm. A means of lowering muscular tension.
   b. Jacobson progressive relaxation, autogenic training, and meditation represent different kinds of relaxation exercises.
4. Imagery.
   a. Involving all of one's senses to create or recreate a performance experience in one's mind.
   b. Psychoneuromuscular theory suggests that brain impulses are being transmitted when athletes imagine their movements without actually performing them.
5. Cognitive techniques/self-talk.
   a. Identifying thoughts and their frequency, content, and valence (i.e., negative or positive) and learning how to manage them in ways that facilitate vs. impede self-acknowledgment and acceptance.
   b. Positive and accurate self-talk is related to self-confidence, and self-confidence is related to success.
6. Concentration and attention: the ability to focus and remain focused on the task at hand without the interference of internal or external stimuli.

G. Special populations.
1. Children: Youth sports is often the spawning ground for subsequent involvement in athletics. Home as well as peer group environments

play a major role in shaping a young athlete's perceptions, beliefs, values, expectations, and experiences in athletics.

2. Adults: Adults participate in recreational athletic activity. Recreational adult athletes may have less overall knowledge about the various aspects of sports participation (i.e., nutrition, rest, exercise, basic physiology, etc.) than athletes who participate in formal athletic programs and as such may be more susceptible to the costs involved in participating in athletics (i.e., injury, etc.).
3. Collegiate: Collegiate athletics has become an important economic and social force in academic institutions. There are both positive and negative consequences for the athlete (i.e., skill acquisition, identity, character development, exploitation, detraction from the educational goal), and the institution (i.e., prestige, community, visibility, alumni support, detraction from educational mission, etc.). It is also important to view the intercollegiate athlete within a developmental context as the tasks and challenges inherent in athletics coincide with the major life tasks and challenges (i.e., identity formation, career exploration, developing and maintaining personal and intimate relationships, morality, etc.) often associated with this age group.
4. Professional: Important to view professional athletics within the context of career development, which suggests, among other things, that people assume career identities, and that job satisfaction/dissatisfaction is a factor in self-esteem and work productivity.

III. Summary
   A. The field of sports psychology is integral to current sports medicine practice.
   B. The primary care team physician and health care team working with the athlete need to be aware of the unique psychological issues and concerns that the athlete may encounter and have a mechanism in place for their prevention and treatment.

Bibliography

American Academy of Pediatrics, Committee on Sports Medicine and Committee on School Health: Organized athletics for preadolescent children, *Pediatrics* 84(3):583-584, 1989.

American Academy of Pediatrics, Committee on Sports Medicine and Fitness: Fitness, activity, and sports participation in the preschool child, *Pediatrics* 9(6):1002-1004, 1992.

Anderson WA et al: A national survey of alcohol and drug use by college athletes, *Phys Sportsmed* 19(2):91-104, 1991.

Begel D: An overview of sports psychiatry, *Am J Psychiatry* 149(5):606-614, 1992.

Coakley J: Sport and socialization, *Exerc Sports Sci Rev* 21:169-200, 1993.

Feigley DA: Psychological burnout in high-level athletes, *Phys Sports Med* 12(10):109-119, 1984.

Finkerton RS, Hinz LD, Barrow JC: The college student-athlete: psychological considerations and interventions, *J Am Coll Health* 37(5):218-226, 1989.

Frazier SE: Mood state profiles of chronic exercises with differing abilities, *Int J Sports Psychol* 19:65-71, 1988.

Hauck ER, Blumenthal JA: Obsessive and compulsive traits in athletes, *Sports Med* 14(4):215-227, 1992.

Kane JE: Personality research: the current controversy and implications for sports studies. In Straub WF, editor: *Sport psychology: an analysis of athlete behavior,* Ithaca, NY, 1978, Mouvement Publications, pp 228-240.

Kelley MJ Jr: Psychological risk factors and sports injuries, *J Sports Med Phys Fitness* 30(2):202-221, 1990.

Kubler-Ross E: On death and dying, New York, MacMillan, 1969.

Maffuli N, Pintore E: Intensive training in young athletes, *Br J Sports Med* 24(4):237-239, 1990.

Mansfield JM, Emans JS: Editors column: Growth in female gymnasts: should training decrease during puberty? *J Pediatr* 122(2):237-240, 1993.

Massimino JH: Sport psychiatry, *Ann Sports Med* 3:55-58, 1987.

Morgan WP, Costill DL: Psychological characteristics of the marathon runner, *J Sports Med Phys Fitness* 12:42-46, 1972.

Morgan WP et al: Personality structure, mood states and performance in elite male distance runners, *Int J Sports Psychol* 247-263, 1988.

Nattiv A, Puffer JC: Lifestyles and health risks of collegiate athletes, *J Fam Pract* 33:585-590, 1991.

Parham WD: The intercollegiate athlete: a 1990's profile, *Counseling Psychol* 21(3):411-429, 1993.

Parham WD: Diversity within intercollegiate athletics: current profile and welcomed opportunity: In Etzel E, Ferrante AP, Dinkney JW, editors: *Counseling college student athletes; issues and interventions,* ed 2. Morgantown, WV, 1996, Fitness Information, Technology, Inc.

Pillemer FG, Micheli LJ: Psychological considerations in youth sports, *Clin Sports Med* 7(3):679-689, 1988.

Puffer JC, McShane JM: Depression and chronic fatigue in the college student-athlete, *Prim Care* 18(2):297-308, 1991.

Rotella JR, Heil J: Psychological aspects of sports medicine. In Reider B, editor: *Sports medicine—the school age athlete,* Philadelphia, 1991, WB Saunders, pp 105-117.

Rowland TW: Exercise fatigue in adolescents: diagnosis of athlete burnout, *Phys Sports Med* 14(9):69-77, 1986.

Smoll FL, Smith RE: Psychology of the young athlete—stress-related maladies and remedial approaches, *Pediatr Clin North Am* 37(5):1021-1046, 1990.

Spielberger CO: Stress and anxiety in sports. In Hackfort D, Spielberger CO, editors: *Anxiety in Sports: An international perspective,* New York, 1989, Hemisphere Publishing, pp 3-17.

Weiss MR, Light Bredemeier BJ: Moral development in sport, *Exerc Sport Sci Rev* 18:331-378, 1990.

Yerkes RM, Dodson JO: The relation of strength of stimulus to rapidity of habit-formation, *J Compar Neurol Psychol* 18:459-482, 1908.

CHAPTER 21

Nutrition in Sports

Ellen J. Coleman, MA, MPH, RD

I. Importance of Nutrition to Athletic Performance
   A. Three primary factors influence athletic performance: genetic endowment, state of training, and nutrition.[23]
      1. Athletes have control over food choices and training but not heredity.
      2. While good diet cannot guarantee athletic success, poor diet can undermine training.
   B. Food provides nutrients that perform one or more physiological or biochemical functions.
      1. Nutrients have three major functions: energy production, tissue growth and repair, and regulation of physiological processes.[23]
      2. Six classes of nutrients are carbohydrates, proteins, fats, vitamins, minerals, and water.[23]
   C. Recommended Dietary Allowances (RDAs): the amount of essential nutrients that are scientifically judged to be adequate to meet known nutrient needs of practically all healthy people.[12] RDAs can be obtained by consuming a variety of foods.[13]
   D. The U.S. Department of Agriculture's Food Pyramid[21] and Dietary Guidelines[20] provide recommendations for the proportions of foods that should be included in a healthy diet. Grain, vegetable, and fruit groups have the highest recommended number of servings and are nutrient-rich sources of carbohydrates.[20]
   E. Nutritional quackery is prevalent in athletics.[19]
      1. Athletes are susceptible to nutritional quackery because they *hope* that nutritional supplements will give them a competitive edge and they *fear* losing.[19]
      2. Factors in the athletic environment help contribute to nutritional quackery[19]: advertising of nutritional products marketed specifically for athletes, recommendations for foods or supplements by misinformed coaches, nutrition misinformation found in leading sports

magazines and books, and dietary habits or recommendations of successful athletes.

II. Energy Systems for Exercise[11]
   A. Adenosine triphosphate-creatine phosphate (ATP-CP) (phosphagen) system sustains all-out effort for 5-8 seconds (a 50-100-m run).
   B. Anaerobic (lactic acid) system sustains exercise lasting for 60 seconds (a 400-m sprint). Only glucose can be used as fuel, and lactic acid accumulates.
   C. Aerobic (oxygen) system provides about 50% of the energy required for exercise lasting 2 minutes; anaerobic and phosphagen systems supply the other 50%.
      1. As exercise time increases, the amount of aerobically produced energy increases.
      2. In addition to glucose, protein and fat may be utilized for fuel.

III. Determinants of Exercise Fuel Usage[11]
   A. Intensity: exercise ≥70% of aerobic capacity is fueled primarily by muscle glycogen and blood glucose.
      1. Fat and carbohydrate are used about equally as fuel during exercise at 40% to 60% of aerobic capacity; fat can only be used as fuel up to about 60% of aerobic capacity.
      2. Fat metabolism cannot supply ATP rapidly enough to support high-intensity exercise; glucose provides more calories per liter of oxygen than fat; lactic acid hinders mobilization of fat.
      3. Muscle glycogen depletion occurs after 90-120 minutes of exercise at 70% to 75% aerobic capacity and is a well-recognized limitation to endurance performance.
   B. Duration: the longer the duration, the greater the contribution of fat as fuel.
      1. It takes about 20 minutes for fat to be available as fuel in the form of free fatty acids.
      2. Fat can supply 60% to 70% of the energy needs for moderate-intensity exercise lasting 4-6 hours.
      3. Blood glucose is the primary source of carbohydrate after 2-3 hours of exercise.
      4. Protein use is minimal (5% to 10% of total calories).
   C. Fitness level.
      1. Endurance training enables athlete to use more fat and less glycogen at same absolute level of exercise.
      2. "Glycogen-sparing" effect enhances endurance; glycogen stores are limited, and fat stores are abundant.
      3. Endurance training enables athletes to store more muscle glycogen and so also improves endurance.
   D. Due to relationship between exercise intensity and duration, muscle glycogen is the primary fuel for most sports.

IV. Carbohydrate Recommendations for Training
   A. Maintaining adequate muscle glycogen stores for training requires a carbohydrate-rich diet.[4]
      1. Athletes should consume 6-10 g of carbohydrate per kg of body weight per day (about 60% to 70% of total calories).[16]
      2. Carbohydrate recommendations = 6 g/kg for 1 hour of training each day, 8 g/kg for 2 hours, and at least 10 g/kg for ≥3 hours.
   B. Athletes who do not consume adequate carbohydrate can experience chronic fatigue due to cumulative depletion of muscle glycogen.[4]
      1. Average American diet only supplies about 5 g/kg (about 46%) carbohydrate.[4]

2. American Dietetic Association Food Exchange Lists can be used to create a high carbohydrate diet.[1]

V. Preexercise Meal Considerations[17]
   A. Overnight fast lowers liver glycogen stores, which can cause hypoglycemia and subsequent fatigue.
   B. Preexercise meal provides energy when athlete exercises for an hour or longer.
      1. Prevents athletes from feeling hungry, which in itself may impair performance.
      2. Elevates blood glucose to provide energy for the exercising muscles.
   C. Preexercise meal recommendations.
      1. Consume a familiar high-carbohydrate meal 1-4 hours before exercise.[17]
      2. Reduce the size of the meal the closer to exercise it is consumed: 300-400 calories an hour before; 700-800 calories 4 hours before.[17]
      3. Avoid high-fiber foods, gas-forming foods, and very salty foods.[23]
      4. Liquid meals (e.g., Ensure or Sustical) empty faster from the stomach than solid meals and help to prevent nausea.[23]

VI. Carbohydrate Feedings During Training and Competition
   A. Carbohydrate ingestion improves performance during endurance exercise lasting >1 hour.[5]
      1. Carbohydrate feedings provide glucose for muscles when their glycogen stores are diminished.[5]
      2. Carbohydrate feedings maintain carbohydrate oxidation, thereby enhancing performance.[5]
      3. Endurance athletes should consume 30-60 g/hr of carbohydrate-rich foods or fluids.[5]
      4. Sports drinks providing 5% to 8% carbohydrate are practical because they replace fluid losses as well.[5]
   B. Athletes competing in multiple events require fluids and carbohydrate-rich foods throughout the day. Failure to consume carbohydrates can cause a deterioration in performance towards end of day.
   C. Carbohydrate recommendations based on time between events:
      1. Less than an hour = water, sports drinks, and diluted fruit juices.
      2. Several hours = fruit, grain products, and liquid meals.
      3. Three hours or more = high-carbohydrate meals.

VII. Carbohydrate Feedings Following Exercise
   A. Replacement of muscle glycogen stores between training sessions necessary to minimize chronic fatigue.[4] Based on time spent training, athletes should consume 6-10 g of carbohydrates per kg daily.[16]
   B. Carbohydrates should be consumed immediately after strenuous training lasting several hours.[7] Delaying carbohydrate intake reduces muscle glycogen synthesis and impairs recovery.[7]
   C. Carbohydrate recommendations after prolonged exercise.
      1. Consume 1.5 g/kg within 30 minutes of exercise and an additional 1.5 g/kg within 2 hours.[6]
      2. High-carbohydrate fluids recommended for initial feeding to promote rehydration.
      3. Particularly important for athletes training several times a day to enhance recovery for second workout.

VIII. Muscle Glycogen Supercompensation: Carbohydrate Loading
   A. Only beneficial for endurance events that exceed 90-120 minutes, such as marathon running.[18]
      1. The greater the preexercise muscle glycogen content, the greater the endurance potential.

   2. Increases muscle glycogen stores by 50% to 100%.[18]
 - B. Six-day regimen consisting of tapered training and dietary carbohydrate manipulation: two phases.[18]
   1. Phase one.
      - a. Training = 90-minute moderately hard exercise session 6 days prior to event. On next 2 days taper training to 40 minutes.
      - b. Diet = 5 g of carbohydrates per kilogram for first 3 days of regimen.
   2. Phase two.
      - a. Training = taper training to 20 minutes for 2 days. Rest the day before event.
      - b. Diet = 10 g of carbohydrates per kilogram for last 3 days of regimen.
 - C. Loading considerations.[18]
   1. Supplements providing 20% to 24% carbohydrate can be added to increase carbohydrate intake in phase two.
   2. Athletes with diabetes and/or high triglyceride levels should obtain medical clearance before loading.

IX. Protein Recommendations
 - A. Athletes require more protein than the RDA of 0.8 g/kg/day.[9]
   1. Protein catabolism predominates during exercise.[23]
   2. Protein synthesis is enhanced in the recovery period.[23]
   3. Regular training increases the efficiency of protein synthesis in recovery.[23]
   4. Increased protein intake is more important during the early phase of strength and endurance training.[23]
 - B. Resistance training promotes synthesis of contractile muscle proteins.[23]
   1. Strength athletes require 50% to 100% more protein than the RDA or 1.2 to 1.7 g/kg/day.[9]
   2. Adequate caloric intake is more important than elevated protein intake to achieve increases in muscle mass.[9]
   3. Increased caloric intake = increased protein intake.[23]
   4. To gain 1 lb of muscle per week (about 100 g of protein) requires only 14 additional g of protein per day.[23]
 - C. Endurance training promotes increases in hemoglobin, myoglobin, and oxidative enzymes in mitochondria.[23]
   1. Endurance athletes require 50% to 75% more protein than the RDA or 1.2 to 1.4 g/kg/day.[9]
   2. When bodily carbohydrate stores are low, muscle protein may supply 5% to 10% of energy for exercise.[23]
   3. The high-carbohydrate diet recommended for endurance athletes has a protein-sparing effect.[23]
   4. Branched-chain amino acids (leucine, isoleucine, and valine) are primary ones utilized for energy during endurance exercise.[23]
 - D. Amino acid/protein supplementation is unnecessary.
   1. Strength and endurance athletes can easily meet protein requirements with a diet supplying 12% to 15% calories from protein.[9]
   2. Average American diet supplies 1.4 g of protein/kg/day.[23]
   3. Strength athletes do not require or benefit from protein supplements.[24]
   4. Excess amino acids that are not converted into new proteins are either burned for energy or stored as fat.[23]
   5. Oral arginine and ornithine promoted to increase muscle mass and decrease body fat by increasing growth hormone; research does not support an ergogenic effect.[24]

6. Further research required to determine if supplementation with branched-chain amino acids improves endurance performance.[23]

X. Fat Recommendations for Health and Performance
  A. The average American diet supplies too much fat (37% of calories) for athletes as well as sedentary people.[13]
    1. High-fat diet increases the risk of cardiovascular disease and certain cancers.[13]
    2. High-fat diet also contributes to obesity, which is associated with a wide range of health problems.[13]
    3. Fat displaces carbohydrate in the diet; muscle glycogen stores cannot be adequately maintained on a high-fat diet.[23]
  B. Dietary fat recommendations to promote health (National Cholesterol Education Program Guidelines).[14]
    1. Dietary fat should provide <30% of total calories.
    2. Saturated fat should comprise <10% of total calories.
    3. Dietary cholesterol intake should be <300 mg/day.
  C. Importance of fat as an exercise fuel.
    1. Endurance training increases the contribution of fat as fuel.[11]
    2. Increased fat utilization enhances endurance performance by sparing muscle glycogen.[11]
    3. Since muscle glycogen is limited and fat stores are abundant, slowing rate of glycogen depletion improves performance in endurance events.[11]
  D. "Fat loading": chronic consumption of a very high–fat diet.
    1. Claimed to improve endurance performance by increasing fat metabolism.
    2. Ability to exercise at ≥70% of aerobic capacity may be impaired due to low muscle glycogen stores.[23]
    3. Potentially dangerous due to protein and potassium losses and increases in serum lipids.[23]
  E. Caffeine ingestion and fat utilization.
    1. Caffeine ingestion prior to exercise augments plasma epinephrine levels and *may* produce a glycogen-sparing effect.[2]
    2. A caffeine intake of 5-9 mg/kg 1 hour before endurance exercise may enhance performance in events >1 hour.[2]
    3. High-caffeine doses (800 mg) produce urinary levels close to International Olympic Committee's (IOC) doping threshold (12 μg/ml of urine).[2]
    4. Side effects: gastrointestinal distress. The diuretic effect of caffeine does not appear to increase thermal stress.[2]
    5. The use of caffeine as an ergogenic aid is controversial—does it violate the ethics of sports?

XI. Vitamin Requirements and Recommendations
  A. Many athletes take vitamin supplements for nutritional insurance and/or to improve their performance.[23]
    1. Advertisements encourage supplement abuse by claiming athletes have higher vitamin requirements.[19]
    2. Exercise does not significantly increase vitamin requirements.[22]
    3. Exception: thiamine is required in proportion to calories. Easily supplied by carbohydrate-rich foods.[22]
  B. Athletes can and should obtain vitamins by eating a variety of foods each day.[13]
    1. Vitamin requirements can be met by eating the minimum recommended number of servings from the Food Guide Pyramid.[21]

2. The vitamin needs of the average person are only about 67% of the RDA.[13]
3. Vitamin deficiencies are rare in industrialized nations.[23]

C. There is a close relationship between vitamin intake and caloric intake: the more eaten, the greater the vitamin intake.[22]
1. Athletes generally eat more than sedentary people, thereby consuming more vitamins.[22]
2. Athletes who limit their caloric intake may be at risk for vitamin deficiencies (e.g., athletes concerned about extra weight affecting performance or about cosmetics).[22]

D. Supplementation at levels exceeding the RDA does not improve performance in well-nourished athletes.[22]
1. Purported ergogenic benefits encourage supplement abuse.[19]
2. At high doses, many vitamins have pharmacological effects and toxicity is a concern.[13]
3. High doses = 10 times the RDA for water-soluble vitamins and 5 times the RDA for fat-soluble vitamins.[13]

E. Athletes should avoid taking vitamin supplements that exceed 100% of the RDA in any 1 day.[13]
1. While there is no evidence that this practice is harmful, there is also no evidence that it is beneficial for most athletes.[23]
2. A supplement supplying no more than 100% of the RDA may be appropriate for athletes with low caloric intakes (e.g., <1200 calories/day).[23]

F. Antioxidant vitamins and muscle damage.
1. Excess production of free radicals, due to intense exercise, may damage muscle cell membrane (via lipid peroxidation) and cause muscle soreness.[8]
2. Several antioxidants (especially vitamin E but also C and beta-carotene) *may* protect against exercise-induced muscle damage but do not improve performance.[8]
3. Research is too preliminary to recommend antioxidant supplementation at this time.[8]

XII. Mineral Requirements and Recommendations

A. Many Americans are not consuming adequate amounts of calcium, iron, zinc, and chromium.[3]
1. Mineral deficiencies to the point of impairing physical performance are rare.[3]
2. A low serum level of minerals usually does not affect performance (exception: iron).[3]
3. Consuming foods rich in calcium and iron helps to ensure adequate intake of other minerals.[23]

B. Athletes in weight control sports are at greatest risk for developing a mineral deficiency.[23]
1. Dietary surveys indicate many of these athletes are not consuming the RDA for iron and calcium.[23]
2. Low intake of calcium and iron suggests inadequate intake of other trace minerals.[23]

C. Adequate calcium intake recommended to help reduce risk of osteoporosis.[15]
1. Until peak bone mass achieved at 30-35 years of age, bone formation exceeds resorption.[15]
2. RDA for children and adults = 800 mg; RDA for ages 11-24 is 1200 mg.[12]

3. National Institutes of Health recommends 1000 mg for postmenopausal women on estrogen and 1500 mg for those not on estrogen.[15]
4. Recommendations for amenorrheic women athletes = 1000 mg if on estrogen and 1500 mg if not.[15]

D. Adequate iron intake recommended to prevent iron-deficiency anemia.
1. RDA for adult men = 10 mg; RDA for women and teenagers of both sexes is 15 mg.[12]
2. Six percent of female population has iron-deficiency anemia; iron deficiency alone is even more prevalent.[23]
3. Iron supplementation improves performance when athlete has iron-deficiency anemia.[3]
4. Iron supplementation does not improve performance when athlete has iron deficiency without anemia.[3]
5. Exercise may increase iron loss via sweating, gastrointestinal bleeding, and hemolysis.[23]

E. Iron recommendations.
1. Periodic evaluation of iron status, especially in menstruating female athletes.[23]
2. Encourage intake of heme (animal) iron sources—better absorbed than nonheme (plant) sources.[23]
3. Consuming heme with nonheme iron sources improves absorption of nonheme iron.[23]
4. Vitamin C improves absorption of nonheme iron; cast iron cookware increases iron content of food.[23]

F. Athletes should avoid taking mineral supplements that exceed 100% of the RDA in any 1 day.[13]
1. Excessive iron supplementation can cause iron overload, especially in susceptible individuals.[23]
2. Of every 1000 Americans, about 2-3 have a genetic predisposition to hemachromatosis.[23]
3. Excessive calcium supplementation can increase risk of kidney-stones in susceptible individuals.[23]
4. Levels associated with toxicity can generally only be achieved by taking supplements.[23]
5. Controlled research does not support claims that chromium picolinate increases muscle mass and decreases body fat.[24]

XIII. Fluid Requirements and Recommendations

A. At rest, average adult requires 2-3 L of water daily (about 1 ml/calorie of energy intake).[23] Water is most essential nutrient since body requires it constantly.

B. Water's most critical function for athletes is the regulation of body temperature.[23]
1. Sweat losses constituting as little as 2% of the body weight impair temperature regulation during prolonged exercise.[23]
2. Three factors contribute to development of heat injuries: increased core temperature, loss of body fluids, and loss of electrolytes.[23]
3. Proper fluid replenishment helps to reduce the risk of heat illnesses.[23]

C. Adequate fluid replacement is the most frequently overlooked performance aid.[23]
1. During prolonged exercise, sweat losses constituting as little as 2% of body weight impair athletic performance due to increased cardiovascular stress.[23]

2. Optimal rate of fluid replacement to reduce body temperature elevation and cardiovascular stress is the rate that most closely matches sweat loss.[5]

D. Inadequate intake is primary obstacle to fluid replacement; thirst is not an adequate guide.[23]
   1. Most athletes replace only 30% to 50% of their fluid losses during exercise.[23]
   2. Necessary to regulate fluid intake by drinking according to schedule rather than by perceived thirst.[23]

E. Hydration guidelines for athletes.
   1. Drink 16 oz (474 ml) 15-30 minutes prior to exercise (hyperhydration).[23]
   2. Drink 4-8 oz (118-237 ml) every 15 minutes during exercise.[23]
   3. Drink 16 oz (474 ml) for every pound of body weight lost after exercise.[23]

F. Electrolyte considerations.
   1. Loss of 1 g of sodium due to 2-lb sweat loss can be replaced by consuming balanced diet (½ teaspoon salt = 1 g of sodium).[23]
   2. Water losses during sweating are proportionally greater than electrolyte losses.[23]
   3. During endurance exercise ≥4 hours, hyponatremia may result from excessive sodium losses or water intake.[23]

G. Fluid replacement beverage considerations.
   1. Water is an appropriate fluid replacement beverage for exercise lasting ≤1 hour.[23]
   2. Sports drinks containing 6% to 8% carbohydrate (about 60-80 calories per 8 oz) may improve performance during exercise >1 hour.[10]
   3. Athletes in endurance events >4 hr should consume fluid replacement drinks containing sodium.[10]
   4. Beverages with >10% carbohydrate (fruit juice, soda) and concentrated fructose drinks are absorbed more slowly and may cause gastrointestinal distress.[10]

References

1. American Diabetes Association, American Dietetic Association: *Exchange lists for meal planning,* Chicago, 1986, American Dietetic Association.
2. Clarkson PM: Nutritional ergogenic aids: caffeine, *Int J Sports Nutr* 3:103-111, 1993.
3. Clarkson PM: Minerals: exercise performance and supplementation in athletes, *J Sports Sci* 9:91-116, 1991.
4. Costill DL: Carbohydrates for exercise: dietary demands for optimal performance, *Int J Sports Med* 9:1-18, 1988.
5. Coyle EF, Montain SJ: Benefits of fluid replacement with carbohydrate during exercise, *Med Sci Sports Exerc Suppl* 24:S324-S330, 1992.
6. Ivy JL et al: Muscle glycogen storage after different amounts of carbohydrate ingestion, *J Appl Physiol* 65:2018-2023, 1988.
7. Ivy JL et al: Muscle glycogen synthesis after exercise: effect of time of carbohydrate ingestion, *J Appl Physiol* 64:1480-1485, 1988.
8. Kanter MM: Free radicals, exercise, and antioxidant supplementation, *Int J Sports Nutr* 4:205-220, 1994.
9. Lemon PRW: Effect of exercise on protein requirements, *J Sports Sci* 9:53-70, 1991.
10. Murray R: The effects of consuming carbohydrate-electrolyte beverages on gastric emptying and fluid absorption during and following exercise, *Sports Med* 4:322-351, 1987.
11. McArdle WD, Katch FI, Katch VL: *Exercise physiology: energy, nutrition, and human performance,* Malvern, PA, 1991, Lea & Febiger.
12. National Research Council: *Recommended Dietary Allowances,* ed 10, Washington, DC, 1989, National Academy Press.
13. National Research Council: *Diet and health: implications for reducing chronic disease risk,* Washington, DC, 1989, National Academy Press.

14. NCEP: Summary of the Second Report of the National Cholesterol Education Program Expert Panel on Detection, Evaluation, and Treatment of High Blood Cholesterol in Adults, *JAMA* 269:3015-3023, 1993.
15. NIH Consensus Development Conference. Optimal calcium intake. Office of Medical Application of Research and National Institute of Arthritis and Musculoskeletal and Skin Disease, 1994, pp 19-20.
16. Position of the American Dietetic Association and The Canadian Dietetic Association: Nutrition for physical fitness and athletic peformance for adults, *J Am Diet Assoc* 93:691-696, 1993.
17. Sherman WM: Pre-event nutrition, *Sports Sci Exch* 2(12):1-6, 1989.
18. Sherman WM: Muscle glycogen supercompensation during the week before athletic competition, *Sports Sci Exch* 2(16): 1989.
19. Short SH, Marquart LF: Sports nutrition fraud, *NY State J Med* 93:112-116, 1993.
20. US Dept of Agriculture, US Dept of Health and Human Services: Nutrition and your health: dietary guidelines for Americans, ed 4, Home and Garden Bulletin no 232, Washington, DC, 1995, US Government Printing Office.
21. US Dept of Agriculture, US Dept of Health and Human Services: *The food guide pyramid,* Home and Garden Bulletin no 252, Washington, DC, 1992, US Government Printing Office.
22. Van Der Beek EJ: Vitamin supplementation and physical exercise performance, *J Sports Sci* 9:77-89, 1991.
23. Williams MH: Nutrition for fitness and sport, ed 4, Dubuque, IA, 1995, Wm C Brown Publishers.
24. Williams MH: Nutritional supplements for strength trained athletes, *Sports Sci Exch* 6(47):1-6, 1993.

CHAPTER 22

Exercise and Menstrual Function

Carol L. Otis, MD

I. Menarche
   A. US average: 12.4 ± 1.2 years; range: 9-17 years; 95% by age 16; 98% by age 18.
   B. Later age at menarche observed in:
      1. Ballerinas: 15.4 ± 1.9 years.
      2. Some athletes training before menarche.
   C. Etiology and causal relationship to training not known.
      1. 1970's Frisch Hypothesis: critical height/weight ratio needed to initiate menstruation.
      2. Other factors also important.
      3. No prospective study has shown that training delays menarche.
   D. Consequences of delayed menarche.
      1. Risk of scoliosis (ballerinas).
      2. Risk of stress fractures (ballerinas).
      3. Risk of low bone mass hypothesized.
      4. Future fertility and menstrual pattern unknown.

II. Menstrual Cycle
   A. Menses normally occurs every 21 to 35 days.
   B. Three phases in the menstrual cycle.
      1. Follicular phase: endometrial lining of uterus grows.
      2. Luteal phase: begins with ovulation. Endometrial lining changes to support a fertilized egg.
      3. Menstruation: without fertilization, endometrial sloughing and menses result.

III. Exercise-Related Changes in Menstrual Cycle
   A. Luteal phase deficiency.
      1. Defined as reduced progesterone secretion during luteal phase. Basal body temperature (BBT) rises. Shortened luteal phase, diminished progesterone secretion, but normal total cycle length.
      2. Etiology, prognosis not known.

3. May be associated with infertility, endometrial hyperplasia, low bone mass.
4. Unknown if it is a phase in development of amenorrhea or a consistent pattern in active women.

B. Anovulation.
1. Definition: absent ovulation. No BBT rise.
2. Variable, unpredictable bleeding patterns: short cycles (<21 days) or long cycles (35-150 days).
3. Perform medical evaluation to determine cause.
4. No studies yet done on bone density.
5. Management: tailor to the individual.
   a. Monthly progestin therapy.
   b. Oral contraceptives.
   c. No therapy: tolerate irregular menses. Monitor for iron depletion, use contraception.
   d. Clomiphene for ovulation induction if pregnancy desired.

C. Primary amenorrhea
1. Workup indicated if:
   a. no spontaneous menstruation by age 14 and absent secondary sex characteristics.
   b. no spontaneous menstruation by age 16 and secondary sex characteristics present.
2. May not be related to athletic activity. Perform full endocrine evaluation.

D. Secondary amenorrhea. Definition varies in research.
1. After 1-3 spontaneous menses, no bleeding for 3-6 months.
2. Pregnancy excluded.
3. Exercise-associated amenorrhea only one of many causes.

IV. Exercise-Associated Amenorrhea (EAA)

A. Prevalence: observed in 2% to 5% of normal population and 3% to 66% of athletes. Reported in women participating in virtually all sports.

B. Cause: unknown, postulated to be reduction of hypothalamic gonadotropin-releasing hormone pulse generator due to negative feedback.

C. Hypothesized predisposing factors.
1. Late menarche.
2. Training prior to menarche.
3. Prior reproductive immaturity; oligomenorrhea, nulliparity.
4. Training factors: mileage, intensity.
5. Body weight.
6. Nutrition.
7. Stress.
8. Age <25.
9. Hormone changes with exercise.

V. Evaluation of Exercise-Associated Amenorrhea

A. EAA is a diagnosis of exclusion. Must rule out other causes before ascribing amenorrhea to exercise alone.

B. History.
1. Pubertal progression.
2. Weight history. Any indication of an eating disorder?
3. Menarche, menstrual pattern. Any relation to training? To injury and layoff?
4. Family pattern of maturation. Family history of osteoporosis, thyroid disease.
5. Exercise: onset, duration, intensity, frequency.

6. Psychosocial factors.
7. Sexual activity.
8. Medications: androgens, oral contraceptives.
9. Other illness: endocrine history, thyroid symptoms.
10. Diet: calcium, protein, iron.
11. Attitude toward problem. Amount known about problem.
12. Gynecological history: molimina, galactorrhea, symptoms of estrogen deficiency or of androgen excess (acne, hair growth), pregnancy history.
13. Injury history: surgery, stress fractures.

C. Physical examination.
   1. Vital signs, general appearance.
   2. Height, weight, consider measuring body composition.
   3. Sexual maturation rating.
   4. Skin: body hair distribution, acne, striae, carotenemia, lanugo hair.
   5. Thyroid.
   6. Breast: discharge.
   7. Pelvic: clitoral size, vaginal moistness, uterine size, ovarian size.

D. Laboratory.
   1. Screening: complete blood count + indices, thyroid-stimulating hormone (thyroxine, triiodothyronine, reverse triiodothyronine), prolactin, pregnancy test.
   2. Progesterone challenge (done only after a negative pregnancy test).
      a. 100-200 mg progesterone IM.
      b. 10 mg Provera PO for 5-14 days.
   3. Positive challenge: rule out cause of unopposed estrogen.
      a. Rule out androgen excess syndrome (PCO) with luteinizing hormone (LH)/follicle-stimulating hormone (FSH) (ratio will be 3 : 1).
      b. Consider measuring androgens (DHEA-S, testosterone) to verify.
      c. Rule out adrenal hyperplasia with cortisol, 17-OH progesterone.
   4. Negative challenge: inadequate estrogen production.
      a. Hypothalamic causes: anorexia, psychogenic (stress) amenorrhea, pituitary failure or masses, hypothalamic masses, EAA, low LH, low FSH.
      b. Ovarian failure, high FSH, low LH.
   5. Imaging tests.
      a. Consider pituitary image if low LH, low FSH (<10), normal prolactin and negative progestin challenge to rule out a pituitary lesion.
         (1) Lateral coned-down view of sella will detect a large pituitary mass in amenorrheic women (normal prolactin).
         (2) Use magnetic resonance imaging (gadolinium) to evaluate pituitary when prolactin is elevated.
      b. Consider pelvic ultrasound to assess uterus and ovaries if inadequate pelvic examination in adolescent. Ovarian size may be normal and not show cysts in androgen excess syndrome (PCO).
      c. Consider bone densitometry to determine risk of osteoporosis in women with hypoestrogenic amenorrhea. Use technique to measure trabecular bone (lumbar spine, Ward's triangle). Reproducibility and precision may be low outside research centers. Precision of 0.5% to 5% is close to rate of observed change in bone mass.
         (1) Dual photon absorptiometry (DPA).

(2) Cat scan (CT).
(3) Dual x-ray absorptiometry (DEXA).

E. Counseling/management.
1. If sexually active, advise that amenorrhea is not reliable contraception. Reinforce "safer sex." Remind woman that first ovulation after amenorrhea occurs before menstruation.
2. Calcium intake: 1500 mg/day elemental calcium maintains calcium balance. Exercise and calcium alone will not prevent bone loss.
   a. Dietary intake.
   b. Supplement; different amounts of calcium in each formulation. $CaCo_3$ highest. Emphasize hydration.
3. Optimize nutrition: increase by 250-1500 calories.
4. Training changes: decrease by 10% to 20%.
5. Weight changes: increase 5% to 10% if underweight.
6. Advise athlete of risk of bone loss.
   a. Decreased bone mineral content only recently described (1984) and researched. Few longitudinal studies done.
   b. Summary to date: 4% trabecular bone lost first year of amenorrhea and similar rates next 2-3 years.
   c. Rate of bone loss similar to bone loss seen after menopause.
   d. Bone mass of athletic women who resume menses spontaneously did not return to normal.
   e. Some bone loss is irreplaceable.
7. Replace estrogen.
   a. Oral contraceptives.
   b. Cyclic estrogen/progesterone therapy. Premarin, 0.625 mg on day 1-25. Provera 10 mg on days 11-25.
   c. Estraderm patch one every 3.5 days for 25 days. Provera 10 mg/day last 10-14 days.
   d. 2 and 3 do not provide contraception.
   e. None of these regimens have been studied in athletic women. In menopausal women and anorectic patients, estrogen is preserved but buildup of bone mass does not occur.

Bibliography

Bullen BA et al: Induction of menstrual disorders by strenuous exercise in untrained women, *N Engl J Med* 312:1349-1353, 1985.

Drinkwater BL et al: Bone mineral content of amenorrheic and eumonorrheic athletes, *N Engl J Med* 311:277-281, 1984.

Drinkwater BL, Bruemner B, Chesnut CH III: Menstrual history as a determinant of current bone density in young athletes, *JAMA* 263:545-548, 1990.

Drinkwater B et al: Bone mineral sensitivity after resumption of menses in amenorrheic athletes, *JAMA* 256:380-382, 1986.

Emans SJ: The athletic adolescent with amenorrhea, *Ped Ann* 13(8):605-612, 1986.

Lelt I: Menstrual problems during adolescence, *Ped Rev* 4(7):203-212, 1983.

Lindberg JS: Increased vertebral bone mass in response to reduced exercise in amenorrheic runners, *West J Med* 146:39-42, 1987.

Lloyd T et al: Women athletes with menstrual irregularities have increased musculoskeletal injuries, *Med Sci Sports Exerc* 18:374-379, 1985.

Loucks AB: Effects of exercise training on the menstrual cycle, *Med Sci Sports Exerc* 22(3):275-279, 1990.

Loucks AB, Horvath SM: Athletic amenorrhea: a review, *Med Sci Sports Exerc* 17(1):56-72, 1985.

Marcus R et al: Menstrual function and bone mass in elite women distance runners, *Ann Intern Med* 102(2):158-163, 1985.

Myburgh KH et al: Low bone density is an etiologic factor for stress fractures in athletes, *Ann Intern Med* 113:754-759, 1990.

Otis CL: Exercise-associated amenorrhea, *Clin Sports Med* 11:351-362, 1992.

Prior JC et al: Spinal bone loss and ovulatory disturbances, *N Engl J Med* 343:1221-1227, 1990.

Puhl J, Puhl B, Harmon C, editors: *The menstrual cycle and physical activity*, Champaign, Ill, 1986, Human Kinetics.

Shangold M: Evaluation and management of menstrual dysfunction in athletes, *JAMA* 263(12):1665-1669, 1990.

Soules MR et al: Luteal phase deficiency: characterization of reproductive hormones over the menstrual cycle, *J Clin Endocrinol Metab* 69:804-812, 1989.

Warren M: Effects of exercise on pubertal progression and reproductive function in girls, *JCEM* 51(5):1150-1157, 1980.

CHAPTER 23

Pregnancy

Raul Artal, MD

Philip J. Buckenmeyer, PhD

Robert A. Wiswell, PhD

I. General Overview
   A. Physical activity patterns of women in reproductive age and pregnancy.
      1. It is recommended that every adult in the United States should participate in 30 minutes or more of moderately intensive physical activity each day, if possible.[30]
      2. 15% of women in reproductive age regularly engage in exercise and most plan to continue with a regular exercise regimen during pregnancy.[34]
      3. Physician's role to advise pregnant patients about limitations, contraindications, potential risks, warning signs, and special concerns.
   B. Guidelines for exercise in pregnancy have been issued by the American College of Obstetricians and Gynecologists (ACOG) and the American College of Sports Medicine (ACSM).

II. Physiological Considerations
   A. Factors associated with pregnancy.
      1. Cardiovascular changes.
         a. Increases in blood volume (40% by end of pregnancy), cardiac output (15% to 20%), stroke volume (increasing 30% by the second trimester), and resting heart rate (approximately 15 bpm; 50% of the increase occurs within the first 8 weeks of gestation).[20]
         b. Mean arterial blood pressure falls during midpregnancy (approximately 10 torr) as a result of a decrease in systemic vascular resistance.[20]

*In summary, this chapter has presented an overview of the current issues pertaining to pregnant women which primary care physicians interested in the sports medicine field might find useful in their practice. Topics dealing with the pregnant athlete include: basic physiological responses to exercise, pre-exercise medical considerations, potential risks of exercise, orthopedic injuries, nutritional needs, exercise prescription, and influence of physical conditioning. The content of this chapter is based upon current guidelines established by the American College of Obstetrics and Gynecology (ACOG) and the American College of Sports Medicine (ACSM).

c. Regional blood flow changes in which blood flow to all tissues is increased with specific increase to the uterus and placenta during the last trimester,[27] as well as considerable increases in blood flow to renal and cutaneous circulation.[20]
d. Hemodynamic changes are specific to body position and can result in supine hypotensive syndrome.[2]

2. Respiratory changes.[7]
   a. Minute ventilation at rest increases by 40% to 50% as a result of increased tidal volume.
   b. Lung compliance increases, and airway resistance decreases.
   c. Early in gestation there is an increase in arterial oxygen tension and a decreased arterial Pco_2. This decrease in Po_2 is normalized by late gestation.
   d. Acid-base balance is maintained in pregnancy.
   e. Oxygen consumption is higher at rest during pregnancy compared to that in age-matched, nonpregnant women.
3. Endocrine changes.[33]
   a. Pregnancy is characterized by a state of reduced peripheral insulin sensitivity and hyperinsulinemia that leads to:
      (1) Increased peripheral glucose utilization.
      (2) Decreased plasma glucose levels.
      (3) Increased tissue storage of glycogen.
      (4) Decreased hepatic glucose production.
   b. Significant increases in total triiodothyronine and thyroxine occur, which may help explain the increase in basal metabolic rate.

B. Physiological responses to exercise and pregnancy.
   1. Maternal response to cardiovascular changes during exercise.
      a. Increase in cardiac output and stroke volume during submaximal exercise.
      b. Splanchnic blood flow decreases approximately 50% during mild to moderate exercise and possibly more with greater intensities. Research suggests that 50% of uterine blood flow must be redistributed before fetus is affected.[40]
      c. Tendency toward hemoconcentration during exercise.[25]
   2. Maternal response to pulmonary changes during exercise:[7]
      a. Respiratory frequency increases with mild exercise compared to nonpregnant controls. No difference between groups at moderate or maximal exercise effort ($Vo_{2\,max}$).
      b. Oxygen consumption, CO_2 production, and tidal volume increase with mild and moderate exercise intensity, with no difference in response between pregnant and nonpregnant women. At $Vo_{2\,max}$, however, there is significantly less oxygen consumption in pregnant women than in nonpregnant women (as indexed per body weight).
      c. Ventilatory equivalent (V_E/Vo_2) significantly differs between pregnant and nonpregnant women at similar exercise intensities, although V_E/Vo_2 is generally higher in pregnant women during exercise.
      d. Respiratory quotient (Vco_2/Vo_2) is significantly greater during higher intensity exercise, suggesting a greater dependence on carbohydrates as the primary fuel source.
   3. Maternal response to body temperature regulation during exercise.
      a. Thermal balance can be maintained during submaximal levels of exercise under mild environmental conditions, particularly by reducing exercise intensity as gestation progresses.
      b. Threshold for fetal teratogenesis is believed to be 39.2°C.[26]

4. Maternal response to hormonal levels during exercise.
   a. Increase in catecholamines may increase frequency and amplitude of contractions and susceptibility to premature labor.[10]
   b. Plasma insulin levels decrease significantly during prolonged exercise.[36]
   c. Ovarian hormones, estradiol and progesterone, increase during exercise, particularly during strenuous exercise.[32]
   d. Exercise training during pregnancy elevates endogenous opioids.[38]
5. Maternal response to substrate utilization during exercise.
   a. Energy demand during exercise may increase 10-fold or more above resting levels depending on activity level.[11]
   b. Prolonged strenuous exercise may induce hypoglycemia more rapidly during pregnancy (i.e., within 45 minutes of continuous exercise at 50-60% $VO_{2\,max}$).[36]
6. Fetal response to substrate availability during exercise.
   a. Glucose is primary fuel source for fetus during pregnancy.[21]
   b. Maternal hypoglycemia, potentially resulting from continuous, vigorous exercise, may place a greater metabolic stress (glucose deficit) on the fetus.

III. Clinical Evaluation
   A. Preexercise considerations.
      1. Screening: patients should be questioned about the following factors.
         a. Absolute contraindications to exercise.[2]
            (1) Pregnancy-induced hypertension.
            (2) Preterm rupture of membranes.
            (3) Preterm labor during the prior or current pregnancy or both.
            (4) Incompetent cervix/cerclage.
            (5) Persistent second- or third-trimester bleeding.
            (6) Intrauterine growth retardation.
         b. Relative contraindications to exercise: these factors deserve careful evaluation and observation but need not be absolutely restrictive.
            (1) Chronic hypertension or active thyroid.
            (2) Cardiovascular disease.
            (3) Pulmonary disease.
            (4) Diabetes mellitus (type 1).
   B. Medical history (checklist of items to consider):

		Family History	
1. Present:	**2. Past:**	**Relative**	**Date**
_____ Vaginal bleeding	_____ Diabetes	_____	_____
_____ Vaginal discharge/odor	_____ Hypertension	_____	_____
_____ Vomiting	_____ Heart disease	_____	_____
_____ Constipation	_____ Rheumatic fever	_____	_____
_____ Headache	_____ Mitral valve prolapse	_____	_____
_____ Abdominal pain	_____ Kidney disease/urinary tract infection	_____	_____
_____ Urinary complaints			
_____ Febrile episode	_____ Nervous and mental problems	_____	_____
_____ Orthopedic problems	_____ Epilepsy	_____	_____
_____ Others	_____ Hepatitis/liver disease	_____	_____
Medications:	_____ Varicosities/phlebitis	_____	_____
List _____________	_____ Thyroid dysfunction	_____	_____

1. Present:	2. Past:	Family History Relative	Date
	_____ Blood transfusions	_____	_____
	_____ Use of tobacco	_____	_____
	_____ RH sensitized	_____	_____
	_____ Tuberculosis	_____	_____
	_____ Asthma	_____	_____
	_____ Allergies (drugs)	_____	_____
	_____ Gynecological surgery	_____	_____
	_____ Hospitalizations	_____	_____
	_____ Anesthetic complications	_____	_____
	_____ Abnormal Pap test results	_____	_____
	_____ Uterine anomaly	_____	_____

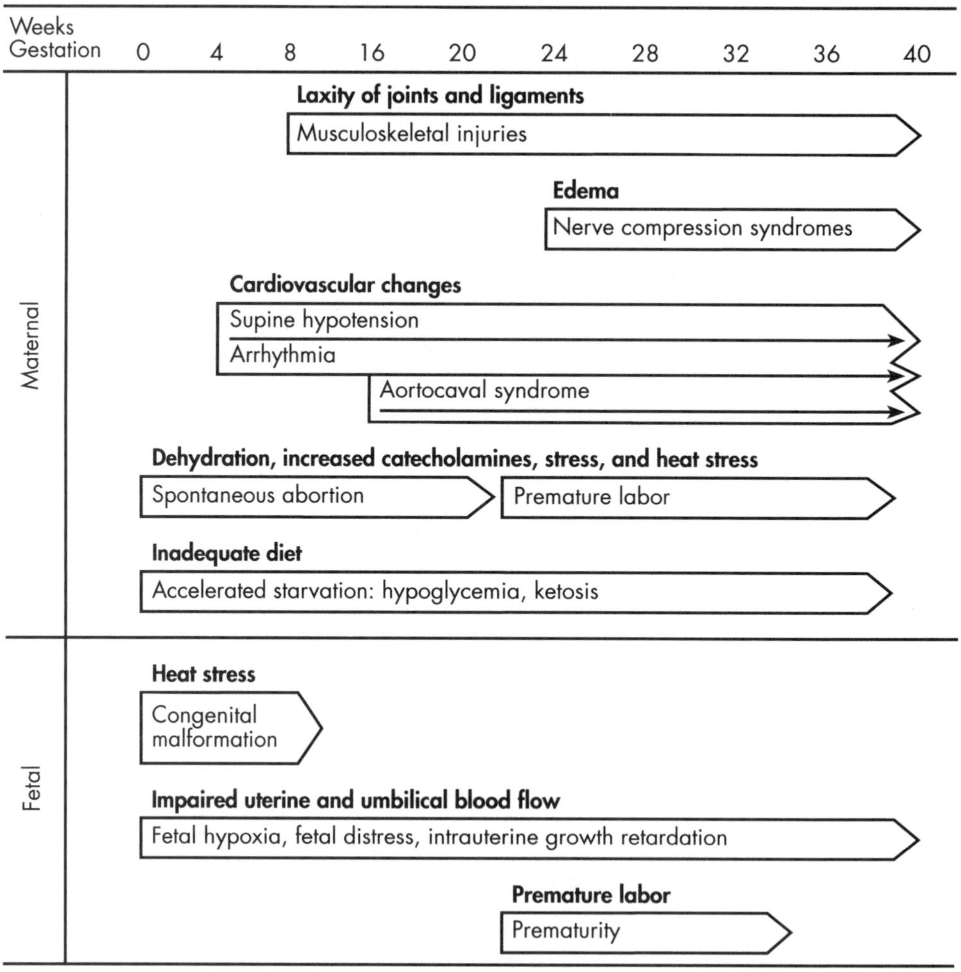

Weeks Gestation 0 4 8 16 20 24 28 32 36 40

Maternal

Laxity of joints and ligaments
Musculoskeletal injuries

Edema
Nerve compression syndromes

Cardiovascular changes
Supine hypotension
Arrhythmia
Aortocaval syndrome

Dehydration, increased catecholamines, stress, and heat stress
Spontaneous abortion
Premature labor

Inadequate diet
Accelerated starvation: hypoglycemia, ketosis

Fetal

Heat stress
Congenital malformation

Impaired uterine and umbilical blood flow
Fetal hypoxia, fetal distress, intrauterine growth retardation

Premature labor
Prematurity

FIGURE 23-1
Potential mechanisms leading to injuries during exercise in pregnancy. (From Artal R et al: Exercise guidelines for pregnancy. In Artal R, Wiswell RA, Drinkwater BL, editors: *Exercise in pregnancy,* ed 2, Baltimore, 1991, Williams & Wilkins.)

C. Laboratory tests: useful in assessing risk in the pregnant woman who wishes to exercise.
   1. Blood type, RH type, antibody screen.
   2. Hematocrit/hemoglobin.
   3. Urine culture/screen.
   4. Diabetes screen.
D. Theoretical risks of exercise in pregnancy (Fig. 23-1).

IV. Orthopedic Injuries Related to Pregnancy[23]
A. Nerve compression syndromes.[18]
   1. Carpal tunnel syndrome.
   2. Ulnar nerve compression.
   3. Tarsal tunnel syndrome.
   4. Peroneal nerve compression.
B. Back pain.
   1. Sacroiliac dysfunction.
   2. Osteitis condensans.
   3. Lumbar disc herniation (rare occurrence).[24]
   4. Meralgia paresthetica.
   5. Spondylolisthesis.
C. Hip pain. Avascular necrosis of femoral head.[14]
D. Pubic pain.
   1. Symphyseal separation.
   2. Symphysitis.
   3. Symphyseal dislocations.
   4. Osteitis pubis.
   5. Pubic stress fracture.
E. Knee and lower leg pain.
   1. Chondromalacia patella.
   2. Edema-induced compartment syndromes.
F. Miscellaneous.
   1. Diastasis recti.
   2. Coccyodynia.

V. Nutritional Concerns of the Pregnant Athlete
A. Requirements.
   1. Caloric intake: at least 300 extra calories per day compared to nonpregnant status; additional calories should meet activity caloric expenditure so that significant weight loss does not occur.[20] These extra calories are believed to suffice during pregnancy since it is assumed that pregnant women also tend to decrease their level of activity during gestation.[29]
      a. Weight gain averages between 10 and 12 kg.
      b. Weight gain of <1.0 kg/month in second and third trimesters is insufficient.[31]
   2. Protein. Additional 10 g of protein or total of 60-100 g/day to maintain 12% protein intake in daily diet.[29]
   3. Iron.
      a. Daily oral supplement of 30 mg of elemental iron.[29]
      b. It has been recommended that an 800 mg total be accumulated in the last half of the pregnancy.
   4. Calcium.
      a. Daily allowance of 1200 mg.[29]
      b. A quart of cow's milk would provide for most calcium and vitamin D needs of pregnancy.
   5. Sodium.
      a. Should adhere to diet composed of natural foods.

b. Processed foods (already seasoned with salt) should be used in moderation.
6. Folic acid.
   a. Dietary need of this nutrient increases with pregnancy.
   b. Should consider having leafy vegetables, oranges, legumes, eggs, whole grain cereals, and wheat germ as part of diet to obtain folic acid.
7. Vitamins.
   a. Need for additional vitamins, beyond the prescribed prenatal vitamins recommended by an obstetrician, remains unclear.
   b. Studies of certain vitamins, like C[17] and E,[1] suggest that supplementation does not provide any significant advantage to exercising subjects who were previously ingesting an adequate amount.
   c. A variety of foods from each of the basic food groups should be sufficient for meeting the nutrient needs of the athlete.
8. Water.
   a. Consumption of 8-12 cups of water daily is suggested for maintenance of normal hydration and expansion of total body water while physically active.
   b. Increase in total body water is important for maintaining normal body temperature during gestation since this is an important determinant of pregnancy outcome.

B. Nutritional risks during pregnancy.[13]
1. Pregravid weight 15% below or 20% above suggested weight for height.
2. Insufficient or excessive rate of weight gain.
3. Age <15 years or >35 years.
4. Presence of social, cultural, religious, psychological, or economic factors that limit or affect adequacy of nutrition.
5. History of low birthweight baby or other obstetrical problems.
6. Chronic disease, such as diabetes, thyroid disorders, or sickle cell disease.
7. Presence of twins or triplets.
8. Pica.
9. Abnormal laboratory values, such as low hemoglobin level, abnormal blood glucose level, albuminuria, and ketonuria.

VI. Exercise Prescription for Pregnant Women.[3,8]

A. Type (mode) of exercise.
1. There is no evidence that any aerobic or anaerobic activity needs to be avoided in healthy pregnant women, except scuba diving.[16] However, some activities have inherent risks (e.g., downhill skiing, contact sports).
2. Activities that increase the probability of even mild abdominal trauma or have unusual balance and agility requirements should be limited or carefully performed and/or monitored.
3. Water exercises are encouraged in pregnancy. Hyperbaric exercise requires caution; scuba diving is contraindicated in pregnancy.

B. Intensity.
1. Intensity of exercise is usually self-monitored in pregnancy. Although pregnant women generally reduce the intensity of their exercise program without specific recommendations, strenuous exercise should be avoided.
2. Clinical monitoring and/or supervision is recommended for women participating in high intensity, competitive exercise.

3. Lower intensity training (50% to 60% of heart rate reserve [HRR]) has been proven successful at increasing the maximal oxygen consumption of pregnant women.
4. Intensity should be modified according to maternal symptoms.

C. Duration.
1. The duration of activity should be based on environmental conditions and prior level of physical condition.
2. Long duration activity should include rehydration during the exercise itself.

D. Frequency: as in the nonpregnant state, should be regular (three to four times per week) as opposed to intermittent activity. However, intermittent activities should not be discouraged since the state of pregnancy lends itself to life-style changes and behavioral modification.

E. Programming.
1. Precautions.[2]
   a. Avoid exercise in supine position after the first trimester.
   b. Avoid motionless standing.
   c. Avoid activities that require significant balancing.
   d. Avoid activities that involve potential for abdominal trauma.
2. Tolerance end points.[10]
   a. Pain of any kind.
   b. Uterine contractions (15-minute intervals or four or more per hour).
   c. Vaginal bleeding.
   d. Dizziness, faintness.
   e. Shortness of breath.
   f. Palpitations, tachycardia.
   g. Nausea/vomiting.
   h. Back pain.
   i. Pubic or hip pain.
   j. Difficulty in walking.
   k. Generalized edema.
   l. Numbness in any part of body.
   m. Visual disturbances.
   n. Decreased fetal activity.

F. Influence of physical conditioning during pregnancy.
1. Outcome issues.
   a. Maternal.[4]
      (1) Women who exercise before pregnancy and continue to do so during pregnancy tend to weigh less, gain less weight, and deliver smaller babies than controls.
      (2) All women, regardless of initial level of physical activity, decrease their activity as pregnancy progresses.
      (3) No information is available to assess whether active women have better pregnancy outcomes than their sedentary counterparts. No information is available on sedentary women.
      (4) Physically fit pregnant women appear to tolerate pain in labor better.
   b. Fetal.
      (1) Research reports suggest that strenuous training programs through pregnancy coupled with a deficient diet may lead to reduced birthweight and intrauterine growth retardation.[28,37]
      (2) Occasional episodes of fetal bradycardia have been recorded with no adverse outcomes; however, the clinical significance is unknown.[9]

2. Trainability.[39]
   a. Similar exercise intensities between untrained and trained pregnant women are perceived as less strenuous to the physically conditioned.
   b. Exercise capacity can be enhanced as a result of training.
   c. Heart rates, at submaximal workloads, can be decreased in trained pregnant.
   d. Submaximal cardiac output and stroke volume is not influenced by low-intensity training.
   e. Low-intensity training does not appear to have any negative maternal cardiovascular effects.

References

1. Aikawa K et al: Effect of exercise endurance training of rodents on vitamin E tissue levels and red blood cell hemolysis, *Biosci Rep* 4:253-257, 1984.
2. American College of Obstetricians and Gynecologists: Exercise during pregnancy and the postpartum period, Technical Bulletin no. 189, Washington, DC, 1994, ACOG.
3. American College of Sports Medicine: *Guidelines for exercise testing and prescription,* ed 4, Philadelphia, 1991, Lea & Febiger.
4. Artal R, Dorey FJ, Kirschbaum TH: Effect of maternal exercise on pregnancy outcome. In Artal R, Wiswell RA, Drinkwater BL, editors: *Exercise in pregnancy,* ed 2, Baltimore, 1991, Williams & Wilkins.
5. Artal R, Posner MD: Fetal responses to maternal exercise. In Artal R, Wiswell RA, Drinkwater BL, editors: *Exercise in pregnancy,* ed 2, Baltimore, 1991, Williams & Wilkins.
6. Artal R, Wiswell RA, Drinkwater BL, editors: *Exercise in pregnancy,* ed 2, Baltimore, Williams & Wilkins, 1991.
7. Artal R et al: Pulmonary responses to exercise in pregnancy. In Artal R, Wiswell RA, Drinkwater BL, editors: *Exercise in pregnancy,* ed 2, Baltimore, 1991, Williams & Wilkins.
8. Artal R et al: Exercise guidelines for pregnancy. In Artal R, Wiswell RA, Drinkwater BL, editors: *Exercise in pregnancy,* ed 2, Baltimore, 1991, Williams & Wilkins.
9. Artal R et al: Fetal bradycardia induced by maternal exercise, *Lancet* 11:258-260, 1984.
10. Artal R et al: Exercise in pregnancy. Maternal cardiovascular and metabolic responses in normal pregnancy, *Am J Obstet Gynecol* 140:123-127, 1981.
11. Astrand PO, Rodahl K: *Textbook of work physiology: physiological basis of exercise,* ed 3, New York, 1986, McGraw-Hill.
12. Berg G, Hammer M, Moeller-Nielsen J: Low back pain during pregnancy, *Obstet Gynecol* 71:71-75, 1988.
13. Butterfield G, King JC: Nutritional needs of physically active women. In Artal R, Wiswell RA, Drinkwater BL, editors: *Exercise in pregnancy,* ed 2, Baltimore, 1991, Williams & Wilkins.
14. Cheng N, Burssens A, Mulier JC: Pregnancy and post-pregnancy avascular necrosis of the femoral head, *Arch Orthop Trauma Surg* 100:199-210, 1982.
15. Danforth DN: Pregnancy and labor from the vantage point of the physical therapist, *Am J Phys Med* 46:653-658, 1967.
16. Fife WP: Effects of diving on pregnancy, *Undersea Med Soc* 36, 1980.
17. Fishbaine B, Butterfield G: Ascorbic acid status of running and sedentary men, *Int J Vitam Nutr Res* 54:273, 1984.
18. Gould JS, Wissinger HA: Carpal tunnel syndrome in pregnancy, *South Med J* 71:144-145, 154, 1978.
19. Hauth JO, Gilstrap LC, Widmer K: Fetal heart rate reactivity before and after maternal jogging during the third trimester, *Am J Obstet Gynecol* 142:545-547, 1982.
20. Hytten FE, Chamberlain G, editors: *Clinical physiology in obstetrics,* Oxford, 1980, Blackwell.
21. Ingermann RI: Control of placental glucose transfer, *Placenta* 8:557-571, 1987.
22. Jarrett JC, Spellacy WN: Jogging during pregnancy: an improved outcome? *Obstet Gynecol* 61:705-709, 1983.
23. Karzel RP, Friedman MJ: Orthopedic injuries in pregnancy. In Artal R, Wiswell RA, Drinkwater BL, editors: *Exercise in pregnancy,* ed 2, Baltimore, 1991, Williams & Wilkins.
24. LaBan MM, Perrin JCS, Latimer FR: Pregnancy and the herniated lumbar disc, *Arch Phys Med Rehabil* 64:319-321, 1983.
25. McMurray RG et al: Pregnancy-induced changes in the maximal physiological responses during swimming, *J Appl Physiol* 71:1454-1459, 1991.
26. Milunsky A et al: Maternal heat exposure and neural tube defects, *JAMA* 268:882-885, 1992.
27. Morton MJ: Maternal hemodynamics in pregnancy. In Artal R, Wiswell RA, Drinkwater BL, editors: *Exercise in pregnancy,* ed 2, Baltimore, 1991, Williams & Wilkins.

28. Naeye RL, Peters E: Working during pregnancy, effects on the fetus, *Pediatrics* 69:724-727, 1982.
29. National Research Council. *Recommended Daily Allowances,* ed 10. Washington, DC, 1989, National Academy of Sciences.
30. Pate RR et al: Physical activity and public health: a recommendation from the Centers for Disease Control and Prevention and the American College of Sports Medicine, *JAMA* 273(5):402-407, 1995.
31. Pitkin RM: Obstetrics and gynecology. In Schneider HA, Anderson CE, Coursin DB, editors: *Nutritional support of medical practice,* Hagerstown, MD, 1977, Harper & Row.
32. Rauramo I, Salminen K, Laatikainen T: Release of beta-endorphin in response to physical exercise in non-pregnant and pregnant women, *Acta Obstet Gynaecol Scand* 65:609-612, 1986.
33. Romem Y, Masaki DI, Artal R: Physiological and endocrine adjustments to pregnancy. In Artal R, Wiswell RA, Drinkwater BL, editors: *Exercise in pregnancy,* ed 2, Baltimore, 1991, Williams & Wilkins.
34. Sady SP, Carpenter MW: Aerobic exercise during pregnancy: special considerations, *Sports Med* 7:357-375, 1989.
35. St John W: Body composition of female college age swimmers. Master's thesis, University of Cincinnati, 1978, p 15.
36. Soultanakis HN: Glucose homeostasis during pregnancy in response to prolonged exercise. Dissertation, University of Southern California Graduate School, 1989.
37. Tafari N, Naeye RL, Gobzie A: Effects of maternal undernutrition and heavy physical work during pregnancy on birth weight, *Br J Obstet Gynaecol* 87:222-226, 1980.
38. Varrassi G, Bazzano C, Edwards T: Effects of physical activity on maternal plasma beta-endorphin levels and perception of pain, *Am J Obstet Gynecol* 160:707-712, 1989.
39. Wallace JP, Wiswell RA: Maternal cardiovascular response to exercise during pregnancy. In Artal R, Wiswell RA, Drinkwater BL, editors: *Exercise in pregnancy,* ed 2, Baltimore, 1991, Williams & Wilkins.
40. Wilkening RB, Meschia G: Fetal oxygen uptake, oxygenation, and acid-base balance as a function of uterine blood flow, *Am J Physiol* 244:H749-H755, 1983.

CHAPTER 24

The Female Athlete Triad

Carol L. Otis, MD

I. Definition
   A. A syndrome of three interrelated medical disorders (disordered eating, amenorrhea, and osteoporosis) described in active women.
   B. Disordered eating: A spectrum of harmful and ineffective methods of weight control that occur in a continuum of severity. These practices range from:
      1. Inadvertently failing to meet basic caloric needs for activity.
      2. Voluntary starvation/fasting.
      3. Binging and purging.
      4. Use of diet pills.
      5. Use of laxatives, diuretics, enemas.
      6. Self-induced vomiting.
      7. Anorexia nervosa.
      8. Bulimia nervosa.
   C. Amenorrhea: can result from any pattern of disordered eating, but anorexia in particular.
      1. Primary amenorrhea.
         a. No menarche in a girl age 16 with secondary sex characteristics.
         b. No menarche in a girl age 14 without secondary characteristics present.
      2. Secondary amenorrhea.
         a. After three spontaneous menses, no menses for 3 consecutive months.
         b. Many medical problems can cause amenorrhea.
   D. Osteoporosis.
      1. A disease characterized by extensive bone loss and risk for fractures.
      2. In certain forms of secondary amenorrhea the lack of ovarian hormones (similar to what occurs at menopause) can result in osteoporosis.

II. Underlying Pathogenesis of the Triad
   A. Pressure to achieve an unrealistically low body weight, body fat percentage, or lean appearance to achieve success in an athletic situation. Pres-

DIAGNOSTIC CRITERIA FOR ANOREXIA NERVOSA

- Refusal to maintain body weight at or above a minimally normal weight for age and height (e.g., weight loss leading to maintenance of body weight <85% of that expected; failure to make expected weight gain during period of growth, leading to body weight <85% of that expected).
- Intense fear of gaining weight or becoming fat, even though underweight.
- Disturbance in the way in which one's body weight or shape is experienced; undue influence of body weight or shape on self-evaluations; denial of the seriousness of the current low body weight.
- In postmenarchal females, amenorrhea (i.e., the absence of at least three consecutive menstrual cycles). A woman is also considered to have amenorrhea if her periods occur only following hormone (e.g., estrogen) administration.

SPECIFY TYPE:

Restricting type—During the episode of anorexia nervosa, the person does not regularly engage in binge eating or purging behavior (i.e., self-induced vomiting or the misuse of laxatives or diuretics).

Binge eating/purging type—During the episode of anorexia nervosa, the person regularly engages in binge eating or purging behavior (i.e., self-induced vomiting or the misuse of laxatives or diuretics).

DIAGNOSTIC CRITERIA FOR BULIMIA NERVOSA

- Recurrent episodes of binge eating. An episode of binge eating is characterized by both of the following:
  —Eating in a discrete period of time (e.g., within any 2-hour period) an amount of food that is definitely larger than most people would eat during a similar period of time and under similar circumstances.
  —A sense of lack of control over eating during the episode (e.g., a feeling that one cannot stop eating or control what or how much one is eating).
- Recurrent inappropriate compensatory behaviors both occur, on average, at least twice a week for 3 months.
- The binge eating and inappropriate compensatory behaviors both occur, on average, at least twice a week for 3 months.
- Self-evaluation is unduly influenced by body shape and weight.
- The disturbance does not occur exclusively during episodes of anorexia nervosa.

SPECIFY TYPE:

Purging type: The person regularly engages in the self-induced vomiting or misuse of laxatives or diuretics.

Nonpurging type: The person uses other inappropriate compensatory behaviors, such as fasting or excessive exercise but does not regularly engage in self-induced vomiting or the misuse of laxatives or diuretics.

Adapted from DSM-IV: *Diagnostic and statistical manual of mental disorders*, Washington, DC, 1994, American Psychiatric Association.

sure is applied by coaches, trainers, peers, self, and parents and is reinforced by societal beliefs.

B. After puberty women naturally gain body fat, normally 20% to 26%, to support reproductive function. Men gain muscle mass and have 14% to 20% body fat. All women are judged by societal standards of attractiveness. The current standard is unrealistically thin.

C. After puberty athletic women, particularly those in sports where a lean (prepubertal) appearance is believed advantageous for performance or judging, are encouraged *to lose weight to improve performance*.

D. After puberty men are encouraged *to gain weight to improve performance.*
E. No scientific evidence exists to support one ideal body weight or body fat percentage for athletic performance. Individual somatotypes, training regime, proper nutrition, genetic endowment, and mental outlook are more important for optimal performance. Each individual has an individual range of weight/body fat percentage that is healthy for him or her.
F. Athletes at most risk for developing the triad are adolescents and young women training in sports at an elite level where appearance or low body weight is emphasized.
G. Adolescence is a vulnerable period characterized by:
   1. Change in body composition, hormonal status.
   2. Change in athletic abilities with change in body.
   3. Pressure to achieve college scholarship, turn professional, or succeed in sports where success occurs before puberty (i.e., gymnastics).
   4. Peer pressure and developmental issues.

III. Pathogenic Weight Control Techniques
A. Faced with pressure to achieve or maintain unrealistically low body weight and or body fat percentage, the active person relies on "pathogenic weight control techniques" in a misguided attempt to lose weight.
B. Are athletes at greater risk?
C. These weight control techniques are harmful, and impair performance. They result in starvation (loss of muscle) and/or loss of body water (dehydration) rather than the desired loss of body fat.
D. Short- and long-term morbidity in many organ systems.
E. Psychological sequelae: depression, low self-esteem, risk for drug use, risk for suicide.
F. Early recognition and intervention important for prognosis.
G. At the extreme end of the spectrum are bulimia nervosa and anorexia nervosa, both associated with acute and chronic morbidity and mortality. These are among the most common and most serious disorders of young adults.

IV. Secondary Amenorrhea
A. Exercise-associated amenorrhea (EAA) is one of the many forms of hypothalamic amenorrhea.
   1. Caused by decreased gonadotropin-releasing hormone pulses to the pituitary.
   2. Anorexia amenorrhea is another form of secondary hypothalamic amenorrhea.
B. EAA is a diagnosis of exclusion. Full individualized evaluation for each woman is needed to rule out other causes.
   1. Workup should include:
      a. Medical and gynecological history, training history, history of weight, 24 hour diet recall, methods of weight control, contraception.
      b. Physical examination: full pelvic, thyroid, breast (galactorrhea?), skin (acne, hair pattern, striae?).
      c. Laboratory tests: thyroid-stimulating hormone, luteinizing hormone, follicle-stimulating hormone, prolactin, complete blood count.
      d. Others include DHEA-S, testosterone, estradiol.
   2. May be reversible by "life-style changes."
      a. Improved nutrition (250-750 calories/day)
      b. Reduction in training intensity (5% to 20%).

      c. Weight gain (5-15 lb).
   3. Other treatment.
      a. Contraception counseling.
      b. Assure 1500 mg of calcium/day.
      c. Consider bone densitometry.
      d. Consider hormone replacement.

V. Osteoporosis
   A. Skeletal accretion occurs until third decade.
   B. Exercise, calcium intake, and genetic and hormonal influences act to determine peak bone mass.
   C. Hypoestrogenemia (with or without nutritional deficits) causes bone loss at any age, not just after menopause.
   D. Bone lost may be irreversible.
   E. Affected young women reach fracture threshold earlier.
   F. Stress fractures may be marker of "premature" osteoporosis.

VI. The Future
   A. Advocate health and realistic body image for young, active women.
   B. Educate coaches, parents, trainers, peers, and women about nutrition, and proper training techniques (Code of Ethics).
   C. Early recognition of "warning signs."
   D. Screening for the triad at preparticipation examinations upon presentation of a clinical problem such as weight change, depression, cardiac symptoms, dehydration, or stress fracture.
   E. Early treatment by multidisciplinary team approach.
   F. Need for research to document etiology, pathogenesis, screening techniques, and therapy.

Bibliography

Brownell KD, Rodin J, Wilmore JH, editors: *Eating, body weight and performance in athletes,* Philadelphia, 1992, Lea & Febiger.

Drinkwater BL et al: Bone mineral density after resumption of menses in amenorrheic athletes, *JAMA* 256:380, 1986.

Nattiv A et al: The female athlete triad. In Agostini R, editor: *Medical and orthopedic issues of active and athletic women,* Philadelphia, 1994, Hanley and Belfus.

Otis CL: Exercise-associated amenorrhea, *Clin Sports Med* 11:351, 1992.

Shangold M et al: Evaluation and management of menstrual dysfunction in athletes, *JAMA* 263:1665, 1990.

Yeager KK et al: The female athlete triad: disordered eating, amenorrhea, osteoporosis [commentary], *Med Sci Sports Exerc* 25:775, 1993.

CHAPTER 25

Osteoporosis

Carol L. Otis, MD

I. Definition
  A. Osteoporosis is a disease "characterized by low bone mass and microarchitectural deterioration, leading to enhanced bone fragility and a consequent increase in fracture risk."[1]
  B. Normal: bone mineral density <1 STD below mean.
  C. Osteopenia: bone mineral density between 1 and 2.5 STD below mean.
  D. Osteoporosis: bone mineral density >2.5 STD below mean.
  E. Severe osteoporosis: bone mineral density >2.5 STD below mean *and* one or more fractures.[6]

II. Scope of problem (National Osteoporosis Foundation 1991)
  A. 25 million U.S. women; 75 million people worldwide.
  B. 1.3 million fractures/year in the United States.
  C. 25% of women >age 60 have spinal fracture.
  D. 32% of women and 17% of men >age 80 have hip fracture.
  E. Post hip fracture: 15% mortality in 3 months. Pain, suffering, life-style change.
  F. Health care costs estimated at $10 billion/year in United States alone.

III. Risk Factors
  A. Caucasian, North European descent, + family history.
  B. Female, fair, small boned, short stature, lean.
  C. Sedentary life-style, immobilization, high caffeine and alcohol use, smoker.
  D. Lack of calcium, vitamin D.
  E. Estrogen or androgen deficiency at any time.
  F. Medication use: glucocorticoids, anticonvulsants, excess thyroid.
  G. Other chronic diseases: rheumatoid arthritis (R.A.), diabetes.

IV. Determinants of Bone Mass
  A. 70% of total = pubertal growth.
  B. Peak trabecular mass achieved by age 30, cortical by age 35.

C. Bone loss.
   1. Decline begins after peak: ? remodeling imbalance.
   2. Rapid decline after menopause.
D. Genetics determines 70% to 80% peak bone mass.
E. Calcium intake protective and additive during growth and development.
F. Hormonal deficiency impairs bone mass, may be irreversible.[3]

V. Role of Exercise
   A. Exercise affects strength and load-bearing capacity of bone by modifying density, distribution, and/or mass.
   B. Principles.
      1. Specificity: site affected is specific to type of exercise.
      2. Overload: training must exceed normal load.
      3. Reversibility: after cessation of training training effect is lost.
      4. Initial values: lowest initial values show most improvement.
      5. Diminishing return: individuals have genetically determined maximums. As maximum is approached, rate of gain slows and plateaus.
   C. Extent of impact of exercise and types of beneficial exercise still being researched.[7]
      1. Weight bearing important.
      2. Loss of bone due to inactivity occurs more rapidly than bone gain.
      3. Muscle mass, strength may have greater effect on bone mass than body weight or body mass index.[12]
   D. Normal hormonal levels needed for effect of exercise to be beneficial.

VI. Young Women (<35 years).
   A. Physiology: Gaining peak bone mass.
      1. In cross-sectional studies of women engaging in weight-bearing activity, bone mass increased 6% to 10% more than in sedentary controls.[11] May have facilitated achieving peak bone mass. Muscle mass may be factor.
      2. In longitudinal studies, (1-2 years) minimal increase seen.[13]
      3. Amenorrheic athletes have lower bone mass.[3,14]
   B. Anorectic women at high risk for osteoporosis and vertebral fractures.[10]
   C. Osteoporosis is one of the disorders of the female athlete triad.[14]

VII. Mature Women (35-50 years).
   A. Lack of data.
   B. Physiology: gradual loss of trabecular bone.
   C. Limited studies show higher bone mass in active women, but few gains with longitudinal exercise program.

VIII. Postmenopausal Women (>50 years).
   A. Physiology: accelerated loss of bone due to hormone deficiency. Estrogen more important than exercise.[8]
   B. Swimmers have bone mass similar to controls.[9] Estrogen users have higher bone mass.

IX. Exercise and Prevention of Hip Fracture
   A. Fewer hip fractures in individuals with higher levels of activity.[2]
   B. Physical activity may help not only with bone mass but also balance, strength, coordination in preventing falls.

X. Exercise Prescription
   A. No prospective studies done to define optimal training programs for bone health. Individually determine goals and capabilities using exercise principles.

B. Specificity: train with weight-bearing activities, emphasize areas at risk for fracture (hip, spine, wrist). Increases in muscle strength and mass may be important and can be trained by resistance training.
   1. Type: weight-bearing (walking, jogging, aerobics, stair climbing, dancing, field sports, racquet sports, court sports) and regional strength training.
   2. Duration: positive effects seen with 30-60 minutes of continuous activity.
   3. Frequency: 3-4 times a week used in studies on sedentary women.
   4. Intensity: unknown, but see overload principle. Medical screening for cardiovascular status may be needed.

C. Overload: must increase over baseline to see effect.

D. Reversibility: gains are rapidly lost.

E. Initial values: benefit proportional to baseline value.

F. Diminishing returns: exercise probably cannot improve beyond genetically determined maximum.

XI. Nutrition[4]

A. Calcium and vitamin D most important.

B. Calcium balance and homeostasis needed.

C. Calcium excretion promoted by alcohol, caffeine, carbonated beverages, protein.

D. Calcium balance can be achieved by increasing calcium intake.

E. Role of other nutrients less defined.

F. Eating disorders may significantly adversely impact peak bone mass.[10]

XII. Calcium

A. Start early. Increases seen in prepubertal children with calcium supplementation at 1000 mg/day.[5]

FOR MORE INFORMATION:

National Osteoporosis Foundation
1150 17th Street N.W., Suite 500
Washington, DC 20036
202-223-2226

Membership and resource manuals, patient educational materials of "The Osteoporosis Report"

Melpomene Institute
1010 University Ave.
St. Paul, MN 55104
612-642-1951 FAX 612-642-1871

Membership, journal, resource packets on osteoporosis and other issues important to active women and girls.

American College of Sports Medicine: Strategic Health Initiative for Women, Sport and Physical Activity
P.O. Box 1440
Indianapolis, IN 46206
317-637-9200

Female Athlete Triad Slide series available for purchase, membership newsletter, information packets on female athlete triad, speaker's bureau directory

B. Achieve adequate intake daily:

Characteristic	Calcium (mg/day)
11-24	1200-1600
Adult	1000
Low estrogen	1500
Pregnancy	1600

C. Calcium alone will not prevent estrogen- or age-related bone loss. Higher levels of calcium are required to maintain calcium balance.

D. Avoid extremes.

References

1. Christiansen C et al: Consensus Development Conference: Prophylaxis and Treatment of Osteoporosis, *Am J Med* 90:107-110, 1991.
2. Cooper D, Barker DJP, Wickham C: Physical activity, muscle strength, and calcium intake in fracture of the proximal femur in Britain, *Br Med J* 297:1443-1446, 1988.
3. Drinkwater BL, Bruemmer B, Chestnut CH: Menstrual history as a determinant of current bone density in young athletes, *JAMA* 263:545-548, 1990.
4. Heaney RP: Nutritional factors in osteoporosis, *Ann Rev Nutr* 13:287-316, 1993.
5. Johnston CC, Miller JZ, Slemenda CW: Calcium supplementation and increases in bone mineral density in children, *N Engl J Med* 327:82-87, 1992.
6. Kanis JA et al: The diagnosis of osteoporosis, *J Bone Miner Res* 9:1137-1141, 1994.
7. Marcus R et al: Osteoporosis and exercise, *Med Sci Sports Exerc* 24:S301-S307, 1992.
8. Notelovitz M et al: Estrogen therapy and variable resistance weight training increases bone mineral in surgically menopausal women, *J Bone Miner Res* 6:583-590, 1991.
9. Orwoll ES et al: The relationship of swimming exercise to bone mass in men and women, *Arch Intern Med* 149:2187-2200, 1989.
10. Rigotti NA et al: Osteoporosis in women with anorexia nervosa, *N Engl J Med* 331:1601-1606, 1984.
11. Risser WL et al: Bone density in eumenorrheic female college athletes, *Med Sci Sports Exerc* 22:570-574, 1990.
12. Snow-Harter C, Bouxsein M, Lewis BT: Muscle strength as a predictor of bone mineral density in young women, *J Bone Miner Res* 5:589-595, 1990.
13. Snow-Harter C et al: Effects of resistance and endurance exercise on bone mineral status of young women, *J Bone Miner Res* 7:761-769, 1992.
14. Yeager K et al: The female athlete triad, *Med Sci Sports Exerc* 25(7):775-777, 1993.

CHAPTER 26

Eating Disorders

Mimi D. Johnson, MD

I. Introduction
   A. Under pressure to excel at their sport, some athletes attempt to lose weight or body fat by developing patterns of disordered eating. These patterns include restricting food intake, binging and purging, and performing compulsive exercise.
   B. This behavior appears to be more common in women than men, with a ratio of 10 : 1.

II. General Principles
   A. There is a spectrum of disordered eating behavior, ranging from restricting food intake only slightly or binging and purging only occasionally, to restricting food intake significantly, as in anorexia nervosa, and binging and purging on a regular basis, as in bulimia nervosa.
   B. Disordered eating of any degree can have adverse health effects, with morbidity and mortality increasing as the severity of the disordered eating behavior increases.
   C. Athletes with disordered eating are at risk for progressing to an eating disorder, and their behavior should be addressed.

III. Prevalence of Disordered Eating Among Athletes
   A. 32% of 182 female college athletes practiced at least one form of disordered eating (vomiting, laxative use, diuretic use, excessive weight loss, diet pill use) daily for at least 1 month.
   B. 62% of 42 female college gymnasts practiced at least one form of disordered eating twice weekly over ≥3 months.
   C. 15.4% of 487 female swimmers aged 9-18 years old engaged in disordered eating behaviors.

IV. Risk Factors in Athletics
   A. Stress, personality, and competitive drive.
      1. Pressure and desire to optimize performance can lead athletes to attempt weight loss, often inappropriately.

2. Pressure to meet weight goals can force an athlete, who lacks the knowledge of how to achieve weight loss in a healthy manner, to resort to disordered eating behaviors.
3. Athletes often have heightened body awareness, which may make them more prone to body image concerns.
4. Personality traits that many competitive athletes have, which are considered positive, are those same traits that we see in persons with eating disorders (i.e., perfectionism, compulsiveness, and high achievement expectations).
5. Athletes block extraneous factors to train, and therefore they can block hunger/feelings as well.
6. Drive for sport can become drive for disordered eating.
7. In the college/elite athlete:
   a. New competitive realm.
   b. Sport is business.
   c. Education is based on performance.

B. Sports at highest risk for development of eating disorders.
1. Athletes of any sport may develop disordered eating behaviors.
2. Sports emphasizing lean appearance that may be judged subjectively: gymnastics, dance, diving, figure skating, and synchronized swimming.
3. Sports emphasizing body leanness for optimal performance: long distance running, swimming, cross-country skiing.
4. Sports utilizing weight classifications: wrestling, judo, tae kwon do, weight lifting, and rowing.

V. Factors Contributing to Development of Disordered Eating

A. Sociocultural factors.
1. The behaviors that contribute to the development of abnormal eating patterns, such as dieting, have become normative for girls and women in Western cultures.
2. Disordered eating is perpetuated by our sociocultural norms that prize thinness.

B. Biological factors.
1. Severe dieting can result in the loss of psychological and physiological cues for satiety.
2. Imbalances in serotonin, norepinephrine, and melatonin activity have been postulated as etiological factors.

C. Psychological factors.
1. Low self-esteem.
   a. Common among athletes with disordered eating.
   b. Athlete's sense of self-esteem may be a reflection of how she feels about her sports performance or other areas of her life.
   c. The athlete may derive her sense of self from external feedback (i.e., performance, appearance), as opposed to internal feedback.
2. Poor coping strategies.
   a. Disordered eating is often an unhealthy attempt to deal with stress. Many of these athletes lack assertiveness skills.
   b. Instead of managing her problems in a healthy way, the athlete may try to manage her weight.
3. Lack of sense of identity.
   a. The athlete may lack a sense of identity outside of being an athlete. She has developed her sense of "who she is" around sports, failing to develop other areas of her life.

4. Family.
   a. Families of women with eating disorders often have difficulty resolving conflict, expressing or tolerating negative emotions, and regulating distance and intimacy among family members, particularly in times of stress.
   b. The women in these families often derive their self-worth as a reflection of others' responses to them, particularly their appearance.
5. Responses to victimization.
   a. 20% to 35% of persons with eating disorders report sexual abuse.
   b. 67% of bulimics report sexual and/or physical abuse.
   c. These etiologies may not be common among athletes with eating disorders but should be considered.

VI. Signs and Symptoms of Disordered Eating Behavior
  A. Warning signals of disordered eating.
    1. Increasing criticism of one's body.
    2. Decrease in food intake at meals.
    3. Preoccupation with food, calories, and weight.
    4. Refusal to eat with other people.
    5. Secretly eating or stealing food.
    6. Bathroom visits after meals.
    7. Compulsive exercise outside of normal training regimen.
    8. Criticism of eating patterns of others.
    9. Inability to relax; always in constant motion.
    10. Very structured daily schedule.
    11. Injury causes abnormal amount of anxiety.
    12. Highly self-critical.
    13. Often prefers to be alone.
  B. Restrictive eating behavior may range from inadvertently failing to meet basal caloric needs to voluntary starvation coupled with extreme exercise regimens. Most athletes who restrict food intake do not meet the criteria for anorexia nervosa.
    1. Physical symptoms associated with food restriction.
       a. Amenorrhea, delayed menarche.
       b. Cold intolerance.
       c. Lightheadedness.
       d. Constipation.
       e. Abdominal bloating.
       f. Fatigue.
       g. Decreased ability to concentrate.
    2. Physical signs associated with food restriction.
       a. Decreased body temperature.
       b. Lanugo
       c. Dry skin, brittle hair/nails.
       d. Decreased fat and muscle.
       e. Bradycardia.
       f. Hypothermia.
       g. Orthostatic blood pressure changes.
    3. Common laboratory findings.
       a. Leukopenia, anemia, thrombocytopenia.
       b. Low-normal to normal follicle-stimulating hormone (FSH) and luteinizing hormone (LH).
       c. (T_3) Low to low-normal triiodothyronine, normal thyroxine (T_4) and thyroid-stimulating hormone (TSH).

d. Cholesterol and serum transaminases may be elevated.
e. Hyponatremia may be seen in fluid overloading.
f. Ketonuria, pyuria, hematuria, elevated urine pH.

4. Electrocardiographic changes.
a. Bradycardia (less than 60 bpm).
b. Low voltage.
c. Low or inverted T waves.
d. Prolonged QT interval (rare but ominous).

C. Binge-purge behavior. The binge-purge cycle is typically exacerbated by dieting. Hunger results in the binge, followed by guilt, which results in the purging behavior.

1. Purging methods.
a. Vomiting.
(1) Does not remove all calories.
(2) Does not relieve hunger.
(3) Results in fluid and electrolyte loss.
b. Laxatives.
(1) Act on large intestines.
(2) Do not affect calories absorbed.
(3) Result in fluid and electrolyte loss.
c. Diuretics.
(1) Act on kidneys.
(2) Do not affect calories absorbed
(3) Result in fluid and electrolyte loss.

2. Physical symptoms associated with purging behavior.
a. Sore throat and chest pain.
b. Bloating and abdominal pain.
c. Fatigue.
d. Constipation/diarrhea.
e. Irregular menses.
f. Face and extremity edema.
g. Depression.

3. Physical signs associated with purging behavior.
a. Parotid gland enlargement.
b. Erosion of dental enamel.
c. Calluses on dorsum of hand.
d. Orthostatic blood pressure.
e. Rarely, esophagitis and Mallory-Weiss tears.

4. Common laboratory findings.
a. Metabolic alkalosis/acidosis.
b. Low potassium.
c. Elevated urine pH, pyuria, proteinuria.
d. Hypocalcemia.

5. Electrocardiographic changes infrequent.

6. Radiographic changes infrequent (mediastinal emphysema).

VII. Effects of Disordered Eating on Performance

A. Impaired performance and increased injury risk.

1. Decreased caloric intake and fluid/electrolyte imbalances can result in decreased endurance, strength, reaction time, speed, and ability to concentrate.

2. Because the body adapts to metabolic changes initially, a decrease in performance may not be evident for some time.

VIII. Evaluation and Treatment

A. Intervention.

1. An athlete with disordered eating may be identified in several ways.
   a. During the preparticipation examination.
   b. Parents may call with concerns.
   c. Coaches, teammates, or trainers may note suspicious behavior.
   d. The athlete may seek help from a nutritionist or psychologist.
2. Approach the athlete gently, not accusingly.
3. Present evidence for concern about the athlete's behavior.
4. Express concern about her health and effect on athletic performance.

B. The multidisciplinary team.
1. Physician monitors medical status, determines sports participation, and coordinates care.
2. Nutritionist provides nutritional guidance.
3. Psychologist or mental health professional addresses psychological issues.
4. Coach, trainer, or exercise physiologist may be important team members.
5. Family must be involved with young athlete living at home.

C. Medical evaluation and treatment.
1. Screening during the preparticipation examination.
   a. Menstrual history.
      (1) Age of menarche.
      (2) Frequency and duration of menstrual periods.
      (3) Date of last menstrual period.
      (4) Use of hormonal therapy.
   b. Nutritional screen.
      (1) 24-hour recall.
      (2) Number of daily meals/snacks.
      (3) List of forbidden foods.
   c. Weight concerns.
      (1) Satisfied with present weight?
      (2) Athlete's perceived ideal weight (is she normal or underweight and thinks she should weigh less?).
      (3) Ever tried to control weight using vomiting, laxatives, diuretics?
   d. Further evaluation.
      (1) If disordered eating is suspected, further evaluation by physician or referral to a nutritionist is appropriate.
      (2) Nutritionist can screen more thoroughly for disordered eating and decide if nutritional counseling alone will suffice.
      (3) If athlete has menstrual dysfunction or has clear signs of an eating disorder, an in-depth medical evaluation should be performed.
2. In-depth medical evaluation.
   a. History.
      (1) Menstrual history.
      (2) Nutritional screen.
      (3) Exercise history.
         (a) Athlete's sports participation.
         (b) Hours spent training per week, in and out of normal training regimen.
      (4) Family history, including weight history.
      (5) Brief psychological history.
         (a) Recent stressors.

(b) General mood, body image, self-esteem.
(6) Past medical history.

b. Review of systems. Cover symptoms of starvation and purging.

c. Physical examination.
(1) Evaluate for signs of starvation and purging.
(2) Blood pressure for orthostasis.
(3) Pelvic examination if irregular/absent menses.
(4) Consider differential diagnoses for eating disorder:
(a) Metabolic disease.
(b) Malignancy.
(c) Inflammatory bowel disease.
(d) Achalasia.
(e) Infection.

d. Laboratory evaluation.
(1) Urinalysis.
(2) Complete blood count and sedimentation rate.
(3) Chemistry panel for electrolytes, calcium, magnesium, and potassium.
(4) Renal, thyroid, liver function tests.
(5) If menses irregular or absent, FSH, prolactin, and pregnancy screen, if indicated.

e. Electrocardiography.
(1) Pulse <50 bpm.
(2) Electrolyte abnormality.
(3) Frequent purging.

f. Positive evaluation.
(1) Determine sports participation.
(a) If athlete losing weight, verbal/written contract with sports participation dependent on weight gain (½ lb/week).
(b) Limit exercise for electrolyte or electrocardiographic abnormalities.
(2) Monitor physical status and laboratory values as needed.
(3) Consider hormone replacement in amenorrheic or oligomenorrheic athlete if there is no other cause of menstrual dysfunction. Bone densitometry may be appropriate.

3. Nutritional evaluation and treatment.

a. Initial evaluation.
(1) Detailed food and weight/height history.
(2) Exercise history.
(3) 3-day food diary to assess caloric, carbohydrate, protein, and nutrient intake.
(4) Body composition measurements.
(5) Estimate caloric intake and needs, and healthy weight range (25% to 50%).
(6) Educate athlete on appropriate weight range, percent body fat, and lean muscle mass.
(7) Emphasize effects of starvation on body composition and muscle loss.

b. Followup visits.
(1) Educate athlete on fueling body.
(2) Individualize recommendations.
(3) Make gradual changes in caloric and nutrient intake.
(4) Measure body composition every 1-2 months for feedback.

4. Psychological evaluation and treatment.
   a. Initial evaluation.
      (1) Identify stressors in athlete's life.
      (2) How does athlete perceive she deals with stress?
      (3) How does she define her eating patterns?
      (4) Consider need for individual vs. group therapy.
   b. Followup treatment.
      (1) Help athlete develop an awareness of her stressors and work on healthy coping strategies, identity issues, self-esteem issues, and assertiveness skills.
      (2) Athlete support group can be helpful.
5. Criteria for hospitalization.
   a. Weight loss >30% of normal.
   b. Cardiac compromise.
   c. Hypotension/dehydration.
   d. Electrolyte abnormalities.
   e. Failure of outpatient treatment.

IX. Prognosis
   A. The athlete with an eating disorder risks medical complications, and possibly death, in addition to being a psychological cripple, controlled by this disorder.
   B. In nonathletes treated for an eating disorder:
      1. 50% do well.
      2. 30% improve but struggle with weight, body image, and relapses.
      3. 20% do poorly.
   C. The causes of death include:
      1. Cardiovascular collapse or arrest (secondary to electrolyte imbalance or ipecac-induced cardiomyopathy).
      2. Sepsis (due to compromised immune function).
      3. Gastric or intestinal perforation.
      4. Suicide.

X. Prevention
   Prevention is the key to addressing this problem.
   A. Athletes, parents, coaches, athletic administrators, training staff, and physicians need to be educated about the risks and warning signs of an eating disorder.
   B. Education of coaches.
      1. Appropriate weight/body composition expectations; the importance of appropriate caloric intake.
      2. How the coach influences athlete's eating behaviors.
      3. Resources for treatment.
   C. Education of athletes.
      1. Appropriate caloric intake.
      2. How to avoid an eating disorder.
      3. Physiological, psychological, nutritional, and performance-affecting effects of disordered eating.
      4. Resources for nutritional or psychological guidance.

Bibliography

Arden MR et al: Alkaline urine is associated with eating disorders, *Am J Dis Child* 145:28-30, 1991.

Amrein PC et al: Hematologic changes in anorexia nervosa, *JAMA* 24:2190-2191, 1979.

Bhanji S, Mattingly D: Anorexia nervosa: some observations on "dieters" and "vomiters", cholesterol and carotene, *Br J Psychiatry* 139:238, 1981.

Bowers TK, Eckert E: Leukopenia in anorexia nervosa: lact of increased risk of infection, *Arch Intern Med* 138:1520, 1978.

Drinkwater BL et al: Bone mineral content of amenorrheic and eumenorrheic athletes, *N Engl J Med* 311:277-281, 1984.

Dubois A et al: Altered gastric emptying and secretion in primary anorexia nervosa, *Gastroenterology* 77:319, 1979.

Dummer GM et al: Pathogenic weight-control behaviors of young competitive swimmers, *Phys Sportsmed* 15:75-86, 1987.

Fohlin L: Body composition, cardiovascular and renal function in adolescent patients with anorexia nervosa, *Acta Paediatr Scand* 268:1-20, 1977.

Fohlin L et al: Function and dimensions of the circulatory system in anorexia nervosa, *Acta Pediatr Scand* 66:11-16, 1978.

Garfinkel PE et al: Body awareness in anorexia nervosa: disturbances in "body image" and "satiety," *Psychosom Med* 40:487, 1978.

Goldberg SJ, Comerci GD, Feldman L: Cardiac output and regional myocardial contraction in anorexia nervosa, *J Adolesc Health Care* 7:15-21, 1988.

Harris RT: Bulimarexia and related serious eating disorders with medical complications, *Ann Intern Med* 99:800-807, 1983.

Hurd HP, Palumbo PJ, Gharid H: Hypothalamic-endocrine dysfunction in anorexia nervosa, *Mayo Clin Proc* 52:711-716, 1977.

Isner JM et al: Anorexia nervosa and sudden death, *Ann Intern Med* 102:49-52, 1985.

Johnson MD: Tailoring the preparticipation exam to female athletes, *Phys Sportsmed* 20:61-72, 1992.

Johnson MD: Disordered eating in active and athletic women, *Clin Sports Med* 13:355-369, 1994.

Kaye WH, Weltzin TE: Neurochemistry of bulimia nervosa, *J Clin Psychol* 52:21-28, 1991.

Kennedy S: Melatonin disturbances in anorexia nervosa and bulimia nervosa, *Int J Eating Disorders* 16:257-265, 1994.

Keys A, Henschel A, Taylor HL: The size and function of the human heart at rest in semi-starvation and in subsequent rehabilitation, *Am Heart J* 55:584-602, 1948.

Kreipe RE, Harris JP: Myocardial impairment resulting from eating disorders, *Pediatr Ann* 21:760-768, 1992.

Levin PA et al: Benign parotid enlargement in bulimia, *Ann Intern Med* 93:827-829, 1980.

Milner MR, McAnarney ER, Klish WJ: Metabolic abnormalities in adolescent patients with anorexia nervosa, *J Adolesc Health Care* 6:191-195, 1985.

Palla B, Litti IF: Medical complications of eating disorders in adolescents, *Pediatrics* 81:613-623, 1988.

Polivy J, Herman CP: Diagnosis and treatment of normal eating, *J Consult Clin Psychol* 55:635-644, 1987.

Pomeroy C, Mitchell JE: Medical issues in the eating disorders. In Bronell KD, Rodin J, Wilmore JH, editors: *Eating, body weight and performance in athletes: disorders of modern society*, Philadelphia, 1992, Lea & Febiger.

Roberts MW, Li S-H: Oral findings in anorexia nervosa and bulimia nervosa: a study of 47 cases, *J Am Dent Assoc* 115:407, 1987.

Root MPP: Persistent, disordered eating as a gender-specific, post-traumatic stress response to sexual assault, *Psychotherapy* 28:96-102, 1991.

Rosen LW, Hough DO: Pathogenic weight-control behaviors of female college gymnasts, *Phys Sportsmed* 16:141-146, 1988.

Rosen LW et al: Pathogenic weight-control behavior in female athletes, *Phys Sportsmed* 14:79-86, 1986.

Russell G: Bulimia nervosa: an ominous variant of anorexia nervosa, *Psychol Med* 9:429-448, 1979.

Silverstein B, Perdup L: The relationship between role concern, preferences for slimness, and symptoms of eating problems among college women, *Sex Roles* 18:101-106, 1988.

Steinhausen H, Rauss-Mason C, Seidel R: Follow-up studies of anorexia nervosa: a review of four decades of outcome research, *Psychol Med* 21:447-454, 1991.

Striegel-Moore RH, Silberstein LR, Rodin J: Toward an understanding of risk factors for bulimia, *Am Psychol* 41:246-263, 1986.

Vigersky RA et al: Hypothalamic dysfunction in secondary amenorrhea associated with simple weight loss, *N Engl J Med* 297:1141-1145, 1977.

Warren MP, VandeWiele RL: Clinical and metabolic features of anorexia, *Am J Obstet Gynecol* 117:435, 1973.

Yates A: Biologic considerations in the etiology of eating disorders, *Pediatr Ann* 21:739-744, 1992.

CHAPTER 27

Growth and Developmental Concerns for Prepubescent and Adolescent Athletes

Suzanne M. Tanner, MD, FACSM

I. Overview
   A. It is advantageous for sports medicine practitioners to gain familiarity with the normal sequence of growth and development of young athletes.
   B. This knowledge allows practitioners to guide youngsters toward appropriate sports, counsel youngsters on setting realistic competitive goals, detect deviations from the norm during preparticipation examinations, counsel children about anticipated maturation events, and serve as a community resource for the design of safe and enjoyable youth sports programs.

II. Appropriate Activities Based on Age
   A. Infancy (0-2 years).
      1. Vision: farsighted.
      2. Balance: limited, based mainly on vision.
      3. Motor skills: mainly reflex.
      4. Recommendations.
         a. Free play in safe, unstructured environment.
         b. Structured exercises do not enhance development.
         c. Swimming programs offer no advantage.
   B. Early childhood (3-5 years). No relation has been found between skill training in early years and later development of sports skills.
      1. Vision.
         a. Not fully mature.
         b. Difficulty tracking moving objects and judging velocity.
      2. Balance: paradoxical decrease at 4-5 years due to overload of integrating visual, proprioceptive, and vestibular cues.
      3. Motor skills: run, kick, hop, throw (20% of 4 year olds), catch (30% of 4 year olds).
      4. Learning:
         a. Short attention span.
         b. Easily distracted due to lack of selective attention.

c. Egocentric learning (self-centered play, learning through trial and error).
d. Need instruction by listening and seeing.
5. Recommendations.
a. Play in a closed system (few variables, constant conditions).
b. Appropriate activities include walking, running, swimming, tumbling, and playing T-ball.
c. Use a flat playing surface.
d. Consider avoiding organized sports. Organized sports may not confer a long-term advantage, and competition is so complex it may interfere with learning skills.

C. Childhood (6-9 years).
1. Vision: tracking of speed and direction of moving object is improved but still difficult (e.g., may judge ball speed but not direction).
2. Balance: automatic.
3. Motor skills.
a. Fundamental motor skills improve.
b. Usually proficient at overhead throw by 6 years.
c. Mature running skill at 8 years.
4. Learning.
a. Short attention span.
b. Easily distracted.
c. May not be able to determine changing offensive and defensive roles.
d. Lack rapid decision-making ability.
e. Need both auditory and visual instruction.
f. Improved cooperation on a team and with playmates since children are less self-centered.
5. Recommendations.
a. Emphasize skill acquisition.
b. Closed-system environment.
c. Appropriate activities include running, swimming, gymnastics.
d. May participate in recreational leagues of contact sports such as soccer and baseball.
e. May begin organized sports with minimal, if any, emphasis on competition.
f. Football, basketball, and hockey may be too complex.

D. Late childhood (10-12 years).
1. Vision: fully developed.
2. Balance: gradually improves, but declines at puberty during peak height velocity ("clumsy teenager").
3. Motor skills: possibly at risk for injury during height spurt.
4. Learning.
a. Able to respond to verbal instruction alone at 11-12 years.
b. Able to integrate information from multiple sources.
5. Recommendations.
a. May begin participation in complex sports such as entry-level football, basketball, and wrestling.
b. Consider basing participation in contact and collision sports on maturation rather than chronological age to decrease injury risk and enhance chance of success for less physically mature children.

E. Guidelines for participation in youth sports. Many physical educators accept the following guidelines. "Readiness" for sports has been defined by R.M. Malina as "the match between a child's level of growth, maturity and development and the task demands presented in competitive sports." The following questions should be answered before encouraging a child to participate in a certain sport.

1. Does the child want to play the sport?
2. Is the child ready socially? Will the child respond to the coach and cooperate with playmates?
3. Is the child ready cognitively? Can the child understand the directions? Is the child's attention span long enough?
4. Is the child physically ready to meet the demands of the sport without a high injury risk and with a fair chance of success?

III. Trainability of Prepubescent Children

A. There is a paucity of data on the effects of intensive training on the child athlete.

B. Definitions.

1. *Trainability:* the magnitude of physiological changes induced by exercise.
2. *Prepubescent:* the period during which a child is at sexual maturation level 1.
3. *Weight lifting:* the use of progressive resistance methods such as barbells, dumbbells, or machines to increase one's ability to exert or resist force.

C. Obstacles to studies.

1. It is difficult to differentiate the effects of training from those of growth and development.
2. Growth may mask training effects. (For example, relative maximum oxygen uptake on a per kilogram basis may decrease as weight increases.)
3. Children may lack discipline required for intense training.
4. Aggressive training may not be employed due to risk of harm to children.
5. Control group needs to be carefully selected. (It may be best to base study comparisons according to maturation level, not just age and sex.)

D. Probable physiological changes from training in prepubescent children.

1. Maximum aerobic power can be increased with training, but perhaps less so than in mature individuals.
2. Anaerobic capacity appears to be trainable regardless of maturation level.
3. Motor skills acquired during childhood are retained longer than parameters such as endurance, anaerobic capacity, and strength.
4. Strength gains are greatest in postpubertal males, but females and prepubertal males may increase strength with weight training.

E. Weight lifting.

1. Risks.
   a. Epiphyseal fractures.
      (1) Case reports exist.
      (2) None in closely supervised studies.
   b. Overuse injuries: lumbar strains are most common.
   c. Supervised weight training may be safer than other sports, such as football.
   d. Burnout, boredom.
2. Benefits.
   a. Improves strength.
   b. Probably improves performance in sports that rely on strength, but coordination and skill acquisition may be greater factors in many sports.

   c. Value in preventing injuries is uncertain.
   d. May gain social skills.
3. Pathogenesis of improved strength in prepubertal children.
   a. Motor learning, rather than muscle hypertrophy, appears to account for strength gains. Weight lifting causes little increase in muscle size in prepubertal children.
   b. Motor learning changes include and increase in motor unit activation in exercising muscles and improved coordination.
4. Possible reasons for great strength gains in boys lifting weights after puberty.
   a. Increased testosterone.
   b. Greater size.
   c. Greater lean mass.
   d. Broader shoulders and bones for muscle attachments.
   e. Larger muscle fibers.
   f. Perhaps gender-related differences in neuromuscular responses.
5. Ages of peak strength gains with weight training.
   a. Girls: age 11.5-12.5 years, during most rapid growth in height.
   b. Boys: age 14.5-15.5 years, ~1 year after growth spurt.
6. Recommended age to begin weight training depends on child's:
   a. Desire to lift weights.
   b. Belief that lifting weights is beneficial.
   c. Maturity to follow instructions.
   d. Discipline to lift weights several days per week.
7. Recommendations for weight-lifting program for prepubescent children.
   a. Program should be well supervised.
   b. Children should use proper size weights (i.e., free weights or small machines).
   c. Avoid major lifts such as clean and jerk, squat lift, and dead lift, which have a greater risk of inducing injury.
   d. Lift with controlled, slow, and smooth technique through a full range of motion.
   e. Balance routine with upper and lower body exercises and pushing and pulling maneuvers.
   f. Exhale while lifting to avoid syncope from Valsalva maneuver.
   g. Sample program for prepubertal child: may perform 15-20 repetitions (one or two sets) for two 20-minute sessions per week. Increase weights by 1 to 3-lb increments.
   h. Sample program for postpubertal child: may perform 8-10 repetitions, three sets, three to four 30 to 60-minute sessions per week.
   i. Use adult or mature spotters.
   j. Weight room should be clean with good lighting.
   k. Warm up prior to lifting.
   l. Perform stretching exercises before and after lifting.

IV. Physiological Changes During Puberty
   A. Hormonal changes (Fig. 27-1).
   B. Timing of normal pubertal events in girls and boys (Table 27-1). Peak height velocity occurs about 2 years earlier in girls than boys, so from age 12-14 years girls may have an advantage over boys in sports in which height is advantageous, such as basketball. Starting at about age 11, girls usually gain more fat than boys, placing girls at a disadvantage in sports in which the body is propelled, such as running.
   C. Sequence of pubertal events (Fig. 27-2).
   D. Determining skeletal age.

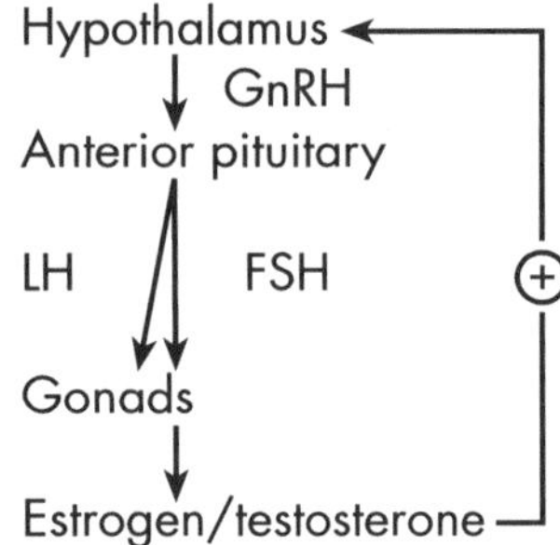

FIG. 27-1.
Hormonal changes in puberty. The hypothalamus synthesizes and secretes the peptide hormone gonadotropin-releasing hormone (GnRH). GnRH is transported to the anterior pituitary gland where it causes production and release of luteinizing hormone (LH) and follicle-stimulating hormone (FSH). LH and FSH circulate in the blood and stimulate the gonads to produce the sex steroids estrogen and testosterone. Before puberty and during adulthood a negative feedback system is operative. During puberty there is increased secretion of GnRH and decreased sensitivity of feedback.

1. May be necessary for determining risk of progression for conditions such as scoliosis.
2. Comparison of a radiograph of a patient's hand with standards for different ages available in radiographic atlases.
3. Radiographic observation of ossification of apophysis of the vertebral ring.
4. Ossification of iliac apophysis.

E. Determining physical maturation: via sexual maturation ratings (Tanner stages) I-V.

V. Definitions of Abnormal Development

A. *Delayed puberty.*
1. Female: lacks evidence of breast development (thelarche) by 13 years.
2. Male: No testicular enlargement by 14.5 years.
3. Individuals who fail to progress normally through puberty.

B. *Primary amenorrhea.*
1. No menarche by 16 years.
2. No menarche for >4 years after thelarche.

TABLE 27-1. Normal Pubertal Events

Event	Girls	Boys
Onset of puberty	10 years (8-14 years)	12 years (9-15 years)
First sign of puberty	Thelarche (breast bud appearance)	Testicular enlargement
Age at peak height velocity	12 years	14 years
Sexual maturation stage at peak height velocity	Stage 2-3	Stage 3-4
Peak weight and strength gain	11.-12.5 years	6 months after peak height velocity
End of growth and maturation	16.5 years	~18-20 years

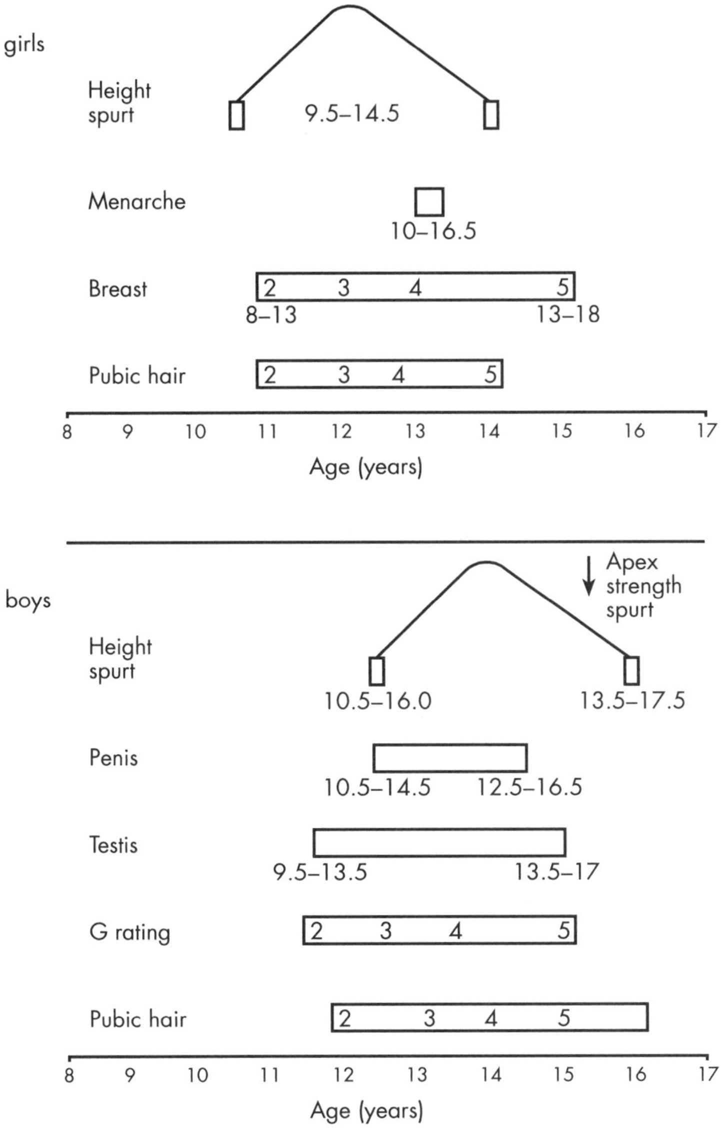

FIG. 27-2.
Sequence of pubertal events. (From Slap GB: Normal physiological and psychosocial growth in the adolescent, *J Adolesc Health Care* 7:135, 1986.)

VI. Clinical Correlations with Sexual Maturation Rating (SMR; Tables 27-2 and 27-3)

VII. Special Conditions
- A. Infant swimming programs.
  - 1. Unproven benefits.
    - a. ↑ parent-child communication.
    - b. Makes infant "water safe" (unlikely).
  - 2. Risks.
    - a. Transmission of giardiasis.
    - b. Water intoxication with seizures.
    - c. False sense of security by parents.
  - 3. American Academy of Pediatrics (AAP) recommendations.
    - a. Parents should understand risks before enrolling infant in classes.

TABLE 27-2. Correlation of Clinical Conditions with Sexual Maturation Rating (SMR)

Clinical Condition	SMR
Hematocrit rise (male)	II-V
Alkaline phosphatase peak	
Female	II
Male	III
Slipped capital femoral epiphysis	II, III
Acne vulgaris	II, III
Appearance of normal male gynecomastia	II, III
Acute worsening of idiopathic scoliosis	II-IV
Menarche (female)	Late III, early IV
Tibial tubercle apophysitis (Osgood-Schlatter condition)	III

b. Follow YMCA guidelines (no total submersion, appropriate water temperature, control fecal contamination!).
c. Instructor to infant ratio should be 1 : 1.
d. Instructor should be trained in cardiopulmonary resuscitation.
e. Physician approval is required for medical conditions.

B. Structured infant exercise programs.
1. No proven benefit.
2. Musculoskeletal injury risk exists.
3. AAP recommendations: encourage parents to provide a safe, nurturing, and minimally structured play environment instead.

C. Atlantoaxial instability in children with Down syndrome.
1. Incidence: 18% of neurologically asymptomatic children with trisomy 21 have cervical anomalies.
2. Types of cervical anomalies:
a. Atlantoaxial instability (12%): ↑ mobility at the articulation of C1 and C2.
b. Abnormal odontoid (6%): hypoplastic, dysplastic.
3. Special Olympic rules: If atlantodens interval is >5 mm in flexion, child is not allowed to participate in activities with risk of spinal in-

TABLE 27-3. Correlation of Hematocrit (50th Percentile) with SMR

	Hematocrit %	
Individual	SMR I	SMR V
Females		
Black	34.0	35.8
Caucasian	35.8	35.9
Males		
Black	34.9	39.3
Caucasian	35.6	40.9

jury such as gymnastics, diving, pentathlon, or butterfly strokes and diving starts in swimming.

4. Arguments against screening with radiographs.
   a. Abnormal radiographs may revert to normal, and normal ones may become abnormal.
   b. Risk of asymptomatic atlantoaxial instability progressing to symptomatic atlantoaxial instability (i.e., with neurological abnormalities) is uncertain.
   c. Identifying symptomatic atlantoaxial instability by history and neurological examination may have greater predictive value of trauma risk.
   d. Efficacy of avoiding certain sports to prevent atlantoaxial instability has never been tested.

D. Risks of distance running in children.
   1. Risks: related mainly to total mileage and number of hours during training.
      a. Musculoskeletal injuries: mainly overuse injuries.
      b. Endocrine: delayed menarche?
      c. Hematologic:
         (1) Iron depletion?
         (2) Main cause may be inadequate nutritional intake.
      d. Thermoregulatory:
         (1) A child's ability to maintain thermal homeostasis is less efficient than that of an adult.
         (2) Concern for events >30 minutes.
      e. Psychological: boredom, burnout.
   2. AAP recommendations.
      a. If children enjoy the activity and are asymptomatic, they may train and participate.
      b. Consider risks listed above when counseling parents.

Bibliography

American Academy of Pediatrics Sports Medicine Committee policy statement draft, Atlantoaxial instability in Down syndrome, 1993.

American Academy of Pediatrics Sports Medicine Committee policy statement, Infant exercise programs, *Pediatrics* 82(5):E3, 1988.

American Academy of Pediatrics Sports Medicine Committee policy statement, Infant swimming programs, 1985.

American Academy of Pediatrics Sports Medicine Committee policy statement, Risks of distance running in children, *Pediatrics* 86(5):799-800, 1990.

Bar-Or O: Physiological perspectives. In *Intensive Participation in Children's Sports,* 1993, Human Kinetics Publishers, pp 127-132.

Bar-Or O: Trainability of the prepubescent child, *Phys Sportsmed* 18(5):65-82, 1989.

Blimkie CJR: Benefits and risks of resistance training in children. In *Intensive Participation in Children's Sports,* 1993, Human Kinetics Publishers, pp 133-165.

Daniel WA: Growth and nutrition of adolescents. In Blum RW, editor: *Adolescent Health Care: Clinical Issues,* New York, 1982, Academic Press.

Dyment PG: Neurodevelopmental milestones: when is a child ready for sports participation. In Sullivan JA, Grana WA, editors: *The Pediatric Athlete,* 1990, American Academy of Orthopaedic Surgeons, pp 27-29.

Greydanus D, McAnarney E: *J Curr Adolesc Med* 2:21-28, 1980.

Mellion MB: Questions parents ask about the young athlete. In *Sports Medicine Secrets,* 1994, Hanley & Belfus, pp 28-32.

Nelson MA: Developmental skills and children's sports, *Phys Sportsmed* 19(2):67-79, 1991.

Risser WL, Risser JMH, Preston D: Weight-training injuries in adolescents, *Am J Dis Child* 144(9):1015-1017, 1990.

Tanner SM: Weighing the risks: strength training for children and adolescents, *Phys Sportsmed* 21(6):104-116, 1993.

CHAPTER 28

Nonsteroidal Antiinflammatory Drugs and Corticosteroids

Jeffrey L. Tanji, MD

Mark E. Batt, MB, BChir

NONSTEROIDAL ANTIINFLAMMATORY DRUGS

I. Introduction
   A. Nonsteroidal antiinflammatory drugs (NSAIDs) are one of the most commonly prescribed medications in the United States (over 100 million prescriptions per year).
   B. Many preparations are approved for over-the-counter dispensing, further expanding their use.
   C. There are numerous drugs of this type; however, only a limited number of general categories of NSAIDs.

II. Effects Common to All NSAIDs
   A. Antiinflammatory.
   B. Analgesic.
   C. Antipyretic.
   D. Platelet inhibitory.

III. Mechanisms of Action
   A. Not all of the mechanisms of action for NSAIDs are known.
   B. Cyclooxygenase inhibition leading to decreased prostaglandin production is the best studied and described mechanism.
   C. Other actions.
      1. Intracellular effects.
      2. Neutrophil inhibition.

IV. Pharmacokinetics
   A. Achieve steady-state levels in blood at 3-4 half-lives.
   B. Half-life varies significantly and is dependent on each individual NSAID.
   C. Clinical response time dependent on half-life of NSAID; generally a 2-3 week trial is necessary.
   D. Most NSAIDs are excreted through the kidneys.

V. Categories of NSAIDs
   A. Salicylates.

1. Acetylsalicylic acid (ASA; aspirin) major drug of this class.
2. Analgesic at low dose, antiinflammatory at high dose.
3. Antipyretic and platelet inhibitory at all doses.
4. Cost very low.
5. Very safe.
6. Ototoxicity and nephrotoxicity an issue at high doses.
7. Other medications in the salicylate class.
   a. Diflunisal.
   b. Tolmetin.
   c. Salsalate.
   d. Trisalicylate.

B. Propionic acids.
1. Ibuprofen is the most commonly used drug of this class.
2. Strongly analgesic, moderately antiinflammatory at all doses.
3. Antipyretic and platelet inhibitory at all doses.
4. Reasonable cost.
5. Very safe.
6. Other medications in this class.
   a. Naproxen.
   b. Ketoprofen.

C. Acetic acids.
1. Indomethacin is the most commonly used drug of this class.
2. Strongly antiinflammatory, moderately analgesic at all doses.
3. Antipyretic and platelet inhibitory at all doses.
4. Reasonable cost.
5. Reasonably safe.
6. Other medications in this class.
   a. Sulindac.
   b. Tulmetin.

D. Oxicams.
1. Piroxicam is the major drug in this class.
2. Long half-life makes single daily dose convenient.

E. Phenylacetic acid.
1. Diclofenac major drug of this class.
2. Similar effects to propionic acid NSAIDs.

VI. Side Effects Common to All NSAIDs

A. Gastrointestinal side effects.
1. NSAID gastropathy is the most common side effect.
2. Dyspepsia, without radiographic or endoscopy findings, is common.
3. Incidence increases with increasing age, concomitant use of corticosteroids or other NSAIDs, smoking, or history of gastrointestinal disorder.
4. Prophylaxis against gastric injury with NSAIDs.
   a. Sucralfate not effective.
   b. H_2-blockers controversial.
   c. Misoprostol has some efficacy.

B. Renal side effects.
1. Acute renal failure, a rare but critical side effect.
2. Prostaglandins play a key role in renal blood flow regulation.
3. At-risk factors for renal toxicity.
   a. Advanced age.
   b. History of renal disease, hypertension.
   c. Hypovolemia.
   d. History of congestive heart failure.

C. Neurological side effects.
  1. Headache.
  2. Tinnitus.
  3. Depression.
  4. All uncommon but usually reported with the acetic acid NSAIDs or high-dose ASA.
D. Skin side effects.
  1. Urticaria.
  2. NSAIDs can provoke allergic reactions in ASA-allergic patients.
    a. Reactive airway disease.
    b. Nasal polyposis.
    c. Rhinitis.

CORTICOSTEROIDS

I. Introduction
  A. Powerful antiinflammatory agents.
  B. Possess glucocorticoid and mineralocorticoid effects.
  C. Generally given topically or by injection and only rare systemically.
    1. Topical use generally for dermatological conditions.
    2. Injection route allows for drug concentration at desired site with fewer systemic effects.
II. Effects of Corticosteroids
  A. Antiinflammatory.
  B. Antipyretic.
  C. Not truly analgesic.
III. Mechanism of Action
  A. Inhibit release of arachidonic acid.
    1. Prostaglandins.
    2. Leukotrienes.
  B. Decrease leukocyte migration.
  C. Stabilize lysosomes.
  D. Limit collagen synthesis and deposition.
  E. Decrease fibroblast proliferation.
IV. Categories of Corticosteroids
  A. Divided into categories by potency and duration of action.
  B. Injectable agents of short duration.
    1. Cortisone.
      a. Low potency.
      b. Not commonly used.
    2. Hydrocortisone.
      a. Low potency.
      b. Commonly used.
  C. Injectable agents of intermediate duration.
    1. Triamcinolone.
      a. Intermediate potency.
      b. Commonly used.
    2. Prednisolone.
      a. Intermediate potency.
      b. Commonly used.
  D. Injectable agents of long duration.
    1. Dexamethasone.
      a. High potency.
      b. Commonly used.

2. Betamethasone.
    a. High potency.
    b. Commonly used.

E. Prednisone is the oral agent of choice.
    1. Given usually in a tapering dose over 1 week to 10 days.
    2. 60 mg initial dose, tapering to 10 mg, then discontinued.
    3. Short duration use minimizes systemic side effects.

V. Side Effects Common to All Agents
   A. Dermatological complications.
      1. Hypopigmentation or hyperpigmentation.
      2. Subcutaneous atrophy.
   B. Musculoskeletal complications.
      1. Ligament rupture.
      2. Tendon rupture.
      3. Steroid "flare."
         a. Pain at injection site.
         b. Caused by precipitation of crystals.
         c. Less common in agents that are fully soluble (dexamethasone).
      4. Can result in systemic symptoms of irritability and insomnia.
      5. Risk of acceleration of osteoarthritis.
      6. Infection is rare.
   C. Side effects of oral use.
      1. Sodium retention.
      2. Reduced carbohydrate tolerance.
      3. Osteoporosis.
      4. Withdrawal.
      5. Peptic ulcer disease.
      6. Myopathy.
      7. Soft tissue breakdown.
      8. Avascular necrosis of the hip.

VI. Common Locations for Injection
   A. Subacromial space of shoulder.
      1. Diagnostic for severity of rotator cuff tendinitis when pain limits strength testing.
      2. Posterior approach.
   B. Lateral or medial epicondyle.
      1. Use low-potency agent.
      2. Caution with regard to skin atrophy.
   C. Carpal tunnel.
   D. Trochanteric bursa.
   E. Knee joint.
   F. Pes anserinus bursa.
   G. Avoid certain areas that are prone to rupture.
      1. Patellar tendon.
      2. Achilles tendon.

Bibliography

Birrer RB: Aspiration and corticosteroid injection, *Phys Sportsmed* 20(12):57-71, 1992.

Graham DY, Agrawal NM, Roth SH: Prevention of NSAID-induced gastric ulcer with misoprostol, *Lancet* 2:1277-1280, 1988.

Kerlan RK, Glousman RE: Injections and techniques in athletic medicine, *Clin Sports Med* 8:541-560, 1989.

Pfenninger JL: Injections of joints and soft tissue: Part I, *Am Fam Phys* 44:1196-1202, 1991.

Pfenninger JL: Injections of joints and soft tissue: Part II, *Am Fam Phys* 44:1690-1701, 1991.

Stankus SJ: Inflammation and the role of anti-inflammatory medications. In Lillegard WA, Rucker KS, editors: *Handbook of Sports Medicine,* Boston, 1993, Andover Medical Publishers.

CHAPTER 29

Banned Substances and Drugs

Wade F. Exum, MD, MBA

I. Drug Control Programs
   A. Drug control implies deterrence and curtailment of the use of performance-enhancing substances in both professional and amateur sports.
   B. Performance-enhancing or "ergogenic" substances.
      1. Used to improve performance or gain unfair competitive advantage.
      2. Ergogenic = work generating (Greek).
   C. Other drugs involved in drug control efforts are the so-called recreational or "street" drugs.
   D. Programs provide for:
      1. Education about the harmful as well as exploitable effects of drugs.
      2. Testing athletes for inappropriate drug use.
      3. Rehabilitation of athletes with identified substance abuse problems.
      4. Research related to performance-enhancing substances or methods.

II. Doping
   A. Definitions.
      1. The word "dope" refers to the stimulating hard liquor that was used in Kaffir religious ceremonies (from the ancient Boer language).
      2. Doping referred to the practice of using a mixture of opium in race horses in the 1800s (Old English dictionary definition).
      3. Modern day doping refers to the practice of using drugs or substances to gain a competitive advantage or to improve athletic performance (practical interpretation of original International Olympic Committee [IOC] Medical Commission definition).
   B. Reasons for prohibiting doping.
      1. Doping poses dangers to the health and well-being of athletes.
      2. Doping tarnishes the image of sports.
      3. Doping creates unfair and unethical physical and/or psychological advantages for users over nonusers.
      4. Doping detracts from fan and participant enjoyment of sport.
      5. Doping threatens support available to sport.

6. Fatalities related to drug use are legend.
   a. The stimulant "trimethyl" caused the first recorded fatality in an athlete in 1886 (a cyclist).
   b. The Danish cyclist Kurt Jensen died in the 1960 Rome Olympics from taking a combination of nicotinic acid and amphetamines.
   c. The 400-m hurdler Dick Howard died from a heroin overdose at the 1960 Olympics.
   d. The British cyclist Tommy Simpson supposedly died from amphetamine ("speed") use during the 1967 Tour de France.
   e. The basketball star Len Bias died from the use of cocaine in 1986.
   f. The football star Lyle Alzado believed prior to his death in 1992 that his fatal brain tumor resulted from the use of anabolic androgenic steroids (AASs) combined with growth hormone (hGH).

C. Many of the above factors prompted the IOC to pass its first resolution against doping in 1962.
   1. The IOC Medical Commission was established in 1967 to control drug use and eliminate drug misuse.
   2. The first Olympic Games drug testing occurred at the 1968 games in Mexico City.
   3. Testing was expanded at the 1976 Montreal games, and AASs were banned.
   4. An effective test was developed for AASs by Dr. Manfred Donike of Germany in the early 1980s and resulted in disqualifications and medal forfeitures for the first time at the 1983 Pan American games.
   5. The IOC's so-called list of banned substances is routinely updated and revised.
      a. The United States Olympic Committee (USOC) has essentially adopted the IOC list intact.
      b. Many amateur sports administrative organizations (i.e., the National Collegiate Athletic Association, the International Powerlifting Association, the Goodwill Games, the World University Games, the Commonwealth Games, the Asian Games, etc.) have adopted modified versions of the list.
      c. Many professional sports have their own drug control policies and practices, but they, too, utilize the concept of banning substances and sanctioning offenders.

D. Techniques for prohibiting doping.
   1. Classes of drugs as well as practices (methods) that are believed or proven to result in unfair competitive advantage are banned.
   2. Restrictions are placed on the use of certain substances that offer advantages only in designated sports or that require monitoring to preclude ergogenic usage.
   3. Penalties are established for infractions related to these prohibitions.

III. Historical Perspectives.

A. Ancient Greek and Roman warriors and competitors used wine, mushrooms, and other substances to calm their nerves or to make them more fierce and aggressive.

B. Incan and native South American mine workers or villagers used coca leaf preparations to ward off fatigue and hunger as early as 300-500 A.D.

C. Aztec athletes used a stimulant derived from cactus plants in the 1400s and 1500s.

D. French cyclists used vin marinari, a concoction containing wine and coca leaf extracts and known as "the wine for athletes," in the late 1800s.

E. Boxers and canal swimmers used a brandy and cocaine mixture as well as strychnine for stimulant effects in the mid- to late 19th century.
F. Earliest recorded reports of drug-taking by athletes in competition.
 1. Swimmers in canal races were charged with taking dope in Amsterdam in 1865.
 2. Coaches and others commonly gave cycle riders a mixture of heroin and cocaine (now known as "speedball") in the late 1800's.
G. Testosterone, the hormone responsible for development of male physical and sexual characteristics, was discovered and developed in the 1930s.
 1. Analogues of this substance, AASs, were developed in the 1950s.
 2. AAS use became widespread in the 1960s after they were shown to result in profound improvements in weightlifting performances.

IV. The IOC Banned Substance List
A. Doping classes.
 1. Stimulants, including caffeine, sympathomimetic amines, cocaine, and certain beta-2 agonists.
 2. Narcotic analgesics, except codeine and certain of its analogues.
 3. Anabolic agents, including AAS and certain beta-2 agonists with marked anabolic activity.
 4. Diuretics and "masking" agents.
 5. Peptide and glycoprotein hormones (i.e., HGH, human chorionic gonadotropin, erythropoietin, and adrenocorticotropic hormone) and their analogues.
B. Doping methods.
 1. Blood doping, including blood transfusions.
 2. Pharmacological, chemical, and/or physical manipulation of the test specimen.
C. Classes of drugs subject to restrictions.
 1. Alcohol: tested for only upon request.
 2. Marijuana: tested for only upon request.
 3. Corticosteroids: permissible only in inhaled or locally injected form with accompanying medical justification.
 4. Local anesthetics, except cocaine: permitted in locally injected form with accompanying medical justification.
 5. Beta blockers: permitted only in sports in which they are not specifically excluded.

V. Laboratory Analyses of Specimens
A. The IOC and College of American Pathologists (CAP) accredit and monitor laboratories that do athletic drug testing (ADT).
B. Urine is the bodily fluid that is currently utilized for ADT.
 1. Specimens are sent to the laboratories utilizing strict chain-of-custody procedures in anonymous (identified by code number only) "split" sample containers which are designated "A" and "B."
 2. Both the "A" and the "B" samples must be shown to contain a banned substance before a positive test result is declared.
  a. The "A" sample constitutes an initial screen.
  b. The "B" sample constitutes a final laboratory analytical result and an automatic appeal.
  c. Non-IOC-accredited laboratories do not necessarily require split specimens.
 3. Blood and other bodily tissue testing have not met with the widespread acceptance that urine testing has sustained.

VI. Penalties or Sanctions
  A. Athletes whose "B" samples prove positive in IOC-based testing have the right to appeal the finding to their sport's governing or administrative bodies.
  B. If athletes with positive tests choose not to appeal or if their appeal is rejected, sanctions can be and usually are levied.
  C. Recommended sanctions.
    1. Class I offense: involve anabolic agents, amphetamine-type and other stimulants, narcotic analgesics, diuretics, hormones, blood doping and manipulation of the test sample, and beta blockers.
      a. Suspension for 2 years for the first offense, depending on the organization involved.
      b. Lifetime ban for any subsequent offense.
    2. Class II offense: involve sympathomimetic amines.
      a. Suspension for a maximum of 3 months for the first offense.
      b. Suspension for 2 years for the second offense.
      c. Lifetime ban for any subsequent offense.

VII. Stimulants
  A. Increase alertness, reduce fatigue, and may increase competitiveness and hostility.
  B. Psychological and physical stimulus to athletic performance as well as detrimental side effects are possible.
  C. Injury risk is increased due to impaired judgment that can result from stimulant use.
  D. Stimulants cause increases in heart rate and blood pressure.
    1. They heighten the potential for dehydration and circulatory compromise during and after vigorous physical activity.
    2. Complications from effects and side effects include risk of cerebral hemorrhage and cardiac irregularities.
  E. Anxiety, insomnia, tremor, aggressiveness, and addiction occur in most abusers.
  F. Medical use is strictly controlled and limited, and there is no justification for use in sport.

VIII. Narcotic Analgesics
  A. Relieve moderate to severe pain and increase pain threshold.
  B. Euphoria, psychological stimulation, a false feeling of invincibility, or illusions of athletic prowess beyond an athlete's innate ability can occur with moderate or high doses.
    1. User may perceive dangerous situations as safe.
    2. Failure to recognize or heed injury are possible.
  C. Physical dependence, addiction, and withdrawal phenomena are associated with narcotic use.
  D. Narcotic overdose.
    1. Always a medical emergency.
    2. Frequently fatal.

IX. Anabolic Agents
  A. Inclusive of the male hormone testosterone as well as its analogues (AASs) and certain beta-2 agonists.
  B. Actions or effects.
    1. Testosterone regulates, promotes, and maintains physical and sexual development in males.
    2. In combination with proper diet and training, these agents can increase muscular size, strength, and endurance.

3. They are believed to speed recovery from injury.
4. Medically, male hormone derivatives are used to:
   a. Stimulate the bone marrow in patients with rare and unusual anemias.
   b. Treat certain types of cancer.
   c. Treat hereditary angioedema.
   d. Treat testosterone deficiency.

C. Side effects and adverse effects.
   1. All users: kidney/liver/heart dysfunction, psychological aberrations, changes in libido, impaired glucose and cholesterol metabolism.
   2. Adult males: acne, testicular atrophy and impotence, gynecomastia, premature baldness, prostate enlargement and prostatitis.
   3. Females: masculinization, hirsutism, deepening of the voice, male-pattern baldness, enlargement of the clitoris, abnormal menstrual cycles.
   4. Adolescents: severe acne, stunted growth.
   5. See chapter 30 for more details.

D. AASs were designated as Schedule III controlled substances by the federal government in 1990.
   1. Improper sale, possession, distribution, or even prescription are now punishable by fine and/or incarceration.
   2. Limited supplies of legitimate AASs have probably fostered black market transactions.

X. Diuretics
   A. Medically used to treat hypertension and fluid retention or overload.
   B. Reasons athletes use or misuse diuretics.
      1. To reduce weight quickly in sports where weight categories are involved.
      2. To produce a more rapid excretion of urine or to dilute the urine in an attempt to minimize the chance of a drug screen revealing the presence of drugs.
   C. Health risks.
      1. Dehydration, volume depletion, hypotension.
      2. Electrolyte imbalance, cardiac irregularities.
      3. Muscle cramps.
      4. Collapse.

XI. Peptide and Glycoprotein Hormones
   A. Function as messengers to stimulate and/or influence bodily functions.
   B. Banned types.
      1. Human chorionic gonadotropin (hCG).
         a. Produced by the placenta in pregnancy to prevent menstruation and maintain the pregnancy.
         b. Used in women to detect pregnancy and to treat some cancers.
         c. Used in men to increase spermatogenesis, counter the development of gynecomastia, and prevent testicular atrophy during AAS use.
         d. Use in males is considered equivalent to the exogenous administration of testosterone.
      2. Adrenocorticotropic hormones (ACTH) or corticotropin.
         a. Stimulates production of glucocorticoid or corticosteroid hormones in the adrenal cortex.
         b. Used in the treatment of rheumatoid arthritis and rheumatic fever, and in the treatment of some dermatological, allergic, and ophthalmic diseases.
         c. Therapeutic value is limited, and it is currently used mainly as a diagnostic tool.

d. Misuse occurs because of the euphoric effect of increased blood levels of corticosteroids.
e. Adverse effects.
   (1) Elevated blood pressure.
   (2) Salt and water retention.
   (3) Increased excretion of potassium and calcium.
   (4) Aggravation of preexisting emotional instabilities or psychotic tendencies.
f. Prolonged use increases the risk of insomnia, allergic reaction, mood swings, personality changes, depression, and even psychosis.

3. Human growth hormone or hGH.
   a. Produced in the pituitary, stimulates growth in all bodily tissues.
   b. Used medically to treat children with primary hGH deficiency (dwarfism).
   c. Excess results in gigantism in children and acromegaly in adults.
   d. Adverse effects.
      (1) Allergic reactions.
      (2) Diabetes mellitus.
      (3) Thyroid disease.
      (4) Menstrual disorders.
      (5) Decreased libido.
      (6) Impotence.
      (7) Shortened life span.
   e. Contamination of some hGH preparations of cadaver origin can cause the fatal neurological condition known as Creutzfeldt-Jakob disease.
4. Erythropoietin (EPO)
   a. Naturally produced in the kidneys to stimulate and regulate the production of red blood cells (RBCs).
   b. Synthetically produced for patients with severe anemia associated with kidney disease, renal dialysis, acquired immunodeficiency syndrome, and cancer.
   c. Can increase aerobic capacity, much like blood doping, for improved performance in endurance athletes.
   d. Adverse effects.
      (1) Dehydration in the setting of excessive RBCs causes thickened, sluggish blood.
      (2) Erythrocythemia with slow blood flow can lead to strokes or heart attacks.

XII. Review
   A. IOC-based programs test athletes for use of specifically listed classes of performance-enhancing substances or methods.
   B. Many professional and other sports organizations have their own drug control policies and programs.
   C. Sanctions for drug offenses vary from organization to organization but can include suspensions, fines, mandated treatment/rehabilitation, probations, and the like.
   D. Further information about drug policy is usually available from individual sports organizations.

Bibliography

Benson MT: *National Collegiate Athletic Association Drug-Testing Education Programs,* Kansas City, KS, 1994-95, NCAA Publishing, pp 1-13.

Exum WF: *U.S. Olympic Committee Drug Education Handbook,* 1995.
Fuentes RJ, Rosenberg JM, Davis A: *Athletic Drug Reference '95,* Research Triangle Park, NC, 1991, Clean Data.
Goldman B, Klatz R: *Death in the Locker Room,* Chicago, 1992, Elite Sports Medicine Publications.
Voy RO: *Drugs, Sport, and Politics,* Champaign, IL, 1991, Leisure Press.
Wadler GI, Hainline B: *Drugs and the Athlete,* Philadelphia, 1989, FA Davis.

CHAPTER **30**

Anabolic-Androgenic Steroids

Troy Reese, PharmD

Wade F. Exum, MD, MBA

I. Introduction
   A. Performance enhancing not a new concept.
      1. Ancient Greek athletes used various substances.[3,12]
         a. Mushrooms.
         b. Caffeine.
         c. Alcohol.
         d. Nitroglycerin.
         e. Opium.
         f. Strychnine.
   B. Today's athletes continue the search for ultimate performance.
      1. Unfortunately, anabolic-androgenic steroids are among some of these agents.
      2. Even with current testing policies and reports of adverse effects, some athletes continue to risk their health, as well as career.

II. History of Anabolic Steroids
   A. Discovery of testosterone.
      1. A naturally occurring hormone, testosterone was first isolated in 1935.
      2. Testosterone has both androgenic (masculinization) and anabolic (tissue-building) properties.
      3. Originally used in chronically ill patients in an attempt to replace lost muscle tissue[11] and to promote a positive nitrogen balance in starvation victims.[14]
   B. Development of synthetic steroids.
      1. An explosion of synthetic compounds were soon developed in an attempt to produce a purely anabolic agent with no androgenic properties.[2]
      2. No purely anabolic agent was discovered, but researchers were able to reduce the androgenic properties.

3. Some of these substances were believed to be used by German soldiers during World War II to increase aggressiveness.[14]

C. Anabolic steroids in sports.
1. Perhaps the first known use of steroids in the sporting arena was in 1954 when a Russian Olympic team reported receiving testosterone products.[7]
2. Their use spread to other countries, including the United States.
3. The International Olympic Committee finally placed a ban on the use of anabolic steroids at the 1976 Summer Olympic Games in Montreal.
4. Although there has been a decline in use, the problem has not been totally eradicated and use continues in athletes and nonathletes alike.

III. Prevalence of Use
A. High school surveys.
1. Various surveys conducted report anabolic steroid use ranging from less than 1% to over 20%.[3,16]
2. One recent survey of Illinois high school students revealed that 1.9% reported using anabolic steroids.[5]
3. A Salt Lake City, Utah, survey showed 3.3% use.[9]
4. A 1988 nationwide survey showed that 6.6% of male high school students reported having used steroids.[16]
5. These surveys also revealed that use is not only by athletes but also by nonathletes wishing to "bulk up" and improve their appearance.

B. Use in athletics.
1. Percentage of use increases when the survey population is limited to athletes.
2. 17% of varsity college athletes responding to a questionnaire reported using steroids.[14]
3. Certain sports (i.e., football, weight lifting, bodybuilding, and track and field) are more likely to report steroid use.[14,16]
4. A 1990 survey of National Football League players reported that 28% of all respondents and 67% of offensive linemen had previously used anabolic steroids.[15]
5. A survey at a major power lifting competition revealed that over half the men and 10% of women reported anabolic steroid use.[15]

IV. Effects on Performance
A. Scientific data.
1. Despite perceptions to the contrary, scientific data studying the effects of anabolic steroids on performance are controversial.
2. Results of studies have been inconsistent.

B. Mechanisms of action.
1. Anticatabolic effects.[6,10,13,14]
a. Due to interaction with cortisol released in response to physical and psychological stress, causing protein degradation and muscle atrophy.
b. Testosterone can displace the corticosteroids from receptor sites, reversing the effects.
2. Anabolic effects.[6,13]
a. Increased protein synthesis.
b. Increase in the release of growth hormone.
3. Motivational effects.
a. Steroids can be considered motivational due to increased aggressive behavior, which can be focused in training sessions.[6,10,14]

b. *Mind over matter:* the suggestion that something may affect performance can mentally spur an athlete to greater achievement. One study showed significant gains in strength, even though the athletes received a placebo.[6,10]

4. Hemodynamic effects.
   a. Some studies show an increase in oxygen uptake.[8,13]
   b. A 1977 study showed increases in cardiac output and stroke volume and a decrease in heart rate.[13]
   c. The increase in aerobic capacity may also be due to an increase in erythropoiesis.[8,10,13]

C. Controversial results.
1. Test parameters have led to conflicting results.
   a. Limited population sizes.
   b. Different anabolic agents.
   c. Varying doses (none supertherapeutic).
   d. Subjects with different skill levels. Greater benefits have been seen in athletes who have reached a plateau prior to starting steroids.[2,6,10]
2. Scientific validity of reports from athletes cannot exist due to:
   a. Lack of controls.
   b. Stacking (taking more than one drug at a time).
   c. Cycling (taking steroids for a period of time, temporarily discontinuing, then beginning a new period of use).
   d. Drug purity not measured.

V. Adverse Effects

A. Overview.
1. An extensive list of adverse effects exists, and these occur to various degrees.
2. Some adverse effects are seen with short-term use, while others occur after years of abuse.
3. Some effects are reversible; others are not.
4. Various factors can influence the occurrence of adverse effects.
   a. Drug used.
   b. Dosage and regimen.
   c. Route of administration: injectable forms of anabolic steroids are associated with fewer adverse effects than oral dosage forms because oral forms pass through the enterohepatic circulation.[10]

B. Cosmetic.
1. Acne usually occurs after at least 4 weeks of use due to an increase in the size and activity of the sebaceous glands. The involved areas include the face, neck, and upper back.[8,13]
2. Changes in hair pattern are often seen with anabolic steroid use.[8,11]
   a. Premature male pattern baldness may be seen in men with the trait. Women may also experience male pattern baldness.
   b. An increase in facial and back hair can occur, especially in women.
3. Gynecomastia (the development of breast tissue in men) can occur as a result of estrogen-like metabolites of some steroids.[6,11]
4. Deepening of the voice in women may result from steroid use.[11]

C. Cardiovascular.
1. Changes in cholesterol profile can lead to coronary heart disease and myocardial infarction.[6,8,11-13]
   a. Increased serum low-density lipoproteins.
   b. Decreased serum high-density lipoproteins.

2. Hyperinsulinemia and impaired glucose tolerance may play a role in decreased high-density lipoproteins.[6,11]
3. Increased blood volume and hypertension are often caused by the sodium-, potassium-, and water-retaining properties of anabolic steroids.[6,11-13]

D. Musculoskeletal system.
1. Premature closure of growth plates of long bones can prevent prepubescent steroid users from reaching full growth potential.[6,8]
2. Changes in muscle-tendon unit increase muscle strength with no corresponding increase in tendon strength, which may result in strains and ruptures.[6,8,12]
3. Sodium and water retention can also weaken muscles, leading to injury.[12]

E. Liver.
1. Hepatotoxicity.
   a. More common with oral forms of steroids due to high first-pass effect.
   b. Jaundice can result due to reduced flow and retention of bile in the biliary capillaries of the hepatic lobules.[11,12]
2. Abnormal liver function tests.
   a. Elevated aspartate transaminase and alanine transaminase levels, usually reversible with discontinuation of steroids.[6,11,14]
   b. Could be early warning sign of liver tumor, which is more serious.
3. Peliosis hepatis has been reported after chronic intermittent use of anabolic steroids.[1,6,11,14] It is characterized by blood-filled lesions in the liver.

F. Reproductive system.[6,8,11,12,14]
1. Oligospermia (decreased numbers of sperm in semen).
2. Azoospermia (absence of sperm in semen).
3. Decreased levels of circulating hormones, including follicle-stimulating hormone (FSH), luteinizing hormone (LH), and testosterone.
4. Testicular atrophy.
5. Infertility.
6. Impotence, usually seen after cessation of use and prior to return to normal function.
7. Irregularities in menstrual cycle.
8. Enlargement of the clitoris.

G. Psychological.
1. Increased aggression can be motivational on the field but can also lead to problems in the user's personal life.[6,8,10,11]
2. Changes in libido, coupled with increased aggression, can result in aggressive sexual behavior.[8,11,12]
3. Postuse depression and dependence have been suggested.[8,16] Symptoms include depressed mood, fatigue, restlessness, anorexia, insomnia, decreased libido, headache, and steroid craving. Decreased muscle size may contribute to signs of dependence because users get "hooked" on the appearance of the steroid body, which fades upon discontinuation.

References

1. Cabasso A: Peliosis hepatis in a young adult bodybuilder, *Med Sci Sports Exerc* 26(1):2-4, 1994.
2. Celotti F, Negri Cesi P: Anabolic steroids: a review of their effects on the muscles, of their possible mechanisms of action and of their use in athletics, *J Steroid Biochem Molec Biol* 43(5):469-477, 1992.
3. Collins LH: Doping in sports, *J Am Acad Phys Assist* 6:465-476, 1993.

4. Fuentes RJ, Rosenberg JM, Davis A: *Athletic Drug Reference '95*, Research Triangle Park, 1995, Clean Data.
5. Gaa GL, Griffith EH, Cahill BR, Tuttle LD: Prevalence of anabolic steroid use among Illinois high school students, *J Athl Train* 29(3):216-222, 1994.
6. Haupt H: Anabolic steroids and growth hormone, *Am J Sports Med* 21(3):468-473, 1993.
7. Hoberman JM, Yesalis CE: The history of synthetic testosterone, *Sci Am* 272(2):76-81, 1995.
8. Lombardo JA, Sickles RT: Medical and performance-enhancing effects of anabolic steroids, *Psychiatr Ann* 22(1):19-23, 1992.
9. Luetkemeier MJ et al: Anabolic-androgenic steroids: prevalence, knowledge, and attitudes in junior and senior high school students, *J Health Ed* 26(1):4-9, 1995.
10. Lukas SE: Current perspectives on anabolic-androgenic steroids abuse, *Tips* 14(2):61-67, 1993.
11. Milhorn HT Jr: Anabolic steroids: another form of drug abuse, *J MSMA*, pp 293-297, Aug 1991.
12. Mottram DR: *Drugs in Sports*, ed 1, Champaign, IL, 1988, Human Kinetics Publishers.
13. VanHelder WP, Kofman E, Tremblay MS: Anabolic steroids in sport, *Can J Sports Sci* 16(4):248-257, 1991.
14. Wadler GI, Hainline B: *Drugs and the Athlete*, ed. 1, Philadelphia, 1989, FA Davis.
15. Yesalis CE: Epidemiology and patterns of anabolic-androgenic steroid use, *Psychiatr Ann* 22(1):7-18, 1992.
16. Yesalis CE, Anderson WA, Buckley WE, Wright JE: Incidence of the nonmedical use of anabolic-androgenic steroids. *National Institute on Drug Abuse* 102:97-112, 1990.

CHAPTER 31

Illicit Drug Use in Sports

William D. Knopp, MD

I. Introduction
   A. Cocaine has drawn much media attention due to the tragic deaths of Len Bias and Don Rogers in 1986.
   B. With the increasing use of illegal drugs in the United States, team physicians should be aware of the drug use patterns among athletes.
   C. This chapter will discuss only illicit drugs and their use in both recreation and performance enhancement.

II. Amphetamines
   A. Description: amphetamines include dextroamphetamine, methamphetamine, phenmetrazine, and methylphenidate, which are all derived from phenylisopropylamine.
   B. Historical perspective.
      1. Phenylisopropylamine was synthesized in 1920 and was used for nasal congestion.
      2. In 1935 amphetamines were used to treat narcolepsy, depression, anxiety, obesity, and hyperactivity in children.
      3. During World War II amphetamines were used by soldiers to reduce fatigue and increase alertness.
      4. Soon after World War II athletes, particularly cyclists, began to use amphetamines to delay fatigue. In 1960 Danish cyclist Kurt Jensen died during the Summer Olympics in Rome from heat exhaustion related to amphetamine use.
      5. In 1967 a male cyclist, Tommy Simpson, died in the Tour de France from cardiac arrest thought to be related to his amphetamine use.
   C. Prevalence of use.
      1. In 1989 Anderson and McKeag found that 3% of athletes at 11 universities had used amphetamines in the past 12 months. This represented a decrease from 8% in their 1985 study.
      2. Mandell reported that professional football players in the 1960s and 1970s used amphetamines extensively, but their use has decreased.

   3. In 1983 Clement surveyed 1687 athletes and found that 10% had used amphetamines.

D. Mechanism of action.
   1. Amphetamines are highly lipid-soluble agents that readily cross the blood-brain barrier and act by increasing the release of dopamine (DA), norepinephrine (NE), and 5-hydroxytryptamine (5-HT).
   2. Inhibit neurotransmitter reuptake.
   3. Inhibit monoamine oxidase (MAO) activity, therefore decreasing the degradation of DA, NE, and 5-HT.
   4. Direct stimulation of postsynaptic receptors.
   5. The above effects cause an increase in body temperature, glucose production, release of free fatty acids, cardiac stimulation, and bronchodilatation.
   6. Eliminated by renal metabolism.

E. Effects on performance.
   1. Due to the legal use of this drug, extensive studies in athletes have been performed.
   2. In 1959 Smith and Beecher found that 75% of swimmers and runners improved their performance with amphetamine use. The runners' times improved by an average of 1%, and in throwing sports distances increased by an average of 4%.
   3. In 1950 Chandler and Blair reported that athletes using amphetamines showed no increase in sprinting speed but did show greater knee extension strength and acceleration and a decrease in fatigue.
   4. In 1959 Haldi and Wynn reported no improvement in times for the 100-yard swim.
   5. In 1963 Golding and Barnard reported no improvement in time or decrease in fatiguability on the treadmill in trained and untrained athletes but they did show a delay in recovery rates for heart rate and blood pressure.
   6. In 1971 Wyndham et al. studied champion cyclists and showed no difference in submaximal or maximal oxygen uptake, heart rate, or minute ventilation in the amphetamine and nonamphetamine groups but the amphetamine group showed significant increases in blood lactate levels. They concluded that these athletes were able to tolerate higher anaerobic activity, suggesting poorer perception of fatigue, overexertion, and heat stress.

F. Therapeutic uses: hyperactivity in children and adults.

G. Dosage and administration.
   1. Primary route is pill or capsule form.
   2. Methamphetamine use has increased dramatically in recent years and may be smoked like crack cocaine.

H. Adverse reactions.
   1. Central nervous system: restlessness, insomnia, addiction, psychosis, tremor, anxiety, dizziness, cerebral hemorrhage.
   2. Cardiovascular.
      a. Cardiac dysrhythmias.
      b. Cardiac ischemia.
   3. Thermoregulation.
      a. Decrease in cutaneous blood flow.
      b. Increase in hypothalamic set point at higher temperature, therefore predisposing to heat stress.
   4. Psychological: high addiction potential.

I. IOC/NCAA rules: banned in all sports.

III. Cocaine
   A. Description: an alkaloid derived from the leaf of the coca plant (*Erythroxylon coca*), which grows in Central and South America.
   B. Historical perspective.
      1. The Incas used it as a mild stimulant by chewing the coca leaf.
      2. Sigmund Freud used it for his patients with depression and various personality disorders but abandoned its use after the addiction potential and lack of efficacy were realized.
      3. Later used as a topical vasoconstrictor and anesthetic on mucous membranes.
      4. In 1986 Len Bias, a basketball player for The University of Maryland, and Cleveland Browns football player Don Rogers died of complications related directly to cocaine abuse.
   C. Prevalence of use.
      1. Anderson and McKeag showed in 1989 that 5% of college athletes had used cocaine in the last 12 months. This was decreased from 17% in their 1985 study.
   H. Adverse reactions.
      1. Central nervous system.
         a. Tremulousness.
         b. Lowered seizure threshold.
         c. Cerebrovascular accident.
         d. Intracerebral hemorrhage.
         e. Physiological dependence.
      2. Cardiovascular.
         a. Hypertension, which increases risk of intracerebral hemorrhage.
         b. Tachycardia and myocardial hypersensitivity, which lowers the threshold for dysrhythmias. Ventricular fibrillation is a common cause of death in persons who use cocaine.
         c. Coronary artery vasospasm and occlusion, leading to myocardial ischemia, infarction, and sometimes death.
      3. Respiratory.
         a. Nasal septal necrosis, sinusitis, rhinitis.
         b. Bronchitis.
         c. Bronchiolitis obliterans.
      4. Psychological.
         a. Psychosis.
         b. Tremendous risk of addiction.
   I. IOC/NCAA rules: illegal in all sports.

IV. Marijuana
   A. Description.
      1. Derived from the hemp plant (*Cannabis sativa*).
      2. The pharmacological agent is tetrahydrocannabinol (THC).
   B. Historical perspective/prevalence of use.
      1. Used as euphoriant in ancient cultures.
      2. U.S. Department of Health and Human Services survey on student drug use from 1975 to 1980 found that one third of students had tried marijuana before entering high school.
      3. Heavy use in U.S. and European youth began in the 1960s, and marijuana continues to be a very popular drug.
      4. McKeag and Anderson showed a decrease in use from 36% in 1985 to 28% in 1989.
   C. Mechanism of action.
      1. A specific yet undefined receptor has been found.

2. Alteration in neuronal cell membranes may account for some of the effect.

D. Effects on performance.
1. Renaud and Cormier found a decrease in the $\dot{V}O_{2\,max}$.
2. Sweating is decreased.
3. No known beneficial effect on athletic performance.

E. Dosage and administration.
1. Smoked in a cigarette or pipe.
2. Less commonly, ingested or may be injected intravenously in a purified form.

F. Therapeutic uses.
1. Used as an antinauseant in terminally ill patients and is available as dronabinol (Marinol).
2. Levonantradol, a homologue of THC, has potential use as an analgesic, antispasmotic, or anticonvulsant.

G. Adverse reactions.
1. Central nervous system.
   a. Impaired motor coordination and decreased muscle strength.
   b. Decreased short-term memory.
   c. Poor concentration and decreased work performance.
2. Cardiovascular.
   a. Tachycardia.
   b. Increased supine blood pressure and decreased standing blood pressure.
3. Male reproduction.
   a. Oligospermia.
   b. Gynecomastia in males.
   c. Decreased plasma testosterone levels.
4. Respiratory: similar to cigarettes.
5. Psychological.
   a. Decreased motivation.
   b. Psychological dependence.
   c. Hallucinations, delusions, and psychosis.

H. IOC/NCAA rules.
1. Not banned by the IOC but is banned by the NCAA.
2. May be detected in the urine 2 to 4 weeks after use due to its high lipid solubility.

V. Narcotics

A. Description: morphine was originally derived from the poppy plant. Codeine and heroin are derived from morphine. Today's synthetic narcotics are variations of the original morphine molecule.

B. Historical perspective/prevalence of use.
1. Have been used for their effects of euphoria and relaxation for millennia.
2. Anderson and McKeag found that in the 12 months prior to the study 28% of athletes in 1985 and 34% in 1989 had used narcotics in some form, either prescription or illicit.

C. Mechanism of action: Narcotic analgesics mimic naturally occurring substances called endorphins and encephalins and bind to opiate receptors.

D. Effects on performance.
1. May be used to mask the pain of injuries, therefore allowing continued participation at the price of further injury.
2. May decrease the perception of exertion and fatigue, but this effect is probably counteracted by the sedative effects.

E. Therapeutic uses.
 1. Pain reduction.
 2. Antitussive.
F. Dosage and administration.
 1. Heroin and opium can be injected or smoked.
 2. Most prescription narcotics are taken orally.
G. Adverse reactions.
 1. Central nervous system.
  a. Physical dependence.
  b. Sedation.
  c. Respiratory depression.
 2. Cardiovascular: bradycardia.
 3. Respiratory: increase in bronchial secretion.
 4. Gastrointestinal.
  a. Nausea.
  b. Constipation.
 5. Psychological: dependence.
 6. Miscellaneous.
  a. Miosis (pupillary).
  b. Diaphoresis.
  c. Anorexia.
  d. Pruritus.
  e. Piloerection.
H. IOC/NCAA rules: all substances are banned by both the IOC and the NCAA.

VI. Barbiturates and Sedatives
A. Description: these substances include barbiturates, meprobamate, glutethimide, methaqualone, and benzodiazepines.
B. History.
 1. Barbiturates were introduced in 1903.
 2. Meprobamate was synthesized in 1957.
 3. Benzodiazepines were formulated in 1960.
C. Prevalence of use.
 1. In 1986 Heitzinger and Heitzinger found that 9% of athletes studied had used tranquilizers at one time.
 2. In 1981 Blythe et al. reported that 3% of athletes studied had used tranquilizers.
D. Mechanism of action.
 1. Benzodiazepines enhance the effect of gamma-aminobutyric acid (GABA) at the GABA receptor, thus increasing the inhibitory effect on the central nervous system by hyperpolarizing and therefore stabilizing cell membranes.
 2. Barbiturates prolong rather than intensify GABA effects, and in high concentrations can be GABA mimetic.
 3. Barbiturates also directly depress excitatory neurons.
E. Effects on performance.
 1. May reduce anxiety and tremor. This may be of particular benefit in sports requiring fine motor control such as archery, riflery, and the biathlon.
 2. The sedative and hypnotic effects have been used in athletes to decrease jet lag or to improve accommodation to time changes with varied success.
F. Therapeutic uses.
 1. Hypnotic.
 2. Sedative.

G. Adverse reactions.
  1. Central nervous system.
    a. Reduction of normal tremor can improve performance in accuracy sports such as archery, riflery, biathalon, etc.
    b. Decrease in motor coordination.
    c. Dependence.
  2. Psychological: dependence.
H. IOC/NCAA rules: all substances banned.

VII. Hallucinogens
A. Description: this group of drugs includes lysergic acid diethylamide (LSD), mescaline, psilocybin, and phencyclidine (PCP).
B. History.
  1. Mescaline and psilocybin are naturally occurring substances in plants and have been used by many cultures for thousands of years.
  2. LSD was synthesized 40 years ago and began to be used recreationally in the 1960s.
  3. PCP was introduced as a "dissociative anesthetic," but its clinical use in humans was rapidly replaced by ketamine.
C. Prevalence of use.
  1. In 1981 Toohey and Corder found that 10% of college athletes had used LSD.
  2. In 1981 Blythe et al. found that 1.5% of the athletes in the universities surveyed had used LSD.
  3. In 1986 Heitzinger and Heitzinger found that 5% of the athletes surveyed had used LSD.
D. Mechanism of action.
  1. LSD appears to bind to presynaptic neurons, inhibiting the release of serotonin.
  2. PCP binds to a receptor similar to the opiate receptor and also appears to block the reuptake of dopamine. The complete mechanism remains undefined.
E. Effects on performance: none of the hallucinogens have any positive effects on performance.
F. Therapeutic uses: none.
G. Dosage and administration.
  1. LSD, mescaline, and psilocybin are taken orally.
  2. PCP can be smoked, snorted, or injected.
H. Adverse reactions.
  1. Central nervous system.
    a. Dizziness, weakness, tremors, nausea, paresthesias.
    b. Visual, auditory hallucinations.
    c. Impairment in thinking, memory, mood, and judgment.
    d. Psychosis.
  2. Cardiovascular: central stimulation of sympathetic nervous system.
I. IOC/NCAA rules: all substances banned.

Bibliography

Anderson WA, McKeag DB: National survey of alcohol and drug use by athletes, *Phys Sportsmed* 19(2):91-104, 1991.

Anderson WA, McKeag DB: The substance use and abuse habits of college student-athletes, (Report No. 2), Mission, KS, 1985, The National Collegiate Athletic Association.

Anderson WA, McKeag DB: Replication of the National study of the substance use and abuse habits of college student-athletes, Mission, KS, 1989, The national Collegiate Athletic Association.

Blythe CS et al: Student athlete questionnaire on use of drugs in athletics, Mission, KS, 1981, The National Collegiate Athletic Association.

Chandler JV, Blair SN: The effect of amphetamines on selected physiological components related to athletic success, *Med Sci Sports Exerc* 12:65-69, 1980.

Golding LA, Barnard JP: The effect of d-amphetamine sulphate on physical performance, *J Sports Med* 3:221-224, 1959.

Haldi J, Wynn W: Action of drugs on efficiency of swimmers, *Res Quarterly* 31:449-553, 1959.

Heitzinger RL, Heitzinger DL: 1981-1986 data collection and analysis: high school, college, professional athletes: alcohol/drug survey, Madison, WI, 1986, Heitzinger and Associates.

Johnston LD, O'Malley PM, Bachman JG: Drug use among American college students and their noncollege-age peers, Washington, DC, 1988, US Dept of Education.

Katzung BG: *Basic and Clinical Pharmacology,* Norwalk, CT, 1992, Appleton and Lange.

Mandell AJ: The Sunday syndrome: A unique pattern of amphetamine use indigenous to American professional football, *Clin Toxicol* 15(2):225-232, 1979.

Mottram DR: *Drugs in Sport,* Champaign, IL, 1988, Human Kinetics Publishers.

Puffer JC, Green GA: Drugs and doping in athletes. In *The Physician's Handbook,* Philadelphia, 1990, Hanley and Belfus, Mosby–Year Book.

Renaud AM, Cormier Y: Acute effects of marijuana smoking on maximal exercise performance, *Med Sci Sports Exerc* 18:685-689, 1986.

Smith GM, Beecher HG: Amphetamine sulphate and athletic performance, *JAMA* 170:542-551, 1959.

Toohey JV, Corder BW: Intercollegiate sports participation and nonmedical drug use, *Bull Narc* 33(3):23-27, 1981.

Wadler GI, Hainline B: *Drugs and the Athlete,* Philadelphia, 1989, FA Davis.*

Wyndham GH, Rogers GG, Benade AJS, and Strydan NB: Physiological effects of the amphetamine during exercise, *S Afr Med J* 45:247-252, 1971.

MUSCULOSKELETAL TOPICS

SHOULDER

CHAPTER 32

Anatomy and Biomechanics of the Shoulder

Todd Jorgenson, MD

I. Overview
   A. Shoulder motion occurs at four sites within the shoulder complex: the sternoclavicular joint, the acromioclavicular joint, the glenohumeral joint, and the scapulothoracic articulation.
   B. All are important to normal shoulder function (Fig. 32-1).
II. Sternoclavicular Joint
   A. True synovial joint.
   B. The only synovial joint connecting the axial skeleton to the arm.
   C. An important joint in overall shoulder motion, it allows 35 degrees of elevation, 35 degrees of translation, and 50 degrees of rotation.
   D. Lacks inherent bony stability, but ligaments stabilize it.
      1. Anterior sternoclavicular ligament resists upward displacement of the clavicle.
      2. Intraarticular disk resists medial displacement of the clavicle.
      3. Posterior sternoclavicular ligament.
      4. Costoclavicular ligament.
      5. Infraclavicular ligament (Fig. 32-2).
III. Acromioclavicular (AC) Joint
   A. The AC joint is a plane joint with 20 to 50 degrees of lateral inclination in the frontal plane.
   B. Very little inherent structural support.
      1. Joint capsule is relatively weak.
      2. Interarticular disk.
      3. AC ligament.
         a. Resists axial rotation.
         b. Resists posterior translation.
         c. Relatively weak.
   D. Joint stability is provided by the coracoclavicular ligaments (conoid and trapezoid).
      1. Strong ligaments.

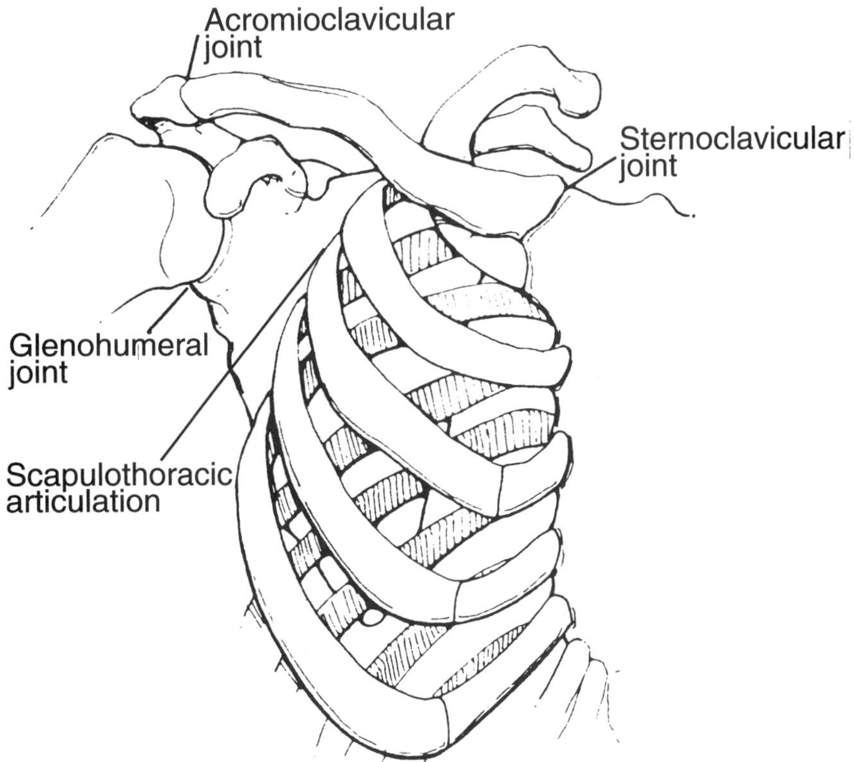

FIGURE 32-1
The articulations of the shoulder joint. (Tibone J, Patek R, Jobe FW, Perry J, Pink M. The Shoulder. In *Orthopedic Sports Medicine* (p. 464) eds. DeLee JC, Drez D. WB Saunders Co. 1994.)

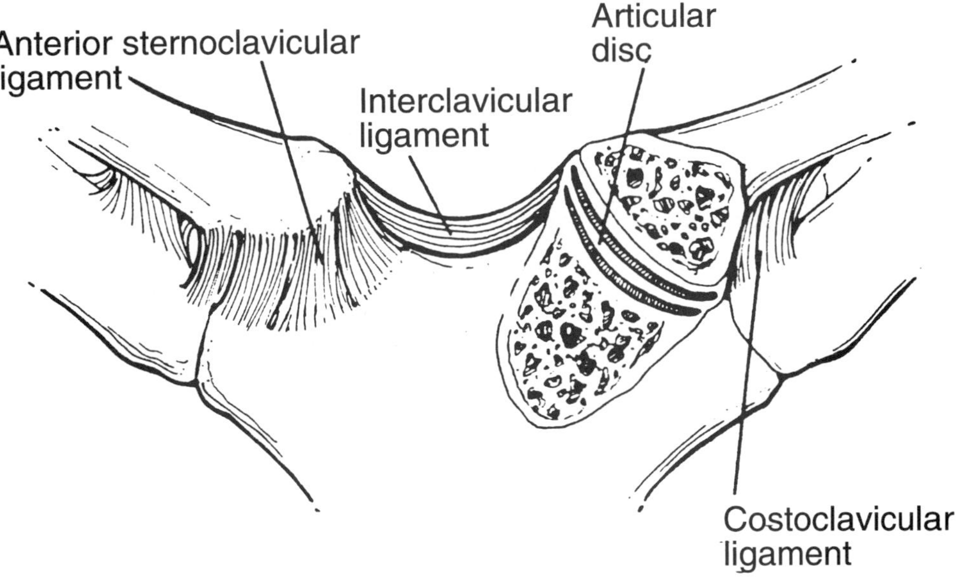

FIGURE 32-2
The demonstration of the anatomy of the sternoclavicular joint. (Tibone J, Patek R, Jobe FW, Perry J, Pink M. The Shoulder. In *Orthopedic Sports Medicine* (p. 464) eds. DeLee JC, Drez D. WB Saunders Co. 1994.)

2. Act to bind clavicle to scapula.
3. Prevent scapular tilt.
4. Limit excess rotation at AC joint.
5. Conoid ligament resists anterior and superior translation.
6. Trapezoid ligament resists axial compression at distal clavicle.

E. Motion at acromioclavicular joint is facilitated by rotation of the S-shaped clavicle.
1. Serves to functionally "lengthen" coracoclavicular ligaments.
2. Allows 20-30 degrees of motion in the vertical, horizontal, and frontal planes.
3. Rotation is necessary to achieve full shoulder elevation (Fig. 32-3).

IV. Glenohumeral Joint
A. The most mobile joint.
B. Delicate balance between functional mobility and adequate stability.
1. Factors contributing to mobility.
a. Minimal bony contact.
(1) Glenoid is slender and shallow.
(2) Average size of glenoid is 41 × 25 mm.
(3) 5 degrees downward tilt of glenoid offers minimal bony support inferiorly.
b. Joint capsule.
(1) Thin and redundant.
(2) Nearly twice the surface area of the humeral head.
2. Factors contributing to stability.
a. Static stabilizers.
(1) Joint capsule.
(a) Offers some stability only at extreme ranges of motion as portions of the capsule become taut.

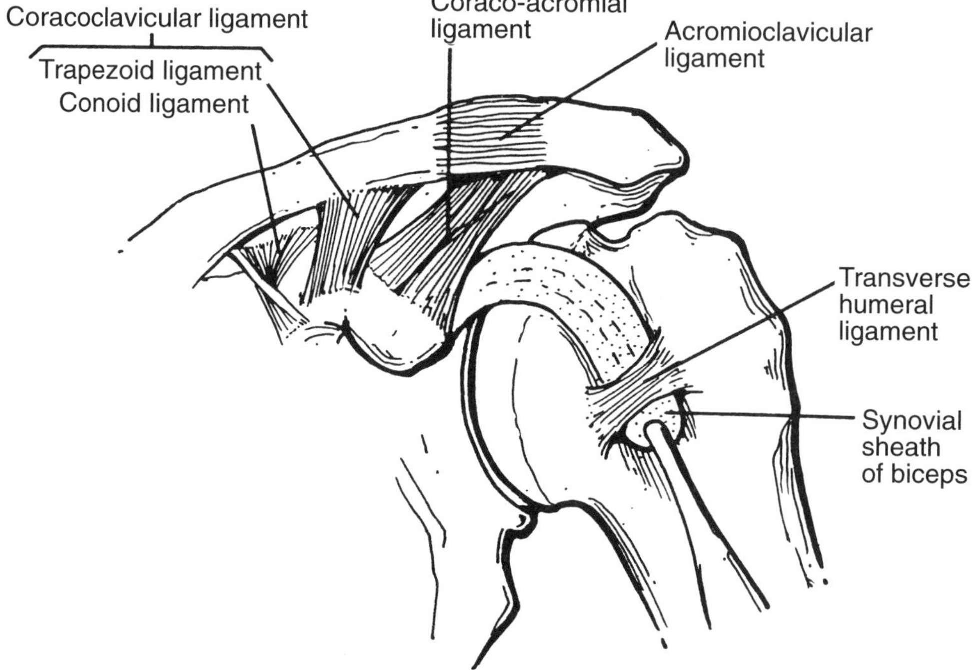

FIGURE 32-3
The demonstration of the anatomy of the acromioclavicular joint. (Tibone J, Patek R, Jobe FW, Perry J, Pink M. The Shoulder. In *Orthopedic Sports Medicine* (p. 465) eds. DeLee JC, Drez D. WB Saunders Co. 1994.)

(2) The glenoid labrum.
  (a) Fibrocartilaginous rim acts to increase the depth and area of the glenoid fossa.
  (b) It increases the humeral head contact area by 75% in the vertical direction and 56% in the transverse direction.
  (c) Adds stability without compromising joint motion.
(3) Glenohumeral ligaments.
  (a) Structural reinforcements of the anterior capsule.
  (b) Formed from folds in the inner wall of the anterior capsule.
  (c) Called upon differentially based on arm position and rotation.
  (d) Designated as superior, middle, and inferior glenohumeral ligaments.
    (i) The superior glenohumeral ligament (SGHL) parallels the biceps tendon. Its primary role is in limiting inferior translation in the adducted arm.
    (ii) The middle glenohumeral ligament (MGHL) arises from the labrum just below the superior glenohumeral ligament and inserts medial to the lesser tuberosity, beneath the subscapularis tendon. Its primary role is to resist external rotation with arms and 45 degrees of abduction.
    (iii) The inferior glenohumeral ligament complex (IGHLC) is the most important of the glenohumeral ligaments anatomically and biomechanically. It originates from the glenoid labrum, inserts into the neck of the humerus, and consists of anterior and posterior bands with an axillary "pouch" in between that forms a "sling." It is the primary restraint to external rotation at 90 degrees abduction. Loss of integrity of the IGHLC is a major cause of anterior glenohumeral instability in throwing athletes (Fig. 32-4).
(4) Negative intraarticular pressure "vacuum effect."
  (a) A significant stabilizing factor to superior/inferior translation in the adducted unloaded arm.
  (b) This effect is lost in the unstable shoulder.

b. Dynamic stabilizers.
  (1) The rotator cuff consists of four muscles that originate on the scapula and insert on the humeral head. Their short, flat, broad tendons fuse intimately with the glenohumeral joint capsule. They are capable of passive as well as dynamic functions.
    (a) Subscapularis.
      (i) Dynamic internal rotator.
      (ii) Passive restraint to external rotation during initial stages of abduction.
    (b) Supraspinatus.
      (i) Dynamic abductor.
    (c) Infraspinatus.
      (i) Dynamic external rotator.
      (ii) Passive restraint to internal rotation.
      (iii) May decrease strain on inferior glenohumeral ligament.
    (d) Teres minor.
      (i) Similar function to infraspinatus (Fig. 32-5).

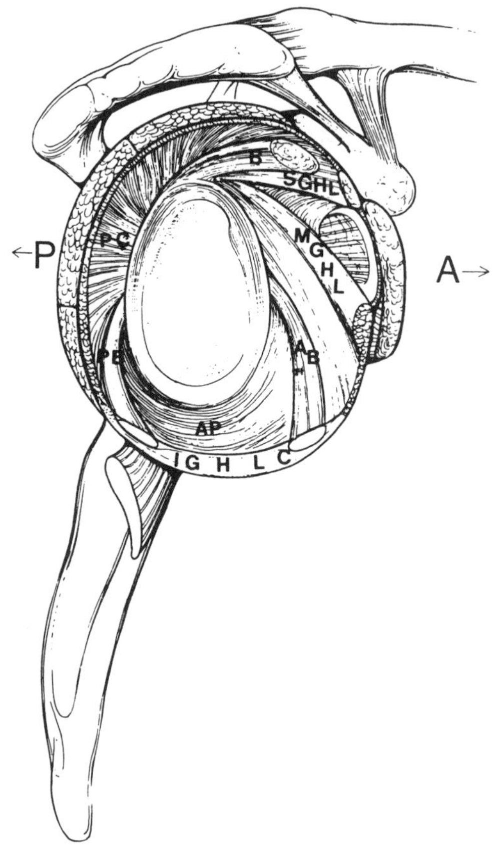

FIGURE 32-4
Anatomical depiction of the glenohumeral ligaments and inferior glenohumeral ligament complex (GHLC). (P = posterior; A = anterior; SGHL = superior glenohumeral ligaments; MGHL = middle glenohumeral ligament.) (Rockwood, CA, Matsen FA, III: *The Shoulder,* WB Saunders Co. 1990.)

(2) The scapular rotators stabilize the glenohumeral joint by positioning the glenoid for optimum bony stability in various positions.
  (a) Trapezius.
    (i) Upper fibers elevate the scapula.
    (ii) Middle fibers retract.
    (iii) Lower fibers depress.
  (b) Levator scapula elevates the scapula.
  (c) Serratus anterior.
    (i) Protraction of scapula.
    (ii) Upward rotation.
    (iii) Depression of scapula (lower fibers).
  (d) Rhomboids.
    (i) Retraction.
    (ii) Elevation.
    (iii) Downward rotation.

V. Scapulothoracic Articulation
  A. Not a true joint.
  B. Scapula rides on the posterior surface of the thoracic cage.
  C. The scapula is suspended by:
    1. AC joint.
    2. Coracoclavicular ligaments.
    3. Surrounding muscular attachments.

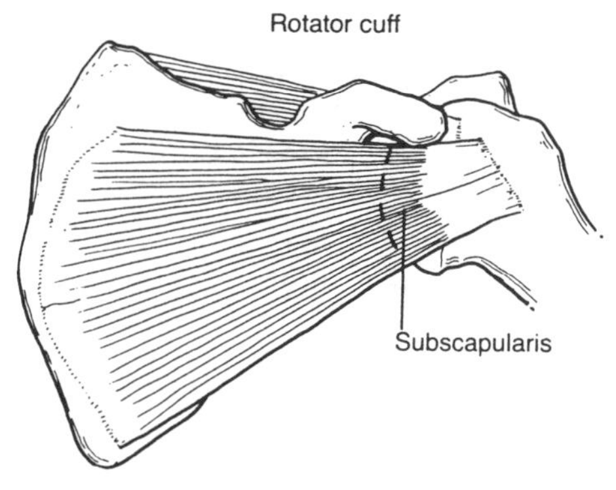

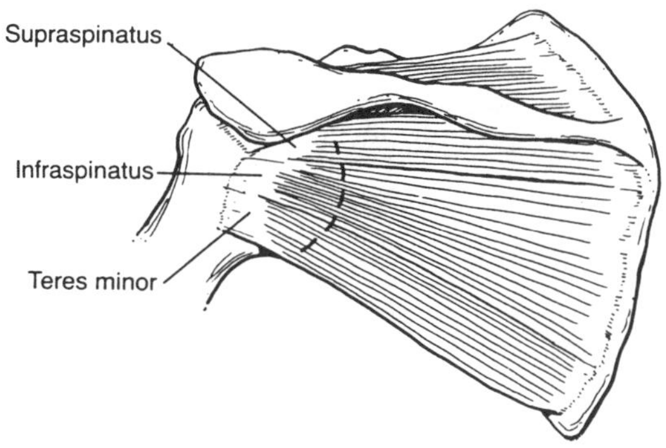

FIGURE 32-5
The four rotator cuff muscles are demonstrated. (Tibone J, Patek R, Jobe FW, Perry J, Pink M. The Shoulder. In *Orthopedic Sports Medicine* (p. 467) eds. DeLee JC, Drez D. WB Saunders Co. 1994.)

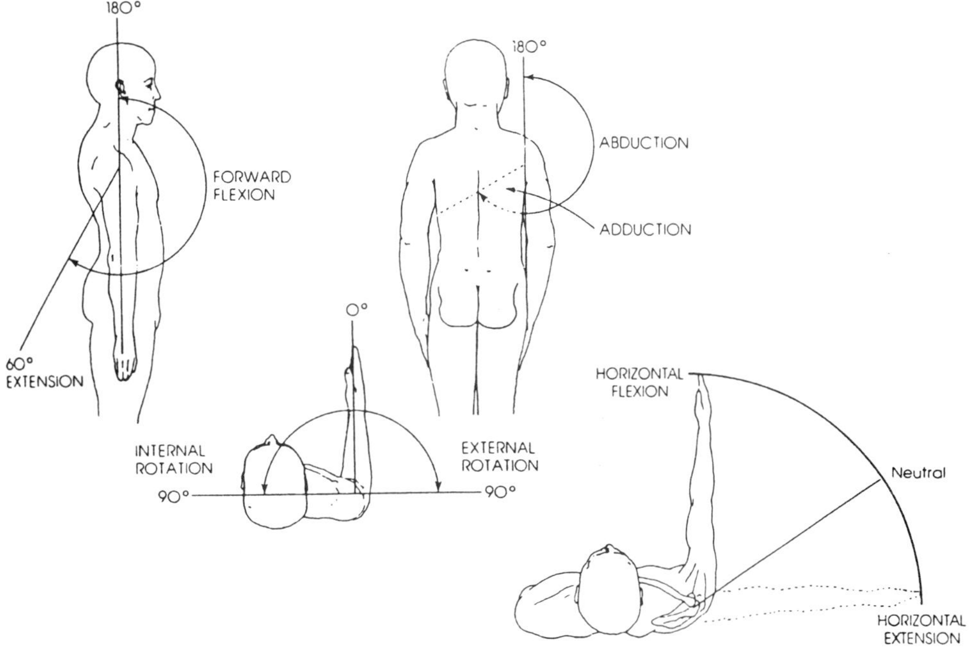

FIGURE 32-6
Ranges in motion of the shoulder complex, including forward flexion, internal-external rotation, abduction, adduction, and horizontal or cross flexion. These motions are all shown in the plane of the body. (From Reid DC: *Sports Injury Assessment and Rehabilitation,* Churchill Livingstone. p. 897.)

D. Scapular motion.
   1. Occurs as an integral component of overall shoulder motion.
   2. Allows increased shoulder mobility.
   3. Facilitates bony support to the glenohumeral joint by positioning the glenoid optimally.

VI. Biomechanics
   A. Shoulder motion (Fig. 32-6, Table 32-1).
   B. Muscles controlling glenohumeral motion.
   C. Muscles controlling scapular motion.
   D. Scapulohumeral rhythm.
      1. Shoulder elevation is the sum of glenohumeral and scapulothoracic motion.
      2. Scapular motion is variable during 0-60 degrees of shoulder elevation (setting stage).

TABLE 32-1. Action and Innervation of Shoulder Muscles

Action	Muscles	Nerve
Abduction	Deltoid	Axillary
	Supraspinatus	Suprascapular
	Infraspinatus	Suprascapular
	Subscapularis	Subscapular
	Teres minor	Axillary
	Biceps (long head)	Musculocutaneous
Adduction	Pectoralis major	Lateral pectoral
	Latissimus dorsi	Thoracodorsal
	Teres major	Subscapular
	Subscapularis	Subscapular
Flexion	Deltoid (anterior fibers)	Axillary
	Pectoralis major	Lateral pectoral
	Coracobrachialis	Musculocutaneous
	Biceps	Musculocutaneous
Extension	Deltoid (posterior fibers)	Axillary
	Latissimus dorsi	Thoracodorsal
	Teres major	Subscapular
	Teres minor	Axillary
	Triceps (long head)	Radial
Horizontal adduction	Pectoralis major	Lateral pectoral
	Deltoid (anterior fibers)	Axillary
Horizontal abduction	Deltoid (posterior fibers)	Axillary
	Teres major	Subscapular
	Teres minor	Axillary
	Infraspinatus	Suprascapular
Internal rotation	Pectoralis major	Lateral pectoral
	Latissimus dorsi	Thoracodorsal
	Deltoid (anterior fibers)	Axillary
	Teres major	Subscapular
	Subscapularis	Subscapular
External rotation	Infraspinatus	Suprascapular
	Teres minor	Axillary
	Deltoid (posterior fibers)	Axillary

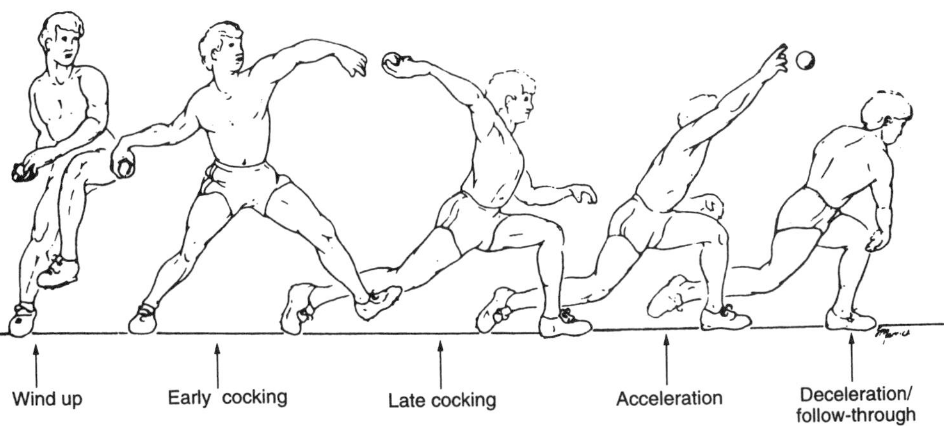

FIGURE 32-7
Five stages of the overhand throwing motion: Stage I. wind-up; Stage II. early cocking; Stage III. late cocking; Stage IV. acceleration; and Stage V. follow-through. (Adapted and reproduced with permission from Glousman RE, Jobe FW, Tibone JE, Moynes D, Antonelli D, Perry J: Dynamic EMG analysis of the throwing shoulder with glenohumeral instability, *J Bone Joint Surg*, 70A:220, 1988.)

TABLE 32-2. Five Phases of Overhand Throwing Motion

Phase	Action ends when	Action
I. Windup	Ball leaves nondominant glove hand.	Deltoid abducts throwing arm.
II. Early cocking	Forward foot hits ground.	Deltoid continues to abduct arm. Infraspinatus and teres minor externally rotate.
III. Late cocking	Shoulder is maximally externally rotated.	Shoulder continues to externally rotate by the infraspinatus and teres minor. Biceps maintains elbow flexion at 90 degrees. The subscapularis begins to decelerate the external rotation.
IV. Acceleration	Ball is released.	Humerus begins to internally rotate by action of the pectoralis major, latissimus dorsi, and triceps.
V. Deceleration/ Follow through	All motion ends.	Eccentric contractions of the teres minor and action of the trapezius, serratus anterior, and rhomboids.

3. Scapular motion is minimal in the 120-180 degree range of shoulder elevation.
4. The sternoclavicular joint, AC joint, and clavicular rotation are important in the 120-180 degree range of shoulder elevation.

E. Biomechanics of overhand throwing (Fig. 32-7, Table 32-2).

Bibliography

Glousman RE et al: Dynamic EMG analysis of the throwing shoulder with glenohumeral instability, *J Bone Joint Surg* 70A:220, 1988.

O'Brien, Arnoczky SP, Warren RF, Rozbruch SR: Developmental anatomy of the shoulder and anatomy of the glenohumeral joint. In Rockwood CA, Matsen FA III, editors: *The Shoulder,* vol. 1, Philadelphia, 1990, WB Saunders pp. 1-33,.

Reid DC: *Sports Injury Assessment and Rehabilitation,* New York, 1992, Churchill Livingstone.

Tibone J et al: The shoulder. In DeLee JC, Drez D, editors: *Orthopaedic Sports Medicine,* Philadelphia, 1994, WB Saunders.

CHAPTER 33

History and Physical Examination of the Shoulder

Greg Hoeksema, MD

I. Introduction
   A. Traditionally, the shoulder has represented a mysterious "black box" for many health care practitioners.
   B. Understanding of basic anatomy and biomechanics discussed in the previous chapter is essential.
   C. Thorough history is the most helpful tool in proper diagnosis of shoulder pathology.
   D. Systematic, simple examination will help to unlock and open the lid to this black box.
      1. Do not overwhelm yourself trying to become familiar with too many different tests.
      2. Vast majority of athletes complaining of shoulder pain will have either rotator cuff pathology (impingement much more frequently than tear), glenohumeral instability, or acromioclavicular (AC) pathology.[3,5,8]
      3. Important to realize these three diagnoses may occur together.
         a. Patient with significant degeneration and spurring of the AC joint can develop a secondary impingement syndrome.
         b. Impingement syndrome in young athletes frequently results from subtle glenohumeral instability.[3,5,8]

II. History
   A. Ascertain hand dominance.
   B. What is the predominant complaint?
      1. Pain is the most common complaint in patients with shoulder pathology.
      2. Other common complaints: noisy joint, decreased range of motion, instability, decreased performance.
   C. Determine level of disability; this may impact treatment approach. For example, the following patients might be approached very differently.
      1. Pain in nondominant shoulder of recreational athlete.

2. Pain in dominant shoulder of an elite athlete that has led to decreased performance.
3. Constant pain in a patient that interrupts sleep nightly.

D. What are/were preferred activities and how often were they performed?
1. Remember, some patients are overhead athletes by occupation (laborer, painter, etc.).
2. Does the patient desire to return to the previous level of performance?
3. Are there new activities or an increase in usual activity?
4. Remember, a frequent historical point of confusion is that there may not be any change in level of activity; repetitive microtrauma is just that, and it may take 10-15 years for a recreational weight lifter to develop AC joint arthritis, for example.

E. Onset of symptoms.
1. Acute onset: almost always macrotrauma.
2. Chronic: classic repetitive microtrauma.
3. Acute on chronic: apparently insignificant macrotrauma can cause significant injury in setting of chronic microtrauma (e.g., rotator cuff tear). Always inquire about prior history of chronic low-grade symptoms in patient with acute injury.
4. What was patient doing at the precise moment when complaint was first noticed?
   a. Impingement syndrome: typically insidious onset in overhead athlete.
   b. Glenohumeral instability: if prodded, patient can usually identify a precise moment when the shoulder became symptomatic. The exception is in the patient with intrinsic laxity/instability of the glenohumeral joint.[3,5,8]
   c. AC pathology: may be acute (AC separation) or insidious (degenerative arthritis).

F. Progression of symptoms over time.
1. Has intensity of pain increased?
2. Has problem decreased performance or caused athlete to stop activity altogether?
3. Does problem occur only with activity or also now at rest?
4. Is there night pain (classically associated with impingement syndrome)?[7]

G. Nature of pain: dull ache versus sharp stabbing.

H. Location of symptoms. Usually, it is difficult for the patient to accurately localize symptoms. Frequently, pain is described as "all over," sometimes anterior, sometimes posterior, or deep inside. Pain of an AC separation, of course, is localized easily.

I. Aggravating factors.
1. Query about specific shoulder positions that aggravate symptoms.
   a. Abduction with external rotation (anterior instability).
   b. All overhead positions (impingement).
   c. Cross-body adduction (AC joint).
2. Query about specific portion of activity that aggravates symptoms.
   a. Extremely useful tool to ferret out specific anatomical location of pathology. Especially useful in:
      (1) Throwing/overhead athletes: cocking phase, acceleration phase, release and deceleration phase, follow through.
      (2) Weight training: what part of which particular exercises cause symptoms or are now avoided by athlete? For example, pa-

tient still lifts weights, but no longer performs military press or gets pain only with deep bench press.

3. Problems with activities of daily living usually indicate more severe pathology.
4. Inability to lie or sleep on affected shoulder common in chronic impingement.

J. Concomitant symptoms.
   1. Neurological: paresthesia, dead-arm sensation, decreased strength.
   2. Noisiness (popping, crunching, grinding): frequent complaint that is very nonspecific and commonly found in patients with no discernible pathology; however, noise or clicking associated with pain is significant.
   3. Decreased range of motion: secondary to pain vs. mechanical block vs. weakness.
   4. Associated chest pain, neck pain, back pain: presence of any of these usually means the shoulder is not the area of primary pathology.
   5. Past medical history.

K. Past history.
   1. Similar symptoms in past. If so, how did they resolve?
   2. Trauma, even very remote historically, can be significant to current complaints.
      a. Remote history of traumatic AC separation (even 10-20 years earlier) may lead to degenerative arthritis of the AC joint with secondary impingement.
      b. Traumatic anterior dislocation of the shoulder in high school football may precipitate problems in patient who takes up tennis 10 years later.

L. Previous treatment regimens.
   1. Medication.
      a. Oral: acetaminophen versus nonsteroidal antiinflammatory drug.
      b. Injected: anesthetics, corticosteroids.
   2. Rest: relative versus absolute.
   3. Physical therapy: have the patient demonstrate exactly what they have been doing.
   4. Ice and/or heat.
   5. Alternative medicine: not uncommon, especially in elite athletes. Herbs, acupuncture, yoga, and the like.
   6. In all of the above, ascertain how much, how often, and for how long. In most cases, you will find there has not been an adequate trial of therapy.

III. Physical Examination

A. Initial examination should begin even before the patient is undressed.
   1. Observe for splinting, lack of arm swing with gait, and the like.
   2. Observe as patient removes shirt to assess for functional disability, decreased motion, pain with motion.
   3. Have female patients in halter style top so bra straps do not interfere with the examination.

B. Visual inspection.
   1. Observe patient from both front and back.
   2. Note any shoulder asymmetry, but keep in mind that patients will frequently carry their dominant shoulder lower than their nondominant shoulder, which can create the illusion of muscular atrophy (Figure 33-1).[9]
   3. Assess for muscular atrophy.
      a. Deltoid, trapezius, biceps usually obvious.

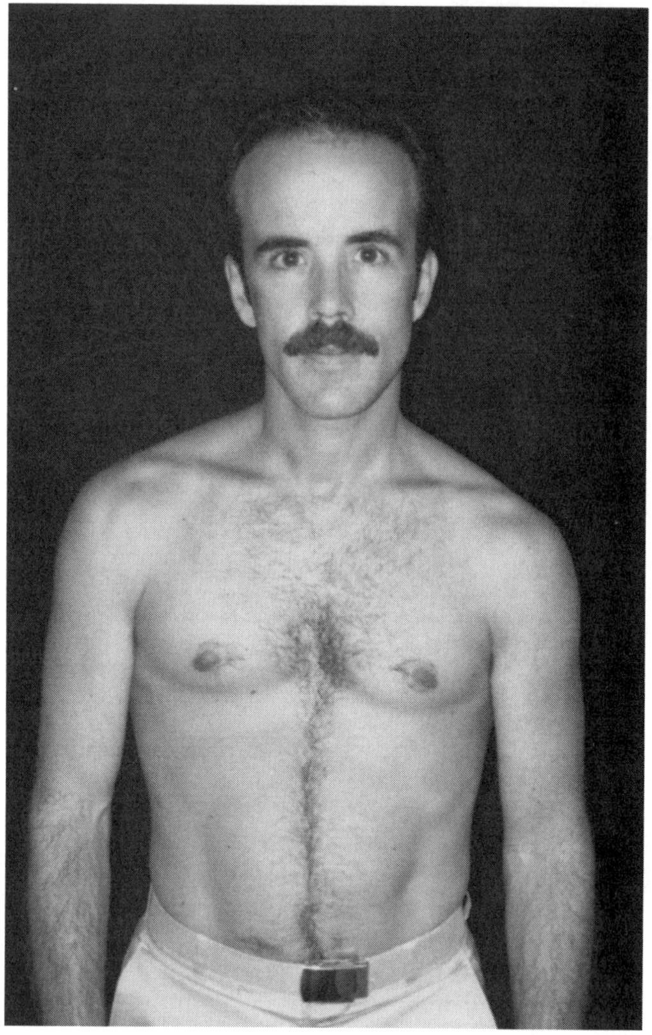

FIGURE 33-1
It is normal to carry the dominant shoulder lower, which can create the appearance of muscular atrophy. Note the apparent asymmetry of the trapezius muscles in this left hand–dominant individual.

   b. Supraspinatus much more subtle because of overlying musculature but important to note.
4. Assess active range of motion.
   a. Forward flexion.
   b. Abduction.
   c. Adduction with internal rotation can be easily assessed by having patient touch thumb as high as possible in the center of back and measuring the difference in centimeters between right and left; this method eliminates the confusion of estimating differences based on thoracic vertebral height and is a useful measurement to assess improvement at followup visits.
   d. External rotation: ensure patient keeps elbows at the side and remember that most throwing athletes will have exaggerated external rotation (and limited internal rotation) in the dominant arm compared to their nondominant arm.[14]
   e. Use the goniometer to make two specific measurements.
      (1) Limit of active range of motion.

(2) Point in the arc of motion that the patient first notes pain: this measurement is extremely useful to compare in followup visits to help assess progress; frequently, patients subjectively will feel unimproved but will have improvement in painless arc of motion.

f. These basic measurements will suffice in assessing the vast majority of patients. Additional motions can be assessed as indicated.

5. Scapulothoracic rhythm.
   a. Observe from behind as patient abducts arms.
   b. Normally, significant scapular lateral rotation on the torso does not begin until approximately 20 degrees of arm abduction and then progresses in a 2 : 1 ratio of humeral motion to scapulothoracic motion.[2]
   c. Scapula rotates to move acromion out of the way of the greater tuberosity of the humerus to prevent impingement and to maintain ideal contractile length of the deltoid as it abducts the arm past 90 degrees.

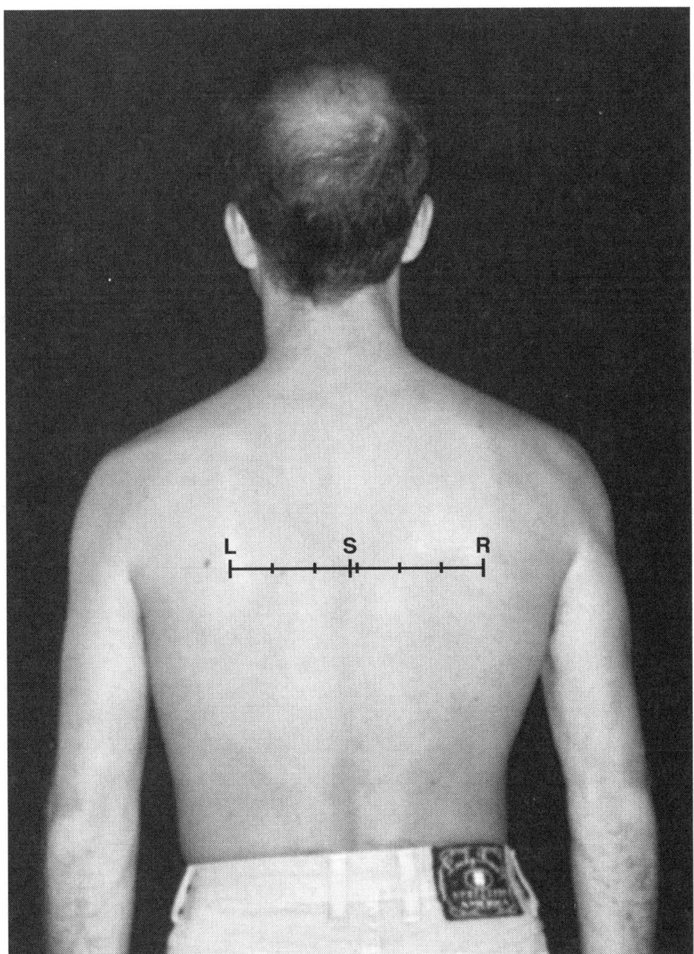

FIGURE 33-2A
Scapulothoracic rhythm can be assessed both dynamically and statically. In panels **A through C,** static measurements from the center of the spine to the inferior tip of the scapula can be compared to the uninjured side to assess for subtle disturbances. Note in this patient how the right scapular lateral rotation is increased in all positions.

d. In chronic impingement, the scapula begins its lateral excursion early and there is an alteration in the usual 2 : 1 ratio of movement.[2,10]
e. Subtle disturbances can be assessed by measuring the distance between the center of the spine and the tip of the scapula in three static positions and then comparing it to the uninvolved side (Figure 33-2, *A-C*).
f. Disturbance of scapulothoracic rhythm is a compensatory, protective mechanism and indicates more severe pathology.
g. Scapular winging can also indicate underlying shoulder pathology.[1,10]
h. Critical to address in any rehabilitation program.

C. Manual inspection.
   1. Muscular strength testing.
      a. With patient's arms at the side and elbows flexed 90 degrees, quickly assess internal/external rotation, and elbow flexion/extension.
      b. Rotator cuff.
         (1) Although we classically assess the rotator cuff using internal and external rotation strength, its main function is to stabilize

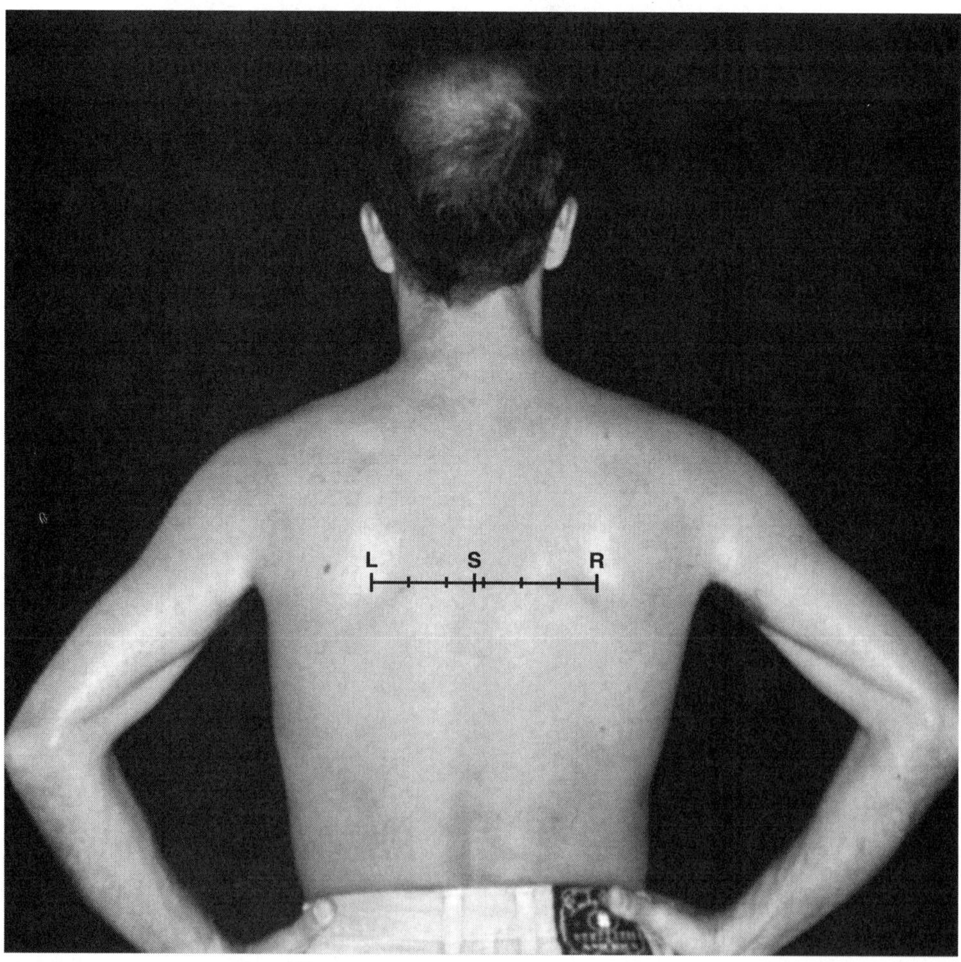

FIGURE 33-2B

the humeral head in the glenoid fossa throughout shoulder range of motion.[2,13,16]

(2) Supraspinatus muscle (Figure 33-3).
  (a) Place arm at 90 degrees of abduction with thumbs pointing downward and bring arm 20 degrees forward of the frontal plane.
  (b) Have patient resist downward force on the arm.[17]
  (c) There should be no clinically discernible difference between dominant/nondominant arms.
  (d) Weakness and/or pain are both considered a positive "supraspinatus test."
  (e) Drop test: passively abduct patient's arm to 90 degrees and then ask the patient to actively hold it there as you let go; inability to do so indicates a large rotator cuff tear.
  (f) The majority of rotator cuff pathology involves the supraspinatus tendon.

(3) Subscapularis muscle is best isolated by having the patient place his/her hand behind the back with palm outward and then pushing the hand away from the back (Figure 33-4). Subscapularis problems are quite unusual.[4]

(4) Infraspinatus and teres minor assist in external rotation.

2. Musculoskeletal palpation.
  a. Clavicle: be sure to palpate both the sternoclavicular and AC joints.
  b. Scapula.
    (1) Follow the spine as it joins to form the acromion.
    (2) Coracoid process is palpable deep and just medial to the anterior deltoid, several centimeters below the clavicle. Pathology in this area is unusual.

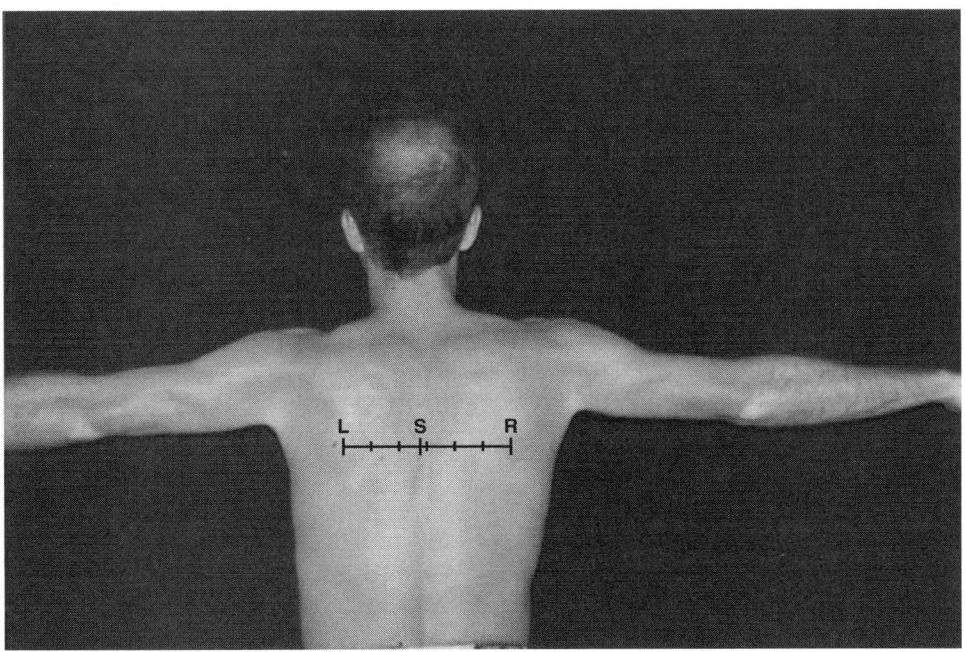

FIGURE 33-2C

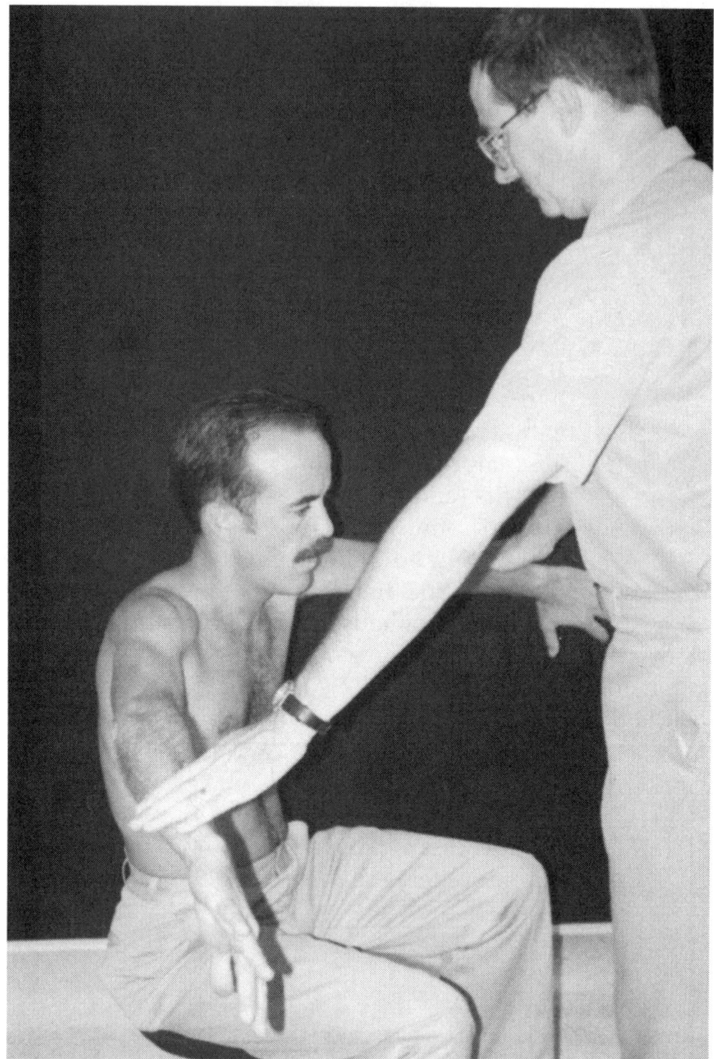

FIGURE 33-3
Test for supraspinatus muscle strength. See text.

c. Humeral head.
   (1) Greater tuberosity easily palpable and tenderness of the supraspinatus tendon can be elicited between the tuberosity and the acromion.
   (2) Bicipital groove and tendon palpable from behind by cupping the humeral head between the examiner's thumb and fingers, and externally rotating the patient's arm. The structures are then easily defined with the tips of the fingers.
      (a) Speed's test: with the elbow extended and the forearm supinated, resist forward flexion of the shoulder at 60 degrees; pain in the area of the proximal tendon is a positive test.
      (b) Yergason's test: pain in the area of the proximal tendon on resisted supination of the forearm with the elbow flexed to 90 degrees.

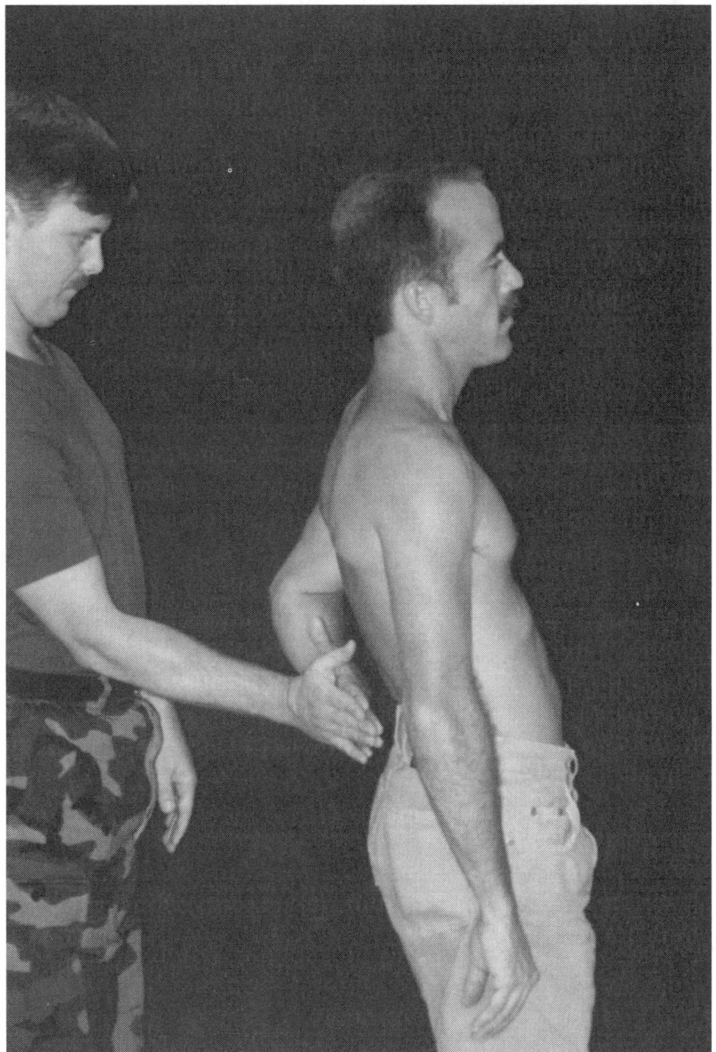

FIGURE 33-4
The subscapularis muscle "lift-off" test. Inability to perform this maneuver is very specific for subscapularis tendon rupture.

(c) Bicipital tendinitis is commonly a subset of impingement syndrome.[12]

3. Glenohumeral joint.
   a. Inferior stability.
      (1) Sulcus sign: appearance of a sulcus just below the acromion when a downward distraction force is placed on the arm in its long axis.
      (2) Grade I to III based on number of centimeters of inferior excursion (i.e., 1 cm = grade I).
      (3) Always compare to other shoulder; grade I sulcus is common finding in normal shoulder.
   b. Anterior/posterior stability.
      (1) Load-shift test (Figure 33-5, *A* and *B*).
         (a) Approach patient from behind and cup humeral head in right hand as noted above for the bicipital groove.

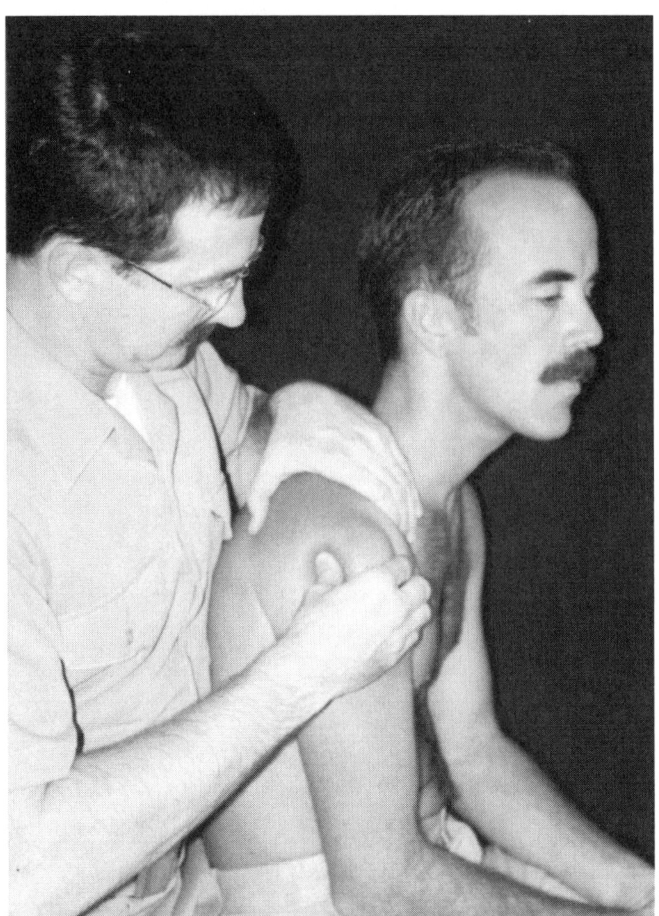

A

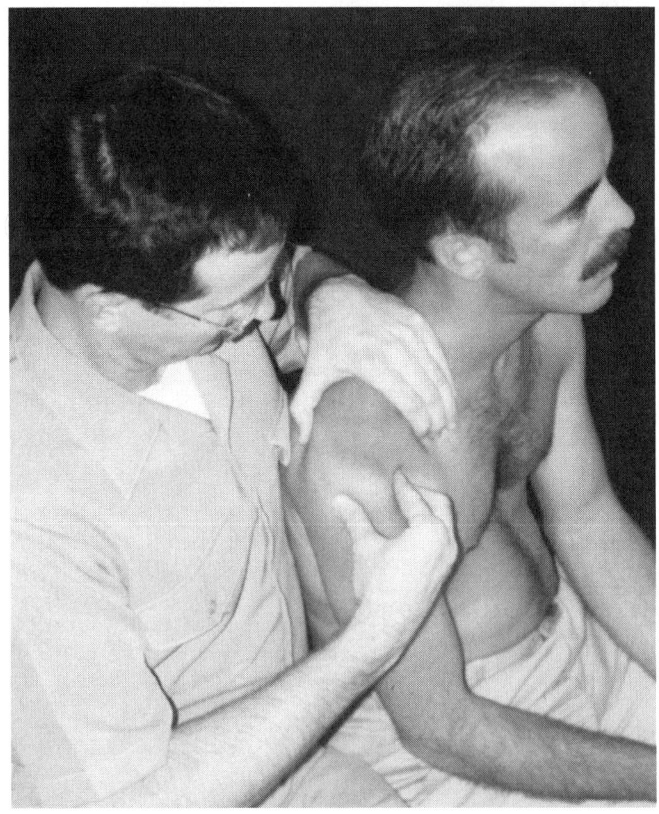

B

FIGURE 33-5A, B

The load-shift test for glenohumeral instability. Compare the position of the humeral head with anterior force **(A)** and posterior force **(B)** in this patient with intrinsic Grade II anterior and posterior instability.

(b) Stabilize scapula by grasping across the top of clavicle, trapezius, and suprascapular area with the left hand.
(c) Apply a forward force on the head of the humerus using the thumb to test for anterior stability.
(d) Apply a posterior force on the head of the humerus using the first two fingers to test for posterior stability.
(e) Remember that the glenoid is slightly anteverted, so use a rolling motion of the head of the humerus; that is, apply slight anteromedial and posterolateral forces on the humeral head.

(2) Apprehension test (Figure 33-6).
(a) Patient in supine position on table.
(b) Place one hand on the table underneath the humeral head to act as fulcrum.

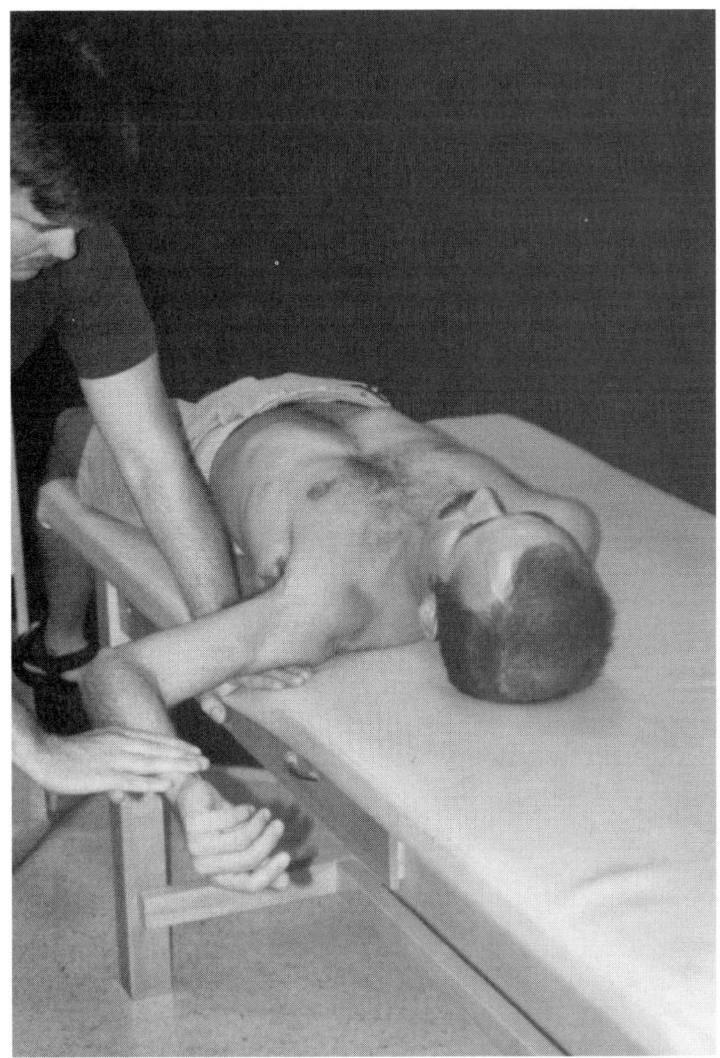

FIGURE 33-6
The apprehension test for anterior glenohumeral instability. The examiner's hand is placed under the humeral head to create a fulcrum; gentle downward force is then applied at the wrist of the abducted, externally rotated arm.

(c) Grasp patient's arm in other hand and move into abduction/external rotation.

(d) Look of apprehension or a feeling of pending dislocation signifies positive test; pain alone does not signify a positive test.

(3) Relocation test (Figure 33-7).

(a) Helps to differentiate between anterior instability and impingement syndrome.

(b) Same technique as apprehension test, except the head of the humerus is stabilized in the glenoid by placing the hand over the anterior aspect of the proximal humerus.

(c) Positive test indicates the patient no longer looks or feels apprehensive and therefore confirms anterior instability.

(4) Grading of anterior/posterior instability.

(a) Grade 1: slight subluxation within fossa.

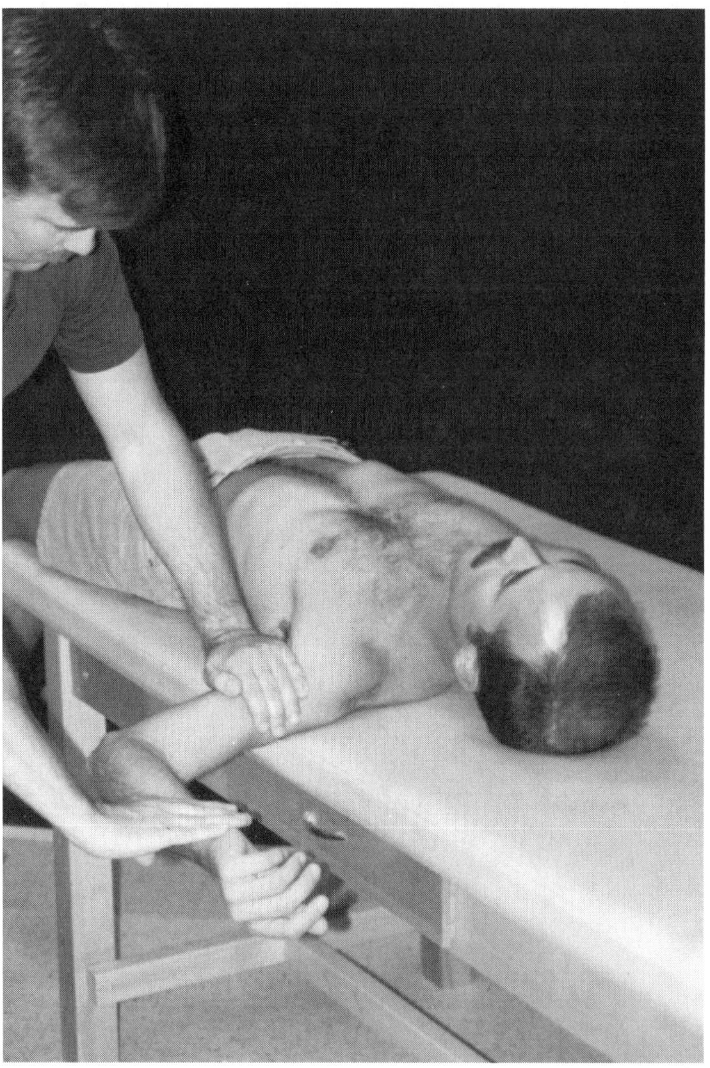

FIGURE 33-7
The relocation test for anterior instability. Note the same technique is used as in the apprehension test, except the hand is now placed on top of the humeral head to stabilize it in the glenoid fossa.

(b) Grade 2: subluxation of part of humeral head out of fossa.
(c) Grade 3: subluxation of head onto glenoid rim.
(d) Grade 4: frank dislocation.

c. Glenoid labrum.
(1) Extremely difficult to assess reliably on clinical grounds.[1]
(2) Labral "clunk" test: akin to McMurray's test of the knee.
(a) Attempt to catch loose labrum between humeral head and glenoid by passively moving arm through superior arc of abduction.
(b) Painful clunk signifies positive test.
(c) Most shoulder clunking does not represent labral pathology.
(3) Subacromial space (impingement syndrome).
(a) There are many different techniques described,[6,11] all of which are based on the functional anatomical pathology; that is, loss of volume of the subacromial space or failure of the rotator cuff to maintain proper seating of the humeral head in the glenoid fossa during abduction.
(b) Thorough history should have already confirmed positive impingement tests in activities of daily living (e.g., "it hurts when I reach for things in the cupboard," "wash my hair," "do overhead press," etc.).
(c) Test clinically by passively abducting arm to 90 degrees and then internally rotate the arm in varying degrees of forward flexion from neutral to 90 degrees (Figure 33-8).
(d) If you have to work too hard to elicit a positive sign, you have the wrong diagnosis!

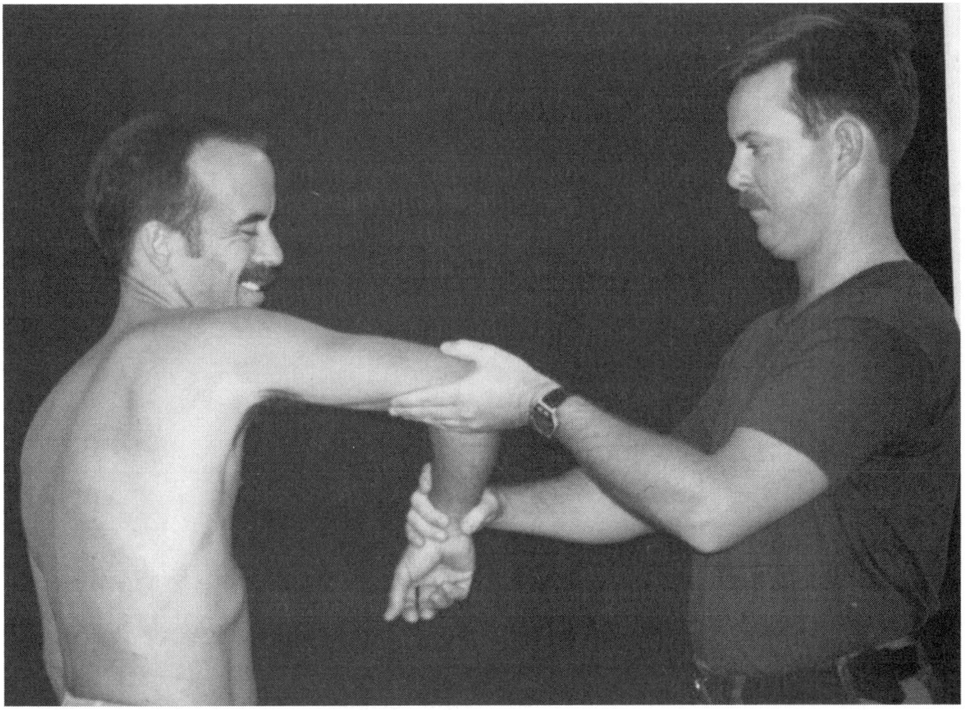

FIGURE 33-8
Impingement test. By abducting the arm to 90 degrees, the greater tuberosity of the humerus is brought into proximity to the acromion. Gentle internal rotation of the arm by downward pressure at the wrist will then elicit pain in the shoulder in a patient with impingement syndrome.

References

1. Andrews JR, Kupferman SP, Dillman CJ: Labral tears in throwing and racquet sports, *Clin Sports Med* 10:901-911, 1991.
2. Calliet R: *Shoulder Pain,* ed 3, Philadelphia, 1991, FA Davis.
3. Fowler PJ, Webster MS: Shoulder pain in highly competitive swimmers, *Orthop Trans* 7:170, 1983.
4. Gerber C, Krushell RJ: Isolated rupture of the tendon of the subscapularis muscle, *J Bone Joint Surg* 73B:389-394, 1991.
5. Glousman RE et al: Dynamic electromyographic analysis of the throwing shoulder with glenohumeral instability, *J Bone Joint Surg* 70A:220-226, 1988.
6. Hawkins RJ, Abrams JS: Impingement syndrome in the absence of rotator cuff tear, *Orthop Clin North Am* 18:373-382, 1992.
7. Hawkins RJ, Murnaghan JP: The shoulder. In Cruess RL, Rennie RJ, editors: *Adult Orthopaedics,* New York, 1984, Churchill Livingstone.
8. Jobe FW et al: An EMG analysis of the shoulder in pitching: a second report, *Am J Sports Med* 12:218-220, 1984.
9. Kendall FP, McCreary EK, Provance PG: *Muscle Testing and Function,* ed 4, Baltimore, 1993, Williams & Wilkins.
10. Miniaci A, Fowler PJ: Impingement in the athlete, *Clin Sports Med* 12:91-110, 1993.
11. Neer CS: Anterior acromioplasty for the chronic impingement syndrome in the shoulder, *J Bone Joint Surg* 54A:42-50, 1972.
12. Neviaser TJ: The role of the biceps tendon in impingement syndrome, *Orthop Clin North Am* 18:383-386, 1987.
13. Perry J: Anatomy and biomechanics of the shoulder in throwing, swimming, gymnastics, and tennis, *Clin Sports Med* 2:247-270, 1983.
14. Plancher KD, Litchfield R, Hawkins RJ: Rehabilitation of the shoulder in tennis players, *Clin Sports Med* 14:111-137, 1995.
15. Poppen NK, Walker PS: Normal and abnormal motion of the shoulder, *J Bone Joint Surg* 58A:195-201, 1976.
16. Sharkey NA, Marder RA: The rotator cuff opposes superior translation of the humeral head, *Am J Sports Med* 23:270-275, 1995.
17. Yocum LA: Assessing the shoulder, *Clin Sports Med* 2:281-289, 1983.

CHAPTER **34**

Impingement Syndrome and Rotator Cuff Injuries

Anthony Saglimbeni, MD

David E.J. Bazzo, MD

IMPINGEMENT SYNDROME

I. Introduction
   A. Impingement is also known as "painful arc syndrome."
   B. It is often the result of the supraspinatus tendon impinging on the caudal surface of the coracoacromial arch.
   C. Impingement is one cause of rotator cuff tendinitis (i.e., inflammation in the cuff).
   D. Traditionally, impingement has been thought of as a mechanical problem, not with the cuff itself, but secondary to the surrounding rigid coracoacromial arch.
   E. The key is to identify the true etiology, so that treatment can be accurately directed.

II. Anatomy and Biomechanics
   A. The shoulder consists of three joints (glenohumeral, acromioclavicular, and sternoclavicular) and one articulation (scapulothoracic).
   B. This configuration allows maximum mobility; however, it predisposes to laxity.
   C. The rotator cuff is one dynamic stabilizer of the shoulder and consists of the supraspinatus, infraspinatus, teres minor, and subscapularis.
   D. The supraspinatus tendon is the most superior in the rotator cuff and inserts onto the greater tubercle. It is impinged by the humeral head against the coracoacromial arch.
   E. The coracoacromial arch consists of the bony coracoid process and acromion, connected by the coracoacromial ligament, whose function is unclear.
   F. Acromial configuration has been classified as type I (flat), type II (curved), or type III (hooked), progressively predisposing to impingement.
   G. The supraspinatus depresses the humeral head in the shallow glenoid fossa.

H. With shoulder elevation the other rotator cuff muscles provide an inferior force on the humerus.
I. Strength imbalance or structural breakdown predisposes to injury.

III. Mechanism

Fu et al.[4] classified impingement as extrinsic (resulting from a problem outside the cuff) or intrinsic (resulting from a problem inside the cuff).

A. Extrinsic.
1. Primary: associated with abnormalities on the underside of the coracoacromial arch, including the acromioclavicular joint. This includes the type I, II, and III classification of Bigliani mentioned above. This is more common in older patients (>40 years old).
2. Secondary: a functional loss of subacromial space due to glenohumeral joint instability. This mechanism is more often seen in younger, more athletic populations. The bicipital tendon may also play a role in preventing superior subluxation of the humeral head, especially in throwing athletes.

B. Intrinsic: when rotator cuff inflammation exists without evidence of extrinsic causes, the etiology is believed to be intrinsic.
1. A critical zone exists where areas of relative hypovascularity coincide with a high frequency of pathology.
2. Another intrinsic cause is angiofibroblastic change from multiple tendon tension overload, resulting in calcification and erosion.

IV. Pathophysiology

A. Whether primary or secondary, impingement results in inflammation (i.e., tendinitis).
B. Furthermore, the zone of relative hypovascularity in the supraspinatus tendon is subject to compression by the humeral head, resulting in degeneration and even tear of the rotator cuff.
C. For this reason the majority of tears are seen within 1 cm of the tendon's insertion, where hypovascularity is greatest.

V. Diagnosis

A. History.
1. Insidious onset of shoulder pain. Often radiates to the arm and is worse at night. May be accompanied by weakness or stiffness.
2. Worsened by overhead activity and lying on the affected side.
3. History of instability.
4. Neurovascular complaints.

B. Physical examination.
1. Palpation for areas of tenderness.
2. Range of motion limitation.
3. Neurovascular assessment.
4. Stability testing may be positive.
5. Provocative maneuvers.
   a. Passive extension with direct rotator cuff tendon palpation shows tenderness.
   b. Pain with resisted abduction or external rotation.
   c. Neer impingement sign: passive flexion with internal rotation.
   d. Hawkins impingement sign: forward flexion to 90 degrees with internal rotation results in greater tuberosity impingement.
   e. Neer impingement test: 3-9 ml of lidocaine injected into the subacromial space resolves symptoms.

C. Diagnostic interventions: plain films should include Neer lateral (or Y view) and Rockwood (outlet) view to define obstruction.

VI. Differential Diagnoses
  A. Rotator cuff tear.
  B. Thoracic outlet syndrome.
  C. Subluxation/instability.
  D. Referred cervical pain.
  E. Bursitis.
  F. Calcific tendinitis.
  G. Adhesive capsulitis.
  H. Arthritis.
  I. Labral tear.
  J. Osteolysis of the clavicle.

VII. Management
  A. Conservative therapy is aimed at reversing inflammation in the rotator cuff.
    1. Relative rest: avoid inciting activities.
    2. Ice.
    3. Systemic nonsteroidal antiinflammatory drugs (NSAIDs).
    4. Injectable steroids if systemic NSAIDs fail.
    5. Restore range of motion with circumduction and pulley exercises early.
    6. Proprioceptive neuromuscular facilitation (PNF) until full painless range of motion is obtained.
    7. Initiate stretching as pain resolves.
    8. Strengthen all shoulder muscles, especially external and internal rotators to improve the efficacy of the dynamic stabilizers. Start with isometric and advance to isotonic or isokinetic exercises. Consider including scapular stabilizers in rehabilitation program.
    9. Ultrasound and iontophoresis may be useful.
    10. If a relapse occurs, an experienced coach, trainer, or physician should review the biomechanics with motion analysis.
    11. Cross-training to maintain remainder of tone function and aerobic fitness.
  B. Surgical.
    1. Arthroscopic procedure for subacromial decompression if conservative therapy for 3-6 months fails.
    2. If instability is the etiology, refer to chapter on instability in shoulder.

ROTATOR CUFF INJURIES

I. Introduction
  A. Aside from impingement, the most common rotator cuff injuries are strains.
  B. Tears are grade 2-3 strains.

II. Mechanisms
  A. The most frequent site of fiber disruption is the supraspinatus at its aforementioned hypovascular area.
  B. Acute tears result from a force applied to the abducted arm.
  C. Chronic tears result from repetitive microtrauma, resulting in inflammation and subsequent thinning and disruption; this is commonly seen in competitive throwers. These people are also predisposed to acute tears by the above mechanism.

III. Diagnosis
  A. History.

1. Acute: history of sustaining some trauma or force. Complaints include pain and inability to abduct.
2. Chronic/degenerative: Pain usually has an indolent onset and in young patients is seen during and after activity. Nocturnal pain is common, and the older athlete often complains of weakness. Pitchers complain of loss of velocity as well.

B. Physical examination.
1. Acute.
   a. Weak abductors with positive drop test (unable to resist adduction force and 90 degree abduction), indicates a tear of the rotator cuff.
   b. Greater tuberosity tenderness.
   c. Pain with abduction from 60-120 degrees.
2. Chronic findings are similar to acute, with the addition of atrophy of the cuff muscles.

C. Diagnostic studies.
1. Plain films are not usually helpful. However, in chronic tears, proximal migration of the humeral head may be evident.
2. Arthrography is rarely used now but will show leakage of dye.
3. If indicated, magnetic resonance imaging and arthroscopy will show defects.
4. Repeat range of motion testing after local anesthetic injection will differentiate limitation due to pain alone versus mechanical disruption and pain.

IV. Differential Diagnoses
   A. Impingement syndrome.
   B. Subluxation/multidirectional instability.

V. Management
   A. Small tears can be treated conservatively with ice, antiinflammatory agents, and rehabilitation as with impingement.
   B. Larger tears require surgical repair, often performed arthroscopically.

Bibliography

Abrams JS: Special shoulder problems in the throwing athlete: pathology, diagnosis, and nonoperative management, *Clin Sports Med* 10(4):839-861, 1991.

Bigliani LU, Morrison DS, April EW: The morphology of the acromion and its relationship to rotator cuff tears, *Orthop Trans* 10:216, 1986.

Frieman BG, Albert TJ, Fenlin JM: Rotator cuff disease: a review of diagnosis, pathophysiology, and current trends in treatment, *Arch Phys Med Rehabil* 75:604-609, 1994.

Fu FH, Harner CD, Klein AH: Shoulder impingement syndrome, a critical review, *Clin Orthop Rel Res* 269:162-173, 1991.

Fu FH, Stone DA: *Sports Injuries: Mechanisms, Prevention, Treatment,* Baltimore, 1994, Williams & Wilkins.

Glousman RE: Instability versus impingement syndrome in the throwing athlete, *Orthop Clin North Am* 24(1):89-99, 1993.

Gold RH, Seeger LL, Yak L: Imaging shoulder impingement, *Skeletal Radiol* 22:555-561, 1993.

Hizon GW: Personal contact.

Mellion MB, Walsh WM, Shelton GL: *The Team Physician's Handbook,* St Louis, 1990, Mosby.

Miniaci A, Fowler PJ: Impingement in the athlete, *Clin Sports Med* 12(1):91-110, 1993.

Neer CS II: Anterior acromioplasty for the chronic impingement syndrome in the shoulder: a preliminary report, *J Bone Joint Surg* 54A:41, 1972.

Neviaser RJ, Neviaser TJ: Observations on impingement, *Clin Orthop Rel Res* 254:60-63, 1990.

Recht MP, Resnick D: Magnetic resonance-imaging studies of the shoulder, *J Bone Joint Surg* 75-A(8):1244-1253, 1993.

Scheib JS: Diagnosis and rehabilitation of the shoulder impingement syndrome in the overhand and throwing athlete, *Rheum Dis Clin North Am* 16(4):971-988, 1990.

Snyder SJ: Rotator cuff lesions, acute and chronic, *Clin Sports Med* 10(3):595-614, 1991.

Zuckerman JD et al: The painful shoulder: Part II. Intrinsic disorders and impingement syndrome, *Am Fam Phys* 43(2):497-512, 1991.

CHAPTER 35

Shoulder Instability

Thomas J. Gill, MD

Lyle J. Micheli, MD

ANTERIOR INSTABILITY

I. Shoulder Anatomy
   A. Shoulder stability.
      1. Result of static and dynamic forces, providing a balance between mobility and stability.
      2. Bony architecture sacrifices stability for motion: most mobile joint in the body.
      3. Wide variation in normal translation of the glenohumeral joint from patient to patient.
   B. Glenoid.
      1. Glenoid able to resist direct force from humeral head.
      2. Small contact area; radius of curvature increased by fibrocartilaginous labrum, allowing more concentric articulation with humeral head. Anterior inferior labrum plays significant role in passive restraint to anterior translation.[3]
      3. Instability due to congenital dysplasia usually presents in adolescence.
      4. Glenoid version: 30 degree retroversion. No consistent association between glenoid version angles and anterior or posterior instability.
      5. Glenoid fractures may result in instability.
   C. Capsule.
      1. Contribute to static stability through selective tightening of the anterior and inferior capsule during humeral abduction and external rotation.
      2. Reinforced by glenohumeral ligaments.
   D. Glenohumeral ligaments: static stabilizers of shoulder; thickenings of the capsule.
      1. Superior: variable. Minor role in inferior instability.
      2. Middle: located across subscapularis tendon. Secondary restraint to anterior instability.

3. Inferior complex: anterior and posterior bands. Most important restraint to anterior, posterior, and inferior translation of the humeral head.
4. Shoulder as a "circle."[7]
   a. For a dislocation to occur, both sides of the glenoid must be disrupted.
   b. Patients with anterior dislocations often have increased posterior translation as well.
   c. Surgery on one side of joint affects stability on the other side.
      (1) Putti-Platt procedure (tightening of anterior capsule) can cause posterior subluxation and instability.

E. Muscles: dynamic stabilizers of shoulder.
   1. Rotator cuff: supraspinatus, infraspinatus, teres minor, subscapularis.
      a. Most important dynamic stabilizers of joint.
      b. Center and compress the humeral head within the glenoid fossa.
   2. Deltoid, latissimus dorsi.
   3. Scapular rotators: trapezius, levator scapulae, rhomboids, serratus anterior.
   4. Position scapula for optimum stability during overhead activity.

II. Pathophysiology
   A. Small defect in either static or dynamic stabilizers can have a cumulative effect on shoulder stability.
   B. Instability complex ("thrower's shoulder, swimmer's shoulder").[3]
      1. Repetitive microtrauma from overhead activity may lead to attenuation of static anterior restraints.
      2. Mild anterior glenohumeral translation then results.
      3. Leads to increased activity by dynamic stabilizers to compensate for this mild instability.
      4. Continued activity causes fatigue of the muscles, leading to further anterior subluxation.
      5. Subluxation allows humeral head to contact the acromion or coracoacromial arch, leading to "secondary impingement."
      6. Secondary impingement may lead to rotator cuff tear.
   C. Anterior dislocation.
      1. Arm forced into abduction, external rotation, and extension.
      2. Humeral head dislocates into subcoracoid position (rarely, subclavicular or intrathoracic).
      3. Instability can be due to widening of rotator interval between supraspinatus and subscapularis.

III. Classification[7]
   A. Etiology.
      1. Traumatic: specific event and mechanism of injury.
      2. Atraumatic: involuntary or voluntary; ligamentous laxity. (Voluntary: ? personality disorder in rare patient.)
      3. Repetitive microtrauma: throwing, swimming, tennis.
      4. Congenital: glenoid dysplasia.
      5. Neuromuscular: Erb's palsy, cerebral palsy, seizures.
   B. Chronology.
      1. Acute: initial event.
      2. Recurrent: repeated episodes.
      3. Chronic (fixed): remains not reduced.
   C. Direction.
      1. Anterior: 95% of shoulder instability; often presents with dislocation.

2. Posterior: present in 2% to 4% of patients with an unstable shoulder; usually subluxation.
3. Inferior: isolated dislocation (luxatio erecta) is rare; usually presents as subluxation in association with anterior or posterior instability.
4. Multidirectional: instability in more than one direction; inferior instability with either anterior or posterior component; rarely, anterior and posterior without inferior component.

D. Degree.
1. Dislocation: humeral head not in contact with glenoid fossa. Causes avulsion of anterior capsule and labrum from glenoid rim (Bankart lesion).
2. Subluxation: increased humeral head translation, causing symptoms.
   a. Usually greater than 50% translation within glenoid.
   b. Increased translation alone does not establish diagnosis of instability; must be associated with appropriate clinical manifestations.
3. Transient/microlabral injury without obvious subluxation, which progresses to subluxation if inferior glenohumeral ligament is affected.

E. "TUBS" and "AMBRI."[8]
1. TUBS: traumatic instability, unidirectional in nature, Bankart lesion present, responds to surgery.
2. AMBRI: atraumatic etiology, multidirectional bilateral involvement, responds to rehabilitation.

IV. History

A. Diagnosis.
1. Instability diagnosed on history and physical examination alone in >90% of cases.[6]

B. Pain.
1. Most common complaint.
2. Often posterior in location due to "check-rein effect."
3. Occurs with overhead activity (impingement syndrome).
4. Instability vs. rotator cuff pathology.
   a. Pain associated with specific phase of overhead activity is likely due to instability. Throwers often complain of painful "clicking" in cockup or acceleration phase.
   b. Pain exacerbated by progressive activity is usually due to rotator cuff tendinitis.
   c. Night pain or rest pain may be due to rotator cuff tear.

C. "Dead arm syndrome."
1. Transient subluxation, giving the sensation that the arm has "gone dead."
2. Most common in throwers.

D. Age.
1. Patients >50 years old may have associated rotator cuff tears.
2. Younger patients more likely to sustain recurrent dislocations.

E. Mechanism of injury: if traumatic dislocation occurred, it is important to determine the magnitude of the traumatic event.
1. The less force required to produce the first dislocation, the more likely that the shoulder will remain unstable.[4]
2. Atraumatic group associated with generalized ligamentous laxity and connective tissue disorders.

V. Physical Examination

A. Inspection.

1. Asymmetry, atrophy, bony deformity.
2. Scapular winging.
3. Wide scarring from previous injury; suggests collagen deficiency.

B. Palpation.
1. Crepitus: subacromial scarring/bursitis, acromioclavicular joint arthritis, glenohumeral arthritis, labral tear, loose bodies.[3]
2. Sternoclavicular joint.
3. Acromioclavicular joint.
4. Anterior acromion: rotator cuff pathology or subacromial bursitis.
5. Bicipital groove.

C. Range of motion.
1. Chronic instability: loss of external rotation.
2. Anterior dislocation: unable to touch opposite shoulder.

D. Apprehension sign.
1. Most sensitive sign of instability.
2. Anxiety/discomfort with arm in abduction and external rotation.
3. Pain without apprehension may be secondary to impingement.

E. Relocation test (Fowler sign):
1. Pain improved by posterior pressure with arm in position of apprehension (abduction, external rotation).
2. Helps differentiate primary impingement from primary instability with secondary impingement.

F. Sulcus sign: depression in skin below acromion when inferior traction is applied to arm.

G. Load testing.
1. With patient supine, arm is placed in abduction and external rotation.
2. Anterior and posterior forces are applied to humeral head by gripping proximal humerus.
3. Amount of translation is then quantified.
   a. Grade I = translation to glenoid rim with no dislocation.
   b. Grade II = dislocation with spontaneous reduction.
   c. Grade III = fixed dislocation.

H. Impingement sign.
1. Abduction and internal rotation of arm elicits pain as greater tuberosity is brought under acromion.
2. Often "secondary impingement" due to primary instability.

I. Neurological examination.
1. Axillary nerve.
   a. Most commonly injured.
   b. Check sensation over lateral deltoid, as well as deltoid strength.
2. Musculocutaneous nerve.
   a. Second most commonly injured nerve.
   b. Assess elbow flexion and sensation over medial aspect of arm and forearm.
3. Rule out cervical radiculopathy or suprascapular nerve entrapment.

J. Examination under anesthesia: should be routine before surgery is initiated.

VI. Radiographic Examination

A. Plain films.
1. True anteroposterior (AP) (in plane of scapula).
2. AP in internal rotation: defines Hill-Sachs lesions.
   a. Impression fracture in posterolateral humeral head by recoil against anterior glenoid rim.

3. Transscapular Y view (perpendicular to plane of scapula).
4. Axillary.
   a. Most important.
   b. Defines bony Bankart lesions. Fractures of glenoid rim.
5. Rule out infection, fracture, or neoplasm.

B. Arthrography: useful to assess rotator cuff.
C. Computed tomography/arthrography.
   1. Helps define glenoid and humeral head integrity.
   2. Contrast outlines labrum.
D. Magnetic resonance imaging.
   1. Labral integrity.
   2. Glenohumeral ligaments.
   3. Rotator cuff.

VII. Reduction Techniques
   A. "Recreate mechanism of injury."
   B. Rowe maneuver.
      1. Gentle manipulation of arm into abduction, external rotation, and extension; have patient "touch opposite ear over head."
      2. Intraarticular lidocaine injection can facilitate reduction.
   C. Double sheet method.
      1. Premedication with narcotic and short-acting benzodiazepine. Muscle relaxation is more important than pain medication and is often amnestic (e.g., morphine and midazolam).
      2. One sheet is placed around chest to stabilize body while a second is placed around the proximal forearm with the elbow in 90 degrees of flexion.
      3. Axial traction is slowly applied with the arm in slight abduction and external rotation. Use with caution in the elderly, as osteopenic bone is more prone to fracture.
   D. Stimson maneuver: patient lies prone, and weights are applied to affected arm hanging off the edge of the table.

VIII. Postreduction Care
   A. Immobilization.
      1. Three weeks in sling. No study has documented association between length of immobilization and recurrent dislocation.[2]
      2. Older patients (>40) have increased incidence of rotator cuff tears and adhesive capsulitis after dislocation;[1] should immobilize for only 10 days.
   B. Early motion: begin range of motion exercises at week 4. Limit abduction to 90 degrees.
   C. Strengthening: begin progressive resistive exercises at week 6. Stress internal rotation for tightening of subscapularis.

IX. Treatment Considerations
   A. Recurrent dislocation.
      1. Age: major risk factor in traumatic group.[5]
         a. <20 years: 90%.
         b. >40 years: 25%.
         c. >50 years: uncommon.
      2. Usually occurs in first 2 years.
      3. Ligamentous laxity. Poor results from surgical treatment in young girls with bilateral laxity.
      4. Connective tissue disorders.
   B. Activity level: stable, strong, pain-free shoulder essential in athletic population (e.g., throwers, swimmers, tennis players, gymnasts).

C. Occupation: manual labor vs. desk work.
D. Dominant extremity.
E. Patient reliability.

X. Nonoperative Treatment
A. Goal: restore strength and range of motion.
B. Relative rest.
1. Avoid causative activity/mechanism (i.e., abduction and external rotation).
2. Nonsteroidal antiinflammatory drugs.
3. Particularly important in athletic population to allow continued conditioning while allowing shoulder to rest.
C. Rotator cuff rehabilitation: emphasis on strengthening internal rotators and regaining external rotation. Tendinitis often presents due to instability-induced impingement and traction of the rotator cuff.
D. Scapular rotators.
1. Stabilize scapula.
2. Often ignored.

XI. Operative Treatment Options
A. Bankart procedure.
1. Addresses pathological lesion (i.e., anchors avulsed anterior capsule back to glenoid rim).
2. If >30% of glenoid is absent, bone grafting is indicated.
3. Hill-Sachs lesions seldom need to be addressed. If persistent instability, the defect can be filled with bone graft or transplantation of the infraspinatus into the lesion.
B. Putti-Platt procedure.
1. Reefing of anterior capsule and subscapularis.
2. Not indicated in athletic population due to loss of external rotation.
C. Capsular shift: indicated when instability is due to patulous capsule and not Bankart lesion.
D. Bristow procedure: transfer of coracoid process to anterior glenoid rim.
E. Eden-Hybbinette procedure: bone graft to anterior glenoid rim.
F. Magnuson-Stack procedure: lateral transfer of the subscapularis tendon.
G. Arthroscopy.
1. Labral debridement may ameliorate pain but not improve stability.
2. Random debridement of loose labral tissue is contraindicated, especially if present below the center of the glenoid. Glenohumeral instability could be exacerbated.
H. Return to sports.
1. Noncontact: 4 months.
2. Contact: 6 months.

POSTERIOR INSTABILITY

I. History
A. Symptoms: often vague.
B. Complaints: similar to anterior instability.
C. Pain: anterior and/or posterior.
D. Instability: seldom a complaint.

II. Physical Examination
A. Range of motion.
1. Chronic instability: loss of passive internal rotation.
2. Posterior dislocation: unable to externally rotate.

B. Palpation: crepitus or "clicking" in 90%.[7]
C. Load test.
D. Apprehension: uncommon.
E. Ligamentous laxity.
   1. Thumb hyperabduction.
   2. Index finger metacarpal-phalangeal joint (MCP) hyperextension.
   3. Elbow hyperextension.
   4. Knee hyperextension.
   5. Hypermobile patella.

III. Pathophysiology of Posterior Instability[7]
A. Capsular laxity/ligamentous laxity.
B. Anatomy.
   1. Humeral head retroversion >40%.
   2. Hypoplastic glenoid.
   3. ? glenoid retroversion >10 degrees.
C. Repetitive microtrauma: seen in followthrough phases of activities such as throwing, swimming free-style, and serving in tennis.

IV. Posterior Dislocation
A. Mechanism.
   1. Direct blow to anterior shoulder.
   2. Flexion, internal rotation, and adduction of arm.
   3. Electric shock, seizures; stronger internal rotators (subscapularis, latissimus dorsi, pectoralis major) overcome weaker external rotators.
   4. Fall on outstretched hand.
B. Clinical findings.
   1. Missed diagnosis in 60% to 80% at first presentation.
   2. Arm held adducted and internally rotated.
   3. Prominent coracoid; posterior bulge.
   4. Marked pain with attempted external rotation or abduction.
   5. Inability to supinate forearm with arm forward flexed.
   6. Pain with resistive testing of rotator cuff.
   7. Recurrent posterior dislocation.
      a. Less frequent than anterior recurrences: 38%.
      b. Patients with recurrent posterior subluxation do not tend to develop recurrent dislocation patterns, as seen with anterior instability.
      c. Age <20 is primary risk factor.
C. Reduction maneuver: lateral traction with arm in internal rotation to disengage head from glenoid, followed by extension and adduction.

V. Radiographic Examination
A. Standard trauma series (AP, Y, axillary).
   1. AP can appear normal.
   2. Axillary view often abandoned due to pain. Most common reason for missed diagnosis.
B. Anterior humeral head often impacted on posterior glenoid rim.
   1. "Reverse Hill-Sachs" lesion.
C. Capsular calcification along posterior capsule and labrum.
D. Bony erosion of posterior glenoid rim.

VI. Nonoperative Treatment
A. Immobilization: 3 weeks.
B. Rehabilitation: strengthen external rotators.

VII. Operative Treatment Options
A. Bone graft: posterior bone augmentation if glenoid deficient or ligamentous laxity present.

B. Soft tissue: anterior vs. posterior capsulorrhaphy.
C. Arthroscopy: main role is diagnostic, not therapeutic.
D. Results: not as reliable as for anterior instability.

MULTIDIRECTIONAL INSTABILITY

I. Definition
   A. Patterns of instability.
      1. Inferior instability is a significant finding in these patients.
      2. Direction of instability.
         a. Anteroinferior > posteroinferior > anterior; posterior and inferior > anteroposterior without inferior.
   B. Continuum: rather than being completely separate entities, there is a continuum between unidirectional instability and multidirectional instability.
II. Etiology
   A. Atraumatic: ligamentous laxity.
   B. Repetitive microtrauma: repetitive activity at extremes of motion.
   C. Traumatic.
III. Clinical Findings
   A. Inferior laxity.
      1. Pain and/or clicking with arm at side.
      2. Subluxation or dislocation with lifting.
      3. Sulcus sign.
   B. Period of disability: Patients with multidirectional instability are disabled for longer periods for a given activity than those with unidirectional instability.
IV. Nonoperative Treatment
   A. Rehabilitation: patients with ligamentous laxity are more likely to respond to rehabilitation than those with traumatic etiologies.
V. Operative Treatment Options
   A. Identify primary direction of instability.
   B. Anterior surgery: most cases of multidirectional instability can be corrected anteriorly.

References

1. Hawkins RJ et al: Anterior dislocation of the shoulder in the older patient, *Clin Orthop* 206:192-195, 1986.
2. Hovelius L: Anterior dislocation of the shoulder in teenagers and young adults, *J Bone Joint Surg* 69A(3):393-399, 1987.
3. Kvitne RS, Jobe FW: The diagnosis and treatment of anterior instability in the throwing athlete, *Clin Orthop* 291:107-123, 1993.
4. Rowe CR: Acute and recurrent anterior dislocation of the shoulder, *Orthop Clin North Am* 11(2):253-270, 1980.
5. Rowe CR, Zarins B, Ciullo JV: Recurrent anterior dislocation of the shoulder after surgical repair, *J Bone Joint Surg* 66A(2):159-168, 1984.
6. Silliman JF, Hawkins JR: Classification and physical diagnosis of instability of the shoulder, *Clin Orthop* 291:7-19, 1993.
7. Skyhar MJ, Warren RF, Altchek DW: Instability of the shoulder. In Nicholas JA, Hershman EB, editors: *The Upper Extremity in Sports Medicine,* St Louis, 1990, Mosby–Year Book, pp 181-212.
8. Thomas SC, Matsen FA: An approach to the repair of glenohumeral ligaments in the management of traumatic anterior glenohumeral instability, *J Bone Joint Surg* 71A(4):506-513, 1989.

CHAPTER 36

Brachial Plexus Injuries

Robert E. Sallis, MD

I. Overview
   A. Injury to the brachial plexus is commonly seen in athletes.
   B. The main focus of this chapter is transient brachial plexopathy, the most common form of injury.
   C. In addition, this chapter discusses thoracic outlet syndrome, acute brachial neuropathy, and backpacker's palsy, all of which can be associated with sports participation.

II. Transient Brachial Plexopathy
   A. Introduction.
      1. Transient brachial plexus injury is a common sports injury.
      2. Most often seen in football. Also seen in wrestling, hockey, basketball, and water sports.
      3. Commonly called "burners," "stingers," "zingers," "hot shots," or "pinched nerves."
   B. Incidence.
      1. Seen in up to 65% of football players during their careers. Recurrent episodes in 57% of players.
      2. Most common in defensive backs.
      3. Frequently not reported to coach, trainer, or team physician.
   C. Mechanism of injury.
      1. Usually caused by blow to player's head, which causes lateral flexion of the cervical spine to the asymptomatic side with concomitant shoulder depression that stretches the nerves of the brachial plexus on the symptomatic side.
      2. May also occur upon lateral flexion toward the symptomatic side, which causes compression of the nerve roots between the shoulder pad and the superior or medial scapula.
   D. Anatomy.
      1. Brachial plexus comprised of C5, C6, C7, C8, and T1 nerve roots.
      2. Nerve roots form three major trunks.
         a. Upper trunk from C5 and C6.

   b. Middle trunk from C7.
   c. Lower trunk from C8 and T1.
3. Nerve trunks pass between the anterior and middle scalene muscles and then under the clavicle, where they divide to eventually form peripheral nerves in the arm.
4. C5 and C6 nerve roots (upper trunk) are most commonly affected.
   a. C5.
      (1) Muscles: deltoid, biceps.
      (2) Numbness: lateral arm.
   b. C6.
      (1) Muscles: biceps, wrist flexors.
      (2) Numbness: thumb, index finger.

E. Signs and symptoms.
1. Sudden burning pain and numbness along the lateral arm, thumb, and index finger.
2. Weakness in the deltoid, biceps, supraspinatus, and infraspinatus (difficulty with shoulder abduction, external rotation, and arm flexion).
3. May have diminished deep tendon reflex at biceps.
4. Symptoms typically resolved within 1 or 2 minutes. Occasionally, player has upper limb paresis that may last months or years or, rarely, can be permanent.

F. Grading of brachial plexus injury.
1. Neuropraxia: mildest form of brachial plexus injury with recovery in minutes to days (includes burners).
2. Axonotmesis: more severe or recurrent injury, which may result in symptoms lasting weeks to months.
3. Neurotmesis: most severe injury, usually resulting in permanent deficit. Rare in sports. Usually seen in auto accidents.

G. Sideline management and return to play.
1. Ensure that more serious injury to neck or shoulder has not occurred, including:
   a. Cervical spine injury.
   b. Clavicle fracture.
   c. Acromioclavicular (AC) separation.
   d. Shoulder dislocation.
   e. Transient quadriplegia.
2. Any athlete with local neck tenderness, a fear of moving the head, or a bony deformity should be immobilized on a spine board and immediately sent for cervical spine radiography.
3. Evaluate sensory and motor function in the affected arm.
   a. Players with persistent pain, weakness, or sensory changes should not return to play.
   b. May return to play if no symptoms, full range of neck motion, and no residual shoulder or arm weakness.
4. Examination should be repeated after the game and during the next week because muscle weakness may appear later. Sensory changes often take longer to develop than motor signs.

H. Further diagnostic evaluation.
1. Should be done on players with persistent symptoms, objective weakness, or sensory loss.
2. Cervical spine radiography, including flexion-extension views to disclose subtle ligamentous instability or partial subluxation.
3. Magnetic resonance imaging (MRI) can show cervical disk herniation or narrowing of the cervical canal.

4. Electromyogram (EMG) can be done to locate site of lesion in players who have persistent weakness. Often abnormalities not seen for 10 to 20 days.
   a. Nerve root lesion: should do MRI of cervical spine to detect disk herniation.
   b. Upper trunk lesion: monitor athlete's progress clinically.
   c. EMG changes may persist for years after symptoms resolve; decisions on return to play are thus best made clinically.

I. Recurrent burners.
   1. No contact sports if any symptoms persist. These need further evaluation as previously described.
   2. Rehabilitation exercises.
      a. Start with passive and active neck flexibility exercises to reestablish normal range of motion (include flexion, extension, lateral flexion, and rotation).
      b. Strengthening program to focus on same movements. Start with isometric exercises and progress to isotonic.
      c. Include shoulder shrugs to strengthen trapezius.
   3. Equipment should be modified to reduce lateral neck motion.
      a. Cowboy collars (heavy plastic collars that attach to shoulder pads and help reduce lateral bending of the neck) and neck rolls.
      b. Shoulder pad lifts (raise shoulder pads up under helmet to reduce lateral bending).
   4. Coach should be informed to look for poor blocking or tackling technique as a possible reason for recurrent burners.

III. Thoracic Outlet Syndrome (TOS)
   A. Introduction.
      1. Implies compression of the neurovascular components, which travel from the neck through the thoracic outlet area and supply the upper extremity.
      2. Can occur in athletes secondary to exertion, as a result of weight training, or as a response to trauma.
      3. TOS is probably an uncommon problem, although a lesser degree of the syndrome may often be seen.
   B. Causes.
      1. Many causes and sites for compression of the neurovascular bundle in the thoracic outlet area have been identified. The most common are:
         a. Compression between the anterior and middle scalene muscles: scalenus anticus syndrome.
         b. Compression between the first rib and clavicle: costoclavicular syndrome.
         c. Compression under a cervical rib: cervical rib syndrome.
         d. Compression under the pectoralis minor muscle and coracoid process with the arm in hyperabduction: hyperabduction syndrome.
         e. Other factors such as poor posture with sagging shoulders or callus formation from fractures of the first rib or clavicle may also contribute.
   C. Symptoms.
      1. May be neurological, venous, arterial, or a combination of these, depending on the nature of the thoracic outlet compression.
         a. Neurological compression symptoms are most common, including:
            (1) Lower trunk of brachial plexus usually affected.
            (2) Pain, paresthesia, and numbness in distribution of the ulnar nerve.

(3) Sensory loss, weakness, and atrophy (late changes).

b. Arterial compression symptoms include claudication, numbness, paresthesia (arm falls asleep), and a cool, pale limb.

c. Venous compression symptoms include pain, edema, and venous engorgement. These symptoms usually begin after exertion and result from thrombosis affecting the subclavian or axillary vein.

D. Diagnosis.

1. Physical examination: several tests that show decrease in the pulse or that reproduce the symptoms or both are used (this indicates a positive test). These tests indicate TOS when positive.

a. Adson's test: done by having the patient take a deep breath and holding it for 10 seconds with neck extended and chin turned toward the affected side. Arm is held at side in slight abduction.

b. Costoclavicular test: done while sitting with shoulders drawn downward and backward.

c. Wright's test: the arm is placed into hyperabduction.

2. Radiography of the neck may show a cervical rib. Chest radiographs also should be obtained to rule out an apical lung lesion (Pancoast tumor), which may be causing compression.

3. Nerve conduction studies, arteriograms, and venograms may be necessary.

E. Treatment.

1. Conservative treatment is usually effective.

a. Rest affected side with sling.

b. Nonsteroidal antiinflammatory drugs, moist heat.

c. Avoid hyperabduction of shoulders.

d. Strengthening program for muscles of the shoulder girdle.

2. Operative treatment is considered after patient does not respond to 4-6 months of conservative treatment.

a. May remove cervical and first ribs and release any abnormal scalene muscle insertion.

b. May excise outer clavicle.

3. Venous thrombosis requires rest and elevation of the affected extremity.

a. Anticoagulation with warfarin sodium for 3 months is recommended.

b. Thrombolytic agents (urokinase or streptokinase) have also been effective.

IV. Other Syndromes

A. Acute brachial neuropathy (brachial plexitis).

1. Rare idiopathic inflammation of the brachial plexus. Onset can be associated with athletic activity, although it is not truly an athletic injury.

2. Symptoms and signs.

a. Intense shoulder pain and paresthesia; tenderness in axilla.

b. Weakness of proximal muscles (mainly deltoid, supraspinatus, infraspinatus, biceps, and triceps) and minimal sensory loss.

c. Laboratory tests show normal results (complete blood count, erythrocyte sedimentation rate, glucose level).

d. EMG *abnormal,* showing diffusely affected plexus.

3. Treatment.

a. Rest (in sling), nonsteroidal antiinflammatory drugs.

b. Rehabilitation exercises when pain resolves.

c. May take weeks to years for recovery.

B. Backpacker's palsy.
   1. Heavy backpack straps compress upper trunk of the brachial plexus. Most commonly occurs on the nondominant side.
   2. Symptoms: usually affects radial and musculocutaneous nerves and produces both motor and sensory deficits.
   3. Treatment is conservative: backpacking should be avoided, and shoulder should be strengthened by exercises.
      a. With chronic symptoms, an EMG may confirm the diagnosis.
      b. A rare refractory case may need surgical decompression.

Acknowledgment

The Medical Editing Department, Kaiser Foundation Research Institute, provided editorial assistance.

Bibliography

Garth WP: Evaluating and treating brachial plexus injuries, *J Musculoskel Med* 11(10):55-67, 1994.

Hershman EB: Brachial plexus injuries, *Clin Sports Med* 9:311-329, 1990.

Hershman EB, Wilbourn AJ, Bergfeld JA: Acute brachial neuropathy in athletes, *Am J Sports Med* 17:655-659, 1989.

Karas SE: Thoracic outlet syndrome, *Clin Sports Med* 9:297-310, 1990.

Markey KL, Di Benedetto M, Curl WW: Upper trunk brachial plexopathy: the stinger syndrome, *Am J Sports Med* 21:650-655, 1993.

Sallis RE, Jones K, Knopp W: Burners: offensive strategy for an underreported injury, *Phys Sportsmed* 20(11):47-55, 1992.

Vereschagin KS et al: Burners: don't overlook or underestimate them, *Phys Sportsmed* 19(9):96-106, 1991.

CHAPTER 37

Rehabilitation of Shoulder Injuries

David B. Richards, MD

W. Benjamin Kibler, MD

I. Overview
   A. The shoulder is the most complex joint in body.
      1. Greatest range of motion (ROM) in all planes.
      2. Inherently unstable.
   B. Rehabilitation requires timely and accurate diagnosis.
      1. History.
      2. Physical examination.
      3. Diagnostic studies.
   C. Injuries (see box on p. 291 for examples).
      1. Macrotrauma.
         a. Acute, single traumatic events.
         b. Can usually define when, where, and how.
      2. Microtrauma.
         a. Result of chronic overload.
         b. Cellular damage fails to heal and leads to tissue damage and failure.
         c. Develops over long period.
   D. Rehabilitation.
      1. Kinetic chain.
         a. A series of "links" beginning with the ground reactive force and progressing to the hand (Figure 37-1).
         b. Muscle mass of shoulder is small. Unable to generate much force. Shoulder functions as a force regulator.
         c. Shoulder rehabilitation should involve the entire kinetic chain.
      2. Phases of rehabilitation.
         a. Acute phase: resolution of symptoms of injury.
         b. Recovery phase: improve ROM, strength, retain neuromuscular firing patterns.
         c. Maintenance phase: force couples, neuromuscular retraining, functional exercises.

COMMON SHOULDER INJURIES

MACROTRAUMA	MICROTRAUMA
Shoulder dislocation	Rotator cuff tendinitis
Acromioclavicular joint separation	Biceps tendinitis
Fractures	Instability
Sternoclavicular joint dislocation	Secondary impingement

II. Injuries
  A. Microtrauma.
    1. Chronic overload.
    2. Inadequate healing.
    3. Biomechanical adaptation.
    4. Develops over time.
  B. Macrotrauma.
    1. Single event.
    2. Instantaneous.
    3. Normal anatomy → abnormal
III. Diagnosis
  A. History and physical examination.
  B. Supporting studies.
IV. Goals of Rehabilitation
  A. Resolve symptoms/signs of injury.
  B. Restore strength and ROM.
  C. Normalize joint kinematics.
  D. Return to competition.
  E. Prevent reinjury.
V. Rehabilitation Phases
  A. Acute phase.

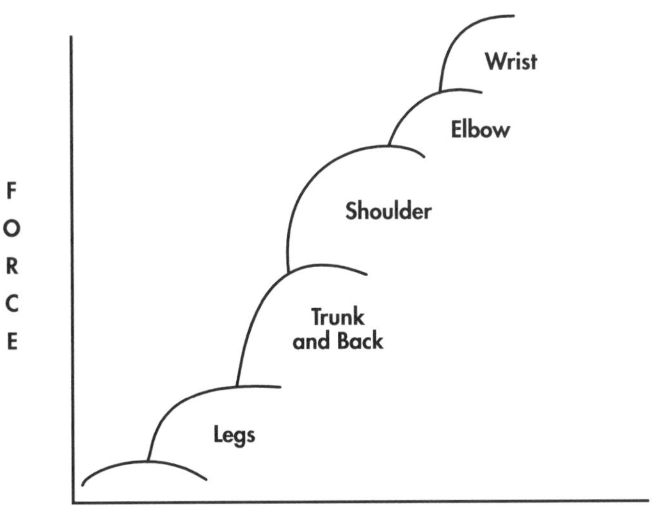

FIGURE 37-1
Normal kinetic chain with each link.

1. Goals.
   a. Decrease pain, swelling.
   b. Improve ROM.
   c. Minimize atrophy.
2. Pain, swelling.
   a. Modalities (ice, heat, electrical stimulation, ultrasound).
   b. Nonsteroidal antiinflammatory drugs.
   c. Bracing.
3. Improve ROM/minimize atrophy.
   a. Mobilize glenohumeral, acromioclavicular, sternoclavicular, and scapulothoracic joints.
   b. Capsular stretching.
   c. Pendulum exercises.
   d. Ropes/pulleys.
   e. Isometrics.
   f. Closed chain/open chain exercises.
4. Criteria for progression.
   a. Full pain-free passive ROM.
   b. Improved strength.

B. Recovery phase.
1. Goals.
   a. Improved strength.
   b. Improved neuromuscular control.
   c. Normal single plane kinematics.
2. Strengthening.
   a. Closed/open chain exercise.
   b. Isokinetics.
   c. Tubing exercises.
   d. Jobe-rotator cuff exercises.
3. Neuromuscular control/kinematics.
   a. Proprioceptive neuromuscular facilitation (PNF) exercises.
   b. Closed chain exercise.
   c. Cocontractions.
   d. Mobilization of all joints around the shoulder.
4. Criteria for progression.
   a. Full pain free active ROM.
   b. Strengthen 75% of the side.
   c. No instability.
   d. Normal scapular motion.

C. Maintenance phase.
1. Goals.
   a. Increase power and endurance.
   b. Improve multiplane neuromuscular control.
2. Power and endurance.
   a. Multiplane exercise.
   b. Isokinetics/isotonics.
3. Neuromuscular control.
   a. Plyometrics.
   b. PNF exercises.
   c. Closed chain exercises (cocontractions).
4. Sport-specific exercises.
   a. Throwing.
   b. Serving.
5. Maintenance.

   a. Maintain flexibility through regular stretching exercises.
   b. Muscle balance.
   c. Overall fitness: aerobic and anaerobic.
6. Criteria for return to play.
   a. Normal kinematics.
   b. Symptom free.
   c. Strength 90% of opposite side.
   d. Completion of sport-specific exercises without symptoms.

Bibliography

AAOS: *Athletic Training and Sports Medicine,* ed 2, Rosemont, IL, 1991, American Academy of Orthopedic Surgeons.

Andrews JR, Harrelson GL: *Physical Rehabilitation of the Injured Athlete,* Philadelphia, 1991, WB Saunders.

Kibler WB, Chandler TJ: Sport specific conditioning, *Am J Sports Med* 22:3, 1994.

Kibler WB: Current concepts of shoulder biomechanics: pathology and treatment, *J Southern Orthop Assoc* 3(3):254-271, 1994.

Kibler WB et al: Current concepts in shoulder rehabilitation. In: *Advances in Operative Orthopaedics,* St. Louis, 1995, Mosby–Year Book.

Pappas AM: *Upper Extremity Injuries in the Athlete,* New York, 1995, Churchill Livingstone.

Petrone F, Nirschl RP: *The Shoulder in the Throwing Athlete,* New York, 1994, McGraw-Hill.

Wilk KE et al: Current concepts in the rehabilitation of the athlete's shoulder, *J Southern Orthop Assoc* 3(3):254-271, 1994.

CHAPTER 38

Anatomy and Biomechanics of the Elbow and Forearm

Michael D. Jackson, MD

Douglas B. McKeag, MD

I. Function.
  A. A ginglymus or diarthrodial (hinge) joint.
  B. Movement provides increased range of motion for the hand and wrist.
  C. Acts to stabilize the proximal upper extremity, allowing skilled or forceful movements of the hands.

II. Functional Anatomy
  A. Osteology (Figure 38-1).
    1. Distal humerus.
      a. Medial epicondyle: site of origin for the flexor pronator muscle group and ulnar collateral ligament.
      b. Lateral epicondyle: site of origin for the extensor muscle group and radial collateral ligament also extensor carpi radialis pelvis of tennis elbow frame.
      c. Trochlea: articulates with the trochlear notch of the ulna.
      d. Capitellum: articulates with the head of the radius.
      e. Coronoid fossa: accommodates coronoid process of the ulna.
      f. Olecranon fossa: accommodates the olecranon process of the ulna.
      g. Radial fossa: accommodates the radial head when elbow is fully flexed.
    2. Proximal radius.
      a. Radial head: articulates with the capitellum and allows pronation and supination of the forearm.
      b. Radial tuberosity: the site of insertion for the biceps tendon.
    3. Proximal ulna.
      a. Olecranon: site of insertion for the triceps.
      b. Coronoid process: site of insertion for the brachialis muscle.
      c. Radial notch: articulates with and aids in stabilization of the radial head.
      d. Trochlear notch: articulates with the trochlea of the humerus.

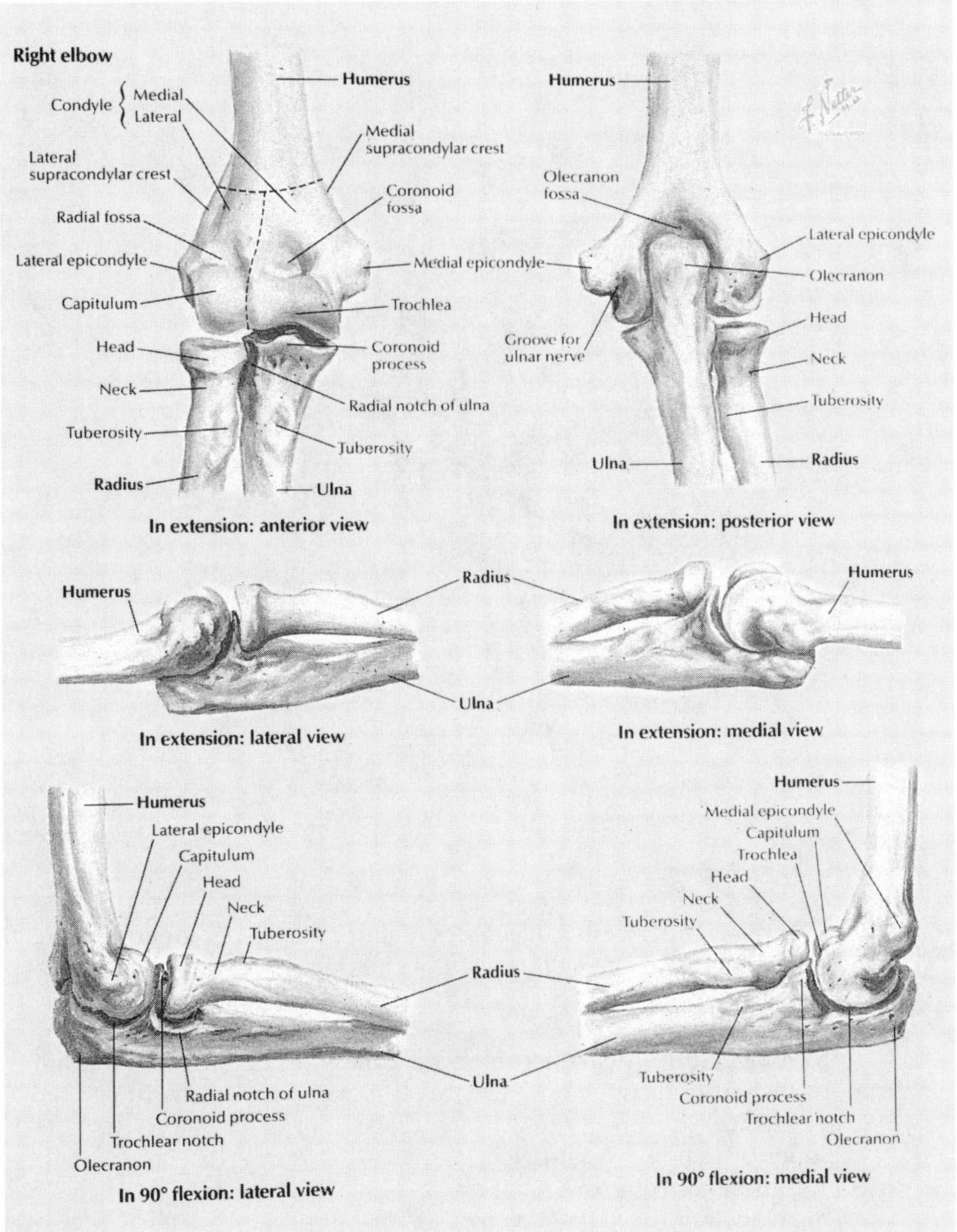

FIGURE 38-1

B. Articulations (Figure 38-2).
   1. Humeroulnar joint.
      a. A modified hinge joint.
      b. Allows approximately 5 degrees of internal and external rotation at the extremes of flexion and extension.[17]
      c. Articulation occurs between the trochlea (distal humerus) and the trochlear notch (proximal ulna).
      d. The distal humerus is rotated anteriorly approximately 30 degrees with respect to its long axis, and the proximal ulna is angled approximately 30 degrees posteriorly with respect to its shaft, there-

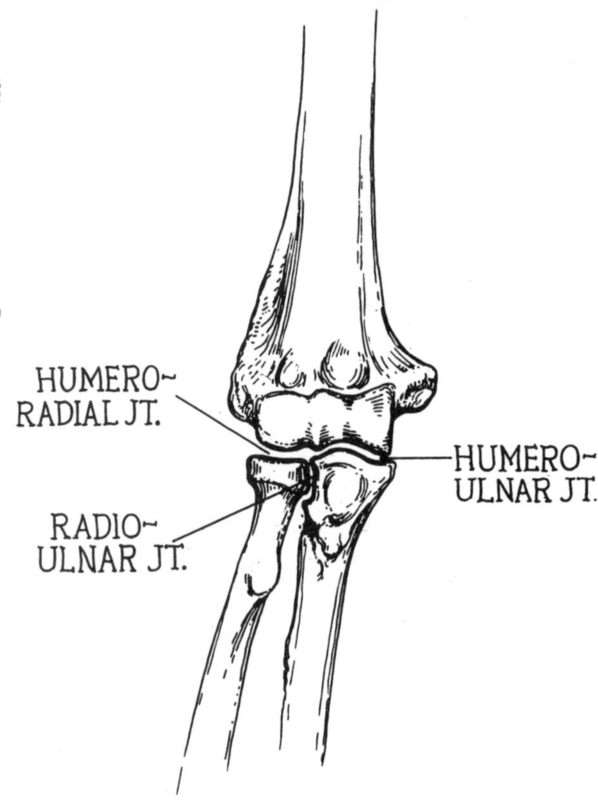

FIGURE 38-2
The three elbow articulations

fore allowing 140-150 degrees of motion at this joint and aiding in stability when the elbow is fully extended.[17]

2. Humeroradial joint.
   a. A hinge/pivot joint.
   b. Articulation occurs between the capitellum and the radial head.
   c. In a fully flexed elbow the radial fossa articulates with the radial head.
3. Superior radioulnar joint.
   a. A uniaxial, diarthrodial joint.
   b. Articulation occurs between the medial rim of the radial head and the radial notch of the ulna.
   c. With pronation and supination the radial head rotates within the annular ligament and radial notch of the ulna.
4. Inferior radioulnar joint.
   a. A uniaxial, diarthrodial joint.
   b. Articulation occurs between the head of the ulna and the ulnar notch at the radius.
   c. With pronation and supination the ulnar notch rotates on the ulnar head of the ulna.

C. Carrying angle.
   1. The valgus angle formed by the longitudinal axes of the upper arm and forearm when the arm is extended in the anatomical position.
   2. Normal angle: approximately 5 degrees in males and 10-15 degrees in females.

D. Ligaments.

1. The medial (ulnar) collateral ligament complex is comprised of three bundles (Figure 38-3).
   a. The anterior bundle originates from the inferior aspect of the medial epicondyle to insert on the medial aspect of the coronoid process.
      (1) This ligament is further divided into an anterior band, which is taut in extension, and a posterior band, which is taut in flexion.[17]
      (2) Compromise of this bundle produces valgus instability of the elbow in all positions except full extension.
   b. Transverse bundle originates from the medial olecranon to insert on the coronoid process. This ligament has no major role in stabilization of the elbow.
   c. Posterior bundle originates from the medial epicondyle to insert on the medial olecranon. This ligament becomes taut when the elbow is flexed ≥90 degrees.
2. Lateral collateral ligament complex consists of four components (Figure 38-4).
   a. Annular ligament encompasses the radial head, thereby stabilizing it in the radial notch of the ulna.
   b. Accessory lateral collateral ligament originates from the inferior aspect of the annular ligament to insert on the tubercle of the supinator crest. This ligament assists in stabilization of the annular ligament during varus stress.
   c. Lateral ulnar collateral ligament originates from the lateral epicondyle to insert on the supinator crest of the ulna. This ligament prevents inferior rotatory subluxation of the humeroulnar joint.

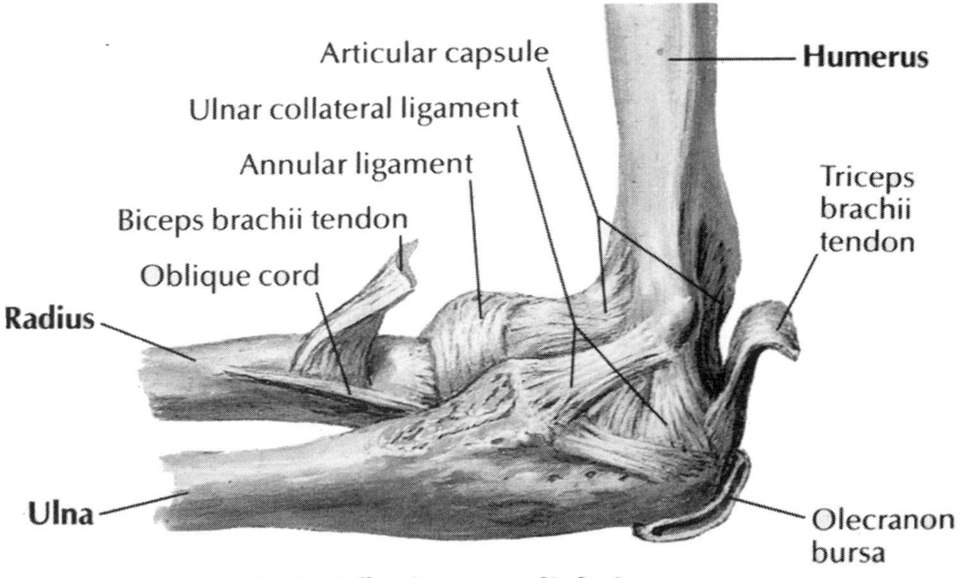

FIGURE 38-3
In 90 degrees flexion: medial view

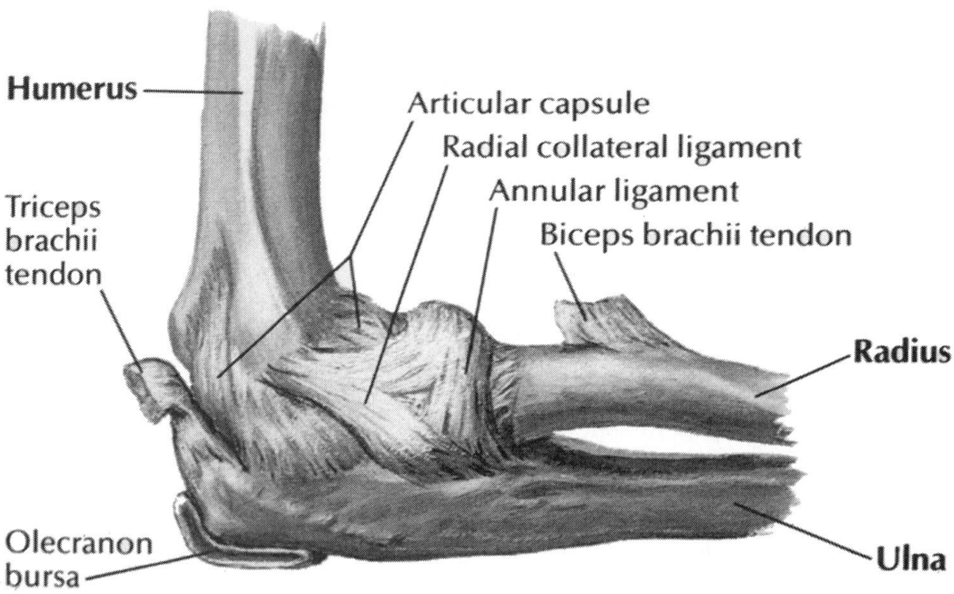

FIGURE 38-4
In 90 degrees flexion: lateral view

   d. Radial collateral ligament originates from the lateral epicondyle to insert into the annular ligament. This ligament provides varus stability to the humeroradial joint and promotes joint stability by maintaining close approximation of the humeral and radial articular surfaces.[11]
   e. Compromise of the lateral ligament complex may result in loss of pronation and supination.

E. There are four groups of muscles that act directly on the elbow.
  1. Flexors.
     a. Biceps brachii originates from the superior rim of the glenoid fossa at the supraglenoid tubercle (long head) and the corocoid process (short head) to insert on the posterior aspect of the radial tuberosity.
        (1) Primary elbow flexor when the forearm is supinated.
        (2) Aids in forearm supination when the elbow is flexed.
        (3) Innervated by musculocutaneous nerve at the C5, C6 root levels.
     b. Brachioradialis originates from the proximal two-thirds of the lateral supracondylar ridge of the humerus and lateral intermuscular septum distal to the spiral groove to insert on the lateral side of the base of the styloid process of the radius.
        (1) Primary role is elbow flexion.
        (2) Innervated by radial nerve at the C5, C6 root levels.
     c. Brachialis originates from the distal half of the anterior aspect of the humerus to insert on the ulnar tuberosity and coronoid process.
        (1) Primary role is elbow flexion in all positions of the forearm.
        (2) Innervated by musculocutaneous nerve at the C5, C6 root levels.

2. Extensors.
   a. Triceps has three heads that take origin from the infraglenoid tuberosity (long head), the posterior aspect of the humerus proximal to the groove for the radial nerve (lateral head), and the posterior aspect of the humerus, distal to the groove for the radial nerve (medial head). It inserts into the posterior surface of the olecranon and the deep fascia of the forearm. Innervated by radial nerve at the C7, C8 root levels.
   b. Anconeus originates from the posterior aspect of the lateral epicondyle to insert on the olecranon. Innervated by radial nerve at the C7, C8 root levels.
3. Extensor supinator group.
   a. Consists of the brachioradialis, extensor carpi radialis longus and brevis, supinator, extensor digitorum, extensor carpi ulnaris, and extensor digiti minimi.
      (1) All originate directly from or in close proximity to the lateral epicondyle.
      (2) Primary roles are extension and supination of the wrist and hand, while also providing dynamic support for the lateral elbow.
      (3) All are innervated by radial nerve from C5-8, T1 nerve roots.
4. Flexor pronator group.
   a. Consists of the pronator teres, flexor carpi radialis, palmaris longus, flexor carpi ulnaris, and flexor digitorum superficialis.
      (1) All originate directly from or in close proximity to the medial epicondyle.
      (2) Primary role is flexion and pronation of the wrist and hand, while secondarily aiding in elbow flexion.
      (3) All except flexi carpi ulnaris (ulnar nerve—C8, T1) are innervated by median nerve from C6-8, T1 nerve roots.

F. Four nerves play a major role in elbow function.
1. Musculocutaneous nerve (Figure 38-5).
   a. Originates from the lateral cord of the brachial plexus at the C5-7 root levels.
   b. After coursing between the biceps and brachialis muscles to pierce the brachial fascia lateral to the biceps tendon, it terminates distally as the lateral antebrachial cutaneous nerve.
   c. Innervates the biceps brachii, brachialis, and corobrachialis.
2. Median nerve (Figure 38-6).
   a. Originates from the lateral and medial cords of the brachial plexus from the C5-8 and T1 root levels.
   b. Courses distally over the anterior medial aspect of the brachium, passing the antecubital fossa medial to the biceps tendon and brachial artery with the anterior interosseous nerve branch arising at the inferior border of the pronator teres.
   c. Innervates the pronator teres, flexor carpi radialis, palmaris longus, flexor digitorum superficialis, abductor pollicis brevis, flexor pollicis brevis (superficial head), lumbricales[6,17] and opponens pollicis. Anterior interosseous branch innervates flexor digitorum profundus,[6,17] flexor pollicis longus, and pronator quadratus.
3. Ulnar nerve (Figure 38-7).
   a. Originates from the medial cord of the brachial plexus from C8 and T1 nerve roots.

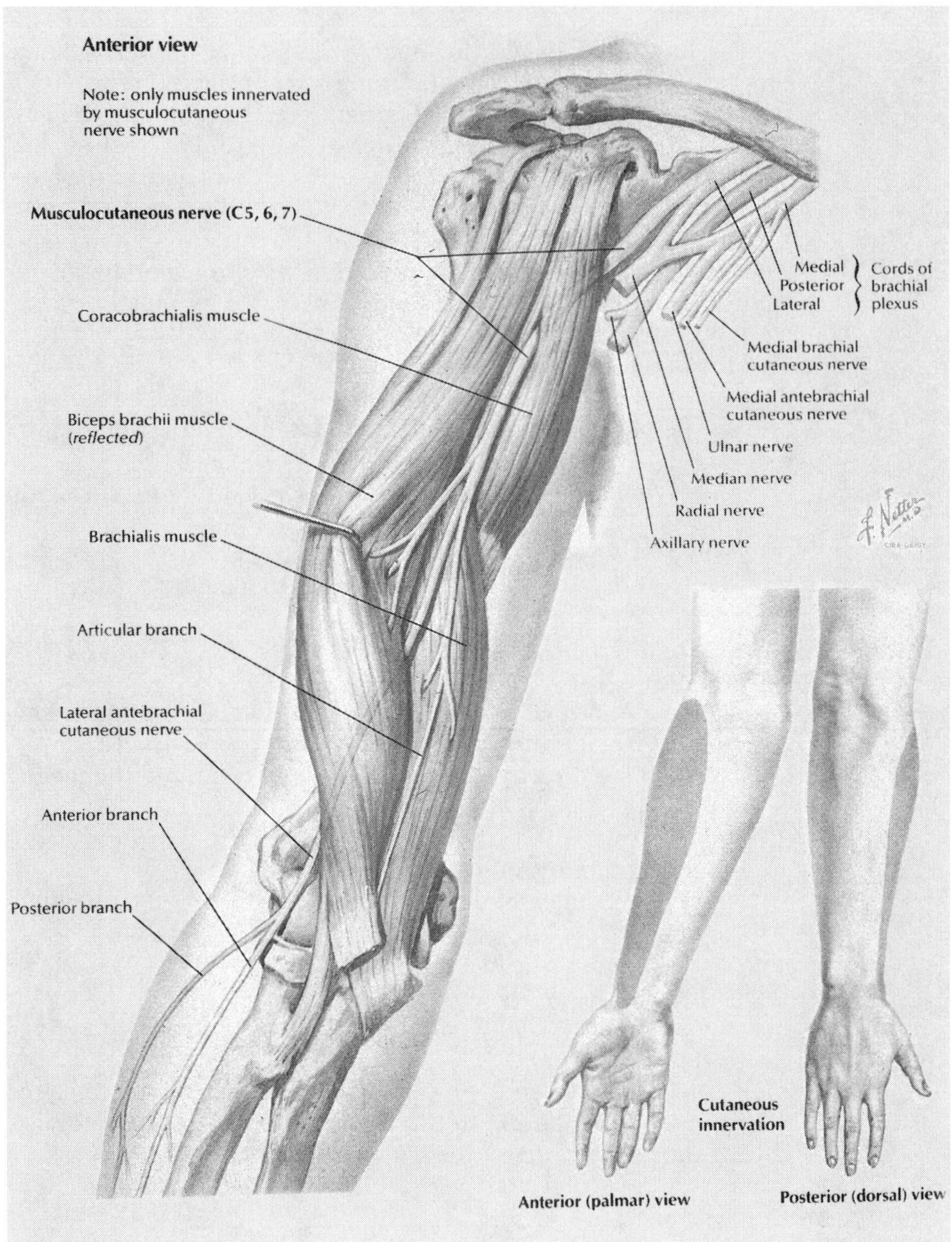

FIGURE 38-5
Musculocutaneous nerve

b. Courses distally from the anterior to posterior compartments of the brachium through the arcade of Struthers, a fascial bridge between the medial head of the triceps and medial intermuscular septum (approximately 8 cm proximal to the medial epicondyle).[17] Continues distally behind the medial epicondyle and through the cubital tunnel where it enters the forearm between the two heads of flexor carpi ulnaris and continues between the flexor carpi ulnaris and flexor digitorum profundus.
c. Innervates the flexor carpi ulnaris, flexor digitorum profundus,[5,11] palmaris brevis, abductor digiti minimi, opponens digiti minimi, flexor digiti minimi, palmar interosseous, dorsal interosseous, lumbricales,[5,11] adductor pollicis, and flexor pollicis brevis (deep head).

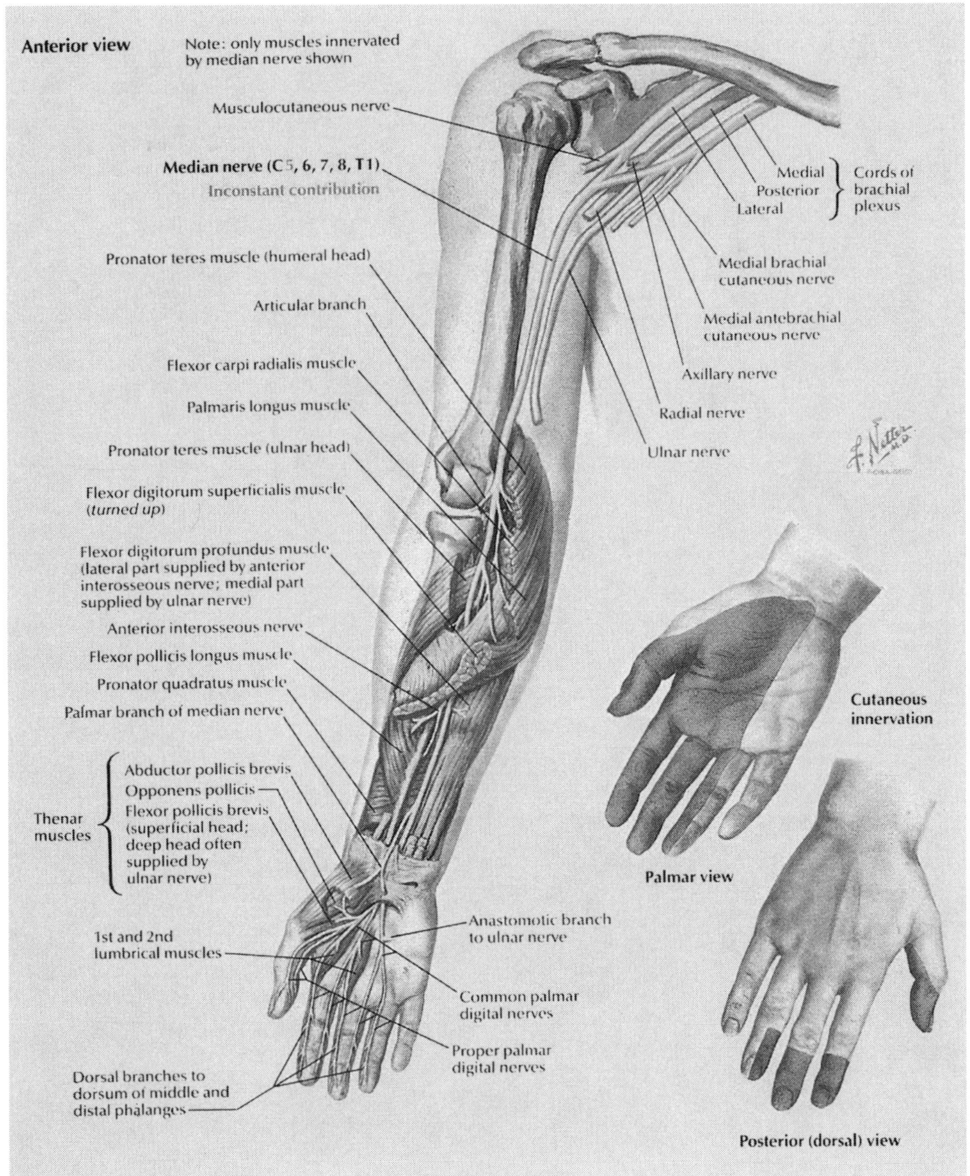

FIGURE 38-6
Median nerve

4. Radial nerve (Figure 38-8).
   a. Originates from the posterior cord of the brachial plexus from the C6, C7, and C8 nerve roots.
   b. Courses laterally through the spiral groove and humerus to pass anterior to the lateral epicondyle, posterior to the brachioradialis and brachialis muscles; divides into posterior interosseous and superficial radial branches at the antecubital fossa.
      (1) Superficial branch continues distally to terminate in the hand.
      (2) Posterior interosseous continues around the posterior lateral aspect of the radius and passes between the two heads of the supinator muscle before dividing into terminal motor branches.
   c. Innervates the triceps, anconeus, brachioradialis, extensor carpi radialis longus and brevis, supinator, extensor carpi ulnaris, exten-

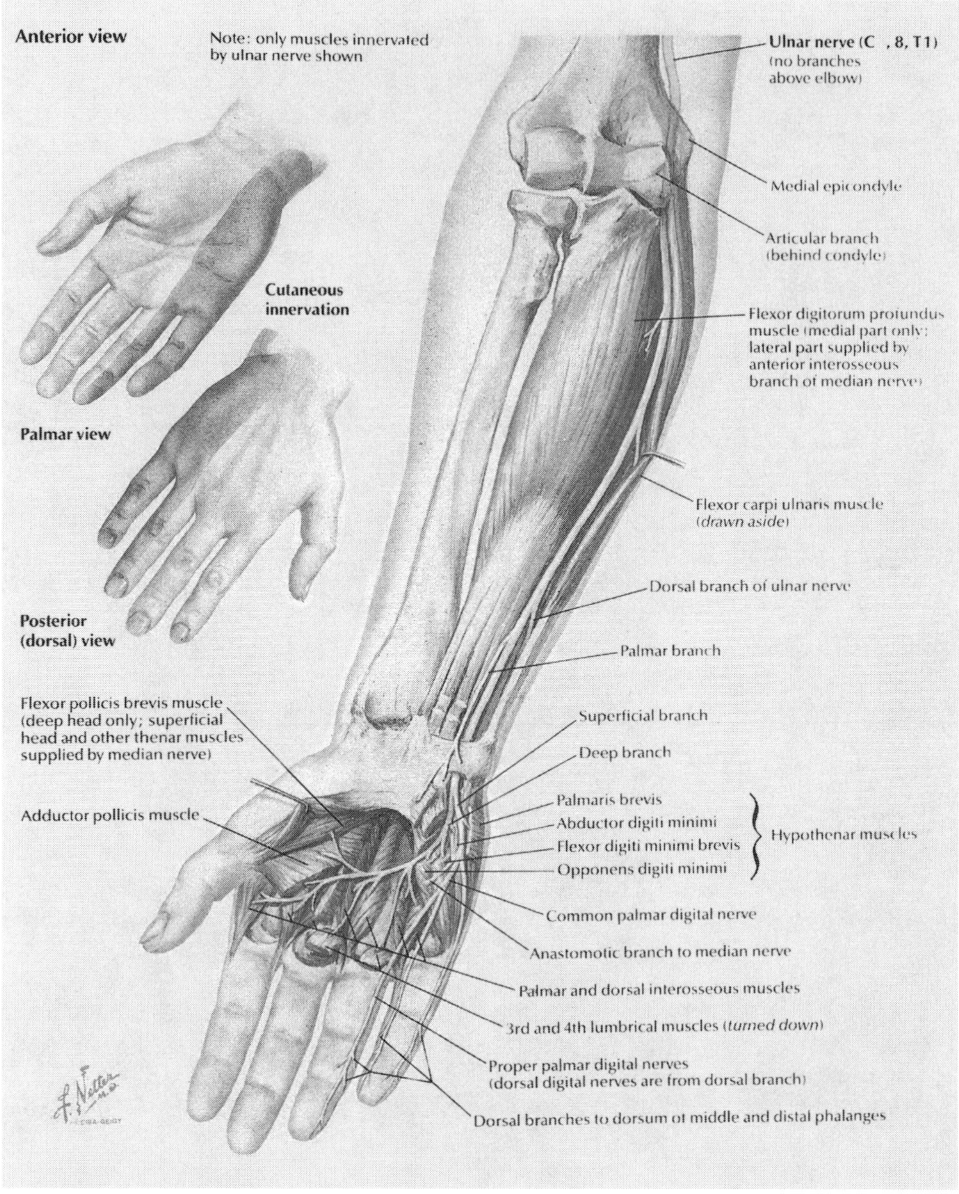

FIGURE 38-7
Ulnar nerve

sor digitorum, extensor digiti minimi, abductor pollicis longus, extensor pollicis longus and brevis, and extensor indices.

G. Five nerves provide cutaneous sensation around the elbow.
   1. Lower lateral cutaneous nerve, a branch from the radial nerve, innervates the anterior and lateral aspect of the forearm.
   2. Posterior cutaneous nerve, a branch from the radial nerve, innervates the posterior central aspect of the arm and forearm.
   3. Lateral antebrachial cutaneous nerve, terminal branch of the musculocutaneous nerve, innervates the lateral aspect of the forearm.
   4. Medial brachial cutaneous nerve and medial antebrachial cutaneous nerve originate from the medial cord of the brachial plexus.
      a. Medial brachial cutaneous innervates the medial aspect of the arm.

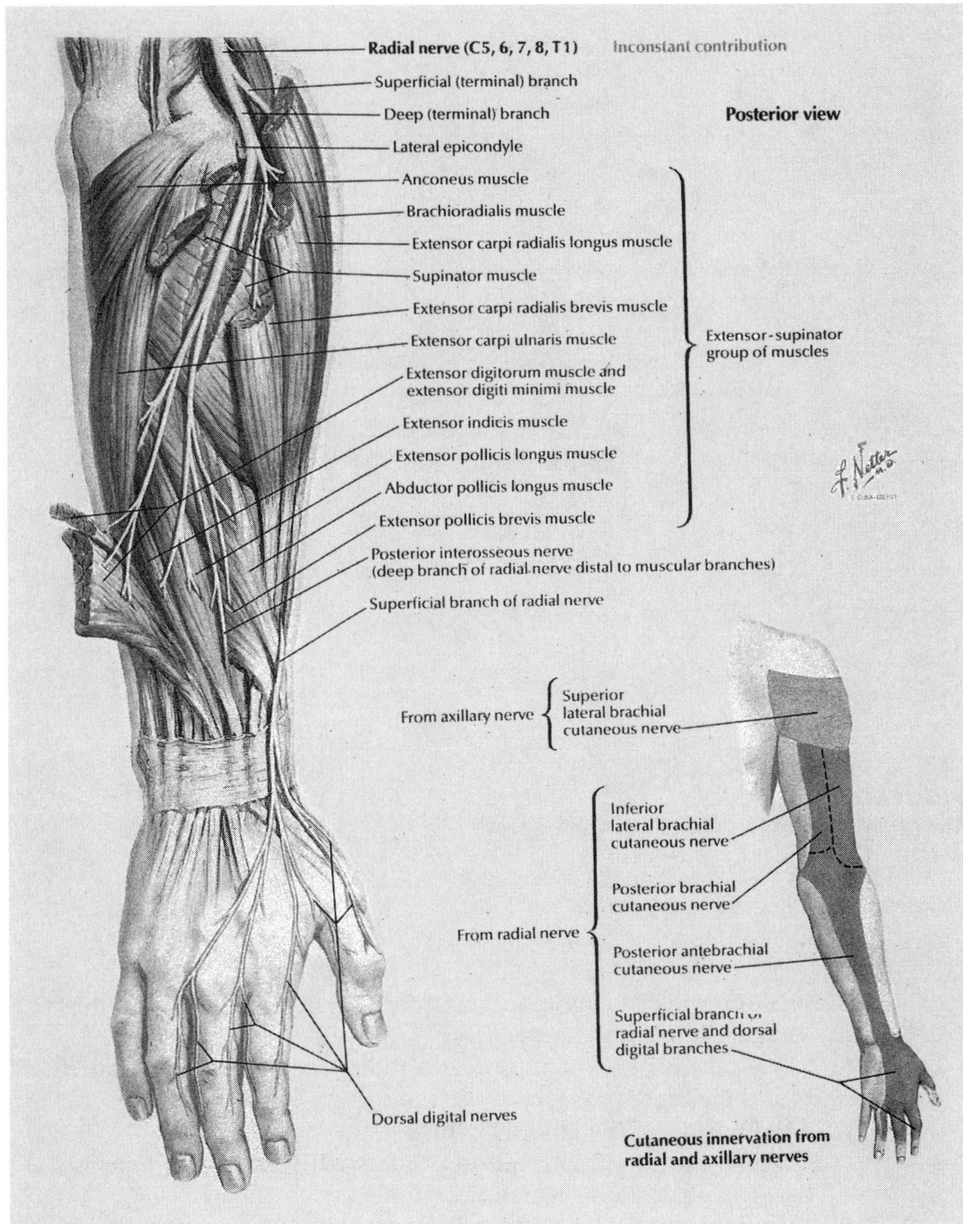

FIGURE 38-8
Radial nerve

b. Medial antebrachial cutaneous innervates the medial aspect of the forearm.

III. Biomechanics

A. The radioulnar-humeral joints are solely involved in flexion and extension of the elbow joints (Figure 38-9).

1. Flexion ranges from 0 (full extension) to approximately 150 degrees.

a. Flexion may be limited by:

(1) The muscle mass of the anterior arm.

(2) Contact of the coronoid process with the coronoid fossa of the humerus.

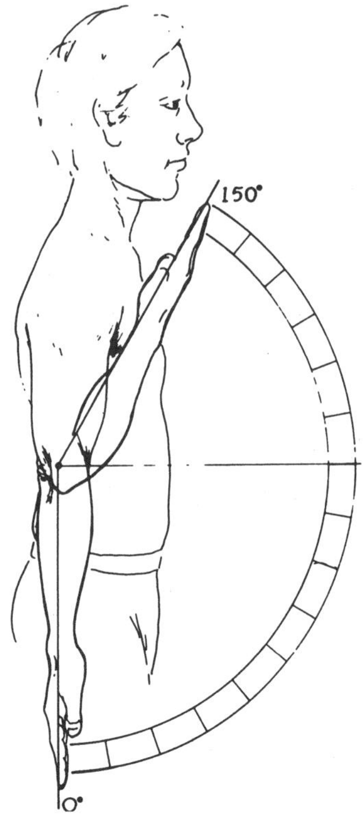

FIGURE 38-9
The elbow range of motion in flexion and extension

2. Extension ranges from approximately 150 (full flexion) to 0 degrees.
    a. Extension may be limited by:
        (1) Tension of the anterior and radioulnar collateral ligament of the elbow.
        (2) Tension of the elbow flexors.
        (3) Contact of the olecranon process with the olecranon fossa on the posterior aspect of the humerus.

B. The radioulnar joints allow pronation and supination of the elbow joint (Figure 38-10).
1. Supination ranges from 0 (full pronation) to approximately 90 degrees.
    a. Supination may be limited by:
        (1) Tension of the volar radioulnar and ulnar collateral ligaments of the wrist.
        (2) Tension of the interosseous membrane (oblique cord and lowest fibers).
        (3) Tension of the forearm pronator muscles.
2. Pronation ranges from 0 (full supination) to approximately 90 degrees.
    a. Pronation may be limited by:
        (1) Tension of the dorsal radioulnar, ulnar collateral, and dorsal radiocarpal ligaments.
        (2) Tension of the lowest fibers of the interosseous membrane.

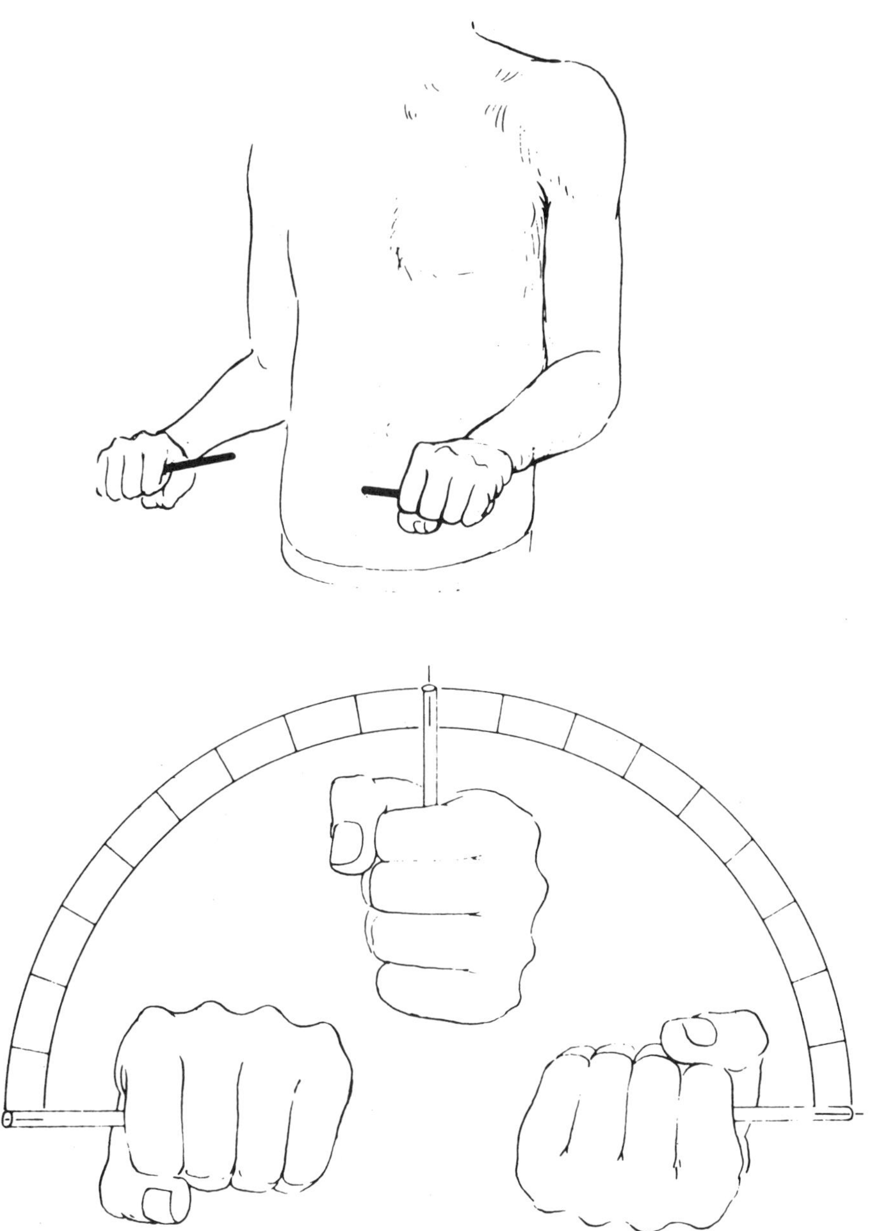

FIGURE 38-10
The elbow range of motion in supination and pronation

Bibliography

Adrian MJ, Cooper JM: *The Biomechanics of Human Movement,* Indianapolis, 1989, Benchmark Press.

Baildon R, Chapman AE: Mechanical properties of a single equivalent muscle producing forearm supination, *J Biomech* 16(10):811-819, 1983.

Berger RA et al: The scapholunate ligament, *J Hand Surg* 7(1):87-91, 1982.

Brand PW et al: Relative tension and potential excursion of muscles in the forearm and hand, *J Hand Surg* 6(3):209-219, 1981.

Daniels L, Worthingham C: *Muscle Testing: Techniques of Manual Examination,* Philadelphia, 1986, WB Saunders.

Hoppenfeld S: *Physical Examination of the Spine and Extremities,* East Norwalk, CT, 1976, Appleton-Century-Crofts.

Johnson C, Glasheen-Wray MB: Effect of forearm abduction of the ulnar collateral ligament, *Phys Ther* 63(5):660-663, 1983.

Kibler WB: Clinical biomechanics of the elbow in tennis: implications for evaluation and diagnosis, *Med Sci Sports Exerc* 26(10):1203-1206, 1994.

Kornecki S: Mechanism of muscular stabilization process in joints, *J Biomech* 25(3):235-245, 1992.

McKeag DB, Hough DO: *Primary Care Sportsmedicine,* Dubuque, 1993, Brown & Benchmark.

Murray BF: Anatomy of the elbow. In Morrey BF, editor: *The Elbow and Its Disorders,* Philadelphia, 1985, WB Saunders, pp 7-40.

Rabinowitz RS et al: The role of the interosseous membrane and triangular fibrocartilage complex in forearm stability, *J Hand Surg* 19(3):385-393, 1994.

Schnatz P, Steiner C: Tennis elbow: a biomechanical and therapeutic approach, *J Am Osteopath Assoc* 93(7):778-788, 1993.

Schneiderman G et al: The interosseous membrane of the forearm: structure and its role in Galezzi fractures, *J Trauma* 35(6):879-885, 1993.

Schuind F et al: The distal radioulnar ligaments: a biomechanical study, *J Hand Surg* 16(6):1106-1114, 1991.

Stewart OJ et al: Influence of resistance, speed of movement, and forearm position on recruitment of the elbow flexors, *Am J Phys Med* 60(4):165-179, 1981.

Stroyan M, Wilk KE: The functional anatomy of the elbow complex, *J Sports Med Phys Fitness* 17(6):279-288, 1993.

CHAPTER 39

History and Physical Examination of the Elbow and Forearm

Michael D. Jackson, MD

Douglas B. McKeag, MD

I. History
  A. A careful history should be obtained. This should be designed to explain and determine the severity of the injury and ultimately its impact on performance.
  B. The chief complaint.
    1. What troubles you most about your elbow?
    2. This may elicit clues in the localization of injury.
  C. Have the patient point to the area causing problems.
    1. Also ask if there is any radiation or paresthesias associated with the pain.
    2. This is helpful in identifying neurological abnormalities.
  D. The mechanism of injury.
    1. How did this injury occur?
    2. Helpful in determining what anatomical structure was injured.
  E. The temporal features.
    1. What was the date of onset or reinjury that initiated this problem?
    2. Was the onset acute or insidious?
    3. What is the duration of symptoms?
    4. How long have the symptoms been improving, worsening, or staying the same?
  F. The character of pain.
    1. Dull, aching, sharp stabbing, burning, numbness, tingling, or paresthesias?
    2. This helps distinguish possible etiologies (i.e., soft tissue, articular cartilage, or neurovascular).
  G. The "how" questions.
    1. How does it bother you now?
    2. How have you treated this?
    3. How do you make it worse?
    4. How do you make it better?
    5. How has the problem interfered with your training program?

H. Impact on the patient's activities. How has this affected your activities of daily living (i.e., personal hygiene, occupational activities, or recreational pursuits)?

II. Physical Examination
   A. Inspection.
      1. Visualize both elbows for comparison. Note muscle hypertrophy, atrophy, swelling, and previous surgical incisions or scars.
      2. Axial alignment.
         a. Note the carrying angle with the arm fully extended.
         b. Normal angle: approximately 5 degrees in males and 10-15 degrees in females.
      3. General appearance.
         a. Note the soft tissue contour of the biceps anteriorly, triceps posteriorly, flexor-pronator muscle group medially, and extensor muscle group laterally.
         b. Muscle or tendon rupture, advanced rheumatoid arthritis, severe swelling, or fracture deformity results in obliteration of these landmarks.
      4. Anterior aspect: inspect the antecubital fossa for soft tissue masses.
      5. Posterior aspect.
         a. Note the area around the olecranon.
         b. Triceps tendon rupture may present as a prominent bony protuberance with an indentation above the tip of the olecranon.
         c. Olecranon bursitis presents as a distended mass under the skin.
         d. Dislocation or subluxation presents as a gross distortion of the contour, typically with a posteriorly prominent displaced proximal ulna.
      6. Medial aspect.
         a. Note the contour of the medial epicondyle.
         b. Nonunion of a medial epicondyle fracture may present as an increased osseous or bony prominence.
         c. Subluxation of the ulnar nerve may be noted anteriorly with flexion while it reduces behind the epicondyle with extension.
      7. Lateral aspect.
         a. Note the presence of effusion or synovitis at the lateral joint line.
         b. Dermal atrophy may be present in individuals who have undergone repeated steroid injections for chronic lateral epicondylitis.
   B. Palpation: bony landmarks (arm abducted and elbow flexed at 90 degrees).
      1. Medial epicondyle: note bony deformities (frequently fractured in children).
      2. Medial supracondylar line of the humerus: bony prominence here may contribute to median nerve compression.
      3. Olecranon.
      4. Ulnar border: palpate from the olecranon down to the ulnar styloid at the wrist.
      5. Olecranon fossa: best palpated with slight extension of the elbow, placing slack on the triceps and thereby exposing a portion of the fossa.
      6. Lateral epicondyle.
      7. Lateral supracondylar line of the humerus: extends almost to the deltoid tuberosity.

8. Radial head.
   a. Palpated with the elbow flexed at 90 degrees, approximately 1 inch distal to the lateral epicondyle just medial and posterior to the wrist extensor muscle group.
   b. Can be felt rotating with pronation and supination.
   c. Pain may indicate synovitis or osteoarthritis.
   d. Dislocation may be congenital or traumatic.
9. Medial epicondyle, olecranon process, and lateral epicondyle form an isosceles triangle when the elbow is flexed 90 degrees (Figure 39-1, *A* and *B*). Disruption of their alignment may indicate fracture and/or dislocation.

C. Soft tissue palpation.
1. Anterior.
   a. Cubital fossa is bordered medially by the pronator teres and laterally by the brachioradialis muscles.
   b. Structures passing medial to lateral through the fossa include:
      (1) Median nerve.
      (2) Brachial artery.
      (3) Biceps tendon.
2. Posterior.
   a. Olecranon bursa may feel boggy and thick if inflamed.
   b. Triceps tendon may be palpated at its insertion on the tip of the olecranon.
3. Medial.
   a. Ulnar nerve may be palpated posterior to the medial epicondyle.
   b. Flexor-pronator muscle group may be tender at its origin if strained.
   c. Medial collateral ligament cannot be palpated directly. Tenderness in this area is indicative of a sprain, which usually results from a sudden valgus stress of the elbow.
4. Lateral.
   a. Wrist extensors are best assessed when the forearm is in neutral position and the wrist is at rest.
   b. Lateral collateral ligament is not directly palpable. Tenderness in this area is indicative of a sprain, which usually results from a varus stress of the elbow.
   c. Annular ligament is difficult to palpate.

D. Range of motion.
1. Flexion: 135 degrees or greater.
   a. Limited by:
      (1) The muscle mass of the anterior arm.
      (2) Contact of the coronoid process with the coronoid fossa.
2. Extension: 0 degrees in males and 0-5 degrees in females.
   a. Limited by:
      (1) Tension of the elbow flexors.
      (2) Tension of the anterior radial and ulnar collateral ligaments.
      (3) Contact of the olecranon process with the olecranon fossa.
3. Supination: 90 degrees.
   a. Limited by:
      (1) Tension of the volar radioulnar and ulnar collateral ligament of the wrist.
      (2) Tension of the interosseous membrane.
      (3) Tension of the forearm pronator muscle.
4. Pronation: 90 degrees.

a. Limited by:
   (1) Tension of the dorsal radioulnar, ulnar collateral, and dorsal radiocarpal ligaments.
   (2) Tension of the lowest fibers of the interosseous membrane.

E. Strength testing.
   1. Strength is assessed with the patient comfortable and the elbow flexed at 90 degrees.
   2. The elbow is supported and stabilized by placing one hand around the posterior aspect just proximal to the joint, while the resisting hand grasps the wrist.
   3. Muscle testing relates to the four motions of the elbow and forearm.
      a. Flexion: patient flexes elbow through range of motion while resistance is applied.
         (1) Biceps tested with forearm supinated.
         (2) Brachialis tested with forearm pronated.
         (3) Brachioradialis tested with forearm in midposition.
      b. Extension: patient extends elbow from the flexed position while resistance is applied. Elbow should be slightly flexed and not locked while resisting motion.
      c. Supination: patient supinates forearm from a pronated position while resistance is applied. Resistance is given on the dorsal surface of the distal radius with counterpressure on the ventral surface of the ulna.

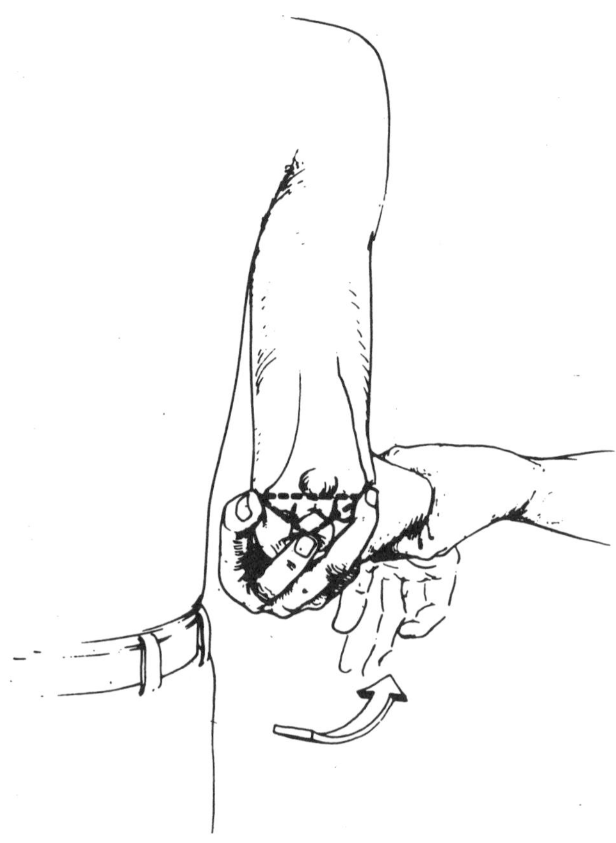

FIGURE 39-1A
When the elbow is flexed, the olecranon and the medial and lateral epicondyles form an isosceles triangle

d. Pronation: patient pronates forearm from a supinated position while resistance is applied. Resistance is given on the palmar surface of the distal radius with counterpressure on the dorsal surface of the ulna.

F. Reflexes.
   1. Biceps reflex.
      a. Elicited on the biceps tendon at the cubital fossa with the patient relaxed, elbow flexed at 90 degrees, and the forearm supported by the examiner.
      b. Evaluates the C5 nerve root.
   2. Brachioradialis reflex.
      a. Elicited on the brachioradialis tendon at the distal end of the radius with the arm positioned in the same manner as for the biceps reflex.
      b. Evaluates the C6 nerve root.
   3. Triceps reflex.
      a. Elicited on the triceps tendon where it crosses the olecranon fossa with the arm supported as in the two previous reflexes, except the shoulder may be forward flexed up to approximately 45 degrees.
      b. Evaluates the C7 nerve root.

G. Special tests.
   1. Ligamentous stability: best detected with the elbow flexed at approximately 30 degrees as this unlocks the olecranon tip from the olecranon fossa.
      a. Varus stress: tests lateral collateral ligament complex stability.
      b. Valgus stress: tests medial collateral ligament complex stability.
   2. Provocative tests.
      a. Lateral epicondylitis.

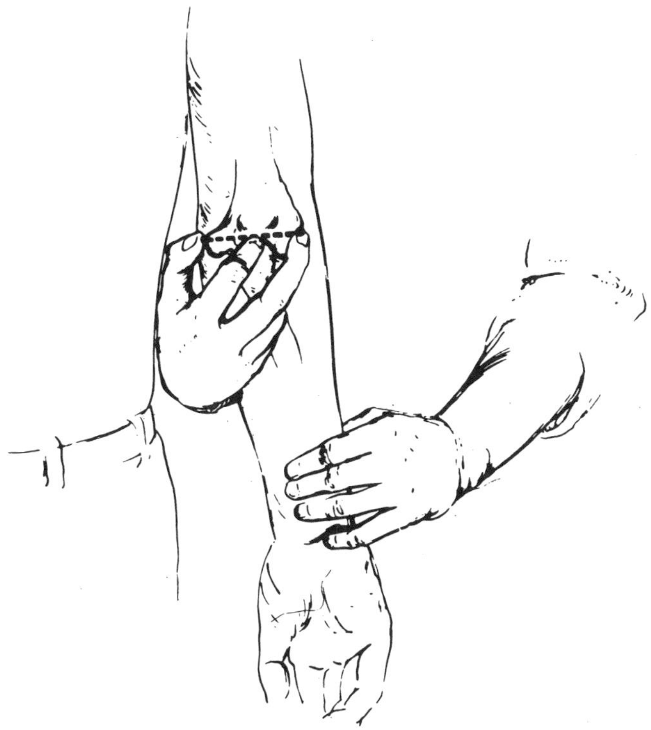

FIGURE 39-1B
When the elbow is extended, the points at the olecranon and the epicondyles lie in a straight line

(1) Resistance to wrist extension.
(2) Resistance to extension of the third digit.
(3) Extension of the elbow with the wrist palmar flexed and the forearm fully pronated.

b. Medial epicondylitis. Extension of the elbow with the wrist dorsiflexed and the forearm fully supinated.

3. Tinel's sign.
   a. Elicited by tapping the area of the ulnar nerve in the groove between the medial epicondyle and the olecranon.
   b. Produces pain that radiates distally in the forearm in the ulnar nerve distribution.

Bibliography

Andrews JR, Harrelson GL: *Physical Rehabilitation of the Injured Athlete,* Philadelphia, 1991, WB Saunders.

Andrews JR, Whiteside JA: Common elbow problems in the athlete, *J Sports Phys Therapy* 17(6):289-295, 1993.

Cabrera JM, McCue FC: Nonosseous athletic injuries of the elbow, forearm, and hand, *Clin Sports Med* 5(4):681-700, 1986.

Cantu RC, Micheli LJ: *ACSM's Guidelines for the Team Physician,* Philadelphia, 1991, Lea & Febiger.

Daniels L, Worthingham C: *Muscle Testing: Techniques of Manual Examination,* Philadelphia, 1986, WB Saunders.

Hoppenfeld S: *Physical Examination of the Spine and Extremities,* East Norwalk, CT, 1976, Appleton-Century-Crofts.

Jobe FW, Nuber G: Throwing injuries of the elbow, *Clin Sports Med* 5(4):621-636, 1986.

Johnson RK: Soft-tissue injuries of the forearm and hand, *Clin Sports Med* 5(4):701-707, 1986.

McKeag DB, Hough DO: *Primary Care Sportsmedicine,* Dubuque, 1993, Brown & Benchmark.

Nicholas JA, Hershman EB: *The Upper Extremity in Sports Medicine,* St Louis, 1990, CV Mosby.

Nirschl RP: Soft tissue injuries about the elbow, *Clin Sports Med* 5(4):637-652, 1986.

Post M: *Physical Examination of the Musculoskeletal System,* Chicago, 1987, Year Book Medical Publishers.

Salter RB: *Textbook of Disorders and Injuries of the Musculoskeletal System,* Baltimore, 1983, Williams & Wilkins.

CHAPTER 40

Injuries About the Elbow

Walter L. Calmbach, MD

Jorge Gomez, MD

I. Lateral Elbow Pain
  A. Lateral epicondylitis.
    1. Mechanism of injury.
      a. Repetitive strain of extensor-supinator muscle mass.
      b. May be a single event or result from a contusion to the lateral epicondyle or chronic overuse.
      c. Affects the extensor carpi radialis brevis most commonly and the extensor carpi radialis longus, the extensor digitorum communis, and the extensor carpi ulnaris less commonly.
    2. Physical examination findings.
      a. Tender at the lateral epicondyle.
      b. Pain with passive wrist flexion.
      c. Pain with active wrist extension (e.g., unable to lift full coffee cup, "Conrad's test").
      d. Pain with full elbow extension.
    3. Diagnosis.
      a. Radiography usually not helpful.
      b. Electromyography usually not necessary.
    4. Differential diagnosis.
      a. Radial nerve entrapment.
        (1) Most commonly at arcade of Frohse.
        (2) Tender 4 cm distal to lateral epicondyle.
      b. Osteochondritis dissecans.
      c. Osteochondrosis of radiocapitellar joint.
      d. Instability at radiocapitellar joint.
      e. Bony tumor.
    5. Treatment.
      a. Relative rest.
      b. Modalities: ice, ultrasound, deep heat.
      c. Wrist-stretching exercises.

d. Strengthening exercises.
   (1) Forearm extensors: power, flexibility, endurance.
   (2) Wrist curls.
   (3) Reverse wrist curls.
   (4) Finger extension (especially the third finger).
e. Nonsteroidal antiinflammatory drugs (NSAIDs): most effective in first 2-3 weeks after injury.
f. Compression strap.
   (1) Proximal to bulk of extensor mass.
   (2) Adjustable to fit conical shape of forearm.
   (3) Prevents full contraction.
g. Corticosteroid injection.
   (1) Controversial.
   (2) No more than three injections in 12 months.
   (3) 0.5 ml betamethasone in 2.0 ml Xylocaine.
   (4) Inject at point of maximal tenderness (i.e., origin of extensor carpi radialis brevis [ECRB]).
   (5) Inject just off the bone.
   (6) Do not enter the substance of the tendon.
   (7) Danger of tendon rupture with repeated injections.

6. Prevention.
   a. Physical.
      (1) Adequate conditioning.
      (2) Warm-up.
      (3) Stretching.
   b. Technique.
      (1) Avoid "leading elbow" with tennis backhand.
      (2) Forearm only partially pronated.
      (3) Forward shoulder lowered.
      (4) Trunk leaning forward.
   c. Equipment.
      (1) Racquet size.
      (2) Racquet weight.
      (3) Grip size: measure from midpalmar crease to tip of fourth finger and between third and fourth fingers.
      (4) String tension: 16 gauge gut strings, 2-3 lb. less than manufacturer's recommendation (i.e., 50-55 lb), lighter, slower tennis balls, slower court.

B. Panner's disease (osteochondrosis of the humeral capitellum).
   1. Mechanism of injury.
      a. Repetitive valgus stress on the elbow causes compressive stress across the radiocapitellar joint.
      b. Usually occurs between 7 and 12 years of age (peak incidence at 9 years); humeral capitellum may be susceptible at this time because of limited blood supply.
      c. Pathophysiology may be similar to Legg-Calvé-Perthes disease of the hip, most common in throwing athletes.
   2. Symptoms.
      a. Fairly sudden onset of lateral elbow pain.
      b. Dull, aching pain, worsened by motion, particularly throwing.
      c. Absence of mechanical symptoms (i.e., locking, catching).
   3. Physical examination findings.
      a. Swelling and tenderness over the lateral elbow.
      b. Mild to moderate limitation of extension (5-20 degrees).

4. Radiology.
   a. Plain films show fragmentation of the capitellum, with alternating areas of sclerosis and rarefaction, and an irregular joint surface.
   b. Further imaging not usually necessary.
5. Treatment.
   a. Treatment is conservative; orthopedic consultation not essential.
   b. Initial treatment includes complete rest from throwing until symptoms subside and range of motion (ROM) returns to normal.
   c. Splinting and sling support for severe pain.
   d. Ice, analgesics.
   e. Active range of motion as pain allows.
   f. Repeat radiography when patient is symptom-free to demonstrate bony remodeling.
   g. May return to play when physical examination and radiography findings are normal (6-12 weeks).
6. Complications.
   a. Condition is self-limited; probability of remodeling leading to a structurally normal joint is excellent.
   b. May result in some limitation of motion.
   c. Long-term disability is rare.

C. Osteochondritis dissecans of the humeral capitellum.
   1. Mechanism of injury.
      a. Represents an island of subchondral bone and its adjacent articular cartilage (osteochondral fragment) that begin to separate from the rest of the humerus.
      b. Repetitive valgus stress on the elbow causes compressive stress across the radiocapitellar joint.
      c. Usually occurs between 10 and 15 years of age.
      d. Most common in throwers and gymnasts.
      e. Etiology unclear; avascular injury is an inconsistent pathological finding. Most common etiological factor is repetitive stress. Genetic susceptibility may be involved.
   2. Symptoms.
      a. Gradual onset of lateral elbow pain.
      b. Dull, aching pain, worsened by motion, particularly throwing.
      c. Locking and catching are common and highly suggestive of articular injury.
   3. Physical examination findings.
      a. Tender at radiocapitellar joint.
      b. Mild to moderate limitation of extension (5 to 20 degrees) in >90% of cases.
      c. Crepitus.
      d. Joint effusion.
   4. Radiology.
      a. Plain films show crescent-shaped region of sclerotic subchondral bone in the humeral capitellum demarcated from the rest of the bone by a rim of lucency. The lesion may involve the entire capitellum. Loose bodies may be seen.
      b. Further imaging often obtained to fully evaluate the articular surface and to look for loose bodies.
   5. Treatment.
      a. Depends on the degree of separation of the osteochondral fragment.

b. Orthopedic consultation usually necessary to fully evaluate the joint surface.
c. Cases with no evidence of separation may be treated conservatively with complete rest for 6-8 weeks, ice, analgesics, active ROM exercise.
d. Repeat plain films at 6-8 weeks to look for evidence of healing.
e. Indications for surgery.
(1) Locking.
(2) Osteochondral fragment separation.
(3) Loose bodies.
(4) Failure of conservative treatment.
6. Complications.
a. Prognosis for return of full function not as good as for osteochondrosis.
b. Articular damage.
c. Early degenerative changes.
d. Limited range of motion.
e. May involve the radial head.
7. Prevention: limit number of pitches.
D. Radial head fractures.
1. Mechanism of injury.
a. Fall on the outstretched hand: axial load with the forearm pronated.
b. Direct blow.
c. May occur in elbow dislocation (~10% of dislocations).
2. Physical examination findings.
a. Tender at radial head.
b. Painful elbow hemarthrosis.
c. Limited range of motion (30-100 degrees).
3. Classification.
a. Type I: marginal fracture without displacement.
b. Type II: marginal fracture with displacement.
c. Type III: comminuted fracture.
d. Type IV: fracture associated with elbow dislocation.
4. Radiology.
a. Anteroposterior, lateral, radiocapitellar views.
b. Posterior fat pad sign (anterior fat pad sign present in some normal patients).
5. Treatment.
a. Type I.
(1) Aspirate hemarthrosis.
(2) Sling for 3 days.
(3) Begin ROM exercises immediately.
(4) Physical therapy to regain full extension.
b. Type II.
(1) Treatment controversial.
(2) Surgery may offer no benefit.
(3) If displaced <2 mm, may treat as type I above.
(4) If displaced >2 mm, → open reduction, internal fixation (ORIF).
(5) Make every effort to preserve radial head.
(6) Excise fracture fragment if mechanical block is present.
c. Type III.
(1) Comminuted fracture of radial head.
(2) If no mechanical block to ROM, consider conservative therapy.
(3) If mechanical block to ROM, consider excision of radial head.

(4) Keep resection proximal to annular ligament.
(5) Consider Silastic implant.
d. Type IV: good results with closed reduction, Type I or II fracture Type III fracture → ORIF.

6. Complications.
a. Unrecognized fractures.
(1) Wrist, especially radioulnar joint.
(2) Capitellum.
(3) Coronoid process.
b. Unrecognized elbow dislocation.
c. Avascular necrosis of radial head.

7. ORIF.
a. Single fracture line.
b. Displaced >3 mm.
c. Diverges >30 degrees from articular surface.

II. Medial Elbow Pain

A. Medial epicondylitis.

1. Mechanism of injury: overuse injury due to repetitive valgus stress, for example, due to:
a. Throwing sports (especially acceleration phase).
b. Racket sports (squash, racketball, tennis).

2. Symptoms.
a. Aching pain.
b. Weak grip.
c. Ulnar nerve paresthesia.

3. Physical examination findings.
a. Tender at medial epicondyle.
b. Increased pain with:
(1) Resisted wrist flexion.
(2) Resisted forearm pronation.
(3) Full elbow flexion.
c. Decreased ROM, especially extension.

4. Radiology: gravity valgus stress film.
a. Widening of epiphyseal lines.
b. Possible fragmentation.

5. Differential diagnosis.
a. Ulnar collateral ligament sprain.
b. Medial apophysitis.
c. Ulnar neuritis.
d. Osteochondritis dissecans.
e. C-spine radiculopathy.
f. Osteoarthritis.

6. Treatment.
a. Relative rest.
b. Modalities: ice, heat, ultrasound.
c. Stretching.
d. Strengthening.
(1) Wrist flexors.
(2) Forearm pronators (pronator teres).
e. Counterforce brace, neutral wrist splint.
f. Return to play with full, painless ROM.

7. Prevention.
a. Adequate conditioning.
b. Warm-up.

c. Stretches.
d. Proper technique (e.g., avoid excessive wrist flexion with tennis serve).

8. Complications.
a. Chronic apophysitis.
b. Epicondylar fracture.

B. Medial apophysitis.

1. Mechanism of injury.
a. True "epicondylitis," in distinction to "medial epicondylitis" in adults, which is actually flexor-pronator tendinitis.
b. Repetitive valgus stress causes traction injury at the medial elbow.
c. Results in inflammation of the growth plate at the medial epicondyle (apophysitis).
d. Occurs in children aged 10-14.
e. Seen in throwing sports, racquet sports.

2. Symptoms.
a. Insidious onset of dull, aching pain.
b. Diminished throwing performance.
c. Weak grip.
d. May have paresthesias in the distribution of the ulnar nerve.

3. Physical examination findings.
a. Little or no swelling.
b. Tender at medial epicondyle.
c. May have mild limitation of extension.
d. Fragment may be palpable if avulsion has occurred.

4. Radiology.
a. Plain films may be normal compared to the uninvolved side or may show widening of the physis, fragmentation of the apophysis, or avulsion of the apophysis.
b. Gravity valgus stress films may reveal separation at the physis.

5. Treatment.
a. Relative rest.
b. Ice, analgesics.
c. Local corticosteroid injections not helpful and not recommended.
d. Active ROM as tolerated.
e. Return to play with full, painless ROM.

6. Complications.
a. Avulsion is most frequent complication but is relatively uncommon.
b. Separation of avulsed fragment >5 mm may require ORIF.
c. Inadequately treated cases may develop chronic apophysitis.

C. Ulnar collateral ligament injuries.

1. History.
a. Acute pain or "pop."
b. Sudden sharp pain over medial elbow.
c. Progressive pain with throwing, unable to continue throwing effectively.

2. Mechanism of injury.
a. Acute valgus stress to flexed elbow, especially during acceleration phase in throwing sports.

3. Physical examination findings.
a. Tender at medial elbow.
b. Pain with valgus stress testing.
c. Valgus laxity.

   d. Swelling at medial elbow.
   e. Decreased ROM, loss of full extension.
4. Radiology.
   a. Plain films.
      (1) Ectopic bone formation in ulnar collateral ligament (UCL).
      (2) Spurring at conoid tubercle.
      (3) Epiphyseal separation.
      (4) Olecranon osteophytes.
      (5) Loose bodies.
      (6) Capitellar osteochondrosis.
      (7) Normal radiography findings do not rule out UCL injury.
   b. Gravity stress films.
   c. Arthrograms: leaking dye from torn capsule.
   d. Magnetic resonance imaging (MRI): complete rupture of UCL.
5. Differential diagnosis.
   a. Medial epicondylitis.
   b. Medial apophysitis.
   c. Ulnar neuritis.
   d. Flexor-pronator muscle tear.
   e. Osteochondritis dissecans.
   f. C-spine radiculopathy.
   g. Osteoarthritis.
6. Treatment.
   a. Relative rest.
   b. Modalities: ice, deep heat, ultrasound.
   c. NSAIDs.
   d. Range of motion exercises.
   e. Strengthening exercises.
   f. Return to play (throwing activities) when no longer tender.
   g. Indications for surgery.
      (1) Instability.
      (2) Chronic UCL insufficiency.
      (3) Unable to throw with maximal force.
      (4) Acute repair of complete ligament rupture (3 degree tear).
      (5) Delayed reconstruction, tendon graft.
7. Prevention.
   a. Adequate conditioning.
   b. Warm-up.
   c. Stretches.
   d. Appropriate technique (e.g., avoid "opening up" too early during acceleration phase of pitch, avoid "round arm" technique in javelin toss).

D. Ulnar neuritis.
1. Mechanism of injury.
   a. Direct blow.
   b. Repetitive elbow flexion.
      (1) Cocking phase in throwing sports.
      (2) Cubital tunnel irritation without elbow instability.
   c. Traction due to dynamic valgus forces (acceleration phase).
   d. Commonly accompanied by medial collateral ligament instability.
   e. Throwing and racquet sport athletes, weight lifters.
2. Symptoms.
   a. Pain at medial elbow.

   b. Onset may be sudden or insidious; neuritis without instability often associated with acute onset after a pitch that acutely stretches the ulnar nerve.
   c. Paresthesias along medial forearm and fourth and fifth fingers.
   d. Decreased throwing or racquet play performance.
3. Physical examination findings.
   a. Soft tissue swelling and tenderness in the vicinity of the cubital tunnel and UCL.
   b. Pressure on the cubital tunnel reproduces the paresthesias (e.g., elbow hyperflexion with wrist extension).
   c. Valgus instability.
   d. Little or no limitation of motion.
   e. Positive Tinel's sign.
   f. Grip weakness, pinch weakness.
4. Differential diagnosis.
   a. Medial epicondylitis.
   b. UCL sprain.
   c. Thoracic outlet syndrome.
   d. C-spine radiculopathy.
   e. Osteoarthritis.
   f. Cubital tunnel mass or ganglion.
   g. Superior sulcus tumor.
5. Treatment.
   a. Complete rest.
   b. Ice, analgesics.
   c. Active ROM as tolerated.
   d. When symptoms subside, advance slowly to full throwing.
   e. Ulnar neuritis associated with medial instability is more difficult to treat.
   f. Surgery should be considered if symptoms do not respond to conservative therapy, or if muscle atrophy develops.
6. Complications.
   a. Persistent neuritis.
   b. Wrist flexor and grip weakness.
7. Prevention.
   a. Limit number of pitches.
   b. Revise pitching mechanics to avoid excessive valgus stress.

III. Posterior Elbow Pain
  A. Elbow dislocation.
    1. Mechanism of injury.
       a. Hyperextension.
       b. Fall on the outstretched arm.
       c. Axial load with the elbow slightly flexed.
       d. Usually causes posterior or posterolateral dislocation.
    2. Concomitant extensive soft tissue damage.
       a. Anterior and posterior capsule.
       b. Collateral ligaments, especially anterior bundle of medial collateral ligament.
       c. Flexor muscle mass, especially brachialis muscle.
    3. Associated fractures.
       a. Radial head fracture (~10% of cases).
       b. Less commonly, fractures of coronoid process, olecranon, medial epicondyle, lateral epicondyle, and, rarely, capitellum.
    4. Physical examination findings.

- a. Obvious deformity, olecranon prominent posteriorly, elbow slightly flexed.
- b. Check vascular integrity: brachial pulse, radial pulse, capillary refill.
- c. Check median nerve function.

5. Radiology.
   - a. Plain films, tomograms.
   - b. No need for MRI, arthrography.
6. Treatment.
   - a. Early reduction.
     - (1) Stabilize distal humerus, apply gentle traction.
     - (2) With forearm supinated, elbow is first extended, then flexed.
     - (3) Redo neurovascular examination after reduction.
     - (4) Check postreduction radiograph.
   - b. Splint.
     - (1) Elbow at 90 degrees of flexion.
     - (2) Forearm full pronation.
     - (3) Early range of motion exercises allowed at 7-10 days.
   - c. If unstable after reduction:
     - (1) Refer to.
     - (2) Cast brace may be applied in a stable position.
     - (3) Extension is adjusted as tolerated.
     - (4) Limit immobilization ≤3 weeks.
   - d. Indications for surgical repair.
     - (1) Irreducible, possibly due to a displaced radial head fracture.
     - (2) Medial instability.
     - (3) Easily redislocated.
7. Complications.
   - a. Stiff elbow, loss of full extension.
     - (1) Avoid prolonged immobilization (<3 weeks).
     - (2) In most cases, may begin ROM within 7-10 days.
   - b. Neurovascular compromise.
     - (1) Especially injury to brachial artery and/or median nerve.
     - (2) Possible Volkmann's ischemic contracture.
   - c. Compartment syndrome.
   - d. Myositis ossificans.
     - (1) Especially after repeated attempts at reduction.
     - (2) Less common if promptly reduced, adequate period of immobilization.
     - (3) Avoid *passive* ROM exercises.
     - (4) Encourage pain-limited active ROM exercises.
     - (5) Must differentiate from calcification of ligaments, capsule.
     - (6) If myositis ossificans occurs, treat with immobilization.
     - (7) No surgical removal of ectopic bone before deposit is mature.
   - e. Recurrent instability.
     - (1) Affects approximately 1% to 2% of cases.
     - (2) Usually due to deficiency of lateral UCL.
     - (3) May be corrected upon surgical reconstruction of lateral UCL.

B. Olecranon fractures.

1. Mechanism of injury.
   - a. Direct trauma.
   - b. Avulsion force due to pull of the triceps.
2. Physical examination findings.
   - a. Posterior elbow tenderness.

      b. Joint effusion.
      c. Swelling over olecranon.
   3. Differential diagnosis.
      a. Traction apophysitis.
         (1) Adolescent patient.
         (2) Repetitive throwing.
         (3) Treat with rest from aggravating activity.
      b. Avulsion of triceps tendon.
      c. Triceps tendinitis.
      d. Olecranon bursitis.
   4. Treatment.
      a. Nondisplaced ($\leq$2 mm).
         (1) Splint elbow at 45 degrees of flexion.
         (2) Begin ROM within 2-3 weeks.
      b. Displaced (>2 mm): ORIF.

C. Triceps tendinitis.
   1. Mechanism of injury.
      a. Overuse injury.
      b. Repetitive elbow extension (e.g., baseball players, carpenters).
   2. Treatment.
      a. Relative rest.
      b. Ice.
      c. NSAIDs.
      d. ROM exercises.
      e. Progressive resistance exercises.
      f. Return to play with full, painless ROM.
      g. Surgery rarely indicated.

D. Triceps avulsion.
   1. Mechanism of injury.
      a. Fall on the outstretched hand.
      b. Direct blow.
         (1) Chronic steroid use.
         (2) Parathyroidism.
      c. Relatively rare.
      d. Rupture usually occurs at tendo-osseous region.
   2. Associated injuries.
      a. Radial head fracture.
      b. Chronic olecranon bursitis.
      c. Systemic medical conditions.
   3. Physical examination findings.
      a. Tender just proximal to olecranon.
      b. Posterior swelling and ecchymosis.
      c. Palpable defect just proximal to olecranon.
   4. Radiology: small bony avulsions seen in 80% of cases.
   5. Treatment.
      a. Immediate reconstructive surgery.
      b. Postoperative immobilization for ~3 weeks.
      c. Elbow: 30-40 degrees flexion.
      d. Good prognosis postoperatively.

E. Olecranon bursitis.
   1. Mechanism of injury.
      a. Acute trauma (e.g., direct blow).
      b. Repetitive trauma (sports, occupation).

2. Physical examination findings.
   a. Superficial swelling over olecranon.
   b. Full range of joint motion, except extreme flexion.
3. Differential diagnosis.
   a. Cellulitis.
   b. Septic arthritis.
   c. Elbow sprain.
   d. Tendinitis.
   e. Crystal arthropathy.
   f. Septic bursitis.
      (1) Pain over olecranon with joint motion.
      (2) Tender to palpation.
      (3) Usually with skin abrasion.
      (4) Aspiration shows purulence, predominantly neutrophils.
      (5) Usually *Staphylococcus aureus* (94%).
      (6) Treatment: incision and drainage, oral antibiotics, intravenous antibiotics if systemic symptoms are present.
4. Treatment.
   a. Steroid injections have no place in acute olecranon bursitis.
   b. Aspiration.
      (1) Diagnostic: bloody, low white blood cell count, predominantly monocytes.
      (2) Therapeutic: distended, uncomfortable, limits ROM, interferes with play.
   c. Sterile conditions, compressive dressing for 48 hours, ice.
5. Prevention.
   a. Elbow pads.
   b. Natural turf.
6. Surgery.
   a. Fibrous tissue formation.
   b. Chronic bursitis.

IV. Anterior Elbow Pain
  A. Coronoid fractures.
    1. Mechanism of injury.
       a. Forceful extension of actively flexed elbow.
       b. Seen in association with elbow dislocation.
    2. Physical examination findings.
       a. Tender in antecubital fossa.
       b. Anterior elbow swelling.
       c. Pain with passive elbow extension.
    3. Radiology.
       a. Anteroposterior, lateral, oblique, radiocapitellar views.
       b. Classification by percentage of coronoid involved:

          Type I: <25%

          Type II: 25% to 50%

          Type III: >50%

    4. Treatment.
       a. Type I.
          (1) Immobilize elbow in splint for 3-4 days.
          (2) Early ROM exercises.
       b. Type II or III.
          (1) ORIF.
          (2) Anatomical reduction of large coronoid fracture.

Bibliography

Bryan W: Baseball. In Reider B, editor: *Sports Medicine: The School-Age Athlete,* Philadelphia, 1991, WB Saunders, pp 447-483.

Carson WG Jr: Overuse injuries of the elbow. In Baker CL Jr, Flandry F, Henderson J, editors: *The Hughston Clinic Sports Medicine Book,* Baltimore, 1995, Williams & Wilkins, pp 324-331.

Graf BK, Lange RH: Osteochondritis dissecans. In Reider B, editor: *Sports Medicine: The School-Age Athlete,* Philadelphia, 1991, WB Saunders, pp 240-254.

Halpern BC: Elbow and arm injuries. In Birrer RB, editor: *Sports Medicine for the Primary Care Physician,* ed 2, Boca Raton, 1994, CRC Press, pp 435-448.

Higgins DL: Fractures about the elbow. In Baker CL Jr, Flandry F, Henderson J, editors: *The Hughston Clinic Sports Medicine Book,* Baltimore, 1995, Williams & Wilkins, pp 312-316.

Hurley JA: Complicated elbow fractures in athletes, *Clin Sports Med* 9(1):39-57, 1990.

Josefsson PO et al: Surgical vs. non-surgical treatment of ligamentous injuries following dislocation of the elbow joint: a randomized, prospective study, *J Bone Joint Surg* 69-A(4):605-608, 1987.

Mehlhoff TL et al: Simple dislocation of the elbow in the adult: results after closed treatment, *J Bone Joint Surg* 70-A(2):244-249, 1988.

Morrey BF, Regan WD: Tendinopathies about the elbow. In DeLee J, Drez D Jr, editors: *Orthopedic Sports Medicine: Principles and Practice,* Philadelphia, 1994, WB Saunders, pp 860-881.

O'Donoghue DH: Injuries of the elbow. In O'Donoghue DH, editor: *Treatment of Injuries to Athletes,* ed 4, Philadelphia, 1984, WB Saunders, pp 221-246.

Roy S, Irvin R: Throwing and tennis injuries to the shoulder and elbow. In Roy S, Irvin R, editors: *Sports Medicine: Prevention, Evaluation, Management, and Rehabilitation,* Englewood Cliffs, 1983, Prentice-Hall, pp 211-227.

Sallis RE: The thrower. In Birrer RB, editor: *Sports Medicine for the Primary Care Physician,* ed 2, Boca Raton, 1994, CRC Press, pp 229-236.

Torg JS et al: Injuries to the upper extremity: elbow. In Torg JS, Shephard RJ, editors: *Current Therapy in Sports Medicine,* ed 3. St Louis, 1995, Mosby–Year Book, pp 104-146.

Watson JT: Fractures of the elbow and forearm, *Clin Sports Med* 9(1):59-83, 1990.

CHAPTER 41

History and Physical Exam

Robert J. Johnson, MD

I. Wrist Injuries
  A. General.
    1. The wrist is capable of motion in three planes and transmits forces from the hand to the forearm, rendering it vulnerable to acute and overuse injuries in many sports.
    2. Severity of wrist injuries is often underestimated by athletes and clinicians. This often leads to underdiagnosis or misdiagnosis and the unfortunate chronic sequelae that may result.
    3. 90% of traumatic wrist injuries are secondary to falls with the wrist dorsiflexed, resisting external forces. Consequently, the wrist is predisposed to compressive injuries dorsally and tension injuries on the volar aspect.
  B. Functional anatomy.
    1. Osseous (Figure 41-1).
      a. Eight carpal bones are divided into two rows of four each.
        (1) Proximal row: scaphoid, lunate, triquetrum, pisiform, forming a smooth arc that articulates with the radius laterally and the fibrocartilaginous complex on the medial side.
        (2) Distal row: trapezium, trapezoid, capitate, hamate, which articulate with the metacarpals and the proximal row.
      b. Second and third carpometacarpal articulations are relatively immobile and serve to stabilize the arched hand.
      c. Scaphoid: only carpal bone to cross midcarpal joint. Stabilizes carpals, but also increases injury risk compared to other carpal bones.
      d. Lunate: transmits forces between capitate and radius.
      e. Triquetrum and hamate.
      f. Trapezium, trapezoid, and capitate: support metacarpals. Saddle-shaped articular surface of trapezium allows thumb apposition and greater range of motion.
      g. Pisiform: sesamoid bone.

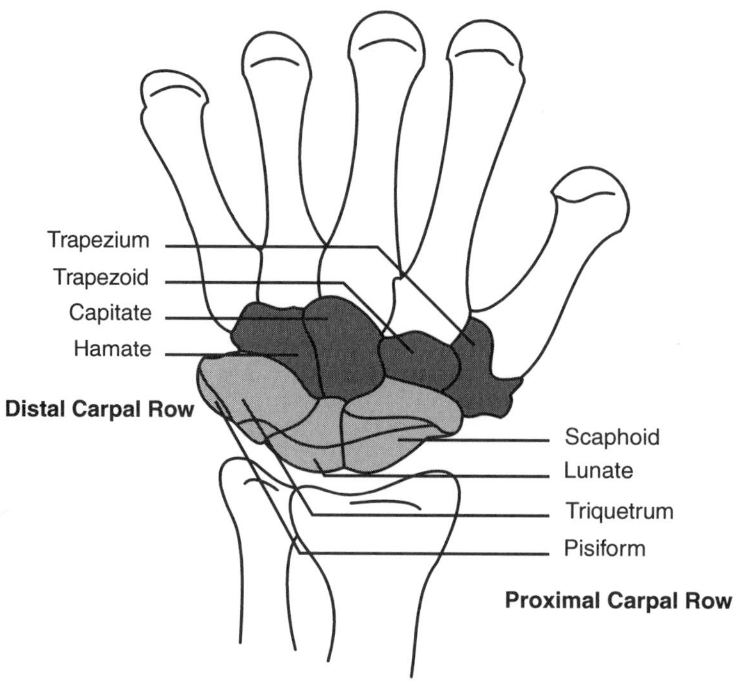

FIGURE 41-1
Carpal bones.

2. Ligamentous anatomy (Figure 41-2).
   a. General configuration is a double inverted V.
   b. Major stabilizing ligaments are radiocapitate, radiotriquetral, and radioscaphoid. As with all volar ligaments, they become taut with wrist extension.
   c. Triangular fibrocartilaginous complex (TFCC) consists of an articular disc (a meniscus homolog), ulnar collateral ligament and dorsal and volar radioulnar ligaments. TFCC serves as a cushion and sta-

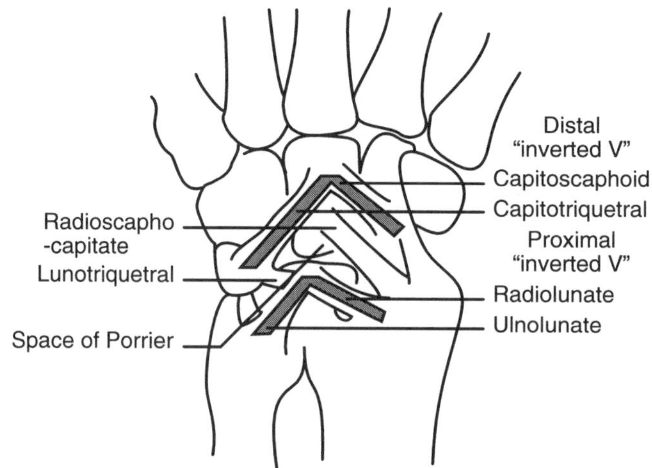

FIGURE 41-2
Ligaments of the volar wrist.

bilizer of the wrist and is symptomatic with either tears or degeneration.

3. Anatomical snuff box.
   a. Formed by the abductor pollicis longus and the extensor pollicis brevis on the radial side and the extensor pollicis longus on the dorsal side.
   b. The scaphoid forms the floor of the "snuff box." Tenderness after trauma suggests scaphoid fracture.
4. Carpal tunnel.
   a. Tunnel contains the tendons of the flexor digitorum profundus and superficialis, the flexor pollicis longus, and the median nerve.
   b. Tunnel rigidity and synovial inflammation combine to increase pressure within the canal to cause symptoms in the distribution of the median nerve.
5. Motor nerve function.
   a. Radial nerve: Wrist extension, thumb extension and abduction.
   b. Median nerve: Wrist flexion, thumb flexion and opposition.
   c. Ulnar nerve: Finger abduction and adduction, thumb adduction.

C. Traumatic wrist injuries.
1. General.
   a. Significant pain and/or swelling suggest significant injury and warrant thorough investigation.
   b. History: Most common mechanism is a fall or collision with the wrist in dorsiflexion.
   c. Physical examination.
      (1) Generally, the greater the swelling, the worse the injury.
      (2) Range of motion limited by pain, swelling, or instability.
      (3) Assess neurovascular status.
2. Osseous injuries.
   a. Scaphoid fractures.
      (1) 70% of all carpal bone injuries.
      (2) Avascular necrosis (AVN) is common due to dependence on a single interosseous blood supply that enters distally and runs proximally.
      (3) The more proximal the fracture, the more delayed the healing.
         (a) Distal one third fractures average 8 weeks to heal (10% of all scaphoid fractures).
         (b) Waist fractures require 3 months (70% of all scaphoid fractures).
         (c) Proximal one third require ≥4 months (20% of all scaphoid fractures).
      (4) Physical examination: pain and/or swelling in the anatomical snuff box and scaphoid tubercle.
      (5) Radiography may be negative initially. Bone scan will be positive in about 72 hours.
      (6) Treatment: if clinically suspicious in spite of negative radiographs, immobilize in a thumb spica cast and reevaluate in 2 weeks. Some hand surgeons recommend the use of a long arm thumb spica cast for waist or proximal fractures to prevent pronation or supination, which may delay or prevent healing. Nondisplaced distal or waist fractures should be casted 8 (distal) to 12 (waist) weeks. Reevaluate every 3-4 weeks with radiography to confirm proper healing.

(7) Return to play: when the fracture is healed >3 months, return possible with protective thumb spica splint for up to 2 months.

b. Trapezoid and trapezium fractures are rare. If nondisplaced, cast for 3-6 weeks. Displaced fractures should be immobilized and an orthopedic surgeon consulted.

c. Lunate: seldom acutely fractured. When associated with negative ulnar variance, may be associated with chronic bony injury known as Kienböck's disease. Orthopedic consultation may be warranted.

d. Triquetrum: second most common carpal fracture. Chip or avulsion fractures can be treated with short arm cast for 4-6 weeks. Nonunion may require surgical excision.

e. Pisiform: usually caused by direct blow to hypothenar eminence. Isolated fractures may be treated with a short arm cast in slight flexion for 3-6 weeks. Comminuted fractures may need surgery; consult an orthopedist.

f. Hamate: fractures of body are uncommon; fractures of the hook are more common, occurring in racquet and club sports during the swing. Check ulnar nerve status in hook injuries. Nondisplaced hook or body fractures casted with wrist in flexion and fourth and fifth metacarpophalangeal (MCP) joints in acute flexion for 3-4 weeks. Displaced hook or body fractures require orthopedic consultation.

g. Capitate: risk of AVN suggests necessity for orthopedic consultation.

3. Ligamentous injuries.

a. Radial ligamentous injuries: most involve ligaments about the scaphoid. If scaphoid lies in abnormal position on radiograph, orthopedic consultation is necessary. Failure to identify these injuries may lead to long-term instability and disability.

b. Ulnar ligamentous injuries: triquetrolunate or triquetrohamate ligaments lead to most instabilities. These, too, require orthopedic consultation.

c. Scapholunate dissociation.

(1) May occur with fall on outstretched hand.

(2) Be suspicious clinically. Initially, scaphoid fracture is ruled out. If patient continues to have pain in area of "snuff box" or toward radioulnar joint, consider this diagnosis. Watson's test may be positive ("click" due to scaphoid subluxation when applying pressure over dorsal radius while pressing on palmar, distal pole of scaphoid and forcing wrist into radial deviation).

(3) Obtain wrist radiographs. Look for increased widening between scaphoid and lunate compared to uninvolved side. If not present, obtain "clenched fist" view as provocative test to accentuate widening between scaphoid and lunate ("Terry Thomas sign").

(4) Conservative treatment is to immobilize 6-12 weeks.

(5) For chronic instability, consider immobilization and/or corticosteroid injection.

(6) For failed conservative therapy for either situation, consult orthopedic surgeon for surgical intervention.

d. Lunate dislocation (dorsal or volar).

(1) Clinically, painful, swollen wrist with lunate palpable in palmar fossa.

(2) Complete dislocation is apparent on lateral wrist radiograph. Remember the normal "teacup" appearance of lunate relative to capitate. Lunate cradles the capitate in the concavity.
(3) Reduce by applying longitudinal traction while extending wrist and applying pressure to volar side of lunate.
(4) Alternatively, splint and consult orthopedic surgeon immediately.

4. TFCC injuries.
   a. Major stabilizer of radioulnar joint; also cushions ulnar axial loads. Dependent on degree of ulnar variance (position of ulnar head in relation to radial articular surface). Positive ulnar variance results in thin TFCC and increased susceptibility to injury.
   b. Physical examination: ulna may be unstable with dorsal subluxation. There may be pain or crepitus with volar compression between ulna and triquetrum. Painful clunk may occur with passive pronation and supination.
   c. Computerized tomography and magnetic resonance imaging are the most reliable methods for evaluating TFCC radiographically. Arthrography may be useful.
   d. Treatment: immobilize 2-3 weeks and reexamine. If pain persists, consider corticosteroid injection. Failure to improve may dictate need for arthroscopy.

D. Overuse injuries.
1. General.
   a. Tendinitis and tenosynovitis can involve any tendon about the wrist. Cause is overdemand, leading to inflammation/hemorrhage, followed by cellular invasion, leading to collagen production, followed by maturation and strengthening.
   b. Physical examination: tendon(s) tender to touch, diffuse swelling over involved tendons, with passive stretching and resisted motion of affected tendons.
   c. Treatment.
      (1) Control inflammation: cryotherapy, nonsteroidal antiinflammatory drugs (NSAIDs), modify activity, corticosteroid injection in sheath may be helpful.
      (2) Splinting/casting may be helpful.
      (3) Modalities.
      (4) Appropriate stretching and strengthening after acute inflammation subsides.
      (5) Gradual return to previous level of activity.
2. Common tendinitis/tenosynovitis syndromes.
   a. de Quervain's tenosynovitis: involves first dorsal compartment, especially abductor pollicis longus and extensor pollicis brevis. Finkelstein's test is positive (thumb grasped by other four fingers during ulnar deviation reproduces pain). Rarely needs surgical release.
   b. Intersection syndrome ("squeaker's wrist"): occurs at intersection of first and second dorsal compartments; more proximal to site of de Quervain's. Common in weight lifters and rowers.
   c. Extensor pollicis longus/brevis tenosynovitis: tendons of second dorsal compartment. Usually occurs in sports requiring repetitive acceleration and deceleration.
   d. Scaphoid impingement syndrome: repetitive forced hyperextension of wrist (weight lifting and gymnastics) causes scaphoid and radius to bump into each other.

e. Common extensor tenosynovitis: fourth compartment syndrome. Painful "goosefoot" swelling over dorsum of wrist.
f. Carpal tunnel syndrome: numbness to first three and one half digits on palmar surface of hand (sensory innervation may be highly variable in distribution in fingers). Positive Phalen's test (symptoms reproduced by wrist flexion) and positive Tinel's sign (45% of the time). Electromyography may be normal 25% of the time. May be treated successfully with splinting and NSAIDs. Persistent cases may need corticosteroid injection or surgery.
g. Ganglions: benign masses filled with viscous fluid, arising most often from dorsal scapholunate ligament, volar radioscaphoid ligament, and sheath of flexor carpi radialis tendon. Probably, traumatically induced with fluid passing through a small opening or weak spot. Treat with rest and consider aspiration and corticosteroid injection. Recurrences may have to be treated with surgical excision.

II. Hand Injuries
  A. Metacarpal fractures.
    1. First metacarpal.
      a. Shaft (uncommon site).
        (1) Base/shaft: usually transverse or oblique.
        (2) Treat conservatively with splint or cast for 2-3 weeks unless angulated. If angulated, consider orthopedic consultation.
      b. Intraarticular.
        (1) Bennett's fracture: base of thumb (fracture/subluxation) fractures and subluxes radially while proximal portion moves dorsally (subluxation related to forces of ligament and muscle attachments).
        (2) Usually needs surgical intervention since reduction is difficult to maintain.
      c. In most cases, return to play (with protection) occurs in 2 weeks.
    2. Metacarpal neck fractures.
      a. Seen in axial load injuries.
      b. Usually result in dorsal angulation (due to shape of metacarpal and force of intrinsic muscles).
      c. Fourth to fifth digits: may tolerate as much as 40-50 degrees of angulation.
      d. Second to third digits: tolerate 10-15 degrees of angulation due to less mobility of second and third digits.
      e. Treatment.
        (1) If there is full range of motion (ROM) of digit without "clawing" (hyperextension of MCP) *and* lack of prominence of metacarpal in palm, treat conservatively with cast or splint (MCP joint flexed 90 degrees) for 2-3 weeks.
        (2) If above criteria not satisfied, obtain orthopedic consultation.
      f. Boxer's fracture.
        (1) Fifth metacarpal neck fracture. Can accept 40-70 degrees of angulation.
        (2) Reduce by flexing MCP to 90 degrees and reverse direction and force of angulation/displacement.
        (3) Treatment: immobilize in ulnar gutter splint incorporating fourth and fifth fingers with MCP flexion 70 degrees for 2 weeks, then early ROM exercises.

3. Metacarpal shaft fractures.
   a. Types: transverse, oblique, and spiral oblique.
   b. Treatment: dependent on fracture location and configuration, degree of displacement, and number of metacarpals involved.
   c. Transverse (due to direct blow or direct axial load).
      (1) Angulation concerns similar to those of metacarpal neck fractures (usually slightly less angulation accepted).
      (2) Fourth to fifth digits: 20-30 degrees of angulation.
      (3) Second to third digits: no angulation.
      (4) Treatment: conservative for those with acceptable angulation. Buddy splint with adjacent finger 2-3 weeks or obtain orthopedic consultation.
   d. Oblique/spiral (usually result in malrotation).
      (1) To check for malrotation, clench fist to look at flexion of all digits.
      (2) Fracture shortening up to 5 mm is acceptable.
      (3) Treatment: cast/splint 2-3 weeks.
      (4) If unacceptable angulation, malrotation, or shortening, obtain orthopedic consultation.

B. Metacarpal dislocations: metacarpal head goes through volar plate, causing buttonholing effect. Longitudinal traction may make the entrapment tighter and convert a simple dislocation into a complex dislocation. Generally, requires surgical reduction.

III. Finger Injuries

A. Distal phalanx fractures.
   1. Usually caused by crush injuries and rarely displaced.
   2. Drain-associated subungual hematomas.
   3. Protective splint is used for symptomatic pain treatment.

B. Distal interphalangeal (DIP) joint injuries.
   1. Mallet finger.
      a. Rupture of extensor digitorum tendon at its insertion on distal phalanx.
      b. Physical examination: inability to actively extend distal phalanx. Characteristic deformity. Radiography may show bony avulsion.
      c. Treatment.
         (1) Bony avulsion: orthopedic consultation if there is volar subluxation or if the fracture involves >30% of joint space. Immobilize straight for 4 weeks.
         (2) No bony avulsion: dorsal splint (or stack splint) in full extension for 8-10 weeks and an additional 6-8 weeks while engaged in sport. Use "no-peek" approach.
   2. Jersey finger.
      a. Avulsion of flexor digitorum usually caused by athlete grabbing a jersey and experiencing sudden pain as distal is forcibly extended while athlete is actively flexing the DIP.
      b. Injury types.
         (1) Avulsion of volar lip of distal phalanx (volar plate intact). Retraction of tendon is limited. Repair by open reduction and internal fixation (ORIF).
         (2) Avulsion of tendon with retraction to hiatus of flexor digitorum sublimis at proximal interphalangeal (PIP) joint. Should be repaired urgently (within 3 weeks). Reconstruction if diagnosis is missed.

(3) Avulsion of tendon with retraction to palm. Acute repair within 7-10 days.

c. Acute injury usually necessitates surgery. Chronically, if athlete is asymptomatic, no treatment is necessary. Joint fusion or tenodesis is necessary if chronic injury is symptomatic (unstable at DIP or hyperextension).

C. Middle phalanx fractures.

1. Stable fractures (usually with palmar angulation).
   a. Buddy tape if nondisplaced, not angulated.
   b. Angulated: immobilize with MCP flexed 70 degrees and the PIP flexed 45 degrees. May permit DIP motion. Buddy tape to prevent rotation. Remove in 3-4 weeks. Protect during athletic activity for an additional 9-10 weeks.
2. Unstable fractures: orthopedic consultation.

D. PIP injuries.

1. Dorsal dislocation.
   a. Hyperextension injury with disruption of volar plate at attachment on middle phalanx. Produces bayonet deformity.
   b. Physical examination and radiography demonstrate deformity.
   c. Reduction: with or without anesthesia. Apply longitudinal traction with slight hyperextension. Thumb of other hand can assist by pushing middle phalanx back into place.
   d. Postreduction: radiograph. Extension block splint or buddy tape for 3 weeks.
2. Volar plate rupture (without dislocation).
   a. Hyperextension injury. Maximal tenderness occurs along volar aspect of PIP. Radiography may show avulsion fragment at base of middle phalanx.
   b. Treat with extension block splint or buddy tape for 3 weeks.
3. PIP fracture-dislocation.
   a. Axial load on partially flexed finger.
   b. Physical examination shows subtle dorsal prominence with pain and swelling at PIP.
   c. Treatment.
      (1) Small fragment: buddy tape for 3 weeks.
      (2) <40% joint surface: closed reduction, extension block splint in 30-60 degrees of flexion for 3 weeks.
      (3) >40% joint surface: orthopedic consultation.
4. Boutonnière deformity (central slip avulsion).
   a. Disruption of central slip of extensor digitorum communis tendon over PIP joint, with migration of lateral bands volar to the axis of the joint. The PIP "herniates" through the "hole."
   b. Second most common closed tendon injury in athletes.
   c. Physical examination: PIP is in 15-30 degrees of flexion, a swollen PIP, and patient cannot actively extend PIP. Radiography may show avulsion fracture at base of middle phalanx.
   d. Treatment: splint in full extension for 4 weeks. Protect during competition for an additional 6-8 weeks. Permit flexion of DIP to help relocated lateral bands to their normal dorsal position. If avulsion fracture involves greater than one third of joint surface, surgery may be necessary.
5. Palmar dislocation: radiography shows volar displacement of middle phalanx. Needs orthopedic consultation since closed reduction is difficult.

6. Collateral ligament tear.
   a. Varus or valgus stress to PIP. Most result in partial tears, but minimal or no instability.
   b. Physical examination shows laxity with varus or valgus stress; stable or unstable with active ROM.
   c. Treatment.
      (1) If lax with stress testing but stable with active ROM, buddy tape to adjacent finger to side of injury for 3 weeks.
      (2) If obvious deformity or unstable with active ROM, surgery is indicated.
7. Proximal phalangeal fractures.
   a. Be cautious in treating these.
   b. Stable: immobilize with wrist in slight extension and MCP at 70 degrees of flexion. Buddy tape. Remove splint in 3-4 weeks and buddy tape until asymptomatic.

E. Skier's thumb (gamekeeper's thumb): Sprain of ulnar collateral ligament of MCP joint.
   1. Hyperabduction of thumb with a lateral stress; usually occurs in a fall while skiing in which ski pole acts as lever arm to increase abduction stress.
   2. Types.
      a. Type 1: torn ligament, nondisplaced.
      b. Type 2: torn ligament, displaced.
      c. Type 3: avulsion fracture, nondisplaced.
      d. Type 4: avulsion fracture, displaced.
   3. Physical examination shows tenderness and swelling over ulnar MCP. Stress with thumb straight and flexed 30 degrees (compare to uninvolved side). Angulation 15 degrees greater than contralateral thumb or 35 degrees absolute indicates ligament disruption.
   4. Treatment.
      a. Partial tear with stable joint: thumb spica cast or splint for 2-4 weeks.
      b. Complete tear: May treat with thumb spica splint for 4 weeks and reevaluate. If still unstable, consider surgery for probable Stener's lesion (a situation in which one end of the torn ulnar collateral ligament lies above the adductor aponeurosis and the other end lies below; may occur in 25% to 50% of complete tears). Some hand surgeons feel a late repair (4 weeks) can be as effective as an early repair.
      c. Avulsion fracture: if displaced >2 mm or rotated, surgery; if nondisplaced, thumb spica cast for 4-6 weeks.

Bibliography

Burton RI, Eaton RG: Common hand injuries in the athlete, *Orthop Clin North Am* 4(3):809-837, 1973.

Culver JE: Instabilities of the wrist, *Clin Sports Med* 5:725-740, 1986.

Culver JE: Injuries of the hand and wrist, *Clin Sports Med* 11(1), 1992.

Hoffman DF, Schaffer TC: Management of common finger injuries, *Am Fam Physician* 43(5):1594-1607, 1991.

Kulund DN, editor: *The Injured Athlete*, ed 2, Philadelphia, 1988, JB Lippincott, pp 371-404.

Newmeyer WJ: *Primary Care of Hand Injuries*, Philadelphia, 1979, Lea & Febiger, pp 9, 93-106.

CHAPTER 42

Wrist and Hand Injuries in Sports

Robert J. Dimeff, MD

I. Anatomy[1,18]

A. Bones.

1. Distal forearm: ulna and radius.
2. Carpal bones: scaphoid, lunate, triquetrum, pisiform, trapezium, trapezoid, capitate, hamate.
3. Metacarpals: I to V from radial to ulnar.
4. Phalanges: 14 per hand—two for each thumb (proximal = 1, distal = 2); three for each finger (proximal = 1, middle = 2, distal = 3).
5. Sesamoids: two at thumb metacarpophalangeal (MCP) joint.

B. Joints.

1. Distal radial ulnar joint (DRUJ): stability maintained by inherent bony anatomy, extrinsic stabilizing structures (interosseous membrane, pronator quadratus, and flexor and extensor carpi ulnaris), and intrinsic stabilizing structure (triangular fibrocartilage complex [TFCC]).[2,5,14]
2. Carpal joints: stability provided by contact surfaces between individual bones, interosseous ligaments (connect carpal bones to each other), and intracapsular ligaments (connect distal radius and ulna to the carpal bones).[3]
   a. Volar intracapsular ligaments are the major stabilizing ligaments of the carpal bones.
   b. Carpal bones of each row are bound tightly to each other by interosseous ligaments.
   c. Proximal carpal row bound tightly to distal radius and ulna; distal carpal row bound tightly to proximal metacarpals.
   d. Little stability between the proximal and distal carpal rows except at the triquetrohamate articulation.
3. Carpometacarpal (CMC) joints: first metacarpal-trapezium articulation is a saddle joint permitting significant thumb motion; other CMC

joints are stabilized by dorsal and volar CMC and interosseous metacarpal ligaments.[1,18]

4. MCP joints: radial and ulnar collateral ligaments (UCL) (lax with MCP extension, taut with MCP flexion); accessory radial and ulnar collateral ligaments, volar accessory ligaments, and transverse metacarpal ligaments also provide MCP stability.[1,18]
5. Proximal interphalangeal (PIP) joint: hinge joint with no abduction/adduction.
   a. Radial and ulnar collateral ligaments, volar plate, accessory collateral ligaments, lateral bands, and oblique retinacular ligaments.
   b. Central slip of extensor mechanism inserts onto dorsal tubercle of middle phalanx.
6. Distal interphalangeal (DIP) joint: hinge joint with no abduction/adduction.[1,18]
   a. Radial and ulnar collateral ligament, volar plate.
   b. Extensor mechanism inserts on dorsal aspect of distal phalanx.

C. Muscle and tendons.
   1. Volar forearm and wrist: flexor carpi radialis (FCR), palmaris longus (PL), flexor carpi ulnaris (FCU), flexor digitorum superficialis (FDS), flexor digitorum profundus (FDP), flexor pollicis longus (FPL).
   2. Dorsal forearm and wrist.
      a. First dorsal compartment: abductor pollicis longus (APL), extensor pollicis brevis (EPB).
      b. Second dorsal compartment: extensor carpi radialis longus (ECRL), extensor carpi radialis brevis (ECRB).
      c. Third dorsal compartment: extensor pollicis longus (EPL).
      d. Fourth dorsal compartment: extensor digitorum communis (EDC), extensor indices (EI).
      e. Fifth dorsal compartment: extensor digiti minimi (EDM).
      f. Sixth dorsal compartment: extensor carpi ulnaris (ECU).
   3. Volar hand: abductor pollicis brevis (APB), flexor pollicis brevis (FPB), opponens pollicis (OP), adductor pollicis (AP), abductor digiti minimi (ADM), flexor digiti minimi (FDM), opponens digiti minimi (ODM), palmaris brevis (PB), lumbricals, palmar interossei.
   4. Dorsal hand: dorsal interossei.

D. Arteries.[1,18]
   1. Radial artery: superficial palmar branch, deep palmar branch (main contributor to deep palmar arch).
   2. Ulnar artery: superficial palmar branch (main contributor to superficial palmar arch), deep palmar branch.
   3. Three palmar metacarpal arteries, four palmar digital arteries.

E. Nerve supply.
   1. Median.
      a. Motor: forearm and wrist—FCR, PL, FDS, FDP (second and third digits), FPL.
      b. Motor: hand—OP, APB, FPD, lumbricals (second and third digits).
      c. Sensory: volar aspect of thumb, radial two and a half digits, and radial two thirds of the palm.
   2. Ulnar.
      a. Motor: forearm and wrist—FCU, FDP (fourth and fifth digits).
      b. Motor: hand—AP, ADM, FDM, ODM, PB, lumbricals (fourth and fifth digits).
      c. Sensory: ulnar third of hand, ulnar one and a half digits.

3. Radial nerve.
   a. Motor: forearm and wrist.
      (1) Radial nerve proper: ECRB and ECRL.
      (2) Posterior interosseous nerve: APL, EPB, EPL, EDC, EI, EDM, and ECU.
   b. Sensory: dorsal radial half of hand and dorsal aspect of thumb.

II. History
   A. Age of patient, handedness, occupation.
   B. Sports participation/position.
   C. Date and mechanism of traumatic injury, location and nature of pain, specific positions or activities that aggravate or relieve symptoms.
   D. History of swelling, bruising, discoloration.
   E. Complaints of loss of motion, clicking, catching, instability.
   F. Paresthesia, weakness, and other neurological complaints.
   G. Risk factors for overuse injuries.
   H. Previous and current treatment.

III. Examination
   A. Inspection: examine contralateral uninjured extremity to provide baseline; observe for swelling, discoloration, deformity, atrophy.
   B. Range of motion (ROM).
      1. Active versus passive.
      2. Observe for symmetrical smooth motion of wrist and digits without shortening, angulation, or rotational deformity.
      3. Normal wrist and hand ROM.
         a. Forearm: 150 degrees of rotation about the ulnar axis at the DRUJ.
         b. Wrist: flexion 80 degrees, extension 70 degrees, ulnar deviation 30 degrees, radial deviation 20 degrees.
         c. Hand:
            (1) MCP fingers: flexion 90 degrees, hyperextension 45 degrees, abduction 20 degrees, adduction 20 degrees (minimal abduction/adduction when MCP flexed).
            (2) MCP thumb: flexion 50 degrees, extension 0 degrees, abduction 70 degrees, adduction 0 degrees.
            (3) PIP fingers: flexion 100 degrees, extension 0 degrees.
            (4) DIP fingers: flexion 90 degrees, hyperextension 20 degrees.
            (5) IP thumb: flexion 90 degrees, hyperextension 20 degrees.
   C. Bony and soft tissue palpation.
      1. Radial styloid process, EPL, EPB, APL, anatomical snuffbox (ulnar margin is EPL tendon and radial margin is composed of EPB and APL tendons).
      2. Scaphoid (ulnar deviation facilitates palpation) with volar tubercle adjacent to FCR tendon, trapezium, tubercle of radius (Lister's tubercle) on dorsal ulnar aspect of radius adjacent to EPL, lunate (flex wrist to facilitate palpation), capitate with a palpable, dorsal depression.
      3. ECRB and ECRL (clenched fist to facilitate palpation), EDC, EI, DRUJ/TFCC, ulnar styloid process, ECU (wrist extension and ulnar deviation to facilitate palpation).
      4. Triquetrum, pisiform (volar ulnar aspect of the hand), hook of the hamate (2-3 cm from the pisiform in a direct line between the pisiform and first web space).
      5. FCU (wrist flexion and ulnar deviation to facilitate palpation), ulnar artery and nerve (deep to FCU), PL (cupping hand facilitates palpation), FCR (wrist flexion and radial deviation to facilitate palpation).

6. Radial artery (radial to FCR tendon), median nerve (deep to FCR tendon).
7. Metacarpals easily palpable, II and III immobile, IV and V mobile.
8. Thenar eminence, hypothenar eminence.
9. MCP joints (MCP flexion facilitates bony palpation), phalanges, IP joints.

D. Special tests.
1. Strength: tendinitis reproduced by active contraction of affected muscle group.
2. Stability test: nerve blocks may be necessary to fully evaluate joint stability.
   a. DRUJ: passive volar and dorsal stress applied to joint.
   b. Watson's test: force applied on distal scaphoid during passive radial deviation may produce palpable and audible clunk.[25]
   c. MCP joints: valgus/varus force to flexed MCP will stress collateral ligaments, MCP hyperextension will stress volar plate.
   d. IP joints: valgus/varus force at various degrees of IP flexion will stress collateral ligaments, IP hyperextension will stress volar plate.
3. TFCC tear: passive wrist extension and ulnar deviation reproduces dorsal ulnar pain and click.
4. Tinel's sign: tapping area of nerve compression reproduces symptoms of carpal tunnel syndrome (median nerve) and Guyon's canal syndrome (ulnar nerve).
5. Phalen's test: passive wrist flexion compresses median nerve and reproduces symptoms of carpal tunnel syndrome.
6. Finkelstein's test: passive ulnar deviation of the wrist with the thumb flexed into the palm reproduces symptoms of inflammation of the first dorsal compartment.
7. Finger flexor tests.
   a. FDS: tendon function intact if patient is able to flex PIP while examiner passively extends other digits.
   b. FDP: tendon function intact if patient can actively flex DIP while examiner passively extends MP and PIP joints of digit being tested.
8. Sensation.
   a. Radial nerve: first dorsal web space; median nerve: volar aspect distal phalanx digit II; ulnar nerve: volar aspect distal phalanx digit V.
   b. C6: volar radial hand; C7: volar middle finger; C8: volar ulnar aspect of hand.

IV. Radiographic Investigations

A. Plain radiographs: posteroanterior (PA), lateral and oblique views of the wrists, hands, and digits.[16]

B. Special views.
1. Wrist: PA with clenched fist, PA with maximum ulnar and radial deviation, true lateral with maximum wrist flexion and extension, scaphoid, carpal tunnel, supination oblique, pisiform triquetral, and carpometacarpal; comparison films with the opposite wrist are often necessary.
2. MP/IP joints: PA with stress of collateral ligaments.

C. Fluoroscopy: dynamic examination to evaluate subtle instability patterns.

D. Triple phase bone scan.

E. Computerized tomography (CT) scan: evaluate carpal bones and DRUJ.
F. Arthrography: evaluation of suspected ligamentous injuries of the wrist.
G. Magnetic resonance imaging (MRI) scan: evaluation of bone, cartilage, extrinsic/intrinsic wrist ligaments, TFCC, and soft tissues about the MCP joints. Must have appropriate magnet, surface coils, software, and radiologist/technician interested in wrist and hand abnormalities; comparison MRI scan often necessary.[6]

V. Overuse Injuries
A. Repetitive microtrauma to a musculoskeletal structure, resulting in overload and breakdown. General treatment includes correction of the underlying etiology, relative rest, rehabilitation exercises, cryotherapy, nonsteroidal antiinflammatory drugs, corticosteroid injection, passive therapeutic modalities, bracing, casting, and, occasionally, surgical intervention.[11,15,19]
B. de Quervain's disease: stenosing tenosynovitis of first dorsal compartment of the wrist (APL and EPB) due to repeated, forceful grasping with ulnar deviation or repetitive use of thumb. Localized pain, swelling, crepitus, and tenderness with a positive Finkelstein's test. Most commonly affects golfers, fishermen, and racquet sports participants. Rule out thumb CMC arthritis, FCR tendinitis, intersection syndrome, scaphoid fracture.[11,15,19]
C. Intersection syndrome: inflammatory response located at the crossing point of the muscles of the first and third dorsal compartments. Tenderness, swelling, and crepitus of the dorsal aspect of the forearm 4-6 cm from radiocarpal joint. Due to repetitive wrist extension and radial deviation and/or thumb extension and abduction; most commonly affects weight lifters, rowers, and canoers.[11,19,26]
D. EPL tenosynovitis: inflammation of the EPL tendon as it passes around Lister's tubercle on the dorsal aspect of the radius. May occur in athletes engaged in repetitive thumb extension and wrist motion. Cortisone injections should be avoided. Surgical treatment includes decompression of the third dorsal compartment with translocation of the EPL tendon to the radial aspect of Lister's tubercle.[11,19,26]
E. EDC, EDM tenosynovitis: dorsal wrist pain, swelling, and tenderness, often history of trauma. Rule out TFCC tear, ECU subluxation, DRUJ instability.[11,19]
F. ECU tendinitis: pain, swelling, tenderness, and, occasionally, crepitus of the dorsal ulnar aspect of the wrist. Most common in sports requiring repetitive wrist motion or racquet sports requiring a snap of the wrist. May be related to underlying TFCC tear or previous traumatic rupture of ECU subsheath causing tendon subluxation. Rule out stress fracture and DRUJ instability.[11,15,19]
G. FCR tenosynovitis: occurs where FCR tendon angles over volar aspect of the scaphoid. Volar radial wrist pain at the base of the thenar eminence reproduced by wrist flexion, radial deviation, and pronation. Rule out scaphoid injury, thumb CMC arthritis, and volar ganglion.[11,19]
H. FCU tendinitis: volar ulnar wrist pain and swelling exacerbated by wrist flexion and ulnar deviation. Most common in golf and racquet sports. Rule out pisotriquetral arthritis; may require excision of the pisiform.[11]
I. TFCC tear: dorsal ulnar wrist pain and clicking increased with wrist extension and ulnar deviation. Caused by repetitive axial loading of the extended wrist, most commonly in gymnasts and weight lifters. Arthrogram or MRI to confirm diagnosis. Degenerative tear associated with

positive ulnar variance (ulnar longer than radius); may require surgical debridement and ulnar shortening.

J. Compressive neuropathies.[27,28]
   1. Median nerve.
      a. Pronator syndrome: compression of median nerve by Struthers' ligament, lacertus fibrosis, pronator teres, or proximal arch of FDS. Insidious onset of proximal volar forearm ache, occasional hand pain, and dysesthesias of the radial three and a half digits.
      b. Anterior interosseous syndrome: activity-related forearm myalgias, discoordination of thumb-index finger pinch, weakness of FDP of the second digit, FPL and pronator quadratus, normal sensation.
      c. Carpal tunnel syndrome: activity-related weakness and dysesthesias of the radial three and a half digits, night pain, and paresthesias. Low incidence in sports, most common in cyclists, throwers, and tennis players.
      d. Palmar cutaneous nerve: dysesthesias of the thenar eminence and proximal palm.
      e. Palmar digital nerve: traumatic neuroma of ulnar digital nerve to the thumb between the sesamoid bone and an external object; most common in bowler's (bowler's thumb) and racquet sports.
   2. Radial nerve.
      a. Posterior interosseous nerve syndrome: vague lateral elbow and forearm pain, weakness of wrist extension and ulnar deviation and MCP extension, normal sensation.
      b. Superficial radial nerve (Wartenberg's disease, cheiralgia paresthetica): dysesthesias of the dorsal radial hand, thumb, and index finger, normal strength; often due to nerve compression by tight wrist bands.
   3. Ulnar nerve: compression of ulnar nerve branches within Guyon's canal, most common in bicyclists due to compression by handlebars. Symptoms localized to ulnar one and a half digits and depend on branch involved: deep branch = motor; superficial branch = sensory; deep and superficial = motor and sensory.

VI. Traumatic Injuries
   A. Fracture: carpal bones.[4,15]
      1. Scaphoid fractures.[4,7,23,24,29]
         a. Most common carpal fracture, usually due to a fall on outstretched hand. Usually present with swelling, decreased wrist extension, and tenderness of the anatomical snuffbox. Radiographs often normal; triple phase bone scan or CT or MRI scan may be helpful in making the diagnosis; alternatively, may treat in thumb spica splint and repeat radiography in 10-21 days.
         b. Proximal third (20% of scaphoid fractures) prone to AVN. Nondisplaced: cast immobilization until healed; displaced: ORIF.
         c. Middle third (70% of scaphoid fractures). Nondisplaced: long arm followed by short arm thumb spica cast for 8-12 weeks until fracture is radiographically healed; displaced >1 mm: ORIF. Athlete may return to play in thumb spica splint; however, surgical fixation with Herbert compression screw may allow early return to participation if the athlete cannot play in a thumb spica splint.[23]
         d. Distal third (10% of scaphoid fractures). Minimally displaced: thumb spica cast for 6-8 weeks; significantly displaced: ORIF.

2. Hamate fractures.
   a. Fracture of the hook due to direct blow to the hyperthenar region or from impact of a racquet handle, golf club, or baseball bat. Localized swelling and tenderness in the area of the hamate. Carpal tunnel or supination oblique radiography, bone scan, CT scan may be necessary for diagnosis. Excision of fragment with return to participation 4-6 weeks versus cast immobilization 4-6 weeks.
   b. Fractures of the body uncommon. Nondisplaced: 6 weeks cast immobilization; displaced: ORIF.
3. Pisiform fractures: direct trauma to hypothenar eminence with local swelling and tenderness. Nondisplaced fractures: 4-6 weeks cast immobilization; displaced or nonunion: surgical excision.
4. Capitate, lunate, triquetrum, trapezium, trapezoid fractures: often difficult to diagnose, may require special radiographic investigations. Nondisplaced: cast immobilization; displaced fractures: ORIF; small, widely displaced fragments should be excised if symptomatic.

B. Fracture: metacarpal bones.[4,8,10,13,20]
1. Base.
   a. Most have minimal or no displacement due to stabilizing effect of intermetacarpal ligaments, intrinsic muscles, and fascia; 4-6 weeks cast/brace with wrist in extension, MCPs in flexion, IPs free.
   b. Metacarpal I.
      (1) Bennett's fracture: fracture/subluxation of the trapezium–first metacarpal joint due to axial blow or adduction stress to the thumb. Surgical fixation usually required due to instability (APL insertion at the base of the metacarpal I causes proximal displacement of metacarpal shaft).
      (2) Rolando's fracture: comminuted articular fracture treated with thumb spica cast for 7 to 10 days; surgical fixation if large, displaced fragments.
   c. Metacarpal V: reverse or "baby" Bennett's fracture due to axial load of fifth digit; fracture fragment held to fourth metacarpal and hamate by intrinsic ligaments; shaft of metacarpal V angulates dorsally; surgical stabilization is required.
2. Shaft: due to direct trauma, axial loading or torsional stress applied to digits, border digits (second and fifth) most commonly affected.
   a. Stable: no rotatory displacement, <2-3 mm of shortening, and satisfactory alignment (less than 20 degrees of dorsal angulation metacarpal II and III, 45 degrees of dorsal angulation metacarpal IV and V); 4-6 weeks short arm cast with return to play in protective orthoses. If athlete cannot play in protective orthoses, surgical fixation will allow earlier return to participation.
   b. Unstable: rotational abnormality, >3 mm of shortening, or unacceptable dorsal angulation; surgical stabilization, early motion, return to play in protective orthoses.
3. Neck: usually due to axial load.
   a. Metacarpal II and III: cast immobilization for 4-6 weeks, may play in protective orthoses; surgical fixation if rotational abnormality or >15 degrees of angulation.
   b. Metacarpal IV and V: cast immobilization for 4-6 weeks, may play in protective orthoses; surgical fixation if significant comminution, extensor lag, unacceptable reduction or malalignment (greater than 40 degrees of angulation) or if unable to participate in orthoses.

C. Fractures: phalangeal.[4,8,10,13,20]
   1. Due to direct impact or torsional stress; swelling, deformity, and tenderness; must assess for rotational malalignment.
   2. Stable: nondisplaced fracture that does not displace under stress; treat with hand-based digital splint for 1-2 weeks, buddy taping for participation, early motion exercises.
   3. Unstable: if displacement or rotational deformity is present or if the fracture displaces under stress, surgical stabilization, splinting, early motion exercises, and return to participation in protective brace.
   4. Articular fracture: if small, nondisplaced and stable, splint for 2-3 weeks with protective bracing for competition. If displacement, rotational deformity, 30% to 40% of joint surface involved, or if the fracture displaces under stress, surgical stabilization, splinting, early motion exercises, and return to participation in protective brace.

D. Sprains, strains, dislocations.
   1. Scapholunate dissociation: volar rotation of scaphoid and dorsal rotation of lunate due to tear of the volar radioscapholunate ligament, usually from a fall on outstretched hand or from a scaphoid nonunion. Pain, swelling, loss of motion, tenderness in the area of the radioscapholunate articulations, positive Watson's test. PA radiography reveals space between scaphoid and lunate >3 mm or two times that of other carpal bones. Lateral radiography reveals scapholunate angle >70 degrees (DISI); normal angle is 30 to 60 degrees. Acute: soft tissue repair and surgical fixation; chronic instability: scapho-trapezio-trapezoidal (S-T-T) fusion.[3,15,16,25]
   2. Ulnar instability: dynamic instability presenting with activity-related pain and clicking at the ulnar aspect of the wrist.[3,15,16]
      a. Triquetrolunate instability: volar rotation of the lunate due to disruption of the triquetrolunate ligament; scapholunate angle less than 30 degrees (PISI), usually requires fluoroscopy to detect. Acute: surgical repair; chronic: lunate triquetral arthrodesis.
      b. Midcarpal instability: capitotriquetroligament elongation or rupture, which causes a dynamic instability pattern; fluoroscopy necessary for diagnosis. Treatment of recalcitrant, chronic instability requires hamate-triquetral arthrodesis.
   3. TFCC tear: traumatic injury as a result of hyperpronation of the forearm with axial loading. Tenderness of the DRUJ and dorsal ulnar wrist pain, which increases at the extremes of wrist extension, pronation and supination, with radiolunar compression, and with dorsal-volar translation of the ulna. Radiography may reveal positive ulnar variance; arthrogram and MRI scan may confirm diagnosis. If relative rest, splinting, and rehabilitation fail to control symptoms, surgical intervention is necessary.[2,5,14,15]
   4. ECU subluxation: rupture of fibroosseous tunnel housing the ECU tendon, usually due to sudden forearm supination with wrist ulnar deviation and volar flexion. Most common in racquet sports, golfers, weight lifters, and bareback riders. In chronic cases, pain is reproduced with ulnar deviation and supination and a palpable subluxing tendon may be present. Acute treatment requires 4-6 weeks of casting with the forearm pronated and wrist extended; surgical reconstruction may be necessary.[15,19,22]
   5. MCP dislocation: forced digit hyperextension causes volar plate avulsion and tearing of collateral ligaments. Most commonly af-

fects the first, second, and fifth digits. Reduce and if stable, immobilize with MCP and IP joints flexed for 3-6 weeks; may return to participation in protective splint. Surgical intervention required for complex, irreducible dislocations.[10,13,21]

6. MCP collateral ligament sprain: due to radial or ulnar deviation stress to a flexed MCP joint; an avulsion fracture may be present. Symptoms include pain, swelling, loss of MCP motion, and point tenderness over the radial or ulnar aspect of the joint, which is increased with radial or ulnar deviation. Radial and ulnar stability must be tested with MCP flexed. Immobilize with 30 degrees of MCP flexion for 3-6 weeks; may participate in protective splint. Fracture involving >20% of the articular surface or with >2 mm displacement requires surgical fixation.[10,21,22]
7. Thumb UCL sprain (skier's thumb): due to abduction stress. Instability with MCP flexion is due to damage to UCL proper; instability at 0 degrees MCP flexion is due to damage to accessory UCL. Treat with thumb spica immobilization for 3-6 weeks; return to participation in protective brace.
   a. Nondisplaced avulsion fracture: immobilize.
   b. Avulsion fracture with >1 mm displacement: surgical stabilization.
   c. Third degree sprain without fracture: immediate or delayed surgical repair may be necessary due to Stener lesion (adductor aponeurosis interposed between torn ends of UCL), which prevents ligament healing.[21]
8. PIP dislocation.[10,12,13,21]
   a. Dorsal: axial load or extension stress to middle phalanx causes disruption of volar plate and tearing of accessory collateral ligaments. Easily reduced by correction of lateral component (if present), axial traction and flexion. Determine radial/ulnar and volar/dorsal stability. Radiograph to rule out fracture. Splint for 1-2 weeks with PIP in 30 degrees of flexion; return to participation in protective brace.
   b. Volar: rare, due to disruption of collateral ligament and central extensor tendon slip. Splint for 3-6 weeks with PIP in extension; return to participation in protective brace. May lead to boutonniére deformity if misdiagnosed and treated as a dorsal dislocation.
9. Boutonniére deformity: rupture of central slip of the extensor tendon over the PIP joint with gradual migration of the lateral bands to the volar aspect of the PIP. Mechanism is forced flexion of actively extended PIP (jammed finger), direct trauma over dorsum of PIP, or volar PIP dislocation. Symptoms include pain, swelling, tenderness over dorsum of PIP, loss of PIP motion, and an extensor lag. Splint with PIP in full extension for 6-8 weeks; may return to participation in protective bracing. If untreated, will lead to flexion contracture of PIP and extension contracture of DIP.[10,12,13,19,21,22]
10. Pseudo-boutonniére deformity: slowly progressive flexion contracture of PIP with unfixed hyperextension of DIP due to calcification and scarring from previous volar plate injury. Treat with extension splint of the PIP; surgical release if flexion contracture >40 degrees.[10,12,13,21,22]
11. Mallet finger: disruption of terminal extensor tendon at its insertion on distal phalanx; the extensor tendon may be stretched or

ruptured or associated with a fracture or a slipped epiphysis. Mechanism is axial load of the fingertip resulting in forced flexion while digit is being actively extended. Symptoms include localized swelling and tenderness and inability to actively extend DIP. Splint with DIP in full extension for 6-8 weeks. Persistent volar subluxation of the distal phalanx or fractures involving greater than 30% of the articular surface may require surgical intervention. May return to participation with protective splinting.[4,12,13,19,21,22]

12. FDP avulsion (Jersey finger): rupture of FDP tendon due to forceful extension of DIP while FDP is actively contracting; most commonly affects fourth digit. Symptoms include pain, swelling, and inability to actively flex PIP joint. Requires surgical repair; may return to participation in boxer-type playing cast if grasping is not essential in sport; maximum gripping activity is delayed until 10-12 weeks postoperatively.[12,13,19,22]
    a. Type I: retraction of tendon into palm—painful, tender, palmar mass, repair within 7-10 days.
    b. Type II: retraction of tendon to PIP joint—repair within 1-3 months.
    c. Type III: avulsion of volar plate with minimal displacement, tendon usually remains attached to the fragment—repair within 3 months.

References

1. Anderson JE: *Grant's Atlas of Anatomy,* ed 9. Baltimore, 1991, Williams & Wilkins.
2. Chidgey LK: TFCC— anatomy and diagnosis. American Society for Surgery of the Hand 1993 Specialty Day, "Injuries of the Wrist—An Update" at the American Academy of Orthopaedic Surgeons 1993 Annual Meeting, San Francisco, Feb 21, 1993.
3. Culver JE: Instabilities of the wrist, *Clin Sports Med* 5(4):725-740, 1986.
4. Culver JE, Anderson TE: Fractures of the hand and wrist in the athlete, *Clin Sports Med* 11(1):101-128, 1992.
5. Dell PC: Traumatic disorders of distal radioulnar joint, *Clin Sports Med* 11(1):141-159, 1992.
6. Fritz RC, Brody GA: MR imaging of the wrist and elbow, *Clin Sports Med* 14(2):315-352, 1994.
7. Gelberman RH: Fractures of the carpal scaphoid—an overview. American Society for Surgery of the Hand 1993 Specialty Day, "Injuries of the Wrist—An Update" at the American Academy of Orthopaedic Surgeons 1993 Annual Meeting, San Francisco, Feb 21, 1993.
8. Hastings H: Management of extra-articular fractures of the phalanges and metacarpals. In Strickland JW, Rettig AC, editors: *Hand Injuries in Athletes,* Philadelphia, 1992, WB Saunders.
9. Hoppenfeld S: *Physical Examination of the Spine and Extremities,* Norwalk, CT, 1976, Appleton-Century-Crofts.
10. Kahler DM, McCue FC: Metacarpalphalangeal and proximal interphalangeal joint injuries of the hand, including the thumb, *Clin Sports Med* 11(1):57-76, 1992.
11. Kiefhaber TR, Stern PJ: Upper extremity tendinitis and overuse syndromes in the athlete, *Clin Sports Med* 11(1):39-56, 1992.
12. Loeb PE et al: The hand: field evaluation and treatment, *Clin Sports Med* 11(1):27-37, 1992.
13. McCue FC, Cabrera JM: Common athletic digital joint injuries of the hand. In Strickland JW, Rettig AC, editors: *Hand Injuries in Athletes,* Philadelphia, 1992, WB Saunders, pp 49-94.
14. Melone CP: Distal radioulnar joint (DRUJ) instability: soft tissue stabilization. American Society for Surgery of the Hand 1993 Specialty Day, "Injuries of the Wrist—An Update" at the American Academy of Orthopaedic Surgeons 1993 Annual Meeting, San Francisco, Feb 21, 1993.
15. Mirabello SC et al: The wrist: field evaluation and treatment, *Clin Sports Med* 11(1):1-25, 1992.
16. Mooney JF, Siegel DB, Koman LA: Ligamentous injuries of the wrist in athletes, *Clin Sports Med* 11(1):129-140, 1992.
17. Palmer AK, Werner FW: Biomechanics of the distal radial ulnar joint, *Clin Orthop* 187:26-35, 1984.
18. Pansky B: *Review of Gross Anatomy,* ed 5, New York, 1984, Macmillan Publishing.
19. Pyne JI, Adams BD: Hand tendon injuries in athletics, *Clin Sports Med* 11(4):833-850, 1992.
20. Rettig AC: Hand injuries in football players. Getting a grip on fractures, *Physician Sportsmed* 19(11):55-64, 1991.

21. Rettig AC: Hand injuries in football players. Soft tissue trauma, *Physician Sportsmed* 19(12):97-107, 1991.
22. Rettig AC: Closed tendon injuries of the hand and wrist in the athlete, *Clin Sports Med* 11(1):77-99, 1992.
23. Rettig AC, Weidenbener EJ, Gloieske R: Alternative management of mid-third scaphoid fractures in the athlete, *Am J Sports Med* 22(5):711-714, 1994.
24. Sypher RV: Indications for ORIF in acute scaphoid fractures. American Society for Surgery of the Hand 1993 Specialty Day, "Injuries of the Wrist—An Update" at the American Academy of Orthopaedic Surgeons 1993 Annual Meeting, San Francisco, Feb 21, 1993.
25. Watson HK, Hempton RF: Limited wrist arthrodesis: the triscaphoid joint, *J Hand Surg* 5:320-327, 1980.
26. Weiker GG: Hand and wrist problems in the gymnast, *Clin Sports Med* 11(1):189-202, 1992.
27. Weinstein SM, Herring SA: Nerve problems and compartment syndromes in the hand, wrist and forearm, *Clin Sports Med* 11(1):161-189, 1992.
28. Whitaker JH, Richardson GA: Compressive neuropathies. In Strickland JW, Rettig AC, editors: *Hand Injuries in Athletes,* Philadelphia, 1992, WB Saunders, pp 209-229.
29. Zemel MP: Carpal fractures. In Strickland JW, Rettig AC, editors: *Hand Injuries in Athletes,* Philadelphia, 1992, WB Saunders, pp 155-173.

CHAPTER 43

Diagnosis and Management of Concussion

Robert Cantu, MD

I. General Overview
   A. Brain injury of singular importance as no regeneration of lost cells.
   B. Concussion is most common brain injury and risk is high in these sports (see box on p. 346).
      1. After initial concussion, chance of recurrence may be increased fourfold.[3]
      2. Severity and duration of functional impairment may be greater with repeated concussions.[4-8,12,17]

II. Definitions of Concussion (no consensus definition)
   A. "A clinical syndrome characterized by immediate and transient posttraumatic impairment of neural function, such as alteration of consciousness, disturbance of vision, equilibrium, etc."[2]
   B. Classification of concussion:
      1. According to duration of posttraumatic amnesia.[9]
      2. According to duration of unconsciousness.[11]
      3. According to both duration of posttraumatic amnesia and duration of unconsciousness[1] (see Tables 43-1[1] and 43-2[10]).

III. Treatment of First Concussion
   A. Grade 1 (mild).
      1. Remove from contest.
      2. If athlete does not have retrograde amnesia and neurological examination at rest and exertion are normal, may consider return to contest after 30 minutes.
   B. Grade 2 (moderate).
      1. Remove from contest.
      2. Send to hospital for neurological evaluation.
      3. May return after asymptomatic for 1 week at rest and exertion.
   C. Grade 3 (severe).
      1. Remove from contest on fracture board with head immobilized if unconscious.

SPORTS ASSOCIATED WITH HIGH RISK OF CONCUSSION

1. Auto racing
2. Boxing
3. Equestrian sports
4. Football
5. Ice hockey
6. Lacrosse
7. Martial arts
8. Motorcycle racing
9. Rugby
10. Skating/Rollerblading
11. Skiing
12. Soccer (goalie)
13. Pole vaulting

2. Send to hospital for neurological evaluation.
3. May return after 1 month if asymptomatic for at least 1 week at rest and exertion.

IV. Treatment of Second Concussion of Season
- A. Grade 1 (mild).
  1. Remove from contest.
  2. May return to play after 2 weeks if asymptomatic for 1 week at rest and exertion.
- B. Grade 2 (moderate).
  1. Remove from contest.
  2. Send to hospital for neurological evaluation.
  3. May return after 1 month if asymptomatic at rest and exertion. Consider terminating the season.
- C. Grade 3 (severe).
  1. Remove from contest on fracture board with head immobilized if unconscious.
  2. Send to hospital for neurological evaluation.
  3. Terminate season; may return to play next season if asymptomatic and diagnostic studies show no evidence of injury.

V. Treatment of Third Concussion of Season
- A. Grade 1 (mild).
  1. Remove from contest.
  2. Terminate season; may return next season if asymptomatic and diagnostic studies show no sign of injury.
- B. Grade 2 (moderate).
  1. Remove from contest.
  2. Send to hospital for neurological evaluation.
  3. Terminate season; may return next season if asymptomatic and diagnostic studies show no sign of injury.

TABLE 43-1. Severity of Concussion

Grade	Duration of Consciousness/Amnesia
Grade 1 (mild)	No loss of consciousness, posttraumatic amnesia <30 minutes
Grade 2 (moderate)	Loss of consciousness <5 minutes or posttraumatic amnesia between 30 minutes and 24 hours
Grade 3 (severe)	Loss of consciousness >5 minutes or posttraumatic amnesia >24 hours

TABLE 43-2. Severity of Concussion (Colorado Medical Society)

Grade	Consciousness/Amnesia Effects
Grade 1	Confusion without amnesia, no loss of consciousness
Grade 2	Confusion with amnesia, no loss of consciousness
Grade 3	Loss of consciousness

VI. Postconcussion Syndrome
- A. Incidence.
  1. True incidence is not known.
- B. Symptoms.
  1. Headache, especially upon exertion.
  2. Fatigue, irritability.
  3. Labyrinthine disturbance.
  4. Impaired memory and concentration.
- C. Neurological signs: usually none.
- D. Correlations: usually correlates well with duration of posttraumatic amnesia.
- E. Evaluation.
  1. Magnetic resonance imaging or computerized tomography of head.
  2. Neuropsychological testing.
  3. Electroencephalography.
- F. Return to competition: must be deferred until all symptoms have abated and diagnostic studies show no sign of injury; otherwise, there is a risk of second impact syndrome.

References

1. Cantu RC: Guidelines for return to contact sports after a cerebral concussion, *Phys Sportsmed* 14(10):75-83, 1986.
2. Committee on Head Injury Nomenclature of the Congress of Neurological Surgeons: Glossary of head injury including some definitions of injury to the cervical spine, *Clin Neurosurg* 12:386, 1966.
3. Gerberich SG et al: Concussion incidences and severity in secondary school varsity football players, *Am J Public Health* 73:1370-1375, Dec 1983.
4. Gronwall D, Wrightson P: Delayed recovery of intellectual function after minor head injury, *Lancet* 2:605-609, Sept 14, 1974.
5. Gronwall D, Wrightson P: Cumulative effect of concussion, *Lancet* 2:995-997, Nov 22, 1975.
6. Gronwall D: Paced auditory serial addition task: a measure of recovery from concussion, *Perpetual and Motor Skills* 4:367-373, 1977.
7. Gronwall D, Wrightson P: Duration of post-traumatic amnesia after mild head injury, *J Clin Neuropsychology* 2:51-60, 1985.
8. Gronwall D, Wrightson P: Memory and information processing capacity closed head injury, *J Neurol Neurosurg Psychiatry* 44:889-895, 1981.
9. Jennet B: Late effects of head injuries. In Critchley M, O'Leary JL, Jennet B, editors: *Scientific Foundations of Neurology*, Philadelphia, 1971, FA Davis, p 441.
10. Kelley JP et al. Concussion in sports: guidelines for the prevention of catastrophic outcome, *JAMA* 266(20):2867-2869, 1991.
11. Maroon JC, Steele PB, Berlin R: Football head and neck injuries: an update, *Clin Neurosurg* 27:414, 1980.
12. Symonds C: Concussion and its sequelae, *Lancet* 1:1-5, Jan 6, 1962.

CHAPTER **44**

Field Management of Head Injuries and Return to Play

Roger L. McCoy II, MD

I. General Overview
   A. Epidemiology.[4]
      1. Estimates are that one in every five high school football players sustains a concussion each season.
      2. Possibly 250,000 concussions per year in high school football alone.
      3. An athlete who has sustained one minor head injury has a fourfold increased risk of having another concussive injury.
   B. Types of head injury.
      1. Scalp/facial trauma.
      2. Skull fractures.
      3. Cerebral concussion.
      4. Cerebral contusion.
      5. Intracranial hemorrhage.
         a. Epidural hemorrhage.
         b. Subdural hemorrhage.
         c. Subarachnoid hemorrhage.
         d. Intracerebral hemorrhage.
      6. Dementia pugilistica.
   C. Mechanisms of head injury.[2]
      1. Blunt trauma can result in injury at the impact site (coup) or at the opposite side of the impact site (contra-coup).
      2. Penetrating objects can also cause severe injury.
      3. Main stress forces generated by trauma include compressive, tensile (negative pressure), and shearing (force applied parallel to a surface).

II. Field Management of Concussion[3,7]
   A. Recognition.
      1. Physician should be active on the sideline, constantly observing players during their activity, as they come on and off the field, and when they are on the sidelines.

2. Any loss of consciousness should be treated as if neck/cervical spine injury is associated, and the athlete should be properly boarded and transferred to the nearest facility.
3. Once an altered state of consciousness has been discovered in an athlete (including the athlete who's been "dinged" or had their "bell rung"), it is wise to keep that athlete nearby; remove the helmet to prevent him or her from returning to play without proper medical release.
4. Symptoms may include headache, dizziness, nausea, unsteadiness, photophobia, blurred or double vision, emotional lability, or mental status changes.
5. Inform the trainer and/or head coach that this athlete has been designated as sustaining a possible concussion and will be out of play for further evaluation on the sideline.
6. Be aware of "the look," as some athletes experience a glazed starry-eyed look after sustaining a mild head injury.

B. Orientation evaluation.
1. Asking the athlete the time, place, person, and situation and circumstances of the injury are fairly easy questions to start out with. Other questions may include: What is your name? What is your date of birth? How old are you? What month, day, or week of the year is it? What is the exact date and what time of day is it?
2. Also, if appropriate, you may ask questions surrounding stadium or athletic location.
3. Ask questions with answers known to you and familiar to the athlete.

C. Memory evaluation.
1. Memory questions may include names of teams and prior contest, present governor or mayor.
2. Recent newsworthy events and details possibly of the contest that are going on as far as players, moves, strategies.
3. Three words and/or three objects at the initial time of questions and at 5 minutes post-initial start of all of the questions.
4. May ask pertinent questions as far as timing of the event, which teams were played the previous week, did our team win last week, which team scored the last points.

D. Concentration evaluation.
1. May do a set of digits and ask the athlete to repeat number of digits backwards, such as 3-1-7, 4-6-8-2, 5-9-3-7-4. Also may ask months of the year in reverse order.
2. May also ask patient to do serial 3s or count back from 100 using 7s or 3s.

E. Cerebellar evaluation.
1. First check cranial nerves II-XII, making sure pupils are symmetrical and reactive.
2. Check for coordination utilizing the athlete's finger to his nose to the examiner's finger random movements and tandem movements using alternating forearm pronation/supination compared to the examiner's similar control movements. Also can check heel-to-toe walking in a straight line with athlete's eyes open and then closed.
3. Checking balance. May also utilize finger-to-nose techniques with the athlete's head tilted back, arms abducted, and heels together (drunk driver's test). Start with Romberg's test with the athlete's eyes open and then closed.

F. Exertional clearance.
   1. After conducting the above tests, it is appropriate to put the patient through some exertional tests for checking reproduction of any symptoms.
   2. Tests may include a 40-yard sprint with five push-ups, five sit-ups, and five knee bends.
   3. Any appearance of headache, dizziness, nausea, unsteadiness, photophobia, blurred or double vision, or any change in emotional lability and mental status with these exercises or continuation/worsening of headache with these exercises should preclude the athlete from play at this time for further evaluation.

III. Return to Competition[3] (See also Table 44-1)
   A. Grade I (mild).
      1. Signs and symptoms include confusion without amnesia and no loss of consciousness.
      2. Remove from contest. Examine immediately and every 5 minutes for the development of amnesia or postconcussive symptoms at rest and with exertion.
      3. Permit return to contest if amnesia does not appear and if no symptoms appear for at least 20 minutes.
   B. Grade II (moderate).
      1. Confusion with amnesia; no loss of consciousness.
      2. Amnesia includes posttraumatic amnesia of events after the impact and the more severe retrograde amnesia of events preceding the impact.
      3. Some clinicians may include brief loss of consciousness in grade II and reserve any prolonged loss of consciousness for grade III; however, brief and prolonged are not well defined at this time.
      4. Remove from contest and disallow return. Examine frequently for signs of evolving intracranial pathology.
      5. Reexamine the next day. Permit return to practice after 1 full week without symptoms.
   C. Grade III (severe).
      1. Includes any loss of consciousness; for most people this includes any brief or prolonged loss.
      2. Transport from field to nearest hospital by ambulance (with cervical spine immobilization if indicated).
      3. Perform thorough neurological evaluation emergently. Admit to hospital if signs of pathology are detected.
      4. If findings are normal, instruct family about overnight observation. Permit return to practice only after 2 full weeks without symptoms.
      5. Prolonged unconsciousness, persistent mental status alterations, worsening postconcussion symptoms, or abnormalities on neurological examination require urgent neurosurgical consultation or transfer to a trauma center.
   D. Second impact syndrome.[5]
      1. Considered aberrant of malignant brain edema syndrome, first described in 1973 and again in 1984 and 1991 as case presentations.
      2. Seen in players not fully recovered from previous head injury.
      3. Considered a variant of malignant brain edema syndrome, first described in 1973,[5] and again in 1984[5] and 1991[8] as case presentations.
      4. Believed due to loss of vascular autoregulation, resulting in vascular engorgement, swelling, herniation, and possibly death.

TABLE 44-1. Grading Concussions in Sports and Guidelines for Return to Play*

Grading		Guidelines		
Severity	**Signs/Symptoms**	**First Concussion**	**Second Concussion**	**Third Concussion**
Grade I (mild)	Confusion without amnesia; no loss of consciousness	May return to play if asymptomatic† at least 20 minutes	Terminate contest/practice; may return to play if asymptomatic† for at least 1 week	Terminate season; may return to play in3 months if asymptomatic†
Grade II (moderate)	Confusion with amnesia‡; no loss of consciousness¶	Terminate contest/practice; may return to play if asymptomatic† for at least 1 week	Consider terminating season, but may return to play if asymptomatic† for 1 month	Terminate season; may return to play next season if asymptomatic†
Grade III (severe)	Loss of consciousness¶	Terminate contest/practice and transport to hospital; may return to play 1 month after 2 consecutive asymptomatic† weeks; conditioning allowed after 1 asymptomatic† week	Terminate season; may return to play next season if asymptomatic†	Terminate season; strongly discourage return to contact/collision sports

Courtesy of Preparticipation Physical Evaluation (monograph). Kansas City, MO, 1992, American Academy of Family Physicians, American Academy of Pediatrics, American Medical Society for Sports Medicine, American Orthopaedic Society for Sports Medicine, American Osteopathic Academy of Sports Medicine.

*These guidelines are not absolute and therefore should not substitute for the clinical judgment of the examining physician.

†No headache, confusion, dizziness, impaired orientation, impaired concentration or memory dysfunction during rest or exertion. (Adapted from Colorado Medical Society: *Report of the Sports Medicine Committee: Guidelines for the Management of Concussion in Sports* [revised]. Denver, 1991, Colorado Medical Society.)

‡Posttraumatic amnesia (amnesia for events following the impact) or more severe retrograde amnesia (amnesia for events preceding the impact).

¶ Some clinicians include "brief" loss of consciousness in Grade II and reserve "prolonged" loss of consciousness for Grade III. However, the definitions of "brief" and "prolonged" are not universally accepted.

E. Postconcussion syndrome.
   1. May follow any concussion and last up to 6 months or longer.
   2. Symptoms include headache (particularly with exertion), dizziness, fatigue, irritability, and impaired memory and concentration.
   3. Symptoms usually resolve spontaneously with time in the majority of patients. Neuropsychological testing has shown rapid recovery curves in 10-15 days in college football athletes.[1]
   4. Athletes should not return to competition until all postconcussion symptoms have resolved.

IV. Indications for Emergency Evaluation
   A. Symptoms.
      1. Nausea and vomiting.
      2. Headache.
      3. Dizziness.
   B. Signs.
      1. Impairment of consciousness (or changes in mental status or behavior, increasing or continued).
      2. Motor activity decreased, unequal or pathological posturing.
      3. Vital signs (changes in ventilation pattern, increasing blood pressure, or decreasing pulse rate).
      4. Seizures.
      5. Pupillary inequality.
   C. Radiological evaluation.
      1. Computerized tomography (CT) scan still indicated for initial evaluation to rule out any acute cerebral hemorrhage.
      2. Magnetic resonance imaging (MRI) gaining favor to help show minor cerebral changes that correlate with postconcussion syndrome. These changes also correlate inversely with neuropsychological testing (i.e., as changes resolve, neuropsychological testing improves).[6]
      3. Skull radiography not always indicated as information may be obtained through the CT scan utilizing bony windows if concern with a particular incident exists.

V. Emergency Treatment
   A. Emergency preparedness.
      1. In contact sports where risks for concussion are possible, the need for an emergency access plan exists.
      2. Emergency medical technicians with ambulance transport should be available in case of emergencies.
   B. Management in a collapsed athlete.
      1. Suspect possible second impact syndrome in unconscious patient and protect the cervical spine.
      2. ABCs of cardiopulmonary resuscitation.
      3. Hyperventilation.
      4. Transport to a medical facility.
      5. Intravenous osmotic diuretic.
      6. CT or MRI for scanning purposes.
      7. Intravenous steroids to reduce intracranial swelling.

References

1. Barth JT et al: Mild head injury in sports: neuropsychological sequelae and recovery of function. In Levin HS, Eisenberg HM, Benton AL, editors: *With Mild Head Injury,* New York, 1989, Oxford, pp 257-275.
2. Cantu RC: Cerebral concussion in sport management and prevention, *Sports Med* 14(1):64-74, 1992.

3. Colorado Medical Society Report of the Sports Medicine Committee: *Guidelines for the Management of Concussion in Sports* (revised), Denver, 1991, Colorado Medical Society.
4. Gerberich SG et al: Concussion incidences and severity in secondary school varsity football players, *Am J Public Health* 73:1370-1375, 1983.
5. LeBlanc KE: Concussions in sports: guidelines for return to competition, *Am Fam Phys* 50(4):801-806, 1994.
6. Levin HS et al: Magnetic resonance imaging and computerized tomography in relation to the neurobehavioral sequelae of mild and moderate head injuries, *J Neurosurg* 66:706-713, 1987.
7. Maddocks DL, Dicker GD, Saling MM: The assessment of orientation following concussion in athletes, *Clin J Sports Med* 5:32-35, 1995.
8. Kelly JP et al: Concussion in sports: guidelines for the prevention of catastrophic outcome, *JAMA* 226(20):2867-2869, 1991.

CHAPTER 45

Anatomy and Biomechanics of the Cervical Spine

Evan S. Bass, MD

I. Anatomy of the Cervical Spine
   A. Bony vertebrae: total of seven (labeled C1 to C7); three have unique features (C1, C2, C7).
      1. General structure of vertebrae (Figure 45-1). The heavy, cylindrical body is the most anterior bony structure and is designed to support weight. Each vertebral body is separated superiorly and inferiorly from the others by an intervertebral disk that assists in bonding the vertebrae to each other as well as in compressing and absorbing shock during weight bearing or axial load. The intervertebral disks also provide rotational and bending flexibility between the bodies of adjoining vertebrae. The vertebral arch is the posteriorly directed bony semicircle that extends from the body of each vertebra to create the large vertebral foramen, through which the spinal cord passes. The arch provides osseous protection for the spinal cord. The transverse processes extend bilaterally, and the spinous process extends posteriorly from the vertebral arch; each serves as a muscular and ligamentous attachment site. Four articular processes (two inferior and two superior) extend from the posterior arch to synovial facet connections with adjacent vertebrae.
      2. Features differentiating cervical vertebrae from thoracic and lumbar vertebrae. The vertebral bodies are thinner in the cervical area and increase in thickness inferiorly down the spine (because of an increasing weight-bearing load). The spinous processes of C3 through C6 are structurally shorter and bifid. Only cervical vertebrae have a foramen transversarium bilaterally in each transverse process, through which the vertebral arteries pass.
      3. Special vertebrae of the cervical spine (C1, C2, and C7).
         a. First cervical vertebra (C1): the atlas. This ring-shaped vertebra has no spinous process and no body. The atlas articulates superiorly and bilaterally with the occipital condyles to form the atlantooccipital

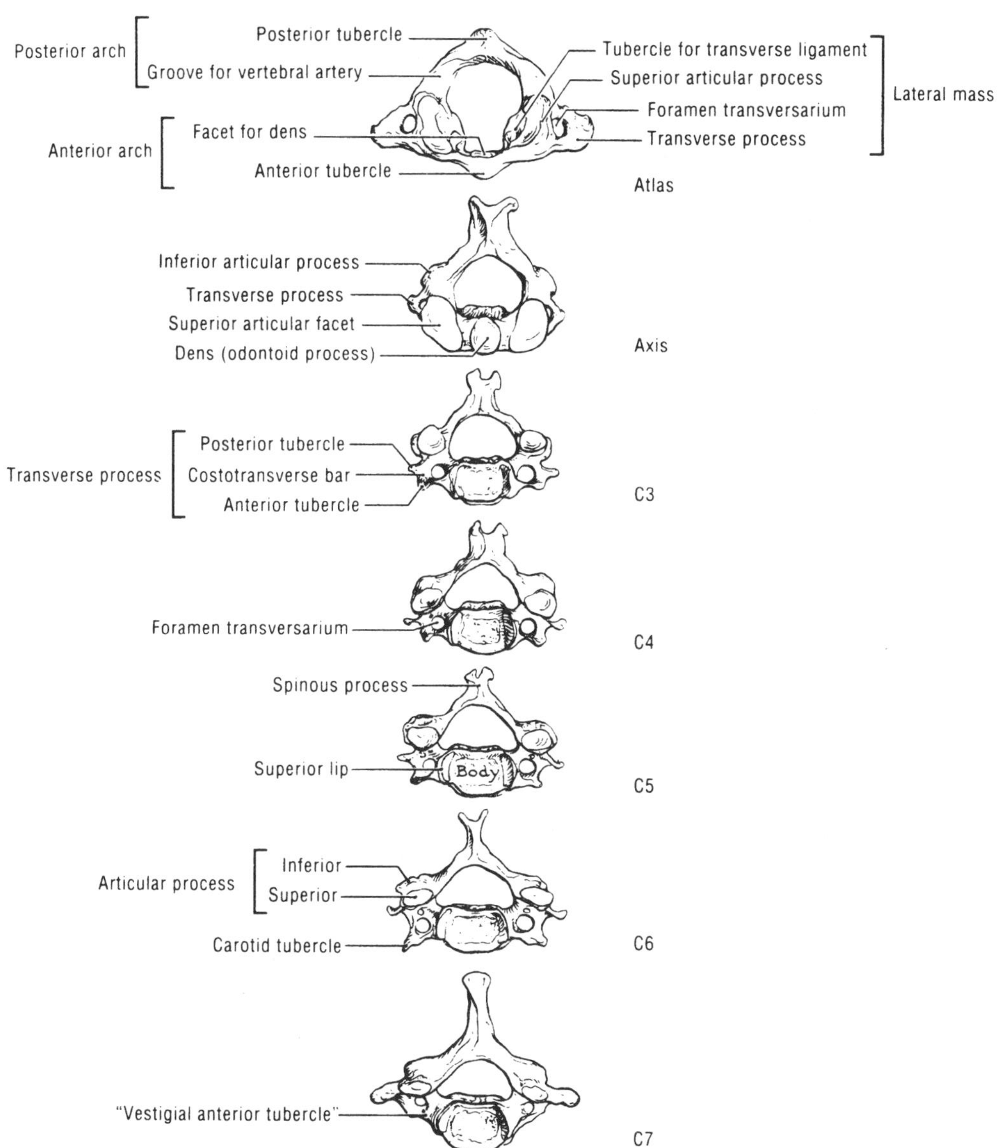

FIGURE 45-1
Drawings of superior aspects of cervical vertebrae. Note that transversaria in C7 are smaller than those of other cervical vertebrae and occasionally are absent. Observe that seventh cervical vertebra has a long spinous process and large transverse processes. C7 is the vertebra prominens. (Reproduced by permission of the author and publisher from Moore KL: *Clinically Oriented Anatomy,* ed. 3, Baltimore, 1992, Williams & Wilkins, p 333.)

joints. Inferiorly, the atlas articulates with the vertebra below it to form the complex atlantoaxial joint (described later in this chapter). Two bony extensions inside the ring structure are the attachment sites of the transverse ligament.

b. Second cervical vertebra (C2): the axis. The axis is the strongest cervical vertebra and has a large bifid spinous process. The axis is easily distinguished from other vertebrae by the presence of the odontoid process or dens, which is a toothlike projection extending upward from the body of the vertebra. The dens projects into the anterior vertebral foramen of C1, where it is held in place by the transverse ligament.

c. Seventh cervical vertebra (C7): the vertebra prominens. C7 is so named because of its large spinous process, which is prominent and palpable through the skin. Large transverse processes coupled with the spinous process make C7 easily distinguishable on radiographs.

B. The articulations of the cervical spine.
   1. Atlantooccipital joints. Bilateral synovial facet joints connect the occipital condyles to the vertebral arch of the atlas.
   2. Atlantoaxial joints. Two lateral synovial facet joints and one synovial rotational joint between the dens of the axis and the anterior tubercle of the atlas.
   3. Intervertebral joints (C2-C7). Each joint has two synovial facet joints connecting the vertebral arches of adjacent vertebrae and one fibrocartilaginous connection between the vertebral bodies (see intervertebral disks).

C. Ligaments and intervertebral disks of the cervical spine.
   1. Structures that support the lower cervical vertebrae (C2-C7).
      a. Intervertebral disks. Each disk is a strong fibrous ring (annulus fibrosis) that encapsulates gelatinous material (nucleus pulposus). The annulus fibrosis provides a strong interconnection between adjacent vertebral bodies, and the nucleus pulposus absorbs axial forces and allows intervertebral flexion, extension, and lateral bending.
      b. Anterior longitudinal ligament. This ligament is attached anteriorly to all vertebral bodies continuously to prevent hyperextension of the neck. Severe hyperextension (from a strong tackle or collision from the rear) can tear this ligament (whiplash injury).
      c. Posterior longitudinal ligaments. These ligaments are attached posteriorly to borders of the intervertebral disks in the vertebral canal to prevent hyperflexion of the neck. They are not as strong as the anterior longitudinal ligament, but additional posterior structures provide support against hyperflexion.
      d. Ligamentum flavum. This ligament connects the posterior arches of adjacent vertebrae and extends continuously in the most posterior portion of the central vertebral canal. The ligamentum flavum is considered an important stabilizer during flexion because of its extreme elasticity.
      e. Interspinous ligaments. These individual ligaments interconnect the spinous processes. They are less developed in the cervical region than in other areas of the spine.
      f. Ligamentum nuchae. This ligament extends continuously along the posterior tip of the spinous processes from the occipital protuberance to the vertebra prominens. It supports the cervical spine and helps maintain the normal lordotic curvature. The ligamentum nuchae is an important site of muscular attachment and can be palpated in the midline posteriorly.
   2. Structures supporting the occipitoatlantoaxial complex.
      a. Cruciform ligament complex. This cross-shaped ligament has laterally directed fibers arising from the atlas to form the transverse ligament, which is the major support securing the dens to the anterior tubercle of the atlas. Rupture of this ligament can allow the dens to pierce the spinal cord. Two vertical projections connect the cruciform ligament complex inferiorly to the atlas and superiorly to the occipital bone.

b. Alar ligaments. These ligaments extend bilaterally from the dens to the occipital condyles of the foramen magnum and limit lateral rotation and flexion of the head.
c. Apical ligament. This ligament extends superiorly from the tip of the dens to the occipital bone and limits flexion of the head.

D. Neural components of the cervical spine.
1. Spinal cord. The spinal cord is encased in the central vertebral canal, which is formed by the bony vertebral arch and body. The cord enlarges at the level of C3 to C6 because of the increased nerve supply necessary for the upper extremities.
2. Nerve roots. The nerve roots project laterally from their origin in the cord and exit between the bodies and transverse processes of adjoining vertebrae. Each nerve is named by the vertebrae it passes above to exit the column, except for nerve C8, which passes below C7 and above the first thoracic vertebra. Useful clinical tests for the neurological components of the cervical spine are presented in Table 45-1.

TABLE 45-1. Neurological Tests for the Cervical Spine Nerve Roots

Action	Muscle(s) Affected	Nerve Root(s) Affected
Motor Function Tests		
Flexion of the head	Many	C1-2
Lateral bending of the head	Many	C3
Shoulder shrug	Trapezius	C4
Shoulder abduction	Deltoid	C5-6
Elbow flexion	Biceps, brachialis	C5-6
Elbow extension	Triceps	C7-8
Wrist extension	Extensor carpi radialis	C6
Finger flexion	Flexor digitorum	C8
Finger abduction	Interosseous muscles	C8-T1
Dermatome Sensory Tests		
Upper neck/occiput		C2
Lower neck		C3
Tip of shoulder		C4
Lateral arm		C5
Thumb		C6
Middle finger		C7
Little finger		C8
Muscle/Tendon Reflex Tests		
Biceps		C5-6
Brachioradialis		C5-6
Triceps		C7-8

3. Phrenic nerve. This nerve is important because it arises from the C3, C4, and C5 nerve roots. Because the phrenic nerve is the sole motor nerve supply to the diaphragm, injuries to the superior cervical spine must be monitored closely for change in respiratory status.

E. Musculature of the cervical spine. The muscles of the cervical spine are closely layered and interwoven, a condition that produces complementary support and dynamic functions. Exact description of these muscles is beyond the scope of this chapter. Table 45-2 lists the musculature on the basis of position in relation to the spine and depth. Table 45-3 groups muscles on the basis of dynamic function. Most cervical muscles receive their innervation from the dorsal rami of the spinal nerves. Some important exceptions are listed in Table 45-4.

F. Vascular structures of the cervical spine. The vertebral arteries pass upward through the foramen transversarium of each vertebra except for C7, through which only accessory veins pass. Upon exiting the cervical spine, the vertebral arteries pass through the foramen magnum and then combine to form the basilar artery. Fractures of the cervical vertebrae, and even prolonged hyperrotation of the head at the atlantoaxial joint, can lead to disrupted blood flow to the posterior fossa of the brain. Small branches from the vertebral arteries supply the spinal structures and spinal cord.

G. Surface anatomy of the cervical spine.
   1. Surface landmarks approximating cervical spine levels.
      a. C1 level: angle of the mandible.
      b. C3 level: hyoid bone.
      c. C4 level: thyroid cartilage.
      d. C6 level: cricoid cartilage.
   2. Palpation of the cervical vertebrae.
      a. The transverse process of the atlas (C1) is palpable between the angle of the mandible and the mastoid process.

TABLE 45-2. Muscles of the Cervical Spine Grouped by Location and Depth

	Positional Relation to Spinal Column		
Depth	**Posterior**	**Anterior**	**Lateral**
Superficial	Trapezius Splenius capitis and splenius cervicis	Sternocleidomastoid	(Superficial and intermediate muscles are not related to support or motion of the cervical spine and function only to position the larynx and mandible)
Intermediate	Erector spinae Iliocostalis cervicis Longissimus cervicis and longissimus capitis Spinalis Semispinalis	Levator scapulae	
Deep	Lower cervical Multifidi Upper cervical Rectus capitis Obliquus capitis	Scalene muscles	Longus colli Longus capitis

TABLE 45-3. Muscles Producing Motion of the Head and Neck

Extension	Flexion	Rotation and Lateral Flexion
Splenius capitis and cervicis Semispinalis capitis and cervicis Longissimus capitis and cervicis Trapezius Interspinalis Rectus capitis posterior major and minor Obliquus capitis superior Sternocleidomastoid (working together)	Sternocleidomastoid (working together) Longus colli and capitis Rectus capitis anterior	Sternocleidomastoid (working independently) Scalene group Splenius capitis and cervicis Longissimus capitis Levator scapulae Longus colli Iliocostalis cervicis Multifidi Intertransversarii Obliquus capitis superior and inferior Rectus capitis lateralis

b. The spinous process of C7 is easily palpable and marks the most inferior border of the cervical spine posteriorly.

II. Biomechanics and Articulations of the Cervical Spine

A. Flexibility: the cervical spine is the most flexible area of the spine and has articulations that allow flexion, extension, lateral bending, and circumduction (all motions combined). To achieve this increased flexibility, however, the bony interlocking of the cervical vertebrae is less than that of other areas of the spine; this, in turn, increases the relative risk of vertebral translation or dislocation in the cervical spine compared with lumbar and thoracic vertebrae.

B. Range of motion of the cervical spine and head.

1. Flexion and extension: full range of motion consists of the cumulative effects of motion at the occipitoatlantoid joint (nodding) and allowed motion of the intervertebral disks and facet joints between the lower vertebrae. About 60 degrees of flexion and 75 degrees of extension are available in the cervical spine. About one third of this motion is through the occipitoatlantoaxial complex, and the remaining motion arises from the intervertebral articulations.
2. Rotation: about 80 degrees of lateral rotation is available to the cervical spine. About 50% of this rotation is derived from the atlantoaxial

TABLE 45-4. Nerve Supply for the Cervical Muscles

Muscle	Innervation
Trapezius	Cranial nerve 11, 3rd and 4th cervical nerves (ventral rami)
Sternocleidomastoid	Cranial nerve 11, 2nd cervical nerve (ventral rami)
Levator scapulae	3rd, 4th, and 5th (dorsal rami) cervical nerves
Other cervical muscles	Usually the dorsal rami of cervical nerves

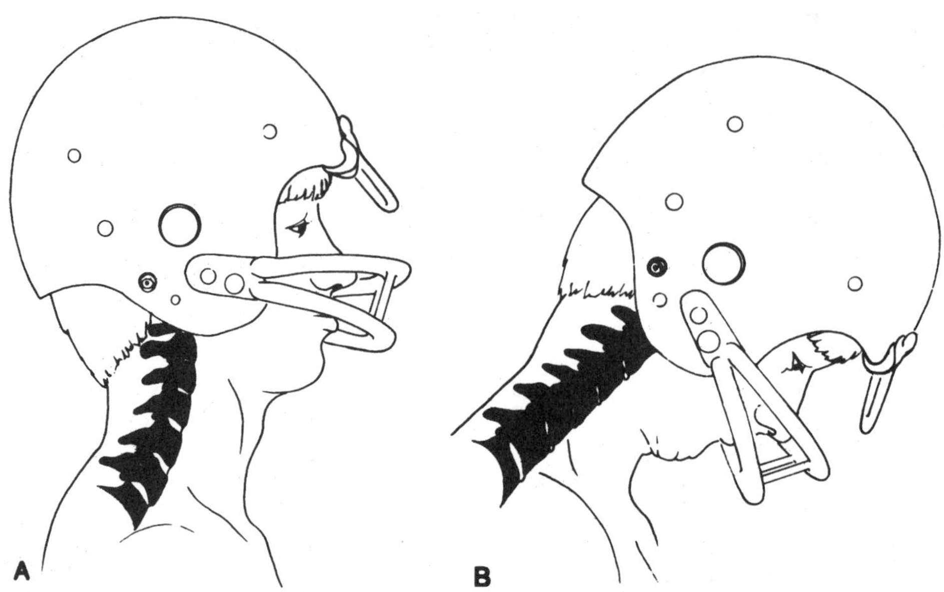

FIGURE 45-2
A, When neck is in the normal upright position, the cervical spine is slightly extended because of natural cervical lordosis. **B,** When the neck is flexed slightly (to about 30 degrees), the cervical spine is straightened and converted into a segmented column. (Reproduced by permission of the author, editor, and publisher from Torg JS, Gennarelli TA: Head and cervical spine injuries. In DeLee JC, Orez D Jr, editors: *Orthopaedic Sports Medicine: Principles and Practice,* Philadelphia, 1994, WB Saunders, pp 417-462.

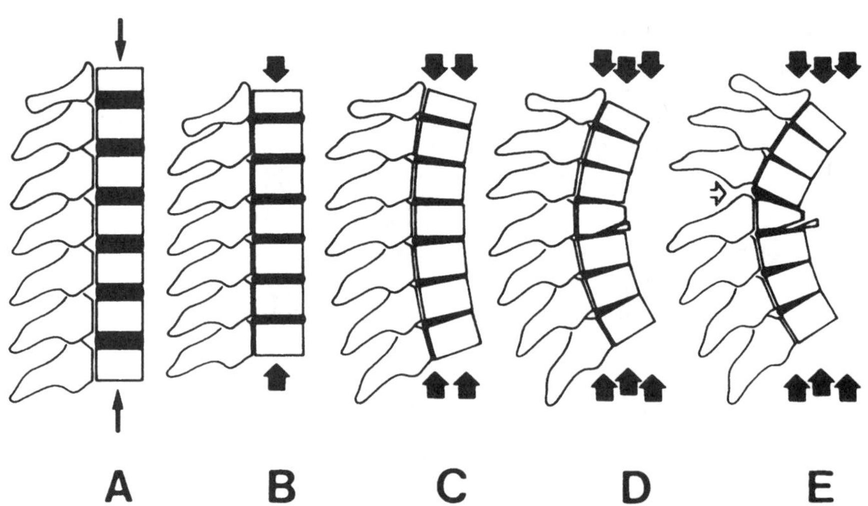

FIGURE 45-3
Biomechanically, the straight cervical spine responds to axial load force like a segmented column. Axial loading of the cervical spine first results in compressive deformation of intervertebral disks (**A** and **B**). As energy input continues and maximum compressive deformation is reached, angular deformation and buckling occur. The spine fails in a flexion mode (**C**) with resulting fracture, subluxation, or dislocation (**D** and **E**). Compressive deformation to failure with resulting fracture, dislocation, or subluxation occurs in as little as 8.4 msec. (Reproduced by permission of the author and publisher from Torg JS et al: The epidemiologic, pathologic, biomechanical, and cinematographic analysis of football-induced cervical spine trauma, *Am J Sports Med* 18:53, 1990.)

joint, and the remaining motions are divided among the intervertebral articulations.

3. Lateral bending: about 60 degrees of lateral bending is available in the cervical spine. Most of this motion is distributed between the intervertebral joints, with the atlantoocipital joint contributing slightly.

C. Load distribution in the cervical spine: most of the weight-bearing capacity is provided by the vertebral bodies and intervertebral disks. The cervical spine achieves natural lordosis of about 30 degrees in the neutral position. In this position an increase downward or axial load upon the head is absorbed by the posterior cervical musculature. However, when the head is forward flexed 20 to 30 degrees, the natural lordosis is lost and the vertebral column straightens to become a stacked, segmented column (Fig. 45-2). Increased axial force is then distributed directly through the vertebral bodies and intervertebral disks. Once maximal compaction of the intervertebral disks is achieved, additional force is absorbed through either fracture or dislocation of the bony vertebrae (Fig. 45-3). The situation is created in contact sports like football or hockey when the athlete may drop the head forward in anticipation of contact. Teaching the proper technique to avoid this event is an essential and effective preventive measure to decrease the incidence of tragic cervical spine injuries.

Acknowledgment

The Medical Editing Department, Kaiser Foundation Research Institute, provided editorial assistance.

Bibliography

Jofe MH, White AA, Panjabi MM: Kinematics. In The Cervical Spine Research Society Editorial Subcommittee, editor: *The Cervical Spine,* Philadelphia, 1983, JB Lippincott, pp 23-35.

Moore KL: Clinically oriented anatomy, ed 3, Baltimore, 1992, Williams & Wilkins, pp 323-372.

Sherk HH, Parke WW: Normal adult anatomy. In The Cervical Spine Research Society Editorial Subcommittee, editor: *The Cervical Spine,* Philadelphia, 1983, JB Lippincott, pp 8-22.

Snell RS: *Clinical Anatomy for Medical Students,* ed 3, Boston, 1986, Little, Brown, pp 919-954.

Torg JS, Gennarelli TA: Head and cervical spine injuries. In DeLee JC, Drez D Jr, editors: *Orthopaedic Sports Medicine: Principles and Practice,* Philadelphia, 1994, WB Saunders, pp 417-462.

Torg JS et al: The epidemiologic, pathologic, biomechanical, and cinematographic analysis of football-induced cervical spine trauma, *Am J Sports Med* 18:53, 1990.

CHAPTER 46

Fractures and Dislocation of the Cervical Spine

Evan S. Bass, MD

I. Clinical Findings in Cervical Spine Fracture or Dislocation
   A. History: mechanism of injury provides valuable clues to diagnosis (specific descriptions of injuries are discussed later in this chapter).
      1. Hyperflexion injuries.
         a. Disruption of posterior ligaments, with or without associated fractures.
         b. Avulsion fractures of the spinous processes (e.g., "clay-shoveler's" fracture of C6 or C7 vertebra).
         c. Wedge or burst vertebral body fractures.
         d. Interlocked facets with dislocation.
      2. Hyperextension injuries.
         a. Rupture of intervertebral disks and/or anterior longitudinal ligament.
         b. Spinal cord compression without fracture.
         c. Compression fracture of posterior elements (e.g., "hangman's" fracture of C2 vertebra).
      3. Axial loading injuries, especially in the flexed forward position ("spearing"). Most common mechanism of cervical spine fractures and dislocation in contact sports, with increased severity if injury also includes a rotational or lateral bending component.
         a. Burst or wedge fractures of the vertebral bodies.
         b. Posterior arch fractures of the atlas (C1).
         c. Interlocked facets with resultant dislocation and/or subluxation.
   B. Neurological symptoms: Not a reliable indicator of severity. Symptoms can range from none to quadriplegia.
   C. Transport of the injured athlete: unfortunately, many injuries are made more severe by poor on-site management. Inquire about and document details on how the injury was managed on site and changes in symptoms that have occurred.

D. Other symptoms: the most common symptom of cervical fracture and/or dislocation is neck pain. Ligamentous instability is usually accompanied by neck pain, which is often exacerbated by flexion and extension.

II. Cervical Spine Radiology

A. Views.*

1. Lateral view: most important view to evaluate for fractures and dislocation. (Special note: These views are to be taken only after other views show no evidence of fracture or dislocation. The patient must initiate flexion and extension without any assistance. The patient is protected from further injury because pain determines the limit of available range of motion.)
2. Anteroposterior (AP) view: to evaluate for sagittally directed fractures, interlocked facets, or spinous process fractures not evident on lateral view.
3. Open mouth AP view: to evaluate integrity of first (atlas) and second (axis) vertebrae, especially the odontoid process.
4. Oblique view(s): used to better evaluate facet dislocation or fractures (C3-C7).
5. Flexion and extension views: obtained to evaluate for possible ligamentous injury and instability in the absence of fracture or dislocation.

B. Interpreting cervical radiography films.

1. Lateral view of the cervical spine.
   a. Count the vertebrae: all seven vertebrae must be seen, or the film must be repeated.
   b. Evaluate five normally smooth lines (Fig. 46-1).
      (1) Prevertebral soft tissues (abnormal widening and/or deviation indicate an underlying hematoma, which may be the only indication of underlying fracture).
      (2) Anterior vertebral bodies.
      (3) Posterior vertebral bodies.
      (4) Spinolaminal line: junction of the laminae with the spinous processes.
      (5) Tips of the spinous processes.
   c. Inspect the first and second vertebrae (Fig. 46-2).
      (1) The distance between the posterior arch of the C1 vertebra and the odontoid process should be no greater than 2.5 mm (in children up to 5.0 mm is acceptable). Greater distances suggest disruption of the transverse ligament (Fig. 46-3).
   d. Inspect the intervertebral spaces for narrowing.
   e. Evaluate cervical lordosis: muscle spasm can decrease natural curvature.
   f. (Optional) Estimate the relative width of the spinal canal: on the lateral view film, the ratio of the height of the spinal canal (the midpoint of the posterior surface of the vertebral body up to the spinolaminar line) divided by the width of the corresponding midvertebral body has been described by Torg and colleagues as a measure of cervical spinal stenosis. A ratio of 0.8 has been suggested to represent significant stenosis; however, the clinical usefulness of this ratio remains controversial, and magnetic resonance imaging (MRI) is recommended if stenosis is suspected.
2. Anteroposterior view of the cervical spine: spinous processes should be in a vertical row with nearly equal interspinous spacing.

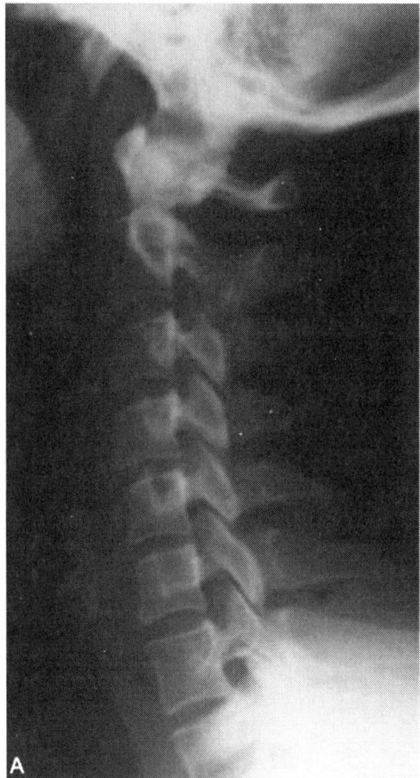

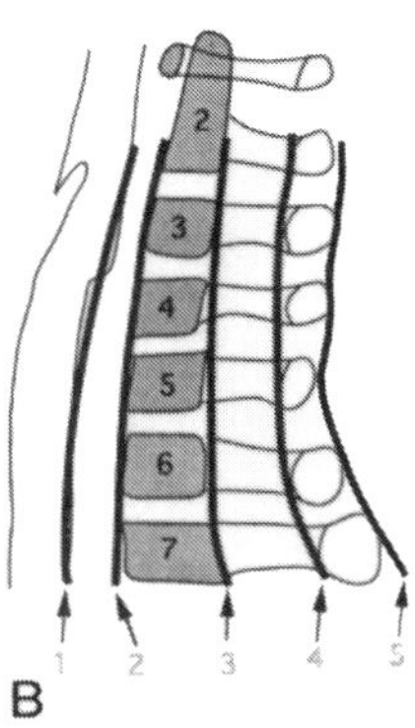

FIGURE 46-1
Normal lateral cervical spine. **A,** Lateral radiograph of normal cervical spine. **B,** Diagrammatic representation of lateral cervical spine showing four parallel lines that should be observed in every such examination. Line 1 is soft tissue line, which is closely applied to posterior border of airway through first four or five body segments and then widens around laryngeal cartilage and runs parallel to remainder of cervical vertebrae. Line 2 demarcates anterior border of cervical vertebral bodies. Line 3 is posterior border of cervical vertebral bodies. Line 4 is drawn by connecting junction of lamina at spinous process, termed the spinolaminal line. This line represents posterior extent of central canal, which contains the spinal cord itself. These lines should be generally smooth and parallel with no abrupt deviations. (Reproduced by permission of the author, editor, and publisher from Helms CA: Trauma. In Brant WE, Helms CA, editors: *Fundamentals of Diagnostic Radiology,* Baltimore, 1994, Williams & Wilkins, pp 886-895.)

a. Local widening (defined as greater than 1½ times the interspinous distances above and below) may indicate interlocking of facets, fracture of the spinous process, or hyperflexion sprain.
b. Malalignment indicates spinous process fracture of interlocked facets.

3. Open mouth AP view (odontoid view).
   a. Visually examine the odontoid process and evaluate for fracture.
   b. The laminae of the atlas and axis should be aligned.
      (1) Malalignment indicates disruption of the bony ring of the axis.
      (2) These fractures are frequently difficult to appreciate on plain radiographs, and computerized tomography (CT) is indicated if there is high suspicion of fracture (pain upon nodding of head).
   c. Distance between the odontoid process and atlas on either side should be equal. Asymmetry is not necessarily an indicator of fracture (possibly fixation of the atlantoaxial joint), but further radiological evaluation is indicated.

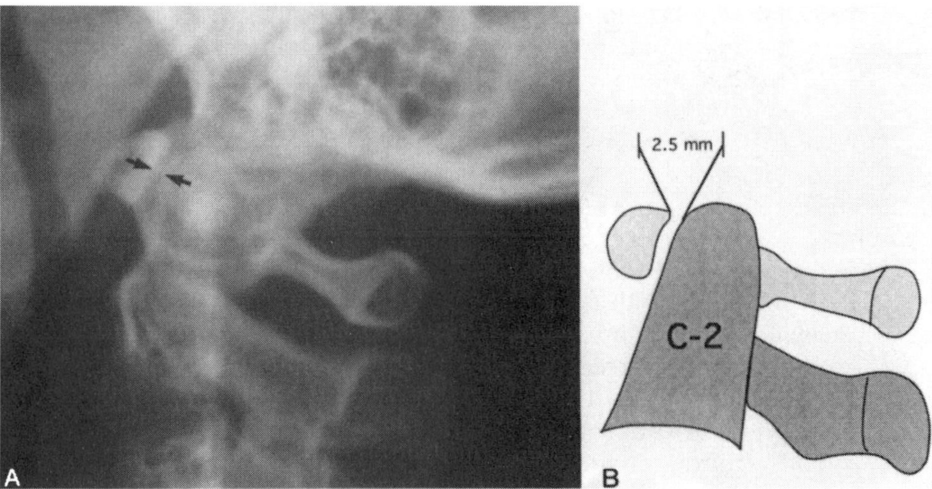

FIGURE 46-2
Normal C1 and C2 vertebrae. Lateral radiograph (**A**) and drawing (**B**) of upper cervical spine show normal distance of anterior arch of C1 <2.5 mm in distance from odontoid process (dens) of C2 (*arrows*). (Reproduced by permission of the author, editor, and publisher from Helms CA: Trauma. In Brant WE, Helms CA, editors: *Fundamentals of Diagnostic Radiology,* Baltimore, 1994, Williams & Wilkins, pp 886-895.)

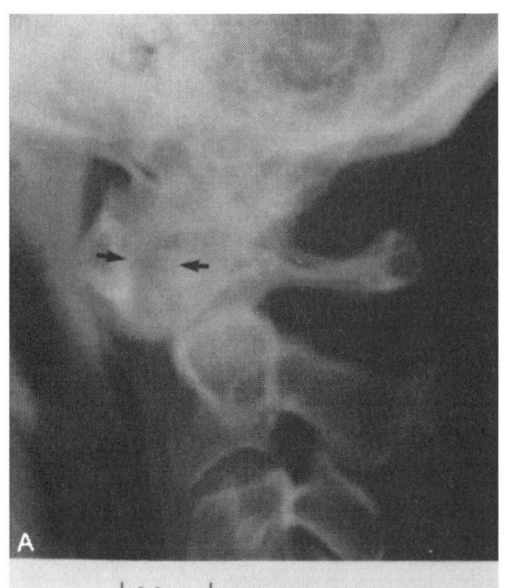

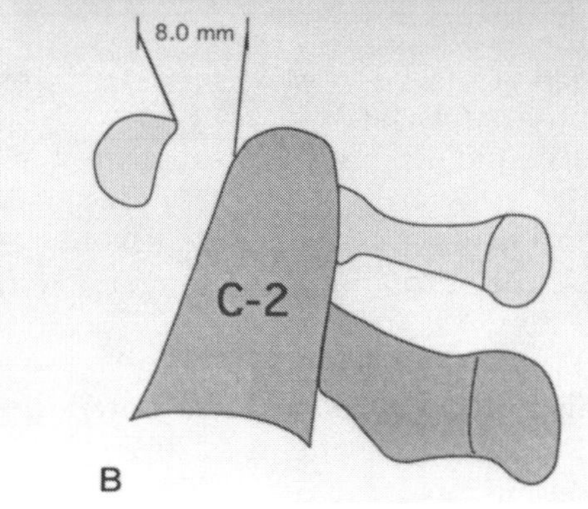

FIGURE 46-3
Cervical vertebrae 1 and 2 dislocation. Lateral radiograph (**A**) and drawing (**B**) of upper cervical spine in patient who experienced trauma to neck show anterior arch of C1 is 9 mm anterior to odontoid process of C2 (*arrows*). This is diagnostic sign of dislocation of C1 on C2 and indicates rupture of transverse ligaments that normally hold these vertebral segments together. (Reproduced by permission of the author, editor, and publisher from Helms CA: Trauma. In Brant WE, Helms CA, editors: *Fundamentals of Diagnostic Radiology,* Baltimore, 1994, Williams & Wilkins, pp 886-895.)

4. Lateral views in flexion and extension of the cervical spine.
   a. Evaluate radiographs for anterior intervertebral disk space narrowing, anterior angulation and displacement, and fanning of the spinous processes.
   b. Instability warrants evaluation by a specialist and aggressive treatment.

III. Fractures, Dislocation, and Subluxation of the Cervical Spine

A. Fractures, dislocation, and subluxation of the cervical spine are consistently associated with football, rugby, hockey, gymnastics, and diving. High school football accounts for generally 30 to 60 injuries annually. Incidence has begun to decrease as better tackling techniques are taught and rules are enforced against using the helmet as a contact weapon. The primary care sports medicine specialist must be alert to types of fractures and dislocation that are detectable on cervical radiographs. Frequently, injuries are described as stable versus unstable, which refers to severity of injury in relation to the spinal cord and is not an indicator of aggressiveness of treatment. Any injury with evidence of fracture or instability warrants immediate consultation with an appropriate specialist.

B. Upper cervical spine (C1-C3) fractures and dislocations.
   1. Transverse ligament rupture.
      a. Caused by forced hyperflexion of the head.
      b. Unstable injury; spinal cord can be impinged by odontoid process.
   2. Fractures of the atlas (C1): Jefferson fracture.
      a. Caused by an axial load onto occipital condyles.
      b. Most commonly seen as bilateral fractures of the posterior arch.
      c. Can also include fractures of the anterior tubercle (burst fracture).
      d. Considered unstable if the overhang of the lateral edges of the atlas over the axis is >7 mm combined, indicating possible transverse ligament rupture.
   3. Fractures of the axis (C2).
      a. Odontoid process fractures can occur due to head impact.
      b. Fracture of the posterior elements of C2 ("hangman's" fracture) generally results from hyperflexion and is seriously unstable.

C. Middle cervical spine (C3-C4) fractures and dislocation: traumatic lesions in this area are rare and are usually not associated with fractures.
   1. Acute intervertebral disk rupture: can have symptoms of transient quadriplegia in the absence of fracture.
   2. Anterior subluxation of C3 upon C4 vertebra.
      a. Seen as instability without fracture on lateral flexion and extension radiographs.
      b. Surgical intervention is frequently necessary.
   3. Facet dislocation.
      a. Can be unilateral or bilateral.
      b. Possible immediate quadriplegia.
      c. Bilateral dislocation has a poor prognosis.

D. Lower cervical spine (C4-C7) fractures and dislocation. Most acute traumatic fractures and dislocation affect this area of the cervical spine. Mechanism of fracture is usually axial loading in the flexed forward position. Dislocation is generally the result of rotational forces in addition to the axial load.
   1. Compression fractures: classified into five types.
      a. Type I: simple wedge or chip from body of vertebra anteriorly. Treated conservatively once stability of ligamentous structures is established. Rare neurological injury.

b. Type II: isolated crush fracture of anterior vertebral body ("teardrop" fracture) with no bone fragments displaced, no posterior bony structures affected, and no neurological symptoms. When ligamentous stability is established, injury may be treated conservatively.
c. Type III: comminuted fracture of the vertebral body with protrusion of fragments into central vertebral canal but no fracture of posterior bony elements. An unstable injury for which surgical stabilization is generally necessary.
d. Type IV: crush fracture with fracture of body in sagittal plane accompanied by a posterior arch fracture. Very unstable and almost always associated with quadriplegia.
e. Type V: combination of a type IV fracture with additional fracture of the posterior arch of an adjoining vertebra. Extremely unstable.

2. Fracture of the spinous process of C6 or C7 vertebra ("clay-shoveler's" fracture).
   a. Caused by a tremendous flexion force on the posterior ligaments, resulting in avulsion of the spinous process.
   b. Generally a stable, harmless fracture in the absence of neurological symptoms.

IV. Return to Play After Cervical Spinal Injury

A. Because of relative lack of research data (most information is anecdotal) and possible medicolegal issues, determining when an athlete should return to play is difficult. The guidelines presented here are neither definite nor complete, and they are presented only to assist the primary care sports physician in answering questions from athletes and parents. Certainly, the decision to return to play in contact sports after a cervical fracture, dislocation, or instability requires thorough discussion between the specialist who treated the injury and the athlete (and parent[s] if the athlete is a minor).

B. Return to play after sprain or strain: return to contact sports is generally possible after the athlete is asymptomatic and has full range of motion and strength. Consider cervical radiography (including flexion and extension views) to rule out cervical instability, if indicated.

C. Return to play after fractures.
   1. Upper cervical fractures (C1 or C2 vertebra): almost all fractures in this area warrant discontinuing contact sports. Surgical fusion affecting these vertebrae also is a contraindication for return to contact sports.
   2. Other cervical fractures.
      a. Compression fractures of a vertebral body. Athletes who have completely healed type I and II fractures, who are asymptomatic, and who have full range of motion and strength can generally return to contact sports. Type III fractures are a relative contraindication for return to contact sports after full healing. Type IV and V fractures are absolute contraindications for return to sports despite full surgical stabilization and healing.
      b. Spinous process or "clay-shoveler's" fracture: the athlete can generally return to contact sports after full healing has occurred, the athlete is asymptomatic, and full range of motion and strength have returned. Cervical radiography, including flexion and extension views, should show complete healing and have no evidence of instability.

D. Return to play after cervical intervertebral disk injury.

1. Treated conservatively: athlete can return to contact sports when asymptomatic and full range of motion and strength have returned.
2. Treated with surgical fusion: athletes who have stable one-level fusion not affecting the C2 vertebra can return to contact sports after full recovery is complete. Spinal fusion affecting more than one level generally is a contraindication for return to contact sports because of the increased stress on the articulation between adjacent vertebrae.

V. Prevention of Cervical Spine Injuries
   A. Rule changes that enforce not using the helmet as a weapon have led to a marked decrease in head and neck injury. The team physician must take an active role to enforce these rule changes.
   B. The team physician must educate players (and parents) about proper tackling techniques and about the severe risks of using the helmet as a weapon.
   C. Check all equipment for proper fit.
   D. Educate players, coaches, trainers, and all assistant personnel in proper approach and handling of a player who may have a neck injury.
   E. Do not hesitate to report all coaches or officials who do not actively promote prevention of injury.

Acknowledgment

The Medical Editing Department, Kaiser Foundation Research Institute, provided editorial assistance.

Bibliography

Cantu RC: Sports medicine aspects of cervical spinal stenosis, *Exerc Sport Sci Rev* 23:399-409, 1995.

Helms CA: Trauma. In Brant WE, Helms CA, editors: *Fundamentals of Diagnostic Radiology*, Baltimore, 1994, Williams & Wilkins, pp 886-895.

Mueller FO, Cantu RC: The annual survey of catastrophic football injuries: 1977-1988, *Exerc Sports Sci Rev* 19:261-268, 1996.

Penning L: Obtaining and interpreting plain films in cervical spine injury. In The Cervical Spine Research Society Editorial Subcommittee: *The Cervical Spine*, Philadelphia, 1983, JB Lippincott, pp 62-95.

Torg JS, Gennarelli TA: Head and cervical spine injuries. In DeLee JC, Drez D Jr, editors: *Orthopaedic Sports Medicine: Principles and Practice*, Philadelphia, 1994, WB Saunders, pp 417-462.

Torg JS et al: The National Football Head and Neck Injury Registry, 14-year report on cervical quadriplegia, 1971 through 1984, *JAMA* 254:3439-3443, 1985.

CHAPTER **47**

Extra-Axial Cervical Spine Injury

James M. Moriarity, MD

I. Anatomy
  A. There are seven cervical vertebrae that connect the thorax to the 15-pound cranium.
    1. These vertebrae provide a wide range of motion, stability, and protection of the brain's connection to the rest of the body via the spinal cord.
    2. The cervical spine also serves as a major anchor to many of the muscles that support the scapula, clavicle, and acromion.
    3. The stability of the spine is the result of an intricate interplay of muscle and ligament that allows mobility as well as providing strength.
  B. Joints of the cervical spine.
    1. C0-C1: the atlantooccipital joints.
      a. Principal motion is flexion and extension.
      b. No rotation.
      c. Lateral movement small.
      d. No disk present.
      e. Synovial articulation.
    2. C1: Atlas.
      a. No vertebral body.
      b. Receives the odontoid process from the axis below and binds it to its anterior arch with the transverse ligament and alar ligament.
    3. C1-C2 (atlantoaxial) joint.
      a. Most mobile articulation of the spine.
      b. Minimal extension/flexion of 10 degrees.
      c. Minimal lateral bending.
      d. Rotation is the greatest of the cervical spine (35 degrees) in each direction.
    4. The atlantoaxial joint is subject to subluxation or dislocation.
      a. 25% of patients with rheumatoid arthritis demonstrate instability of this joint.

   b. 40% of patients with Down syndrome are subject to atlantoaxial dislocations/subluxation and should be screened with cervical spine films prior to participation in gymnastics, diving, swimming the butterfly stroke, high jump, pentathlon, and soccer.
   c. Atlanto-dens interval (ADI) of <4 mm in children and <3 mm in adults is considered normal. An ADI of 6.5-11 mm is highly associated with neurological symptoms and subject to C1-C2 fusion.
5. C2: Axis.
   a. Has a vertebral body that is superiorly extended by the odontoid process.
   b. The odontoid process acts as a pivot for the rotation of the atlas above.
   c. The superior articulating facets are oriented horizontally to facilitate rotation.
   d. The inferior articulating facets are oriented obliquely and permit little rotation.
6. Uncovertebral joints of Luschka.
   a. Pairs of joints beginning with C2-C3 and inferiorly to C6-C7.
   b. Each vertebral body when viewed from above is shaped like a bucket seat and receives the body from above with a relatively tight fit.
   c. Has a synovial lining and functions like a joint.
   d. Subject to same degenerative and traumatic changes that afflict other joints.
   e. The uncovertebral joints permit flexion and extension and limited rotation and resist lateral glide of adjacent vertebral bodies.
7. Facet joints.
   a. 14 pairs of facet joints (apophyseal).
   b. Superior articulating process face upward, dorsal, and medial.
   c. Inferior articulating process face downward, ventral, and lateral.
   d. The facet joints are oriented obliquely to the horizontal and sagittal plane, permitting neck motions of flexion, extension, and lateral bending. Minimal rotation occurs but due to the obliquely oriented position of the facet joints; some rotation occurs with lateral bending.
   e. Greatest motion is in flexion and extension at C5-6, then C4-5 and C6-7.
   f. The facets are highly innervated structures.
   g. The two posterior columns of paired facet joints together with the anterior vertebral body column form a strong tripod of biomechanical support.
   h. All the joints in the neck contain meniscoid elements with similar structure and function as the menisci of the knee.

C. Transverse processes.
   1. Contain foramina for the passage of the vertebral arteries.
   2. Rotation of spine past 50 degrees leads to kinking of the artery and symptoms of vertebral basilar (VB) syndrome.
   3. Symptoms of VB syndrome include visual disturbances, nausea, vertigo, tinnitus, and, on occasion, complete syncope termed "drop attacks."

D. Cervical nerves.
   1. Eight pairs of cervical nerves.
   2. With exception of C1, exit through the intervertebral foramina. C2

nerve root exits in the C1-C2 interforaminal space. C8 exits through the C7-T1 space.
3. C1 exits through the atlas-occipital membrane.

E. Intervertebral disks.
1. Make up 25% of the height of the cervical spine.
2. No disk between atlas and occiput, atlas and axis.
3. The wedge shape of the disk with a greater anterior width is what gives the cervical spine its lordotic curve.
4. Nucleus pulposus is 80% water in young individuals and is largely uncompressible. The nucleus may deform in shape in response to compressive forces.
5. The annulus fibrosus retains the nucleus. It is made up of strong interlacing fibers of collagen and is attached to the vertebral bodies by Sharpey's fibers. It is thicker anteriorly and weaker postero-laterally. The water content of the disk is reduced by 20% with aging.

II. Examination of the Cervical Spine
A. Range of motion.
1. Flexion.
   a. 80-90 degrees with most of the flexion occurring at the C4-C7 level.
   b. Upper cervical spine flexion is manifested as "nodding." Lower cervical spine flexion is "bowing."
   c. Isolated flexion movement can occur between C0-C1 (nodding), whereas flexion of any other vertebrae results in movement of adjacent vertebrae.
   d. In flexion the disk widens posteriorly and narrows anteriorly.
   e. The intervertebral foramina are 30% larger in flexion.
2. Extension.
   a. Limited by ligament tightness to 70 degrees.
   b. No anatomical block to extension, accounting for greater ligament injury in whiplash injury.
   c. C0-C1 has most extension motion followed by C4-C7.
   d. Extension narrows the intervertebral foramina and loads the facet joints.
3. Lateral bending.
   a. Varies from 20-45 degrees right and left.
   b. Mostly occurs at the atlantooccipital joint and C1-C2. The facet joints contribute a small amount.
4. Rotation.
   a. 70-90 degrees each direction.
   b. Always occurs with some flexion owing to the inclination of the facet joints.
   c. 50% of rotation occurs at the C1-C2 joint.
   d. Facet joints also permit rotation.
5. Retraction.
   a. Forward and backward gliding of spine on same horizontal plane.
   b. Backward gliding simultaneously causes upper cervical spine flexion with lower cervical spine extension. Forward gliding reverses process.
   c. Greater flexion of neck can be achieved from backward gliding position.

B. Nerve root myotomes (Table 47-1).
C. Dermatomes: there is a great deal of overlap within the dermatomes.

TABLE 47-1. Nerve Root Myotomes

Nerve Root	Muscle Action
C1-C2	Nodding of head
C3	Lateral bending of neck
C4	Shoulder shrugging
C5	Shoulder abduction
C6	Arm flexion, wrist extension
C7	Arm extension, wrist flexion

D. Special tests.
  1. Lhermitte's sign: patient sits in long leg position on examination table. Neck is flexed, and the trunk is flexed forward. A positive sign is present if the patient experiences a sharp pain down the spine and into the upper and lower limbs. A positive test indicates dural irritation.
  2. Spurling's maneuver (foraminal compression test): axial compression of the head in a neutral, left lateral, or right lateral position elicits radicular pain symptoms or localized pain in the neck.
  3. Distraction test: performed on patients with radicular symptoms. With the patient in a lying position the examiner slightly flexes the neck and applies traction to the head. If pain is relieved, the test is positive for foraminal encroachment.

E. Reflexes, nerve root, disk space test (Table 47-2).

F. Landmarks.
  C1: transverse process anterior and inferior to mastoid.
  C2: posterior to angle of jaw.
  C7: most prominent spinous process of neck.

III. Cervical Spine Abnormalities and Return to Play
  A. Congenital conditions.
    1. Odontoid abnormalities involving agenesis, hypoplasia, or os odontoideum are absolute contraindications to contact sports.
    2. Spina bifida occulta is not a contraindication to contact sport.

TABLE 47-2. Nerve Root, Disk Space, Reflex, and Myotome

Nerve Root	Disk Space	Reflex	Muscle	Action
C5	C4-5	Biceps	Deltoid	Shoulder abduction
C6	C5-6	Brachioradialis	Biceps	Elbow flexion
C7	C6-7	Triceps	Triceps	Elbow extension
C8	C7-T1	None	Flexor digitorum	Finger flexion
T1	T1-2	None	Hand intrinsics	Finger adduction(?), abduction

3. Atlantooccipital fusion is a contraindication to contact sport.
4. Klippel-Feil anomaly is congenital fusion of two or more cervical vertebrae.
   a. Type I anomaly describes mass fusion of the cervical and upper thoracic vertebrae and precludes contact sport.
   b. Type II anomaly describes fusion in one or two adjacent vertebrae only. Participation is judged on the presence of associated instability, disk disease, and level of fusion.

B. Developmental conditions.
   1. "Spear-tackler's spine": defined as loss or reversal of the normal lordotic curve of the cervical vertebral column, which predisposes an athlete to axial loading.
   2. Cervical stenoses: cervical stenosis as a cause of transient sensory and motor loss in athletes has received attention as a possible preventative discovery on physical examination.
   3. Cervical stenosis is defined as a Pavlov ratio of <0.8 on lateral cervical spine radiography. A more precise definition is the loss of cerebrospinal fluid cushion surrounding the spinal cord as defined by magnetic resonance imaging (MRI).
   4. 92% of all *symptomatic* reported cases of transient neurapraxia and transient quadriplegia have a Pavlov ratio of <0.8.
      a. 12% of *asymptomatic* controls are <0.8.
      b. 48% of *asymptomatic* professional and 45% of college football athletes have a ratio of <0.8. This disparity is due to the larger vertebral body size seen in these athletes.
   5. For a player who sustains transient neurapraxia with a ratio of <0.8, there is a relative contraindication to return until an evaluation is undertaken and all responsible parties are appraised of the theoretical risk of further competition.
   6. Absolute contraindications to return to competition for players with transient neurapraxia are when it is associated with:
      a. Ligamentous instability of the spine.
      b. Intervertebral disk disease.
      c. Degenerative changes.
      d. MRI evidence of cord defects or swelling.
      e. Symptoms >36 hours.
      f. More than one recurrence.

C. Traumatic conditions.
   1. Upper cervical spine trauma to C1-C2 resulting in fracture or instability is a contraindication to contact activities.
   2. Lower cervical spine trauma.
      a. Instability of lower cervical segments manifested by horizontal displacement >3.5 mm or angulation >11 degrees of adjacent vertebrae is a contraindication to contact activities.
      b. Acute fractures are contraindications to contact sport. Healed fractures must be judged individually with consideration given to location, type, instability, and associated complications.
      c. Intervertebral disk injury is a relative contraindication to contact activities if:
         i. The herniation is central and acute.
         ii. An acute or chronic herniation results in neurological findings or limited neck range of motion.
         iii. Herniation coexists with symptomatic neurapraxia and spinal stenoses.

d. No contraindication exists for resolved disk herniation treated conservatively or surgically, provided that the patient is asymptomatic and neurologically intact.

Bibliography

Carroll C, McAffee P, Ruler L: Whiplash injury, *J Musculoskeletal Med* 9(6):97-113, 1992.

Kurzweil P, Jackson D: Low back pain in recreational athletes, *J Musculoskeletal Med* 9(1):24-40, 1992.

Magee D: *Orthopedic Physical Assessment*, Philadelphia, WB Saunders, 1987.

Maricic M, Gall E: Which therapy for cervical arthritis, *J Musculoskeletal Med* 6(10):67-77, 1989.

McKenzie RA: *The Cervical and Thoracic Spine*, New Zealand, Spinal Publications.

Mooney V: Office evaluation of low back disorders, *J Musculoskeletal Med* 6(9):18-35, 1989.

Mooney V: Indications for surgery in low back pain, *J Musculoskeletal Med* 7(2):61-85, 1990.

Pizzutillo P: Adolescent spondylosis and spondylolisthesis, *J Musculoskeletal Med* 6(4):88-104, 1989.

Reid D: *Sports Injury Assessment and Rehabilitation*, New York, 1992, Churchill Livingstone.

Torg J: *Athletic Injuries to the Head, Neck, and Face*, ed. 2, St Louis, 1991, Mosby–Year Book.

Torg J, Gennarelli T: Head and cervical spine injuries. In DeLee J, Orez D: *Orthopedic Sports Medicine*, Philadelphia, 1994, WB Saunders.

Weiker G: Evaluation and treatment of common spine and trunk problems, *Clin Sports Med* July, pp 399-419, 1989.

CHAPTER **48**

Cervical Spine Injuries: On-Field Management

Andrew W. Nichols, MD

I. Introduction
  A. Prevalence and demographics of cervical spine injury.[3]
    1. Between 6,000 and 10,000 individuals sustain cervical spinal cord injuries in the United States annually.
    2. Of such injuries 55% to 75% occur as a result of motor vehicle accidents or accidental falls.
    3. Many of the remaining injuries occur during both supervised and unsupervised sports and recreational activities. High risk sports include diving, trampolining, skiing, football, wrestling, gymnastics, hockey, and surfing.
    4. Only a small fraction of athletic neck injuries result in permanent neurological sequelae. However, if improperly handled, an unstable spinal condition may be converted into a permanent neurological injury.
  B. Cervical spine injury sites and types.[7]
    1. Potential structures of the cervical spine that may be injured include the bony vertebrae, intervertebral disks, anulus fibrosus, ligaments, spinal cord, nerve roots, peripheral nerves, or any combination of these structures.
    2. The various types of athletic injury that may affect the cervical spine include brachial plexus neurapraxia, stable cervical strain, muscular strain, brachial plexus axonotmesis, intervertebral disk injury with or without neurological deficit, stable cervical fracture without neurological deficit, subluxations or dislocations with or without neurological deficit, unstable fractures with or without neurological deficit, quadriplegia, and death.

II. Initial On-Field Evaluation
  A. Initial presentation syndromes of various injuries.[3-5]
    1. Unstable cervical spine injury: neck pain or stiffness; often neurological examination is normal. The presence of *bilateral* symptoms or

lower extremity involvement may suggest the presence of an unstable cervical spine injury.
2. Bony cervical vertebral injury: intense neck pain and tenderness over cervical spine with or without neurological deficit.
3. Cervical ligamentous disruption: the onset of symptoms is often insidious; often only cervical stiffness occurs initially, due to secondary muscular spasm.
4. Transient quadriparesis: sudden partial or complete quadriparesis often associated with paresthesias and dysesthesias, typically without neck pain; symptoms usually resolve without intervention.
5. Burning hands syndrome (central cord contusion): *bilateral* upper extremity paresthesias and weakness (may affect lower extremities but to a lesser degree); symptoms usually resolve without intervention. Neck pain is typically *absent.*
6. "Burner" or "stinger": sudden *unilateral* upper extremity ache, burning sensation, or weakness; symptoms tend to resolve without intervention.

B. Principles of on-field management of suspected cervical injury.
1. Emergency preparedness is paramount.
2. Team physician or trainer should "captain" the medical team during the process of evaluation and initial management.
3. Medical team should practice techniques at least annually.
4. Readily available equipment should include spine board, stretcher, equipment for cardiopulmonary resuscitation, bolt cutters, knife blades, and a telephone for communications.
5. Ambulance services should be readily available for transport of an injured individual to a hospital emergency facility that is equipped to manage a severe spinal injury.
6. The immediate objective is to preserve neurological function by protecting the cervical spine from further damage. An estimated 50% of neurological deficits are created *after* the initial traumatic episode.[2]

C. Evaluation of the conscious athlete with a suspected cervical injury (Figure 48-1).
1. History and physical examination.
   a. Evaluate airway, breathing, and circulation (ABC), while immobilizing the neck.
   b. If the airway is obstructed, remove the mouthpiece and perform the "jaw-thrust" maneuver rather than the "head-tilt" maneuver, so as to maintain the integrity of the cervical spine.
   c. The helmet should not be removed unless it becomes necessary for the performance of resuscitative efforts. The airway may usually be adequately accessed by simply removing the face mask. A scalpel blade or pocketknife will effectively cut the plastic loops that attach the face mask to the helmet shell, allowing the rescuer to flip the face mask upward. Older style helmets often require boltcutters for removal of the entire face mask.
   d. The individual should be questioned to determine:
      (1) The mechanism of injury.
      (2) The presence of cervical pain.
      (3) The presence of neurological symptoms, including paresthesias, dysesthesias, and weakness.
      (4) Any prior history of neck injuries.
   e. Palpate for cervical tenderness.

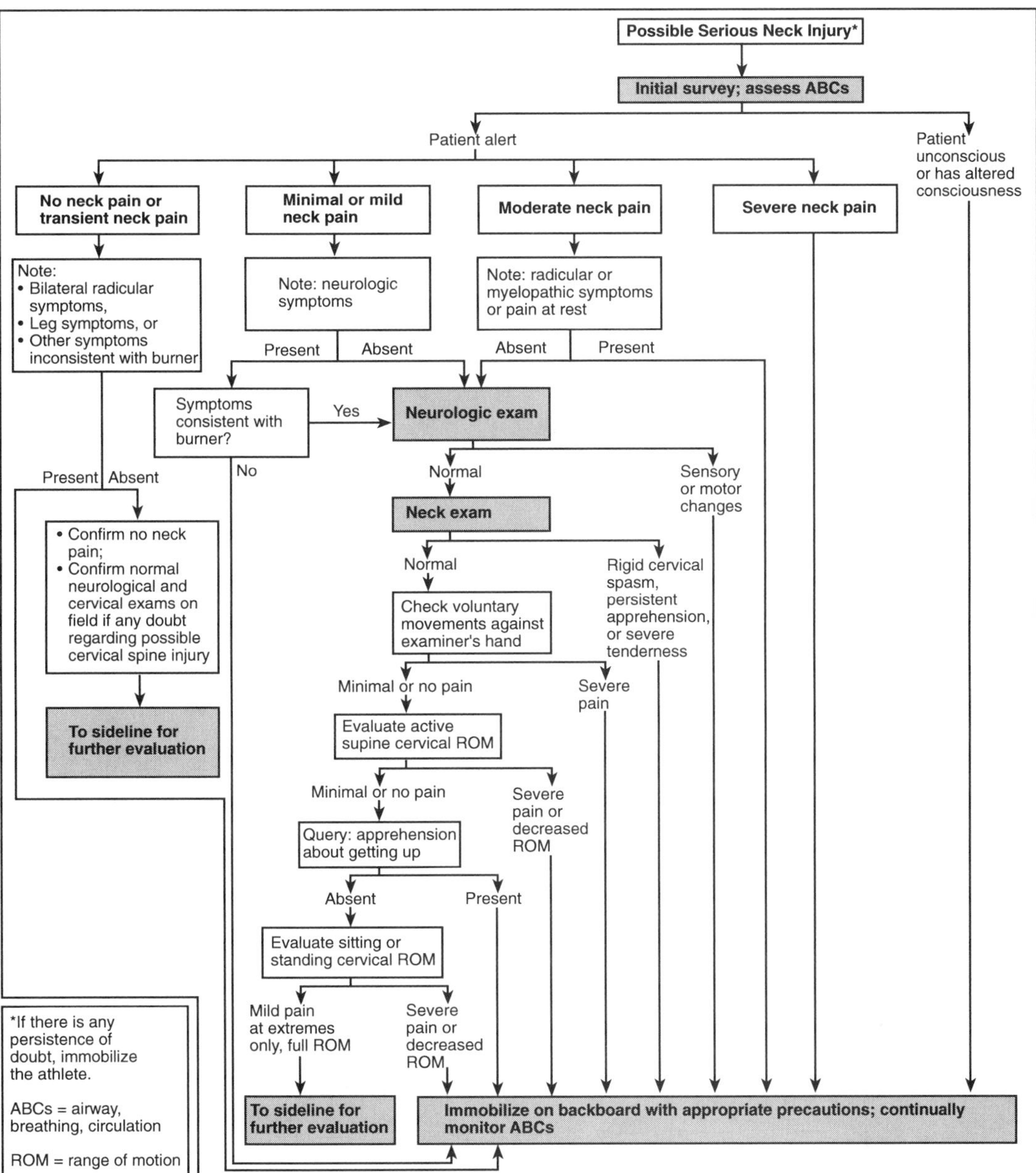

FIGURE 48-1
On-field process of assessing neck injuries. (Reproduced from Anderson C: Neck injuries, *Physician Sportsmed* 21:26, 1993, with permission.)

f. Perform a brief gross neurological examination of all four extremities by asking the injured individual to move his or her fingers and toes. Sensation should also be grossly checked.
g. If the player is intact neurologically and cervical pain and tenderness are absent, active motion of the neck may then be tested.

2. Mode of transport of the injured individual.
   a. The presence of any of the following should prompt full cervical immobilization and transport to emergency facilities on a spine board:
      (1) Abnormal mentation.
      (2) Neurological signs or symptoms.

(3) Cervical pain or tenderness.

(4) Cervical pain, stiffness, or neurological symptoms that develop during active cervical motion.

b. The absence of these findings indicates that it is safe for the injured individual to ambulate with assistance to the sideline for further evaluation.

3. Procedure of spinal immobilization for transport.

a. The medical team leader should direct all actions of the medical team while maintaining rigid head control. It is particularly important to avoid cervical flexion or extension.

b. Ideally, four members of the medical team are present to "log roll" the player onto a full length spine board for transport. The individual who provides the head and neck immobilization should use the "cross-arm" technique of stabilization if the player needs to be turned from the prone to the supine position. During this maneuver, this person's arms "unwind" while maintaining cervical traction.

c. Assistants located at the shoulders, hips, and knees should log roll the individual *toward* them and directly onto the spine board at the medical team leader's direction.

d. Once placed supine on the spine board, the head and spine should be secured to the board by the use of tape and lightweight bolsters. If the player is wearing a helmet, this should be left in place until it has been radiographically determined in an emergency facility that there is no injury to the cervical spine. Satisfactory lateral radiographs can usually be obtained with the football helmet still in place.

D. Evaluation of the unconscious athlete with a suspected cervical injury.

1. The cervical spine should be immobilized while the airway, breathing, and circulation (ABC) are assessed.

2. If the airway is obstructed, the "jaw-thrust" maneuver should be used rather than the "head-tilt" maneuver.

3. Full cervical spine precautions must be maintained with the use of a spine board, and the individual should be transported to an emergency facility equipped to manage unstable cervical injuries.

III. Sideline Evaluation

A. Expanded history and physical examination.

1. Attempt gentle active cervical motion so that the player may respond to pain by stopping motion. Motions should include "head nod," "chin-to-chest," and "chin-to-shoulder." If the range of motion is limited or if moderate to severe pain develops, the cervical spine should be immobilized and the player should be transported for radiography.

2. The presence of rapid onset muscle spasm is ominous and should also prompt full cervical spine precautions. On the other hand, moderate to severe neck stiffness and pain, which often develop from a cervical strain, should not appear for 1 to 2 days after the injury.

3. If active motion without resistance is tolerated, gentle resistance should then be applied by the examiner's hand.

4. If this action fails to produce pain, gentle passive range of motion may be tested.

5. Cervical tenderness is often best elicited in the supine position with the neck slightly extended. The presence of severe tenderness, especially if localized over vertebral bodies or if associated with neurological symptoms or severe spasm, is cause for great concern. Mild ten-

derness over the paraspinal muscles or spinous processes is generally much less worrisome.

B. Return to play may be permitted once the following conditions are met:
   1. Normal neurological examination.
   2. Full, pain-free, active cervical range-of-motion.
   3. Intact sensory function, motor function, and deep tendon reflexes.
   4. The absence of pain with axial compression.
   5. The absence of torticollis.
   6. The absence of dysesthesias.
   7. The athlete perceives that he or she is able to return to play.
   8. A sport-specific "functional" sideline examination does not reveal abnormalities.
   9. The athlete can be continuously observed after return to play.

IV. Further Clinical Evaluation
   A. As previously noted, the football helmet should not be removed until the player has reached the emergency facility and radiography has demonstrated the absence of bony injury to the cervical spine. Further, the helmet should be removed only by personnel who are familiar with the correct procedure. Jostling and pulling of the helmet during the extraction process present high potential for inducing further trauma.
   B. Satisfactory cervical spine and skull radiographs can usually be obtained with the football helmet in place.
   C. Procedure for the removal of a football helmet in the presence of a potential cervical injury.[6]
      1. As the head, neck, and helmet are manually stabilized, the chin strap is cut.
      2. While maintaining spine stability, the cheek pads, located inside the helmet, are removed by sliding the flat edge of a screwdriver or bandage scissors under the snaps that fasten the pad to the inner surface of the shell.
      3. As one person continues to stabilize the head and neck and another steadies the chin, the person stabilizing the head inserts his or her index fingers into the helmet ear holes and pulls laterally and longitudinally to spread the helmet and ease it off.
      4. Should a rocking motion become necessary, this must be coordinated by the two individuals.
   D. Radiographic evaluation.
      1. The importance of obtaining cervical radiographs is underscored by one study in which 32% of college freshman football players were found to have abnormalities on routine cervical spine radiography. Many could not recall prior injury.[1]
      2. Plain film radiographs should include lateral (with and without the helmet in place), anteroposterior, obliques, odontoid (open mouth view), swimmer's (if necessary), and flexion/extension views (if concern exists about stability and ligamentous disruption).
      3. Computerized tomography is especially useful to identify occult fractures in the axial plane and disk injuries and to assess and visualize the relationship of a bony injury to the spinal cord.
      4. Magnetic resonance imaging can identify cord contusions and nerve root displacement.
   E. Differentiating between injuries to nerve roots, brachial plexus, and the spinal cord.[4]
      1. Nerve root injury: pain radiates into a specific dermatome.
      2. Brachial plexus injury: persistent pain in an entire upper extremity,

sensory disturbances in multiple dermatomes, or weakness in more than one muscle.
3. Spinal cord injury: *bilateral* symptoms that often affect the lower extremities are associated with long tract signs or occur with bowel and bladder disturbances.
4. Electromyography may reliably help to distinguish between these etiologies.

V. Conclusion
   A. Injury prevention.
      1. In football most episodes of catastrophic neck injury result from initiating contact with the head.
      2. The American Football Coaches Association emphasizes that the purpose of the helmet is to protect the wearer and is not to be used as a weapon. They recommend further that greater emphasis needs to be placed by players, coaches, and officials to eliminate "spearing," "butting," and "ramming."
   B. Once a neck injury has occurred, the primary goal of the athletic medical team should be to prevent further injury.
   C. The athletic medical team must have a rehearsed "game plan" of how to efficiently and safely manage a catastrophic neck injury. Adequate preparation requires having the necessary equipment on hand, a means of transport, and ample training and practice on the part of the medical team.

References

1. Albright JP et al: Head and neck injuries in football: an eight year analysis, *Am J Sports Med* 13:147-152, 1985.
2. American Academy of Pediatrics Committee on Sports Medicine and Fitness: Head and neck injuries. In Dyment PG (ed): *Sports Medicine: Health Care for Young Athletes,* ed 2, Elk Grove Village, IL, 1991, American Academy of Pediatrics, pp 236-249.
3. Anderson C: Neck injuries: backboard, bench, or return to play? *Physician Sportsmed* 21:23-34, 1993.
4. Bailes JE, Maroon JC: Management of cervical spine injuries in athletes, *Clin Sports Med* 8:43-58, 1989.
5. Fourre M: On-site management of cervical spine injuries, *Physician Sportsmed* 19:53-56, 1991.
6. The National Collegiate Athletic Association: Guidelines for helmet fitting and removal in athletics. In: *1994-5 NCAA Sports Medicine Handbook,* Overland Park, KS, 1994, The National Collegiate Athletic Association, pp 65-66.
7. Torg JS: *Athletic Injuries to the Head, Neck, and Face,* St Louis, MO, 1991, Mosby–Year Book, pp 426-437.

CHAPTER 49

Low Back Pain

Robert J. Johnson, MD

I. Epidemiology
   A. Incidence/prevalence.
      1. Lifetime prevalence = 60% to 80%.
      2. Annual incidence = 5% (range 1% to 20%); 60% to 85% recurrence, usually in first year.
      3. Peak age incidence = 24-45 years.
      4. Cost to **us** >$50 billion/year.
   B. The workforce.
      1. Leading cause of disability in people <45 years old.
      2. Third leading cause of disability in people >45 years old.
      3. Number one reason for osteopathic and chiropractic visits.
      4. Second leading cause for visits to primary care physician offices.
      5. 40% of workers' compensation claims.
      6. 2% of national workforce has compensable back injury each year.
      7. 25% of disability costs due to low back pain.
      8. 25 million workers lose 1 or more days of work annually due to low back pain.
      9. Disability claims for low back pain increased by 2800% between 1957 and 1976 during a time in which incidence of back pain was unchanged.
   C. The sports side of back pain.
      1. General.
         a. 10% of all sports injuries involve the back.
         b. Most are self-limited, and individuals so affected never appear in your office.
         c. Almost 25% of adolescents with back pain in excess of 2-3 weeks will have structural abnormalities, most involving the pars interarticularis.
      2. Football.
         a. 6% of high school players have low back pain.

b. 30% of college players have low back pain.
c. National Football League: 12% of practice and game time is lost each season due to low back pain.

3. Basketball.
   a. Second or third most common anatomical site of injury.
   b. Position: center is most commonly injured.
   c. 15% incidence of time loss.
4. Golf.
   a. Most common injury in amateur golfers.
   b. Second most common injury in professional golfers.
5. Dance.
   a. Fourth most common injury among general dance population.
   b. Ballet: leading site of injury (San Francisco Ballet, 1990).
   c. Second most common injury site in aerobic dance.
6. Gymnastics: pars interarticularis injury.
   a. 10% incidence in female gymnasts.
   b. This incidence is four times greater than in the general population.
7. Tennis.
   a. 4% male professional players miss at least one tournament due to low back pain.
   b. 10% junior players have low back pain.
   c. 43% male tennis players have lumbar disk herniation.
8. Weight lifting: most common site of injury.
9. Swimming: 600,000 lumbar rotatory movements per year.

D. Low back pain risk factors.
1. Age: risk increases until age 50; then relative risk for men decreases.
2. Gender: Incidence of low back pain is higher in men until age 60 when the incidence (frequency) is equal.
3. Genetic: no known genetic antecedent.
4. Anthropometric factors.
   a. Spinal canal size and shape: no correlation (?).
   b. Obesity and height: role uncertain; may be mildly contributory.
5. Spinal posture: weak to nonexistent correlation.
6. Physical fitness: Unfit individuals have a greater risk than fit individuals.
7. Environmental factors: Strong association between cigarette smoking and low back pain.
8. Workplace factors.
   a. Risk increased in those who lift, bend, twist.
   b. Sedentary: associated with increased risk.
   c. Vibration: increased risk for low back pain.
9. Psychosocial factors (most important risk factors).
   a. Job dissatisfaction.
   b. View of injury as compensable.
   c. Psychological dysfunction: depression, anxiety, hypochondriasis.
   d. Poor health habits.
   e. Less appealing work environment.
   f. Poor ratings by supervisors.
   g. History of prior disability.

E. Predictability of low back disability.
1. Physical and diagnostic factors: diagnosis had little impact on disability. 90% of those with compensable low back pain have nonspecific diagnosis.

2. Acute treatment: little effect, but unnecessary; unproven interventions *may prolong* disability.
3. Muscle strength/endurance: Preemployment lifting evaluation has decreased injury rate when work capacity matched with tasks.
4. Psychologic status: MMPI characterization—hypochondriasis, hysteria, depression ("inverted V").
5. Work environment: job dissatisfaction, unpleasant work conditions, repetitive or menial tasks; interaction between worker and supervisor is most important determinant.
6. Compensation and perception of injury: potent predictor; engagement of attorney implies poor prognosis.
7. Demographics: associated with decreased income, lower education level, lower levels of physical activity.

F. Duration of disability and return to work.
   1. Disability >6 months = 50% chance.
   2. Disability of 1 year = 20% chance.
   3. Disability >2 years = 0% chance.

II. History
   A. Pertinent questions.
      1. Usual historical data.
      2. Usual activity, sport, pastime?
      3. Initiating event?
      4. Sites and boundaries of pain?
      5. Radiation?
      6. Is the pain deep? Superficial? Shooting? Burning? Aching?
      7. Paresthesia or anesthesia?
      8. Aggravating activities?
      9. Activities that relieve pain?
      10. Is pain improving? Worsening?
      11. Pain while sleeping?
      12. Any problems with voiding?
      13. Postures that improve or exacerbate pain?
      14. Worse in A.M.? P.M.? As the day progresses?
      15. Medications? Associated medical problems?
   B. Mechanisms of musculoskeletal pain.
      1. Constant ache: inflammatory process.
      2. Pain on movement: noxious mechanical stimuli (stretch, pressure, crush).
      3. Pain accumulates with activity: repeated mechanical stress, inflammatory process, degenerative disk.
      4. Pain increases with sustained posture: fatigue in muscle support, gradual creep of tissues may stress affected part of motor unit.
      5. Latent nerve root pain: movement has produced an acute and temporary neurapraxia.

III. Physical Examination
   A. Observation.
      1. Gait.
      2. Attitude (tense, lethargic, bored, etc.).
      3. Spinal posture.
      4. Step deformity in lumbar spine (spondylolisthesis).
   B. Palpation
      1. Bony.
      2. Soft tissue.

C. Range of motion, patient standing.
   1. Observe differences, asymmetry, willingness of patient to perform movements.
   2. Consider "overpressure" if tolerable pain.
   3. Hold position additional 10-20 seconds to see if symptoms increase.
   4. Forward flexion (maximum is 40-60 degrees). Measurement between spinous processes increases 7-8 cm when taken between T12 and S1. Note how far patient is able to bend forward (midthigh, knees, midtibia, floor) and compare to straight leg raising test.
   5. Extension (20-35 degrees). Hold for 10-20 seconds.
   6. Lateral flexion (15-20 degrees). Observe lumbar curve for smooth motion and curve to side of motion. Angulation suggest hypomobility of lumbar spine.
   7. Rotation (3-18 degrees). Stabilize pelvis to prevent pelvic rotation.
   8. Consider combination movements: lateral flexion in flexion, lateral flexion in extension, flexion and rotation, and extension and rotation.
   9. One-legged stance to observe for Trendelenburg sign.

D. Passive movements (+/−).

E. Resisted movements. Patient seated. Test forward flexion, extension, side flexion, rotation.

F. Special tests.
   1. Straight leg raising test (Lasègue's test). Unilateral leg raise is complete at 70 degrees. Positive test is one that duplicates radicular pain.
   2. Neck flexion + straight leg (Brudzinski's sign).
   3. Ankle dorsiflexion + straight leg (Bragard's test).
   4. Bilateral straight leg raise: pain at <70 degrees suggests sacroiliac pain; pain at >70 degrees suggests lumbar pain.
   5. Crossover test: raising "well leg" causes radicular pain in opposite leg.
   6. Femoral nerve traction test: patient lies on unaffected side with hip and knee flexed. Passively flex knee of affected leg while gently extending hip. This puts traction on nerve roots at the midlumbar area (L2-L4). A positive test is pain.
   7. "Bowstring" test: sciatic nerve.
   8. Sitting root test: sciatic nerve.
   9. Reflexes.
      a. Patellar (L3-L4).
      b. Medial hamstrings (L5-S1).
      c. Lateral hamstrings (S1-S2).
      d. Posterior tibial (L4-L5).
      e. Achilles (L5-S1).
   10. Sensory examination.
   11. One-legged hyperextension test: positive test suggests pars interarticularis injury.
   12. Motor examination.
      a. L2-L3: hip flexors, adductors.
      b. L3-L4: knee extension (quadriceps).
      c. L4-L5, S1: foot dorsiflexion, foot inversion, plantar flexion.

IV. Treatment of Musculoligamentous Low Back Pain

A. The dilemma.
   1. ". . . few treatments for low back pain have proven to be more effective than placebo" (Deyo, Nachemson).

2. "Abnormal diagnostic behavior by physicians leads to abnormal illness behavior on the part of the patient; then the patient's illness behavior begins to influence the doctor's treatment decisions" (Nachemson).
3. "Back pain is not the epidemic. Back pain treatment, back pain disability, and related spending is" (Bigos).
4. "Physicians are doing too much to patients" (Bigos).
   a. Overtesting.
   b. Overtreatment.
   c. Endless treatment.
   d. Ineffective conservative treatment.
   e. Inappropriate surgery.

B. Prognosis of low back pain (regardless of treatment or diagnosis).
   1. 70% are improved in <1 week.
   2. 70% are asymptomatic in <1 month.
   3. 90% are asymptomatic in 6-12 weeks.

C. Treatment principles ("three Es").
   1. **E**xercise: early controlled motion, exercise to quota (exercise to a specific time limit rather than to a symptom, such as pain).
   2. **E**ducation: 94% of those with good understanding of back and back pain returned to work; only 33% of those with poor understanding returned to work.
   3. **E**ncouragement: Minimize medication use.

D. Agency for Health Care Policy and Research Recommendations (1995).
   1. As much activity as tolerated.
   2. Early return to work.
   3. Manipulation (within first 3-4 weeks).

E. Specific treatment for low back pain.
   1. Rest (remember, it's a four-letter word): study in primary care showed those with no rest returned to usual activities 42% faster than patients on bedrest. If rest is prescribed, place a specific time limit.
   2. Ice (therapeutic) vs. heat (symptomatic).
   3. Exercise: in randomized trials, physical therapy was no more efficacious than increasing activity. General endurance training, stretching, strengthening of back extensors, abdominal, and lower extremity muscles are *probably* efficacious.
   4. Activity: *MOVE!*
   5. Medications.
      a. Nonsteroidal antiinflammatory drugs (NSAIDs) (if effective, due to analgesic properties; acetaminophen is likely to be as effective).
      b. Muscle relaxants: no proven efficacy other than central nervous system depression.
      c. Antidepressants: chronic pain situation.
   6. Traction: no proven benefit.
   7. Return to work (be creative).

F. Hints of behavioral disturbance.
   1. Widespread superficial tenderness to touch.
   2. Widespread tenderness not fitting normal anatomical distribution.
   3. Low back pain on axial loading.
   4. Pain with passive trunk rotation.
   5. Distracted straight leg raising test.
   6. Altered sensation that is nonanatomical.
   7. Motor weakness that is nonanatomical.

G. Prevention strategies.
   1. Primary prevention.
      a. Attempts to determine factors that cause disabling low back pain and creation of programs to prevent these situations have had modest impact at best.
      b. Include fitness and worksite changes.
   2. Secondary.
      a. Short term: effective.
      b. Long term: uncertain effect.
      c. Preventing recurrence: minimal.
   3. Tertiary.
      a. Pertains to those who have become disabled.
      b. Goal is to return individual to function and have individual accept residual impairment.
      c. Results are highly variable.

V. Problems of the Lumbar Spine
A. Herniated nucleus pulposus.
   1. Characteristics.
      a. Most common in those 30-50 years old.
      b. L5-S1 is most common (90%). Cauda equina syndrome occurs in 0.24% to 2%.
      c. Progressive paresis/unrelenting pain: 5% to 20%.
   2. Etiology: abnormality in annulus fibrosus, degenerative tears of annulus lead to bulging nucleus pulposus. Increased pressure within disk space, especially with flexion and rotation, causing the material to migrate posteriorly. Repeated activity may cause the material to encroach on nerve roots.
   3. Symptoms.
      a. Pain caused by annular nerve irritation, inflammatory response, nerve root compression.
      b. Neurological: unilateral or bilateral paresthesias exacerbated by sitting, riding in car, bending or twisting. Relieved by knee flexion, fetal position, prone position with stomach supported.
   4. Signs.
      a. Positive straight leg raise test, positive bowstring test, other neurological tests as outlined in the physical examination section.
      b. Increased pain with flexion activities.
   5. Differential diagnosis: remember other causes such as infection, tumor, inflammatory condition, degenerative disease, musculoskeletal ligamentous injury, intraabdominal and retroperitoneal causes.
   6. Radiographic evaluation.
      a. Computerized tomography (CT): 36% abnormalities in asymptomatic people (Wiesel, 1984); best to evaluate bony abnormalities, canal size and shape, lateral recesses, and facet joints.
      b. Myelography: 24% abnormalities in asymptomatic people (Hitselberg, 1968).
      c. Diskography: 37% abnormalities in asymptomatic people (Holt, 1968).
   7. Noncompressive (biochemical) radiculopathy.
      a. Nonneurogenic mediators (PLA_2).
      b. Neurogenic mediators (substance P).
      c. Autoimmune response.
   8. Treatment.
      a. Conservative.

(1) Spontaneous resolution without surgery due to foreign body granulation tissue, fragment dehydration.
(2) Largest herniations resolve the most.

b. Measures.
(1) Activity as tolerated.
(2) Anecdotal reports of prednisone use for 4-5 days.
(3) Control symptoms.
(4) Exercise.

c. Surgical.
(1) 75% to 90% recover without surgery.
(2) 10% to 17% need surgery.
(3) Indications: Progressive neurological deficit, cauda equina syndrome, recurrent radiculopathy with neurological symptoms.

B. Spondylolysis: stress injury of the pars interarticularis.
1. Epidemiology.
a. 5% to 8% in general population.
b. Occurs in gymnasts, dancers, football linemen and linebackers, competitive divers, weight lifters, pole vaulters.
c. Unusual before age 5.
d. Defects most often occur in those 5-10 years of age, most of whom are asymptomatic.
e. 85% occur at L5, 15% at L4, rarely occurring at higher lumbar levels.
2. Mechanism of injury.
a. Associated with extension, rotation, bending activities.
b. No evidence of congenital occurrence.
3. Scope of injury.
a. Pars stress injury (stress fracture of the pars, no changes on standard radiographs; positive bone scan or single photon emission computerized tomography scan).
b. Unilateral spondylolysis.
c. Bilateral spondylolysis.
4. Symptoms.
a. Pain adjacent to midline structures.
b. Increased pain with extension, rotation activities.
5. Signs.
a. One-finger, almost midline, pain.
b. Pain with extension.
c. Positive one-legged hyperextension test.
6. Radiography: may be negative or "scotty dog" appearance on oblique film.
7. Treatment.
a. Mild symptoms: modification or mild restriction of exacerbating activities, abdominal strengthening, hamstring stretching.
b. Moderate to severe symptoms: cessation of all exacerbating activities (may require 6-12 weeks), abdominal strengthening, hamstring stretching; consider antilordotic brace (?).
c. After pain-free interval, gradual return to previous level of activity.
d. Antilordotic braces are used by some, but this approach is not a uniform treatment mode.

C. Spondylolisthesis: sliding of one vertebra over another, usually due to loss of stabilizing effect of pars interarticularis (bilateral spondylolysis).

1. Mechanism of injury: same as that of spondylolysis. Sports of involvement are similar.
2. Symptoms: similar to those of spondylolysis; significant spondylolisthesis may also have neurological symptoms.
3. Signs: in addition to those found in spondylolysis, a "step-off" may be noted in the lumbar spine.
4. Scope of injury.
   a. Grade I: 25% slip.
   b. Grade II: 50% slip.
   c. Grade III: 75% slip.
   d. Grade IV: 100% slip.
   e. Spondylolisthesis may be completely asymptomatic and an incidental finding on radiography.
5. Radiography: lateral film demonstrates the "slip" of one vertebra on another.
6. Treatment.
   a. Asymptomatic (usually grade I-II).
      (1) No activity restriction.
      (2) Abdominal strengthening and hamstring stretching as in pars injuries.
   b. Symptomatic (usually greater than grade II).
      (1) Modify or restrict activities based on symptoms.
      (2) Hamstring stretch, abdominal strengthening.
      (3) Antilordotic brace (+/−).
      (4) Surgery for progressing spondylolisthesis or neurological symptoms, usually grade II or greater. Symptomatic "slips" must be monitored by interval radiographs to determine if they are progressing.

D. Facet syndrome.
1. Characteristics.
   a. Most common in degenerative disk disease.
   b. Radicular pain.
   c. Pathophysiology: as joints degenerate, disk spaces narrow, causing facet joints to sublux posteriorly. This narrows intervertebral foramen, leading to impingement on nerve.
2. Symptoms.
   a. Similar to radiculopathy associated with disk herniation.
   b. More diffuse back pain may also be present.
3. Signs.
   a. Findings of nerve root impingement.
   b. Increased muscle spasm in paravertebral muscles.
4. Radiography.
   a. Oblique films may show narrowed foramina.
   b. CT may show narrowed foramina.
5. Treatment.
   a. Symptom-limited activity.
   b. NSAIDs or corticosteroids to reduce edema of neural elements.
   c. Facet injections (corticosteroids).
   d. Surgery for resistant problems.

E. Ankylosing spondylitis.
1. Characteristics.
   a. 1% prevalence.
   b. Autoimmune disease.
   c. Involves sacroiliac joint.

2. Symptoms.
   a. Insidious onset, ages 15-35.
   b. Symptoms >3 months.
   c. AM stiffness.
   d. Pain usually improves with exercise.
3. Signs.
   a. Back pain.
   b. 20% have peripheral joint involvement.
   c. Enthesopathies are common (plantar fasciitis, Achilles tendinitis, costochondritis).
   d. Extraskeletal involvement of eyes, lungs, heart may occur.
   e. HLA-B27 positive, seropositive.
4. Radiography: sacroiliac (S-I) joints show blurring and patchy sclerosis of joint margins. Usually bilateral.
5. Changes occur in lumbar spine that are radiographically evident and may cause restricted motion of lumbar spine.
6. Treatment.
   a. Maintain posture to minimize kyphotic changes.
   b. NSAIDs and corticosteroids typically ease pain.

F. Piriformis syndrome.
1. Characteristics.
   a. Irritation of sciatic nerve as it exits beneath piriformis muscle.
   b. Caused by nerve irritation by hypertrophied or spastic muscle.
   c. Trauma may be implicated in half of cases.
2. Examination.
   a. Lumbar spine has normal range of motion in spite of significant pain.
   b. Sciatic notch tenderness.
   c. Positive or negative straight-leg raising (SLR) test.
   d. Active external rotation and passive internal rotation of hip trigger symptoms.
3. Difficult diagnosis because it is difficult to confirm by testing and examination. Symptoms closely mimic disk herniation.
4. Treatment.
   a. Conservative rest-ice-compression-elevation (R-I-C-E) measures.
   b. Stretching of hip abductors.
   c. Consider corticosteroid injection at site of pain.
   d. Rarely, surgical decompression is necessary.

Bibliography

Alexander MJL: Biomechanical aspects of lumbar spine injuries in athletes: a review, *Can J Appl Sport Sci* 10(1):1-20, 1985.

Brigham CD, Schafer MF: Low back pain in athletes, *Adv Sports Med Fitness,* 1:145-182, 1988.

Cacayorin ED, Hichhauser L, Petro GR: Lumbar and thoracic spine in the athlete: radiographic evaluation, *Clin Sports Med* 6(4):767-783, 1987.

Deusinger RH: Biomechanical considerations for clinical application with low back pain, *Clin Sports Med* 8(4):703-715, 1989.

Deyo RA: Conservative therapy for low back pain: Distinguishing useful from useless therapy, *JAMA* 250:1057, 1983.

Flemming JE: *The Spine in Sports: Spondylolysis and Spondylolisthesis in the Athlete,* Philadelphia, 1990, Hanley and Belfus.

Hitselberger WE, Witten RM: Abnormal myelograms in asymptomatic patients, *J Neurosurg* 28:204-206, 1968.

Holt EP, Jr: The question of lumbar discography, *J Bone Joint Surg* 50:720, 1968.

Kraus DR, Shapiro D: The symptomatic lumbar spine in the athlete, *Clin Sports Med* 8(1):59-69, 1989.

Nachemson AL: Newest knowledge of low back pain: A critical look, *Clin Ortho & Related Research* 279:8-20, 1992.
Spencer CW, Jackson DW: Back injuries in the athlete, *Clin Sports Med* 2(1):191-215, 1983.
Stanitski CL: Management of sports injuries in children and adolescents, *Orthop Clin North Am* 19(4):689-697, 1988.
Symposium: Assessment and management of back pain in the physically active individual, *ACSM* June 1994.
Wiesel SW, Tsourmas N, Feffer HL, et al: A study of computer-assisted tomography: The incidence of positive CAT scans in an asymptomatic group of patients, *Spine* 9:59-551, 1984.
Wilhite J, Huurman WW: Thoracic and lumbosacral spine. In Mellion M, Walsh WM, Shelton G, editors: *The Team Physician's Handbook,* Philadelphia, 1990, Hanley and Belfus, pp 374-400.

CHAPTER 50

Spondylolysis and Spondylolisthesis

Peter G. Gerbino II, MD

Lyle J. Micheli, MD

I. Definitions
   A. Spondylolysis: nondisplaced stress or traumatic fracture of the pars interarticularis.[35,37]
   B. Spondylolisthesis: "vertebral sliding."[13] Displaced spondylolysis or other circumstance leading to forward displacement of one vertebral segment upon its subjacent neighbor.[23]
   C. Prespondylolytic stress reaction[3]: repetitive cyclic loading of pars interarticularis leading to increased isotope uptake by ^{99}Tc bone scan but preceding actual stress fracture.
   D. Spondyloptosis: complete dislocation of one vertebral segment upon another.

II. Classification
   A. Spondylolytic process.
      1. Repetitive cyclic loading (hyperextension).
      2. Prespondylolytic pars interarticularis stress reaction.
      3. Spondylolysis (unilateral or bilateral).
      4. Spondylolisthesis (stable or progressive).
      5. Spondyloptosis.
   B. Spondylolisthesis.
      1. Grading by percent slip.[14]
         a. Grade I: ≤25%.
         b. Grade II: 25% to 50%.
         c. Grade III: 50% to 75%.
         d. Grade IV: 75% to 100%.
      2. Grading by slip angle.[2]
         a. Predicts propensity for progression.
         b. Measure angle between inferior endplate of upper vertebra and superior endplate of lower vertebra.
         c. Greater than 50 degrees in skeletally immature patient indicates high risk for progression.

3. Grading by morphological types of spondylolisthesis.[36]
   a. Dysplastic: true developmental deficiency of lumbar facet or posterior element architecture, permitting facilitated displacement.
   b. Isthmic: bilateral pars interarticularis deficiency or fracture permitting motion.
      (1) Lytic: a pars stress fracture.
      (2) Elongation: stress remodeling of the pars.[10]
      (3) Acute: traumatic fracture of the pars.
   c. Degenerative: facet joint arthrosis and distortion leading to vertebral displacement.
   d. Traumatic: acute fracture of the posterior elements other than the pars, permitting displacement.
   e. Pathological: underlying disease state leading to posterior element fracture or attenuation and displacement.

III. Etiology
   A. True etiology is unknown.
   B. Incidence in general population is approximately 5%.[28]
   C. Heredity is involved as a predisposing factor in some patients.
      1. Alaskan Native Americans have a 50% incidence in their general population.[32]
      2. Coincidence of spondylolysis among first degree family members is 50%.[38]
      3. Increased incidence in patients with spina bifida occulta, scoliosis, laminar defects, and transitional vertebrae.[5,22,29]
   D. Spondylolysis in athletes is different from general population.
      1. Familial coexistence rate is unknown but felt to be less than in general population.
      2. Frequency of coexistent spinal abnormalities is unknown.
      3. Incidence in gymnasts is 11%.[12]
      4. Spondylolysis in athletes is a pars interarticularis stress fracture.
         a. Sports with hyperextension maneuvers involve the greatest risk.
            (1) Gymnastics.[3,15]
            (2) Football.[18]
            (3) Dancing.[11,20]
            (4) Figure skating.[19]
         b. Patients who are unable to walk from birth never develop spondylolysis.[27]
   E. Factors that cause slippage as opposed to nondisplaced stress fracture are unknown.

IV. Clinical Findings (Athletes)
   A. History.
      1. Athlete ≤18 years old with low back pain complaint has a 45% likelihood of having spondylolytic etiology.[21]
      2. If hyperextension of the lumbar spine is part of the sport, the incidence increases.
      3. Hyperextension maneuvers in sports lead to increased pain.
   B. Physical examination.
      1. Gait is antalgic or normal.
      2. Lumbar musculature and hamstrings are tight. Hyperlordosis is common.[6]
      3. Lumbar spine extension exacerbates symptoms.
      4. Buttock or thigh pain may be present.[16]
      5. Sciatica is a rare finding in adolescents.[34]

6. With spondylolisthesis, there may be hyperlordosis and "heart-shaped" buttocks.[9]
7. Adults may have sciatica, neurological findings, or exercise-induced claudication.[8]

V. Diagnostic Imaging
 A. Plain radiographs.
  1. Anteroposterior: check for spina bifida occulta, scoliosis, transitional vertebra.
  2. Lateral: inspect disc heights, lordosis, obvious spondylolysis or spondylolisthesis. Standing lateral view best brings out spondylolisthesis slip angle and displacement.[2]
  3. Obliques: check "scotty dog" of Lachapele. Look for pars interarticularis fracture elongation, or sclerosis. Determine whether condition is unilateral or bilateral.[30]
 B. Technetium bone scan.
  1. Standard bone scan inadequate.
  2. Single photon emission computerized tomography (SPECT) bone scan is specific for early stress reaction in pars.[1,4,24,26,29]
  3. Low uptake in a radiographically obvious spondylolysis indicates long-standing fibrous nonunion and poorer healing potential.
 C. Computerized tomography (CT) can show detail of fracture. Gives best detail of facet arthrosis and spinal stenosis.
 D. Magnetic resonance imaging: Hypointense at pars stress area on T1 image. May replace SPECT bone scan for primary diagnosis in future.[39]

VI. Treatment
 A. Goals.
  1. Prespondylolytic pars stress reaction.
   a. Resolution of pain.
   b. Healing of pars.
   c. Strengthening of pars.
  2. Spondylolysis.
   a. Resolution of pain.
   b. Healing of pars fracture with bony union.
   c. Healing of pars fracture with fibrous union if bony union not possible.
  3. Spondylolisthesis.
   a. Resolution of pain.
   b. Prevention of progression.
   c. Healing of fracture rarely possible.
 B. Protocol.
  1. Prespondylolytic stress reaction and spondylolysis.
   a. Boston overlapping brace in 0-degrees lordosis, 23 hours per day.[17,31]
   b. Physical therapy for hamstring stretching. Lumbar flexibility in brace at first, out of brace as symptoms resolve.
   c. Avoid sports at first. Advance to full participation in brace as symptoms resolve.
   d. Continue bracing up to 6 to 9 months as necessary to heal pars.
   e. May need repeat SPECT bone scan or CT scan to monitor healing.
   f. Electromagnetic field treatment for persistent nonunion may be used. No data yet available on efficacy.[25]
  2. Spondylolisthesis.
   a. Boston overlapping brace in 0-degree lordosis, 23 hours per day.

b. Physical therapy for hamstring stretching. Lumbar flexibility in brace at first, out of brace as symptoms resolve.
c. Continue bracing until fracture symptoms resolve. Ensure that there is no progression of slip.
d. Bony union unnecessary for full return to sports.
3. Spondylolisthesis with progression or persistent pain.
a. Spinal fusion in situ.[7,33]
b. Spinal fusion with hardware and possible reduction.[9]
c. Direct repair of pars defect.[7]
4. Future considerations.
a. Greater use of pars repair rather than fusion.
b. Electrical stimulation to enhance union of pars defect.[25]

VII. Conclusions
A. Spondylolysis in athletes is a stress fracture caused by repetitive hyperextension.
B. The fracture can be treated and healing may be facilitated by immobilization in a rigid antilordotic brace.
C. Adults may also have degenerative disks, facet arthrosis, or spinal stenosis confounding treatment.

References

1. Bellah RD et al: Low-back pain in adolescent athletes: detection of stress injury to the pars interarticularis with SPECT, *Radiology* 180:509-512, 1991.
2. Boxall D et al: Management of severe spondylolisthesis in children and adolescents, *J Bone Joint Surg* 61A(4):479-495, 1979.
3. Cirillo JV, Jackson DW: Pars interarticularis stress reaction, spondylolysis, and spondylolisthesis in gymnasts, *Clin Sports Med* 4(1):95-110, 1985.
4. Collier BD et al: Painful spondylolysis or spondylolisthesis studied by radiography and single-photon emission computed tomography, *Radiology* 154(1):207-211, 1985.
5. Cowell MJ, Cowell HR: The incidence of spina bifida occulta in idiopathic scoliosis, *Clin Orthop* 118:16-18, 1976.
6. Gerbino PG, Micheli LJ: Back injuries in the young athlete, *Clin Sports Med* 14(3):571-590, 1995.
7. Hardcastle PH: Repair of spondylolysis in young fast bowlers, *J Bone Joint Surg* 75B(3):398-402, 1993.
8. Harris IE, Weinstein SL: Long-term follow-up of patients with grade III and IV spondylolisthesis, *J Bone Joint Surg* 69A(7):960-969, 1987.
9. Hensinger RN: Spondylolysis and spondylolisthesis in children. In Floman Y, ed: *Disorders of the Lumbar Spine*, Rockville, MD, 1990, Aspen Publishers.
10. Hensinger RN, Lang JR, MacEwen GD: Surgical management of spondylolisthesis in children and adolescents, *Spine* 1(4):207-216, 1976.
11. Ireland ML, Micheli LJ: Bilateral stress fracture of the lumbar pedicles in a ballet dancer, *J Bone Joint Surg* 69A:140-142, 1987.
12. Jackson DW, Wiltse LL, Cirincoine RJ: Spondylolysis in the female gymnast, *Clin Orthop* 117:68, 1976.
13. Kilian H: De spondylolisthesis gravissimae pelvangustiae caussa nuper detecta. Commentario Anatomico-Obstetrica. Bonn, 1854, Georgii.
14. Meyerding HW: Spondylolisthesis, *Surg Gynecol Obstet* 54:371, 1932.
15. Micheli LJ: Back injuries in gymnastics, *Clin Sports Med* 4(1):85-92, 1985.
16. Micheli LJ: Low back pain in the adolescent: differential diagnosis, *Am J Sports Med* 7:362-364, 1979.
17. Micheli LJ, Hall JE, Miller ME: Use of modified Boston brace for back injuries in athletes, *Am J Sports Med* 8:351-356, 1980.
18. Micheli LJ, Kasser JR: Case Report 6: painful spondylolysis in a young football player. In Hochschuler SH, ed: *The Spine in Sports*, Philadelphia, 1990, Hanley and Belfus.
19. Micheli LJ, McCarthy C: Figure skating. In Watkins RG, ed: *The Spine in Sports*, St Louis, Mosby–Year Book, pp 557-563, 1996.
20. Micheli LJ, Micheli ER: Back injuries in dancers. In Shell CG, ed: *The 1984 Olympic Scientific Congress Proceedings, Vol 8: The Dancer as Athlete*, Champaign, IL, 1986, Human Kinetics Publishers.
21. Micheli LJ, Wood R: Back pain in young athletes. Significant differences from adults in causes and patterns, *Arch Pediatr Adolesc Med* 149:15-18, 1995.

22. Miki T et al: Congenital laminar defect of the upper lumbar spine associated with pars defect. A report of eleven cases, *Spine* 16(3):353-355, 1991.
23. Neugebauer F: Aetiologic der Sogenncanten spondylolisthesis, *Arch Gynak Munchen* 35:375, 1882.
24. Papanicolaou N et al: Bone scintigraphy and radiography in young athletes with low back pain, *Am J Radiol* 145:1039-1044, 1985.
25. Pettine KA, Salib RN, Walker SG: External electrical stimulation and bracing for treatment of spondylolysis. A case report, *Spine* 18(4):436-439, 1993.
26. Rosen PR, Micheli LJ, Treves S: Early scintigraphic diagnosis of bone stress and fractures in athletic adolescents, *Pediatrics* 70(1):11-15, 1982.
27. Rosenberg NJ, Bargar WL, Freidman B: The incidence of spondylolysis and spondylolisthesis in nonambulatory patients, *Spine* 6(1):35-38, 1981.
28. Rowe GG, Roche MB: The etiology of separate neural arch, *J Bone Joint Surg* 35A(1):102-110, 1953.
29. Shands AR, Bundens WD: Congenital deformities of the spine. Analysis of the roentgenograms of 700 children, *Bull Hosp Joint Dis* 17(2):110, 1956.
30. Sherman FC, Wilkinson RH, Hall JE: Reactive sclerosis of a pedicle and spondylolysis in the lumbar spine, *J Bone Joint Surg* 59A(1):49-56, 1977.
31. Steiner ME, Micheli LJ: Treatment of symptomatic spondylolysis and spondylolisthesis with the modified Boston brace, *Spine* 10:937-943, 1985.
32. Stewart TD: The age incidence of neural-arch defects in Alaskan natives, considered from the standpoint of etiology, *J Bone Joint Surg* 35A(4):937-950, 1953.
33. Stinson JT: Spondylolysis and spondylolisthesis in the athlete, *Clin Sports Med* 12(3):517-528, 1993.
34. Turner RH, Bianco AJ Jr: Spondylolysis and spondylolisthesis in children and teenagers, *J Bone Joint Surg* 53A(7):1298-1306, 1971.
35. Wiltse LL: The etiology of spondylolisthesis, *J Bone Joint Surg* 44A(3):539-560, 1962.
36. Wiltse LL, Newman PH, Macnab I: Classification of spondylolysis and spondylolisthesis, *Clin Orthop* 117:23-29, 1976.
37. Wiltse LL, Widell EH Jr, Jackson DW: Fatigue fracture. The bone lesion in isthmic spondylolisthesis, *J Bone Joint Surg* 57A(1):17-22, 1975.
38. Wynne-Davies R, Scott JH: Inheritance and spondylolisthesis: a radiographic family survey, *J Bone Joint Surg* 61B(3):301-305, 1979.
39. Yamane T, Yoshida T, Mimatsu K: Early diagnosis of lumbar spondylolysis by MRI, *J Bone Joint Surg* 75B(5):764-768, 1993.

CHAPTER 51

Lumbar Spine Pain: Rehabilitation and Return to Play

Andrew J. Cole, MD, FACSM

Stanley A. Herring, MD, FACSM

I. Background
   A. Epidemiology of lumbar spine sports injuries.
      1. Most frequent site of injury: Gymnastics, football, weightlifting, wrestling, dance, rowing, swimming, amateur golf, ballet.*
      2. Second most frequent site of injury: professional golf, aerobic dance.[17,18,47]
      3. Less frequent but statistically significant: general dance, skating, tennis, baseball, jogging, cycling, basketball.[13,20,21,28,42,58]
      4. Time lost from sports participation.
         a. Football: 12% incidence of spine injuries necessitating time loss.[48]
         b. Basketball: 15% of missed playing time of centers due to low back pain.[58]
         c. Tennis: 40% of men's professional tennis tour players missed at least one tournament because of back pain.[20]
   B. Epidemiology of lumbar spine pain: implications.[26]
      1. 60% to 90% lifetime incidence and 5% annual incidence.
      2. Peak incidence at 40 years old; 12% to 26% of children and adolescents experience low back pain.
      3. 90% of cases resolve without medical attention in 6-12 weeks, 40% to 50% are symptom free within 1 week, and 75% with sciatica have relief of pain at 6 months.
      4. 70% to 90% of patients have recurrent episodes.
      5. Therefore, although there may be *symptomatic* improvement, anatomical and functional changes may persist that increase the chance of reinjury. The anatomical structures and functional deficits that develop with sports-related injuries of the lumbar spine are the same as for the general population. The musculoskeletal demands that sports activity creates may precipitate more significant symptoms. A comprehensive rehabilitation program must be initiated immediately so

*References 9, 17, 18, 22, 26, 29, 31, 42-44, 52.

that all aspects of an athlete's entire injury complex are thoroughly rehabilitated and return to competition can occur rapidly and safely. The rehabilitation program is based on an understanding of the unique biomechanical stresses placed on the lumbar spine and its entire kinetic chain by any given individual sport.[26]

C. Why rehabilitate?[25]
 1. To most rapidly resolve the clinical symptoms and signs created by the primary lumbar spine injury so that active treatment can be initiated and the deleterious effects of inactivity minimized. Prolonged bedrest results in decreases in muscle strength, flexibility, cardiovascular fitness, bone density, and disk nutrition as well as increased spinal segmental stiffness and depression.[6,55]
 2. To restore function, return to sport and minimize the chance of a recurrence by rehabilitating both the primary site of injury and any secondary sites of dysfunction.
  a. ≤70% loss in trunk musculature strength after 6 months of lumbosacral pain.[40]
  b. Thus rehabilitation continues beyond the resolution of symptoms so that all other aspects of the injury complex are fully rehabilitated including normalizing flexibility, strength, power, and endurance.
  c. The single best predictor for a new injury during athletic activity is a history of a previous injury.[3,4,19,38,45]
 3. To create a *pre*habilitation program based on the *re*habilitation program so that optimum physiological and biomechanical fitness can be maintained and risk of future injury minimized.[34]

II. Factors Influencing Rehabilitation Program Design and Progression[26,27,51]
 A. There are few lumbar spine physical examination tests that specifically define the precise structure or structures that have been injured and/or are painful.
 B. The initial assessment is really a functional diagnosis because it is based on the history, physical examination, and recognition of specific reproducible patterns of painful motion.
 C. Initial treatment techniques seek to minimize pain by avoiding painful patterns of movement while expanding nonpainful patterns.
 D. Reduction of pain is a very important guide to help measure treatment success. If the athlete fails to progress or reaches a plateau during rehabilitation, reevaluation is imperative.
  1. Further diagnostic testing (imaging, electrodiagnostic testing) may be required so that specific pain control techniques can be utilized and the rehabilitation program advanced.
   a. Change of physical therapy techniques. (See section III).
   b. Addition or change in oral medication. (See section III).
   c. A fluoroscopically guided contrast-enhanced diagnostic and therapeutic spinal injection procedure (e.g., facet, selective nerve root, epidural, or sacroiliac joint injection). If done under fluoroscopic guidance with contrast enhancement, the injection is *both* diagnostic (the precisely placed local anesthetic anesthetizes the presumed painful structure) and therapeutic (the steroid [and possibly the anesthetic] decreases or eliminates pain that is mediated by inflammation).[7,10,11,16,57]
  2. Distinguish between low back pain and low back pain disability.[50] Low back pain disability syndrome is a product of the painful musculoskeletal injury and the athlete's adaptation to it (i.e., significant

psychosocial overlay exists). Consider psychological intervention in addition to physical therapeutic treatment.

III. The Rehabilitation Program[26]
   A. Rehabilitation principles apply to all spine disorders in the acute, subacute, and chronic settings for both nonsurgical and surgical patients.
   B. A comprehensive rehabilitation program ensures that rehabilitation progresses beyond the absence of symptoms since absence of symptoms does not necessarily imply normal function.
      1. A comprehensive rehabilitation program corrects soft-tissue inflexibilities, strength, endurance and power in the involved spinal segments and the entire kinetic chain.
      2. The program also provides education and training for posture, body mechanics, proprioception, and a supervised return to sport.
   C. No one component of the rehabilitation program should be used in isolation, but rather in concert with other appropriate components.
   D. Acute phase.
      1. Education: proper body mechanics for movement and activities of daily living; natural history of spine injury.[30]
      2. Physical modalities: little benefit if used in isolation.[14,33]
         a. Superficial cold and heat: decreases spasm and pain.[32] Ice packs, gel packs (cold); heating pads, hydrocollator packs, whirlpool (heat): penetrates to a depth of only 2 cm.
         b. Deep heat (diathermy): decreases spasm and pain, increases collagen distensibility (helping to improve flexibility).[8] Ultrasound most commonly; microwave and shortwave rarely used due to increased risks, equipment costs, and portability difficulties.
         c. Therapeutic electricity: decreases spasm, edema, and pain.[56]
            (1) High-voltage pulsed galvanic stimulation (HVPGS).
            (2) Transcutaneous electric nerve stimulation (TENS).
      3. Medications: permit early and more rapid progression of rehabilitation by decreasing pain and/or inflammation.[46]
         a. Nonsteroidal antiinflammatory drugs (NSAIDs): see Chapter 28. Studies do not specifically demonstrate efficacy for low back pain.[26]
         b. Nonnarcotic and narcotic: acetaminophen plus NSAID enhances analgesia. Narcotics for more severe acute pain: at an adequate dose for pain relief on a time-contingent basis. Rarely a role for prolonged use of narcotics.
         c. Muscle relaxants: studies do not clearly show efficacy for low back pain.[26] Central effect causes lethargy that can inhibit ability to participate in rehabilitation and interfere with the cognitive learning that is needed with patient education phase.
         d. Corticosteroids: pain relief from antiinflammatory action. Oral or injected. (See section II.D.1.c.)
      4. Manual therapy[50]: helps to modulate pain, provides early controlled motion and stresses to the injured lumbar spine segments.
      5. Mechanical therapy/traction: may provide pain relief by intervertebral distraction, stretching muscle and other soft tissue structures and providing a period of relative rest. If symptoms are diskogenic, apply traction in prone position to unload disk; if primarily posterior element pain, apply traction in supine position to unload posterior elements.[26]
         a. Horizontal split table traction: traction force at least 25% of body weight to distract vertebral bodies.

b. Autotraction: patient controls amount and direction of traction force.
c. Inversion gravity traction: potential side effects include hypertension, tachycardia, gastrointestinal reflux, and berry aneurysm rupture.

6. Therapeutic exercise: begins during acute phase due to deleterious effects of prolonged bedrest—more than 2 days. (See section I.C.1.)[26]
 a. Determine initial movement pattern depending on presumed pathology, pain pattern, and pain centralization (McKenzie method[41,53]).
  (1) Extension bias: most commonly diskogenic pathology with decrease in symptoms with repetitive extension on motion pattern testing and centralization of pain with extension. Extension exercises may reduce intradiskal pressure, allow anterior migration of the nucleus pulposus, and increase mechanoreceptor input, activating the pain gate mechanism. May increase symptoms if large central herniation, foraminal stenosis, or foraminal herniation present. Cardiovascular fitness may be initiated with aquatic stabilization training, cross-country ski machine or other aerobic activity that places the spine in neutral to extension bias.[12]
  (2) Flexion bias (Williams' Exercises[5]): most commonly posterior element pain with decrease in symptoms with repetitive flexion on motion pattern testing and centralization of pain with flexion. Flexion exercises may reduce facet joint compressive forces and provide stretch to the lumbar musculature, ligaments and myofascial structures. May increase intradiskal pressure and exacerbate diskogenic symptoms. Cardiovascular fitness may be initiated with aquatic stabilization training, stationary bicycle in slight lumbar flexion, stair climbing, or other aerobic activity that places the spine in neutral to flexion bias.[12]

E. Subacute phase.
 1. Connective tissue: manual soft tissue techniques that increase soft tissue distensibility along lines of physiological stress, promoting proper alignment of collagen fibers during remodeling and healing.[1,24,33] Affect both creep and plastic deformation of the connective tissue.[37,54]
 2. Myofascial system: myofascial release techniques apply pressure and shear forces to the fascial layers, improving elasticity and freedom of movement and decreasing pain.[2,23]
  a. Fascia absorbs shock, transmits mechanical force, and exchanges metabolites from fibrous elements to the circulatory and lymphatic systems. It separates and supports muscles, allowing for independent muscle function as well as coordinated multimuscular function.
  b. Loss of normal fascial gliding and increased cross-linking of fibers result in loss of myofascial system mobility and secondary loss of spinal segmental articular mobility and lower extremity flexibility.
 3. Mobilization: restores optimal *joint* mobility by applying forces at *individually targeted specific* motion segment levels (vs. connective tissue and myofascial system techniques that restore *soft tissue* mobility).[15,35,36,39]
  a. Graded I-V, depending on depth and force of applied load. Grade I, II: oscillations; grade III, IV: larger amplitude forces that move joint into its restricted range of motion and provide stretch; grade

V: manipulation that is low amplitude and high velocity and takes the joint to its end range of physiological motion.[2]

4. Exercise: dynamic lumbar stabilization training.[48,49]
   a. Goals.
      (1) Control pain.
      (2) Gain dynamic control of segmental spine and kinetic chain forces, particularly torque.
      (3) Optimize soft tissue repair and regeneration.
      (4) Eliminate repetitive motion segment injury and minimize the chance of an acute dynamic overload.
   b. Concepts.
      (1) Neutral spine: the initial training position that is the least painful and most biomechanically sound because it is the loose-packed position that decreases tension on ligaments and joints, allows more balanced segmental force distribution between disk and facet joints, is close to the center of reaction, allows movement into flexion and extension quickly, and provides the greatest functional stability with axial loading.
      (2) Muscle "fusion": Engram (cortically preprogrammed automatic multimuscular movement patterns activated without conscious control) for neutral spine position is developed through a specific set of stabilization exercises so that the athlete can recruit the spinal muscular stabilizers quickly and automatically.
      (3) Flexibility training allows the athlete to assume the neutral position so that strength can then be developed to help maintain the correct neutral position during both static and dynamic conditions.
      (4) While maintaining neutral position, exercises progress from static (e.g., supine and/or prone) to dynamic (e.g., standing, jumping, and other motions). Graded challenges to the neutral position are created first by gravity then by the therapist and or assistive devices (e.g., a Swiss ball). These challenges progress from predictable to unpredictable (e.g., simulating a blindside hit during football). Sports-specific retraining occurs by breaking down the required motion during sport to its individual component motions and the neutral position trained for each. Finally, the components are reassembled so that the entire sporting motion occurs using dynamic stabilization techniques.
5. Cardiovascular fitness: provides aerobic fitness required for sports. Cross-training in neutral spine position can help maintain fitness while protecting a healing motion segment. Aquatic rehabilitation can completely unload the spine if performed in deep water. The athlete is then transitioned to progressively shallower training locations so that graded gravitational forces are applied to the spine.[12,13]

IV. Return to Play[25]
   A. Criteria.
      1. No symptoms or signs of the clinical injury.
      2. Negative provocative testing of the injury site.
      3. Full pain-free range of motion.
      4. Normal flexibility.
      5. Normal strength and strength balance.
      6. Good general fitness.

7. Normal sports mechanics.
8. Ability to demonstrate sports-specific skills.

B. Depending on level of sports participation (e.g., high school vs. professional) and time of the season the injury occurs, some flexibility in the criteria is possible and should be based on sound clinical judgment.

References

1. Andriacchi T et al: Ligament injury and repair. In Woo SL-Y, Buckwalter JA, editors: *Injury and Repair of the Musculoskeletal Soft Tissues,* Park Ridge, IL, 1988, American Academy of Orthopaedic Surgeons.
2. Basmajian JV, Nyberg R, editors: *Rational Manual Therapies,* Baltimore, 1993, Williams & Wilkins.
3. Bender et al: Factors affecting the occurrence of knee injuries, *J Assoc Physical Mental Rehabil* 18:130, 1964.
4. Blyth CS, Mueller FU: Football injury survey: Part 1. When and where players get hurt, *Phys Sportsmed* 2:45, 1974.
5. Bogduk N: Lumbar dorsal ramus syndrome, *Med J Aust* 2:537, 1980.
6. Bortz W: The disuse syndrome, *West J Med* 141:169, 1984.
7. Cole AJ, Dreyfuss P, Stratton SA: The sacroiliac joint: a review, *Crit Rev Concepts,* in press.
8. Cole AJ, Eagleston RE: The use of ultrasound, shortwave and microwave diathermy for rehabilitation of sports injuries, *Phys Sportsmed* 22(2):77-88, 1994.
9. Cole AJ, Eagleston RE, Moschetti ML: Spine injuries in the competitive swimmer, *Sports Med Digest* 16(1):1-3, 1994.
10. Cole AJ, Herring SA: Role of the physiatrist in management of musculoskeletal pain. In Tollison DJ, editor: *The Handbook of Pain Management,* ed 2, Philadelphia, 1994, Williams & Wilkins, pp 85-95.
11. Cole AJ, Herring SA, editors: *The Low Back Pain Handbook: A Guide for the Primary Care Clinician,* Philadelphia, Hanley & Belfus, in press.
12. Cole AJ, Moschetti ML, Eagleston RE: Spine pain: aquatic rehabilitation strategies, *J Back Musculoskel Rehab* 4(4):319-320, 1994.
13. Cole AJ et al: Spine injuries in runners: a functional approach, *J Back Musculoskel Rehab* 5(4): 317-340, 1995.
14. Deyo R: Conservative therapy for low back pain: distinguishing useful from useless therapy, *JAMA* 250:1057, 1983.
15. DiFablo RP: Efficacy of manual therapy, *Phys Ther* 72:853, 1992.
16. Dreyfuss P, Dreyer S, Cole AJ: Zygapophyseal joint injection techniques. In Weinstein S, editor: *Physical Medicine and Rehabilitation Clinics of North America,* Philadelphia, WB Saunders, 6(4):715-741, 1995.
17. Duda M: Golf injuries: they really do happen, *Phys Sportsmed* 15:191, 1987.
18. Duda M: Golfers use exercise to get back in the swing, *Phys Sportsmed* 17:109, 1989.
19. Elkstrand J, Gillquist J: Soccer injuries and their mechanisms: a prospective study, *Med Sci Sports Exerc* 15:267, 1983.
20. Feeler LC: Racquet sports, *Spine* 4:337, 1990.
21. Fortin JP, Roberts D: Competitive figure skating injuries, *Arch Phys Med Rehabil* 68:642, 1987.
22. Gibbs R: Personal communication, 1993.
23. Greenman PE: *Principles of Manual Medicine,* Baltimore, 1989, Williams & Wilkins.
24. Herring SA: Rehabilitation of muscle injuries, *Med Sci Sports Exerc* 22:453, 1990.
25. Herring SA, Kibler WB: A framework for rehabilitation, in press.
26. Herring SA, Weinstein SM: Assessment of nonsurgical management of athletic low back injury. In Nicholas JA, Hershman EB, editors: *The Lower Extremity and Spine,* vol 2, ed 2, St Louis, 1995, Mosby.
27. Herring SA, Weinstein SM: Low back pain and injury prevention and the role of physical therapy for acute low back pain injury, in press.
28. Hochschuler SH, editor: Spinal injuries in sports, *Spine State Art Rev* 4:1990.
29. Hoshina H: Spondylosis in athletes, *Phys Sportsmed* 8:75, 1980.
30. Jackson CP: Historic perspectives on patient education and its place in acute spinal disorders. In Mayer TG, Mooney V, Gatchel RJ, editors: *Contemporary Conservative Care for Painful Spinal Disorders,* Philadelphia, 1991, Lea & Febiger.
31. Jackson DW: Low back pain in young athletes: evaluation of stress reactions and discogenic problems, *Am J Sports Med* 7:364, 1979.
32. Kaul MP, Herring SA: Superficial heat and cold, *Phys Sportsmed* 22(12):65, 1994.
33. Kellet J: Acute soft tissue injuries—a review of the literature, *Med Sci Sports Exerc* 18:489, 1986.
34. Kibler WB, Herring SA: Formulating a rehabilitation program. In Griffin LY, editor: *Rehabilitation of the Injured Knee,* ed 2, St Louis, 1995, Mosby.

35. Koes BW et al: Randomized clinical trial of manipulative therapy and physiotherapy for persistent back and neck complaints: results of one-year follow-up, *BMJ* 304:601, 1992.
36. Koes BW et al: The effectiveness of manual therapy, physiotherapy, and treatment by the general practitioner for nonspecific back and neck complaints: a randomized clinical trial, *Spine* 17:28, 1992.
37. Lee M: Mechanics of spinal joint manipulation in the thoracic and lumbar spine: a theoretical study of posteroanterior force techniques, *Clin Biomech* 4:249, 1989.
38. Lysens et al: The predictability of sports injuries, *Sports Med* 1:6, 1984.
39. MacDonald RS, Bell CMJ: An open controlled assessment of osteopathic manipulation in nonspecific low back pain, *Spine* 15:364, 1990.
40. Mayer T et al: Qualification of lumbar function. II. Sagittal plane trunk strength in chronic low back pain patients, *Spine* 10:765, 1985.
41. McKenzie RA: *The Lumbar Spine, Mechanical Diagnosis, and Therapy,* Walkance, New Zealand, 1981, Spinal Publications.
42. Micheli LJ: Back injuries in dancers, *Clin Sports Med* 2:473, 1983.
43. Micheli LJ: Back injuries in gymnastics, *Clin Sports Med* 4:85, 1985.
44. Mutoh Y, Takamoto M, Miyashita M: Chronic injuries of elite competitive swimmers, divers, water polo players, and synchronized swimmers. In Ungerechts BE, Wilke K, Reischle K, editors: *Swimming Science V,* vol 18, Champaign, IL, 1988, Human Kinetics Books.
45. Robey JM, Blyth CS, Mueller FD: Athletic injuries: application of epidemiologic methods, *JAMA* 217:184, 1971.
46. Robinson JP, Brown PB: Medications in low back pain. In Kraft GH, Herring SA, editors: *Low Back Pain,* Philadelphia, 1991, WB Saunders.
47. Rothenberger LA: Prevalence and types of injuries in aerobic dancers, *Am J Sports Med* 16:403, 1988.
48. Saal JA: Rehabilitation of sports-related lumbar spine injuries. In Saal JA, editor: *Physical Medicine in Rehabilitation: State of the Art Reviews: Spine,* Philadelphia, 1987, Hanley & Belfus.
49. Saal JA: Dynamic muscular stabilization in the nonoperative treatment of lumbar pain syndromes, *Orthop Rev* 19:691, 1990.
50. Shelton JL, Robinson JP: Physiological aspects of chronic back pain. In Herring SA, editor: *Low Back Pain,* Philadelphia, 1991, WB Saunders, pp 127-144.
51. Spitzer W, LaBlank F, Dupuis M: Scientific approach to the assessment and management of activity related spinal disorders: a monograph for clinicians. Report of the Quebec task force of spinal disorders, *Spine* 12(7S):S1-S59, 1987.
52. Staniski CL: Low back pain in young athletes, *Phys Sportsmed* 10:77, 1982.
53. Stankovic R, Johnell O: Conservative treatment of acute low-back pain: a prospective randomized trial—McKenzie method of treatment versus patient education in "mini back school," *Spine* 15:120, 1990.
54. Threlkeld AJ: The effects of manual therapy on connective tissue, *Phys Ther* 72:893, 1992.
55. Urban J, McMullin J: Swelling pressure of lumbar intervertebral discs: influence of the age, spinal level, composition, and degeneration, *Spine* 13:179, 1988.
56. Windsor RE, Lester JP, Herring SA: Electrical stimulation in clinical practice, *Phys Sportsmed* 21:85-93, 1993.
57. Woodward JL et al: Epidural procedures in spine pain management. In Lennard TA, editor: *Physiatric Procedures in Clinical Practice,* Philadelphia, 1995, Hanley & Belfus.
58. Yost JG Jr, Elfieldt HJ: Basketball injuries. In Nicholas JA, Hershman EB, editors: *The Lower Extremity and Spine in Sports Medicine,* St Louis, 1986, Mosby.

CHAPTER 52

Knee Anatomy and Mechanisms of Injury

David V. Anderson, MD

I. Introduction
   A. Knee injuries are among the most common of all sports medicine injuries. Many sports medicine physicians devote nearly 70% of their training to studying and treating patients who have injured or symptomatic knees. A thorough understanding of the functional anatomy and its relationship to the mechanisms of injury is essential for satisfactory management of knee injuries.
   B. Anatomy varies by size and strength of structures. Most structures have multiple functions. Understanding that form follows function allows an examiner to predict which anatomic structures are damaged by knowing which function was being taxed at injury.

II. Bony Anatomy
   A. General overview.
      1. Mechanically, the knee has two mutually exclusive functions: stability when extended and under the stresses of body weight, and mobility necessary for walking and orientation of the foot and leg to the ground.
      2. The knee is composed of two functional joints: the femorotibial and the femoropatellar.
   B. Femoral condyles.
      1. Primary motion is flexion and extension on its transverse axis.
      2. Secondary motion is axial rotation when the knee is flexed.
      3. When the knee is flexed, side-to-side movements occur because of ligament laxity or "play." Instability is indicated by side-to-side motion when the knee is fully extended.
      4. Coupled rolling and gliding form the basic motion (Fig. 52-1).
   C. Tibial plateau.
      1. Reciprocally curved surfaces separated by a blunt eminence with medial and lateral spines extending anterior to posterior.
      2. The eminence is one of the factors preventing rotation in extension.

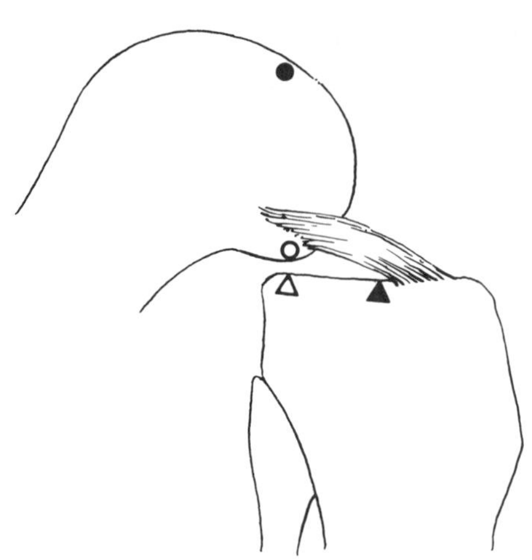
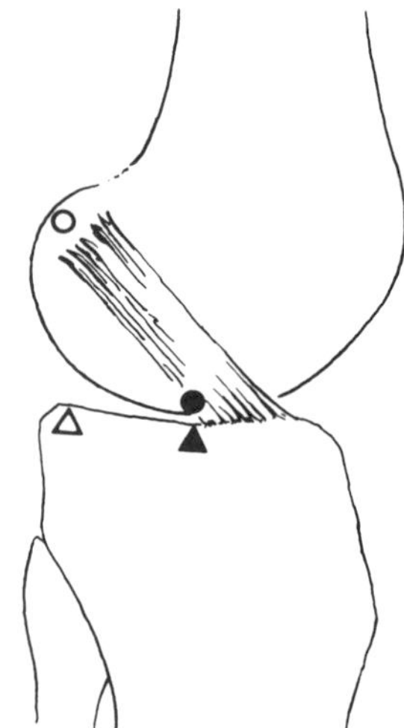

FIGURE 52-1
Femoral condyle rolling and gliding with flexion.

3. The lateral tibial plateau is convex in the anteroposterior plane, which allows the lateral femoral condyle to move further backwards and causes automatic internal tibial rotation with flexion.

D. Patella.

1. Sesamoid bone with two concave surfaces (i.e., facets) separated by a vertical ridge. The patella is embedded in the extensor mechanism, which increases its efficiency by 1½ times.
2. By fitting into the vertical trochlea and intercondylar notch, the patella redirects the superolateral force of the quadriceps pull into a vertical force.
3. The suprapatellar pouch and lateral recesses unfold to allow the patella to move. Adhesions restrict this motion.
4. The lateral trochlear pillar is higher than the medial pillar, which resists lateral dislocation in extension and in slight degrees of flexion (Fig. 52-2).

E. Proximal tibiofibular joint.

1. Has its own synovial cavity.
2. Stability provided by bony architecture.
3. Anterolateral dislocation is most common and is due to a fall on an inverted foot (skating injury).
4. Posterior dislocation due to direct trauma (often with tibia fracture).

III. Cruciate Ligaments

A. General overview.

1. These ligaments form the axes for knee rotation and link rotation with flexion/extension.
2. The length and orientation of the cruciate ligaments determine the shape and function of the knee.

B. Anterior cruciate ligament (ACL).

1. Three bands—anteromedial, posterolateral, and intermediate—run inferiorly, anteriorly, and medially from high on the back of the lateral intercondylar notch to just lateral to the medial tibial eminence (Fig. 52-3).
2. The primary restraint to anterior tibial subluxation.

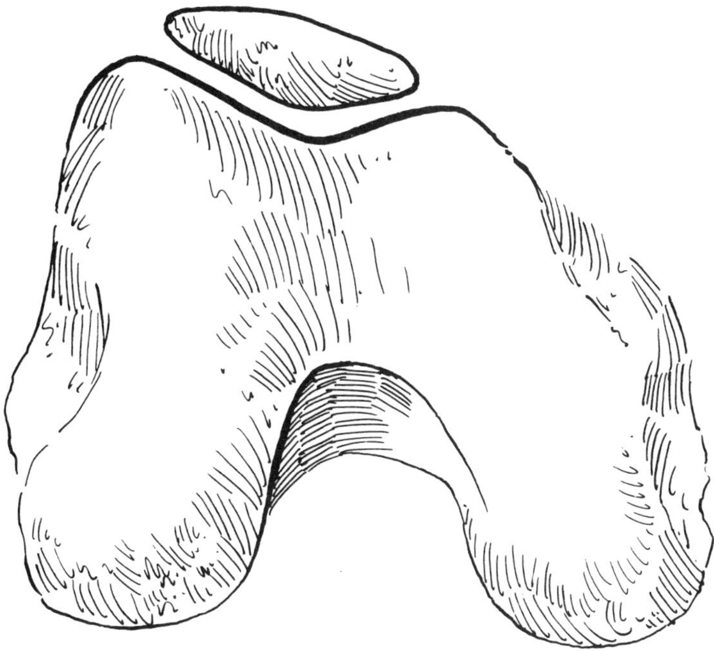

FIGURE 52-2
Patellofemoral joint.

3. Tighter with the knee in full extension (posterolateral band) and looser in midflexion. Some fibers (intermediate band) are always tight.
4. Uncoils from the posterior cruciate ligament (PCL) in external rotation, resulting in looseness until stretched by the medial side of

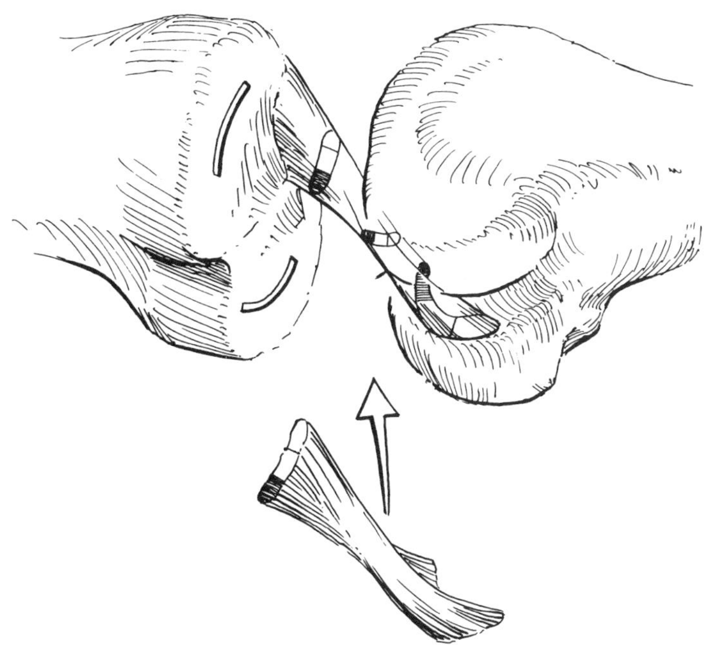

FIGURE 52-3
ACL bands and orientation.

the lateral femoral condyle; tightens in internal rotation (Fig. 52-4).

5. Pulls the femur anteriorly while the condyle rolls posteriorly during flexion (without the ACL the posterior menisci are under increased stress; Fig. 52-5).
6. Mechanisms of injury.
    (1) Loads applied when the ligaments are under maximum tension result in greatest strain.
    (2) The ACL is the most common disabling knee injury in athletes; 70% of all ACL injuries occur during jumping (gymnasts, basketball) and cutting of cleats or skis.
    (3) Noncontact, deceleration-valgus-external rotation injury is the usual mechanism of injury (especially in women).
    (4) Forced hyperextension and deceleration-internal rotation are less common mechanisms, which can also injure the PCL.
    (5) Tibial spine avulsions are associated with ACL tears in children <13 years of age.
    (6) Half of ACL tears are associated with a clinically significant meniscal tear.

C. PCL (Fig. 52-6).
    1. A fan-shaped ligament that runs inferiorly, posteriorly, and laterally from the front of the medial intercondylar notch to just lateral to the posterior tibial plateau.
    2. The primary restraint to posterior tibial subluxation and a secondary restraint to medial instability.
    3. Vertically oriented and tighter in flexion; horizontal and looser in extension.
    4. Pulls the femur posteriorly while the condyle rolls anteriorly during extension (absence of PCL leads to a 25% increase in loads on the patellofemoral joint).
    5. Mechanisms of injury.

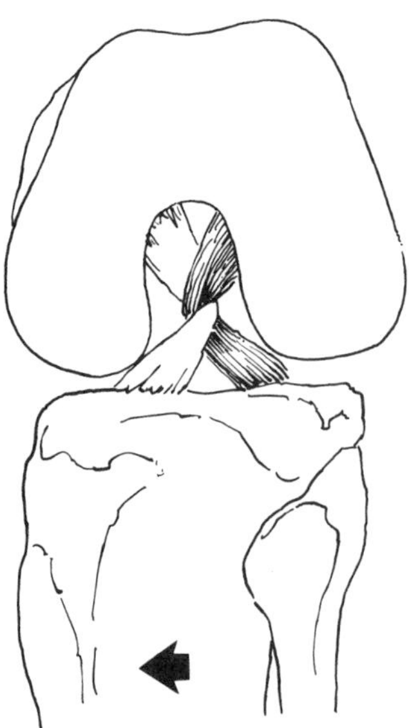

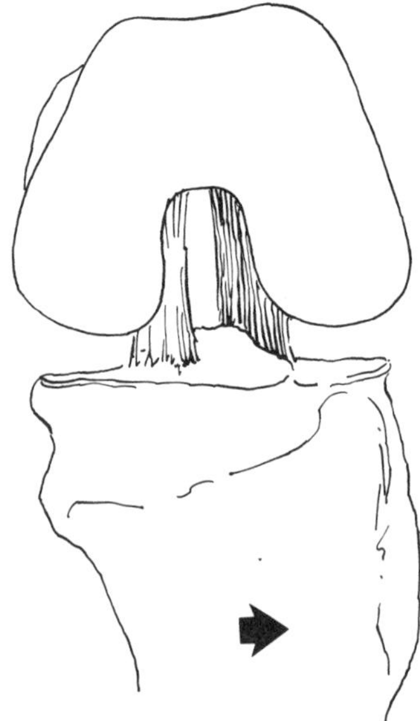

FIGURE 52-4
Exaggerated view of cruciate ligaments torsion with tibial rotation.

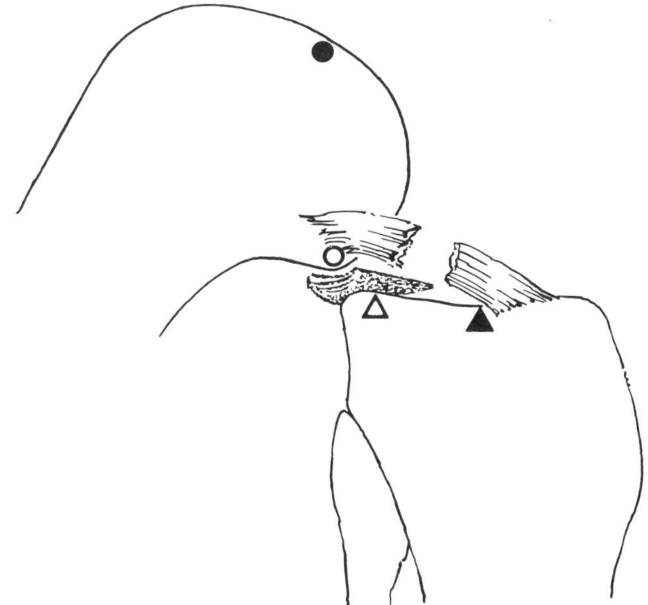

FIGURE 52-5
Increased posterior meniscus stress with loss of ACL.

(1) Direct blow to the front of the tibia with the knee flexed (i.e., car dashboard) is the most frequent cause of PCL injuries.
(2) Hyperflexion (sliding) is a common mechanism during athletics.
(3) Often not associated with meniscal injuries, but often are associated with articular cartilage damage.
(4) The cruciates are about twice as stiff as the collaterals; young ligaments are stronger and stiffer than old ligaments.

IV. Collateral Ligaments
  A. General overview.
    1. These ligaments strengthen the articular capsule medially and laterally to provide transverse stability of the knee. They run obliquely and uncoil upon internal rotation of the tibia and coil or tighten upon external rotation (opposite the cruciates).
    2. Most of the collateral fibers become tight in extension and loose in flexion. This elastic reserve allows axial rotation and accounts for normal laxity.
  B. Medial collateral ligament (Fig. 52-6).
    1. Attaches on the postero-superior aspect of the medial femoral condyle and runs antero-inferiorly to the upper end of the tibia.
    2. Maximum tension at full extension, minimal between 25 and 80 degrees.
    3. Abduction stress increases tension at increasing degrees of flexion.
    4. Mechanisms of injury.
      (1) Noncontact valgus stress with external rotation: grade I, II.
      (2) Contact valgus stress with or without external rotation: grade III.
  C. Lateral collateral ligament (LCL; Fig. 52-7).
    1. Attaches posterosuperiorly on the lateral femoral condyle and runs obliquely to attach anterior to the fibula styloid.
    2. Primary restraint to varus stress in extension.

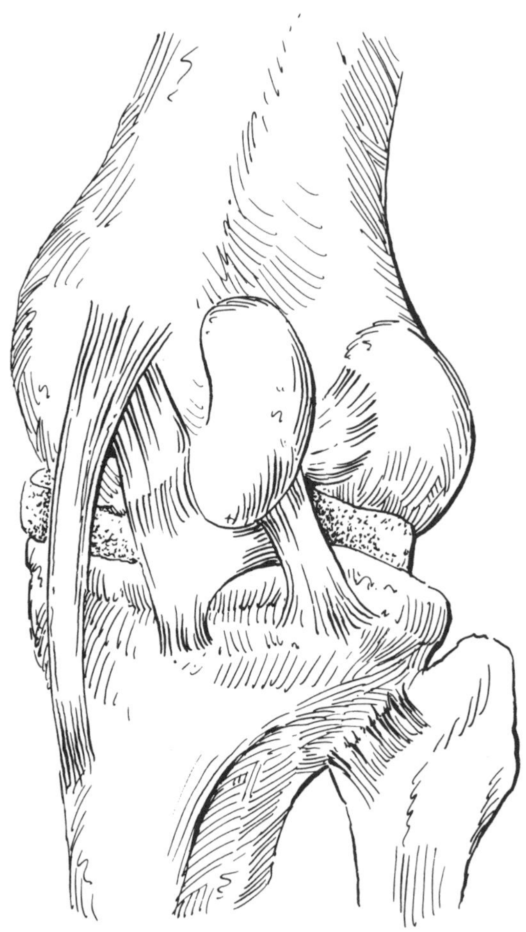

FIGURE 52-6
PCL, MCL, posterior oblique ligament.

3. Adduction stress increases tension to peak at 70 degrees flexion.
4. Structurally weakest of the four main ligaments but works in conjunction with the posterolateral corner to prevent varus and external rotation.
5. Mechanisms of injury.
    (1) Contact varus stress.
    (2) Uncommon; may represent subtle knee dislocations.
    (3) High associated incidence of peroneal nerve injuries.
    (4) Most LCL injuries are in combination with PCL or ACL injuries.

V. Capsular Ligaments
  A. General overview.
    1. The posterior capsule resists the natural tendency for increases in knee hyperextension while standing in full extension or recurvatum.
    2. The collateral and capsular structures, which are parallel to one another, are synergistic and are often injured simultaneously or become progressively lax (i.e., stretched out) following acute injuries.
  B. Posterior oblique ligament (Fig. 52-6).
    1. Attaches the posterior medial meniscus to the tibia and femur.
    2. Resists external rotation.
    3. Restrains posterior drawer in internal rotation.

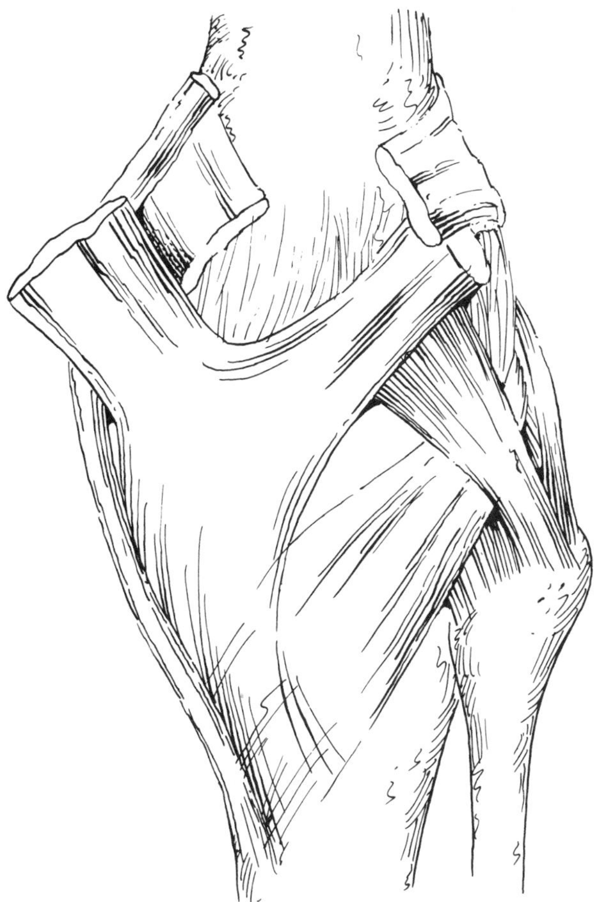

FIGURE 52-7
Arcuate complex, LCL.

C. Arcuate popliteal ligament complex (posterolateral corner; Fig. 52-7).
   1. Reinforcing ligament of the lateral side. Injury results in posterolateral rotary instability.
   2. Attaches to the posterior horn of the lateral meniscus.
   3. The most important secondary restraint to posterior tibial subluxation.
   4. Important as tension receptors for proprioceptive feedback.

D. Mechanisms of injury.
   (1) Blow to the anteromedial tibia, which causes knee hyperextension, is a mechanism for posterolateral corner tear; ACL is often torn also.
   (2) Noncontact, hyperextension external rotation with varus force is a mechanism for posterolateral injury.
   (3) Contact to the lower lateral thigh or upper tibia injures the posteromedial corner.

VI. Meniscus

A. General overview (Fig. 52-8).
   1. The meniscus are shaped to allow for load bearing, joint stability, and shock absorption.
   2. During rotation the menisci displace with the femur (opposite the direction of the tibia). The peripheral one third is vascularized and can heal if stable.

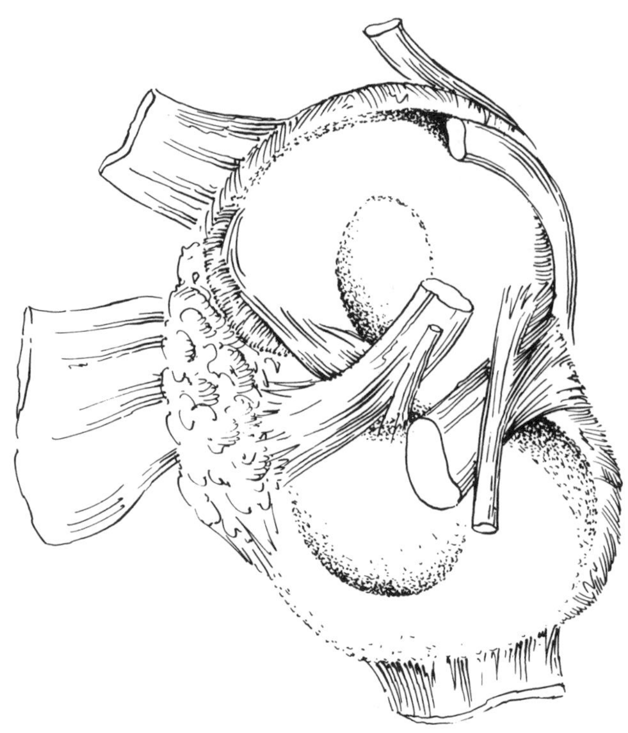

FIGURE 52-8
Superior view of menisci, fatpad.

B. Mechanisms of injury.
   (1) Combined valgus and external rotation, where the posterior horn of the medial meniscus is trapped by the posterior condyles.
   (2) Forced extension of the knee where one of the menisci fails to move forward with the femur.
   (3) Most circumferential tears (including bucket handle tears) are associated with a torn ACL.

VII. Muscles
   A. General overview.
      1. Several muscles "line" the collateral ligaments, forming "active ligaments" that stabilize the knee to varus/valgus stresses.
      2. The lateral collateral ligament is assisted by the iliotibial tract, and the medial collateral ligament is assisted by the sartorius, gracilis, and the semitendinosus (pes anserinus).
   B. Quadriceps.
      1. Oriented in axial deviation of about 10-15 degrees: the Q angle.
      2. Are synergistic with the PCL.
      3. Rectus femoris, vastus intermedius and medialis internally rotate the freely mobile tibia but externally rotate the femur when the tibia is fixed (increasing the Q angle).
      4. The distal transverse part of the vastus medialis counteracts the rotary force that results from the Q angle.
   C. Hamstrings.
      1. Biceps femoris, semimembranosus, semitendinosus, sartorius, gracilis, and the popliteus.
      2. Except popliteus and short head of the biceps, all are hip extensors.

3. Synergistic with the ACL and are often injured in conjunction with it (especially the biceps).

D. Iliotibial tract (IT band).
1. Originates from the lateral iliac crest to insert as a fibrous band onto the lateral intermuscular septum and Gerdy's tubercle.
2. Contributes to the lateral patellofemoral ligament of the knee.
3. Functions as an extensor with the knee in extension and a flexor with the knee in flexion.

E. Mechanisms of injury.
(1) Violent contractions against resistance (falls, running downhill).
(2) Violent side-to-side stresses, which also stress the collaterals.
(3) Active extension with the foot planted in internal rotation is a frequent mechanism of patellar dislocation.
(4) Flexion and extension over the lateral epicondyle irritate the IT band (e.g., running).

VIII. Anterior Soft Tissues

A. General overview.
1. There are three synovial folds: suprapatellar, medial patellar, and lateral patellar.
2. The medial fold is most likely of all to become symptomatic (plica syndrome).
3. The anterior fatpad is rich in small vessels and nerve endings.
4. There are several bursae of note including the prepatellar and pes anserinus bursae, which lubricate areas of repetitive friction, and the semimembranosus bursa, which under conditions of increased knee fluid forms the "Baker's cyst."

B. Mechanisms of injury.
(1) Direct blow to flexed knee can lead to inflammation of all anterior soft tissue structures.
(2) Subtle hyperextension (running downhill) can pinch the fatpad or irritate a plica.
(3) Overuse and malalignment can cause bursal and tendon inflammation.

Acknowledgment

The Medical Editing Department, Kaiser Foundation Research Institute, provided editorial assistance.

Bibliography

DeLee JC, Drez D: *Orthopedic Sports Medicine, Principles and Practice,* Philadelphia, 1994, WB Saunders.

Kapanji IA: *The Physiology of the Joints,* Vol Two, *Lower Limb,* Edinburgh/London/New York, 1970, Churchill Livingstone.

Kulund DN: *The Injured Athlete,* Philadelphia, 1988, JB Lippincott.

Mueller W: *The Knee, Form Function, and Ligament Reconstruction,* New York/Berlin/Heidelberg, 1983, Springer-Verlag.

Orthopedic Knowledge Update, vol 4, Park Ridge, Il, 1993, AAOS.

CHAPTER **53**

Knee Ligament Injuries

James G. Garrick, MD

I. Ligaments (Sprains)
  A. Anterior cruciate ligament (ACL).
    1. Anatomy and biomechanics.
      a. Anterior, central tibia to medial aspect of lateral femoral condyle.
      b. Primary function to limit anterior tibial displacement.
      c. Major secondary restraint limiting internal rotation.
      d. Minor secondary restraint to varus-valgus angulation in full extension.
    2. Injuries.
      a. Most common in football, basketball, soccer, women's gymnastics, volleyball, and downhill skiing. Female rates are greater than male rates in soccer and basketball.
      b. Appears to be most common in teens and 20s (may be secondary to sport participation during these years).
      c. Mechanism(s): Cutting, deceleration, hyperextension.
        (1) Most are noncontact injuries.
        (2) Contact injuries usually involve other structures (e.g., "terrible triad of O'Donoghue": ACL, medial collateral ligament [MCL], medial meniscus).
      d. Meniscus injuries of some magnitude (identified by magnetic resonance imaging [MRI] or arthroscopy) in >60%.
      e. Evidence of subchondral bone injury (by MRI) in >50% (? significance).
      f. History.
        (1) Heard/felt "pop" or "snap."
        (2) Sensation of knee "going out": "knuckle sign."
        (3) Sense of "instability."
        (4) Modest early swelling: significant effusion at 24 hours.
        (5) Pain—which may initially be minimal—in anterior knee (behind patellar tendon): posterolateral joint line.

(6) Usually able to bear weight with moderate comfort.
(7) Avoid full extension while bearing weight.

g. Examination.
(1) Effusion: usually not tense.
(2) Tenderness.
(A) Medial or lateral joint line with meniscal tear.
(B) Anterolateral tibial plateau with avulsion fracture.
(C) Anterior jointling (on either side of patellar tendon).
(3) Stability: measure amount of excursion and firmness of "endpoint" and compare to contralateral knee.
(4) Drawer test (at 90 degrees of flexion) will fail to identify 50% of complete ACL tears.
(a) If positive = ACL sprain.
(b) If negative = meaningless.
(5) Lachmann test ("drawer test" with knee flexed 15 degrees): KT-1000 difference of >3 mm.
(a) If positive = ACL sprain.
(b) False negative rate = 5% to 10%; depends on skill of examiner.
(6) Pivot shift: "jerk" test.
(a) Meaningful only if positive.
(b) Difficult to perform with painful effusion.

h. Special tests.
(1) X-rays: avulsion fracture of anterolateral tibial plateau; diagnostic.
(2) Arthrogram: accuracy highly dependent on skill of arthrographer.
(3) MRI: approximately 90% accuracy.
(4) Examination under anesthesia: ? overkill.
(5) Arthroscopy: 100% accuracy ("gold standard").

i. Treatment: Orthopedic referral.
(a) Rehabilitation.
(b) Surgical reconstruction.
i. Usually delay 3-5 weeks to lessen likelihood of fibrosis and loss of motion.
ii. Immediate if impingement from displaced meniscal tear.
iii. Success of stabilization of joint with reconstructive procedures is relatively unaffected by the time elapsed between injury and definitive surgery.

3. Complications/problems.
a. Long-term degenerative joint disease is more closely associated with meniscal pathology than instability.
b. Continued uncontrolled instability episodes increase the risk of meniscal injury and (possibly) degenerative joint disease.
c. Successful surgical management requires a substantial commitment to an extensive postoperative rehabilitative regimen lasting a minimum of 2-3 months.
d. A sequela of ACL injuries may be an enhanced likelihood of chondromalacia of the patella, which (some believe) is further enhanced by the use of bone–tendon–bone grafts using the patellar tendon.

B. Posterior cruciate ligament (PCL).
1. Anatomy and biomechanics.
a. Extends from posterior central tibia to lateral aspect of medial femoral condyle.

b. Primary function to limit posterior tibial displacement.
c. Major secondary restraint to external tibial rotation.
2. Injuries.
a. Far less common than ACL injuries.
b. Vehicular trauma may be bigger source than sports (proximal tibia strikes dashboard).
c. Usually contact injury: blow to proximal, anterior tibia.
d. May be noncontact from hyperextension.
3. History.
a. Magnitude of injury may seem modest.
b. Fall on anterior tibia or struck in anterior tibia.
c. May or may not feel "pop."
d. Initial swelling may be minimal with isolated PCL injury; increases by 48 hours.
e. May be able to bear weight comfortably.
f. Reluctant to fully extend.
g. ? sense of "instability."
4. Examination.
a. Effusion variable and partially a function of injury to other structures.
b. Popliteal tenderness.
c. Stability: if positive = PCL sprain; if negative = may be due to quadriceps contraction/protective spasm.
(1) "Sag" test: compare to contralateral.
(a) Supine with knee flexed 90 degrees and relaxed with foot on examination table. Proximal tibia displaced posteriorly.
(b) Supine with hip and knee each flexed 90 degrees and heel supported by examiner. Posterior displacement of proximal tibia.
(2) Posterior drawer test: measure posterior excursion and firmness of "end point."
5. Special tests.
a. Radiography: may show avulsion of tibial attachment.
b. MRI: less accurate than for ACL.
c. Arthroscopy: less definitive than for ACL.
6. Treatment: orthopaedic referral.
(1) Rehabilitation.
(2) Surgical repair if ligament avulsed with tibial attachment.

C. MCL.
1. Anatomy and biomechanics.
a. Deep layer is thickened medial capsule.
b. Superficial layer.
(1) From adductor tubercle to anteromedial tibia.
(2) Inserts nearly at level of tibial tuberosity.
(3) Major medial stabilizing structure.
2. Injuries.
a. Most common in football and skiing.
b. Injury usually requires outside force (blow to outside/lateral side of knee; e.g., clipping in football).
c. In skiing occurs without direct blow.
d. Usually initially painful.
e. All become more painful with time (and swelling).
f. More severe sprains accompanied by a sensation of instability ("bends the wrong way," "loose," etc.).

g. History.
   (1) Struck from lateral side.
   (2) Feels/hears pop or snap.
   (3) Immediate medial pain: with complete tears (grade III sprains) pain may disappear within minutes; partial tears often more painful.
   (4) Usually initially falls to ground: complete tears may allow painless walking and even running minutes after injury; complaints of instability, not pain.
   (5) Knee "stiffens up" within hours.
h. Examination.
   (1) Medial swelling.
   (2) Effusion may be minimal.
   (3) May be medial ecchymosis (if >24 hours old).
   (4) Medial instability (opening) when stressed in 20 degrees of flexion.
      (a) Opens with firm end point: grade II.
      (b) Opens with soft end point: grade III.
i. Special tests.
   (1) Radiography/stress radiography: may reveal epiphyseal fracture (tibia or femur). Remember; most high school football players have "open" epiphyses.
   (2) MRI: overkill.
   (3) Examination under anesthesia: overkill.
j. Treatment.
   (1) Grade III sprains: refer to orthopedic surgeon. Most will be treated with protective bracing and rehabilitation.
   (2) Grade I and II sprains.
      (a) Hinged brace for protection: "locked" to limit painful motion.
      (b) Quadriceps strength and endurance program.
k. Complications.
   (1) More severe injuries may involve ACL and medial meniscus (O'Donoghue's triad).
   (2) Misdiagnosis of epiphyseal fracture.
      (a) Either can result in positive "instability tests."
      (b) Epiphyseal injuries usually more painful.
      (c) May not be visible on standard radiography.
   (3) Residual, *functional,* instability rare if adequately rehabilitated.

D. Lateral collateral ligament.
   1. Anatomy.
      a. Ligament extends from lateral femoral epicondyle to head of fibula: ligament is a discrete, extracapsular structure.
   2. Injuries.
      a. Isolated injuries are *rare.*
      b. Injuries usually the result of knee dislocations.
         (1) An orthopedic emergency as major vascular injuries common.
         (2) Cruciate ligaments and peroneal nerve often injured.

II. Patella.
   A. Anatomy.
      1. Patella is located within the quadriceps tendon.
      2. The tendency to displace laterally is an anatomical reality.
      3. Lateral displacement is thwarted by:
         a. The groove between the femoral condyles (femoral trochlea).

b. The medial retinaculum (capsule).
c. The vastus medialis muscle (component of the quadriceps).

B. Injuries.
1. Dislocation.
a. Occurs more frequently in females than males.
b. Always occurs laterally (absent prior surgical intervention).
c. Usually the result of intrinsic forces: does not require a direct blow or outside force.
d. First-time dislocations may be among the most impressive (to the patient) of knee injuries.
e. First-time dislocations are usually accompanied by significant soft tissue injuries (medial retinacular and vastus medialis muscle tears).
f. First-time dislocations are often accompanied by intraarticular fracture of the articular surfaces of the patella or lateral femoral condyle.
g. Most dislocations spontaneously reduce when the knee is extended.
h. History.
(1) Knee flexed (10-40 degrees), quadriceps actively contracting, foot externally rotated (as with "cutting" to the opposite direction).
(2) "Ripping, tearing, grinding" sensation: usually described in colorful, expansive terms by the patient.
(3) Immediate disability; unable/unwilling to arise and bear weight.
(4) Immediate and significant swelling: patient may describe watching the knee enlarge.
(5) Because the dislocation usually reduces spontaneously with extension of the knee, patient is usually unaware of exactly what happened.
i. Examination.
(1) Large, tense, tender effusion (all lessened with subsequent dislocations).
(2) Tenderness of medial retinaculum, vastus medialis, and adductor tubercle.
(3) Unable/unwilling to actively extend knee the terminal 10-15 degrees.
(4) Medial ecchymosis may be present after 12-18 hours.
(5) NOTE: If patella is dislocated at time of examination and fails to reduce with gentle pressure and extension of the knee, the reduction may be blocked by an intraarticular fracture fragment. Don't force it!
j. Treatment.
(1) Refer first-time dislocations to orthopedic surgeon.
(2) Immobilize in 10 degrees of flexion with knee immobilizer.
(3) Ice and compression wrap.
(4) At 48 hours begin removing immobilizer 3-4 times per day for active range of motion exercises.
(5) Begin isometric quadriceps contractions as soon as possible. Electrical muscle stimulation daily: electrodes over vastus medialis. (Up to 2 hours per day: rental unit for home use.)
(6) Discontinue immobilizer with 0-90 degrees of comfortable, active motion: replace with patellar stabilizing brace to be worn during all weight-bearing activities and for athletics for 3-6 months.

Bibliography

Arendt E, Dick R: Knee injury patterns among men and women in collegiate basketball and soccer, 23(6):694-701, 1995.

Caborn DN, Johnson BM: The natural history of the anterior cruciate ligament-deficient knee, *Clin Sports Med* 12(4):625-636, 1993.

Daniel DM, Fritschy D: Anterior cruciate ligament injuries. In Delee JC, Drez D, editors: *Orthopedic Sports Medicine: Principles and Practice,* vol 2, Philadelphia, 1994, WB Saunders, pp 1313-1360.

Levandowski R: Knee injuries. In Birrer RB, editor: *Sports Medicine for the Primary Care Physician,* Boca Raton, 1994, CRC Press, pp 505-530.

Reid DC: Knee ligament injuries. In *Sports Injury Assessment and Rehabilitation,* New York, 1992, Churchill Livingstone, pp 437-550.

Walsh WM: Knee injuries. In Mellion MB et al, editors: *The Team Physicians Handbook,* Philadelphia, 1990, Hanley and Belfus, pp 414-439.

Zarins B, Fish DN: Knee ligament injuries. In Nicholas JA, Hershman EB, editors: *The Lower Extremity and Spine in Sports Medicine,* St Louis, 1995, Mosby–Year Book, pp 825-864.

CHAPTER 54

Meniscal Injuries

James G. Garrick, MD

I. Anatomy and Biomechanics
  A. Fibrocartilage.
    1. Blood supply only to peripheral one third.
    2. Interstitial "degeneration" over time (seen on magnetic resonance imaging [MRI]).
  B. Meniscal functions.
    1. Enhance nutrition of articular cartilage.
    2. Contribute (minimally) to stability.
    3. Redistribute force (pressure on articular surface of tibia from femoral condyles). Lateral meniscus "bears more weight" than medial meniscus.

II. Injuries
  A. Isolated injuries nearly always occur while weight bearing.
    1. Medial meniscus: "cutting" (i.e., tibial rotation while weight bearing in a partially flexed position)—football, soccer, basketball, etc.
    2. Lateral meniscus: often the result of rotation while in the maximally flexed position (squatting)—wrestling.
  B. Combination injuries: Greater than 60% of anterior cruciate ligament injuries involve meniscal lesions.
    1. Initial injury: lateral more common than medial.
    2. Chronic injuries: medial may be more common than lateral.
  C. Types of meniscal tears: all more likely to involve posterior portions of the menisci.
    1. Bucket handle tears.
      a. Medial more common than lateral.
      b. Prone to cause locking.
      c. More common in younger athletes.
    2. Flap tears.
      a. May start as small, peripheral bucket handle–type tears, then "fracture" radially.
      b. May cause impingement but usually not prolonged locking.

3. Radial tears.
   a. Increased incidence with age?
   b. Lateral more common than medial.
4. Horizontal (degenerative) tears.
   a. Likelihood increases with age.
   b. Less likely to cause locking/impingement.

III. History
   A. Acute tears (nondegenerative).
      1. Memorable specific incident.
      2. Hears/feels "snap" or "pop."
      3. May fall.
      4. May be accompanied by immediate locking: displaced bucket handle tear. (NOTE: True locking occurs suddenly and "unlocks" just as suddenly. Difficulty extending the knee after a prolonged period of sitting is *not* locking.)
      5. Usually results in an effusion within 24 hours.
   B. Degenerative tears.
      1. Usually in older athletes (>40 years).
      2. Onset may involve minimal trauma.
      3. Recurrent joint line discomfort with athletic activities.
      4. Usually recurrent effusions.
      5. May have minimal "impingement" episodes.
      6. Inability or unwillingness to assume squatting position.

IV. Physical Examination
   A. Range of motion may be restricted by:
      1. Presence of an effusion.
      2. Impinging meniscal fragment. Meniscal impingement rarely limits flexion—nearly always extension. (Flexion may be limited by the presence of an effusion.)
   B. Tenderness.
      1. Medial joint line for medial meniscus.
      2. Lateral joint line for lateral meniscus.
      3. Meniscal impingement test (i.e., digital pressure on meniscal attachment while flexing or extending the knee).
   C. Provocative tests (McMurray, Apley, etc.).
      1. All are maneuvers designed to entrap (lock) a torn meniscal fragment.
      2. Most require full flexion/hyperflexion of the knee.
      3. Most are impossible (as originally described) in the presence of an effusion (which inhibits flexion).
      4. All are uncomfortable in the acutely injured knee.

V. Special Tests
   A. Arthrograms: success depends on skill of examiner. More meaningful if positive than if negative.
   B. MRI: gold standard.
      1. "Interstitial degeneration" may be clinically meaningless.
      2. One third of asymptomatic adults with negative knee examinations are believed to have frank meniscal tears based on MRI.

VI. Treatment
   A. Meniscal tears are treated operatively (excised or repaired) because they are *symptomatic,* not because they *exist.*
   B. If "locked," attempt to "unlock."
      1. Extend from the flexed position with rotation in valgus or medial meniscus and varus for lateral meniscus.
      2. Success may be enhanced with local anesthesia.

C. Rehabilitation (concentrate on quadriceps).
   1. Discourage hyperflexion.
   2. Avoid rotation and varus/valgus stresses.

D. Orthopedic referral.
   1. Vertical tears (bucket handle variety) in the peripheral one third may be surgically repaired.
   2. In cruciate-deficient knee, meniscal repairs are believed to have a higher level of success if the knee is stabilized (reconstructed).

Bibliography

DeHaven KE, Bronstein RD: Injuries to the menisci of the knee. In Nicholas JA, Hershman EB, editors: *The Lower Extremity and Spine in Sports Medicine,* St Louis, 1995, Mosby–Year Book, pp 813-824.

Fu FH, Baratz M: Meniscus injuries. In Delee JC, Drez D, editors: *Orthopedic Sports Medicine: Principles and Practice,* vol 2, Philadelphia, 1994, WB Saunders, pp 1146-1162.

Levandowski R: Knee injuries. In Birrer RB, editor: *Sports Medicine for the Primary Care Physician,* Boca Raton, 1994, CRC Press, pp 505-530.

Reid DC: Internal derangement and other selected lesions of the knee. In *Sports Injury Assessment and Rehabilitation,* New York, 1992, Churchill Livingstone, pp 301-345.

Thompson WO, Fu FH: The meniscus in the cruciate ligament-deficient knee, *Clin Sports Med* 12(4):625-636, 1993.

Walsh WM: Knee injuries. In Mellion MB et al, editors: *The Team Physician's Handbook,* Philadelphia, 1990, Hanley and Belfus, pp 414-439.

CHAPTER **55**

Anterior Knee Pain and Overuse

J. Michael Wieting, DO, MEd

Douglas B. McKeag, MD, MS

I. Introduction
  A. Scope of problem.
    1. Anterior knee pain is one of the most common musculoskeletal complaints of children, adolescents, and adults, especially among physically active persons.
    2. According to Garrick, of 16,748 patients presenting to the family physician with musculoskeletal problems, 11.3% had anterior knee pain.[9]
    3. May affect as many as 25% of all athletes.[21]
    4. More common in females.[20]
    5. A very common problem known by many names, including chondromalacia patella, anterior knee pain, patellofemoral dysfunction, patellalgia, patellar compression syndrome.
  B. Nature of the problem.
    1. Because of a frequent lack of an easily identifiable objective pathological cause, anterior knee pain is difficult to evaluate, diagnose, and therefore treat, causing frustration for the physician and the patient/athlete.
    2. Commonly only subjective; the fact that there is often no objective finding does not rule out genuine pain.
    3. Encompasses a wide variety of potential problems, from short duration acute symptoms, to chronic symptoms with accompanying psychological factors.[13]

II. Anatomy of Anterior Knee Pain
  A. Knee joint: general considerations.
    1. A synovial hinged joint, allowing flexion and extension.
    2. Depends on numerous supporting ligaments and tendons for stability.
  B. Patella (see Figure 55-1).
    1. Triangle-shaped bone with a downwardly directed apex.

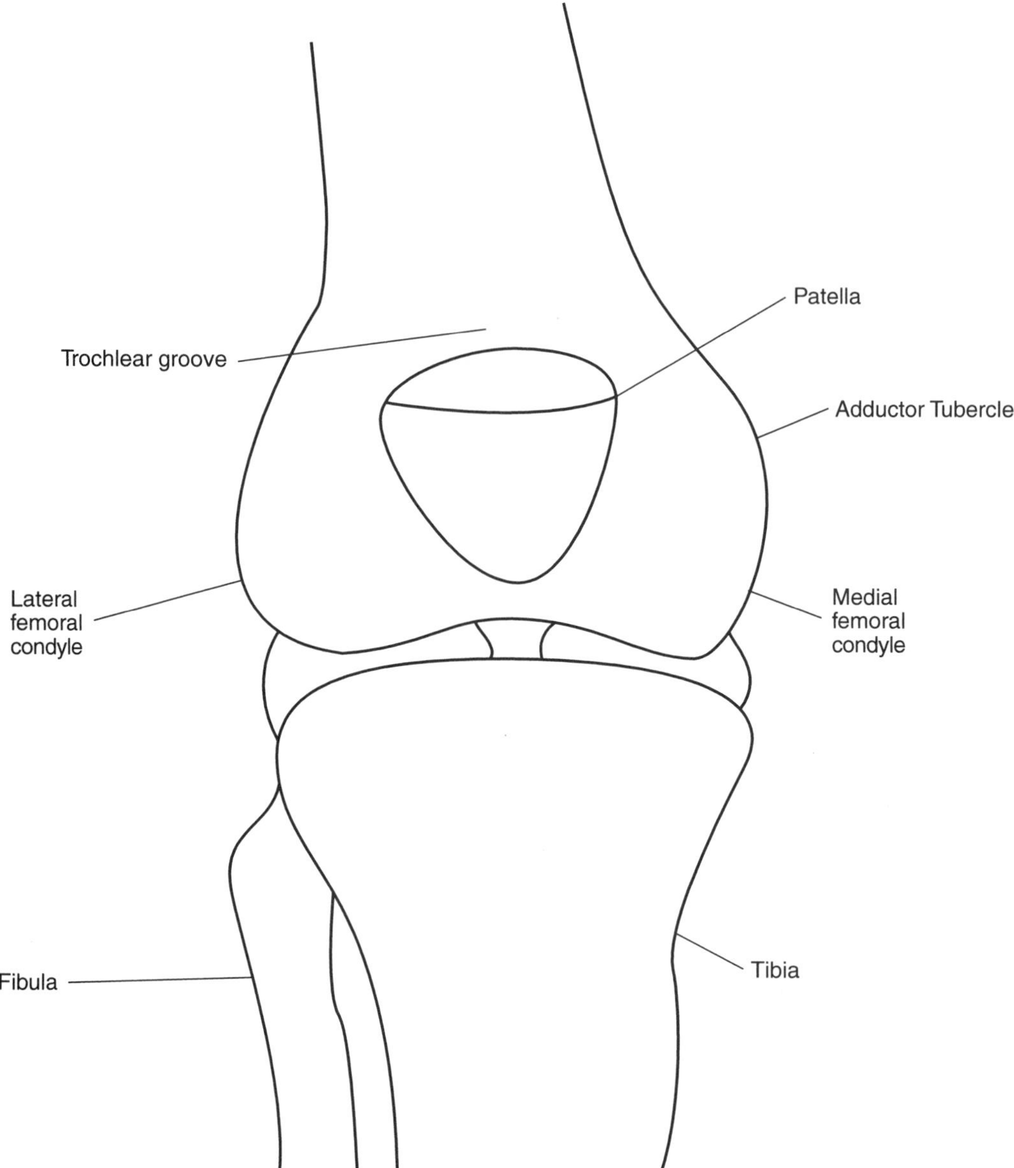

FIGURE 55-1
Anteroposterior view of bony anatomy of the knee.

2. Uppermost part is smooth for articulation with the trochlea (distal articulating surface) of the femur.[14]
3. Largest sesamoid bone lies in and interrupts the quadriceps tendon, holding it forward.
4. Protects the knee from direct trauma and provides a fulcrum for the quadriceps in extension.

C. Functional knee motion on the patella.
   1. Patella movement is constrained medially by the vastus medialis oblique (VMO), laterally by the vastus lateralis and the iliotibial band.[2]
   2. The patella femoral ligament, the patellotibial ligament, and the retinaculum restrict patellar movement.[10]
   3. Knee extension causes the patella to rest against the suprapatellar fat pad.

CAUSES OF ANTERIOR KNEE PAIN

INTRINSIC

- Abnormality of articular cartilage or subchondral bone
- Poor healing after trauma

EXTRINSIC

- VMO wasting
- Patellar position, shape, or instability
- Femoral rotation
- Tibial torsion
- Medial facet overuse

4. Knee flexion causes the patella to enter the trochlea of femur; contact with the trochlea varies with the amount of flexion.
   a. At 20-30 degrees of knee flexion, the trochlea is engaged.[22]
   b. At 90 degrees of flexion the patella enters the condylar fossa and contacts the lateral and medial femoral facets.[22]
   c. The medial facets of the patella contact the articulating surface of femoral condyles at 130-135 degrees of knee flexion.[22]

III. Biomechanics and Pathophysiology of Anterior Knee Pain
  A. A multifactorial problem, not due solely to the patella.
  B. Dominant factor is chronic overloading.
  C. Causes of anterior knee pain.
    1. Intrinsic factors (see box above).
    2. Extrinsic factors (see Table 55-1).
  D. Structural causes of anterior knee pain.
    1. At the patella.
      a. Enhances quadriceps mechanical advantage, stabilizes and protects patellar tendon, and minimizes forces placed on the femoral condyles.[10]
      b. Increases knee extension force by 50%.[10]
      c. Q angle (created by a line from the anterior superior iliac spine to the midpatella and a line from the midpatella to the tibial tubercle with knee fully extended; average is 14 degrees for males and 17 degrees for females) increase can indicate abnormal patellar tracking.
    2. At the patellofemoral joint.
      a. Patellofemoral cartilage designed for load bearing (with horizontal surface, interwoven central, and vertical deep fibrils).[21] (See Tables 55-1 and 55-2.)
      b. In full knee extension, lower patellar border contacts suprapatellar fat pad; patella moves proximally with a lateral shift (limited by lateral retinaculum).

TABLE 55-1. Patellofemoral Weight Bearing with Activity[21]

Activity	Weight Bearing
Walking	0.5 × body weight
Ascending or descending stairs	3.3 × body weight
Squatting	6.0 × body weight

TABLE 55-2. Patellofemoral Weight Bearing with Range of Motion[21]

Motion	Weight Bearing
5 degrees of flexion	30% body weight
30 degrees of flexion	2 × body weight
45 degrees of flexion	3 × body weight
75 degrees of flexion	6 × body weight

c. With increasing knee flexion, tibia internally rotates and patella moves upward creating a "high unit load."[21]

3. At the femur.
   a. Femoral torsion can increase patellofemoral contact pressure, resulting in conformational changes in the distal femur.[21]
   b. Femoral anteversion (twist of femur around its long axis—normal is 18 degrees, pain associated with greater than 20 degrees) associated with increased incidence of osteoarthritis and patellofemoral dysfunction.[6]
4. Muscle or ligament pathology in the lower extremity causes abnormal (uneven or excessive) forces, damaging patellar articular cartilage and resulting in inflammation.

IV. History
   A. Family history of anterior knee pain may be positive.
   B. Trauma.
      1. Specific known event. Note:
         a. Position of leg.
         b. Popping or clicking.
         c. Swelling.
      2. Unknown: most common.
   C. History of overuse: recent increase or other change in exercise or training program.
   D. Pain: symptom, not diagnosis.[20]
      1. Usually activity related.
         a. During activity could indicate structural problems, abnormal patellar tracking, or patellar subluxation.
         b. After activity could indicate inflammation.
      2. Nature.
         a. Vague, nonspecific, dull, aching, and stiff (most common); in two thirds of cases, bilateral.
         b. Sharp (consider loose bodies or synovial impingement).
         c. Point tenderness: consider trauma.
      3. Onset.
         a. Insidious: often an inflammatory disorder (i.e., patellar tendinitis, etc.).
         b. Sudden: associated with trauma (patellar dislocation, subluxation, etc.).
      4. Exacerbating factors.
         a. Increase in activity (e.g., stair climbing, uphill running, deep kneebends, squatting, etc.).
         b. After prolonged sitting with knee flexion ("theatre sign"): due to synovial plica being pulled tightly over femoral condyles.

E. Knee insecurity, feeling of "giving way": may indicate patellofemoral instability.[7]
   1. With turning likely due to ligamentous or meniscal injury.[7]
   2. With ascending stairs or descending incline likely a patellar or peripatellar lesion.[7]
F. Questionnaire.
   1. Kujala and associates developed a questionnaire to objectively evaluate and score subjective symptoms and functional limitations in patellofemoral disorders and relate them to objective imaging findings.[15]
   2. Gives valuable information about etiology of anterior knee pain (i.e., patellar lateralization, quadriceps function) and its imaging correlations.

V. Physical Examination
   A. General.
      1. Methodical.
      2. If possible, patient barefoot and dressed in shorts.
   B. Observation.
      1. Standing (note posture), sitting, and supine.
      2. Gait (walking and running).
         a. Normal.
         b. On heels.
         c. Inverted or everted.
      3. Note foot position and shape.
      4. Note lower extremity edema or malalignment.
      5. Genu varus or valgus.
      6. Pelvic obliquity.
      7. Q angles.
         a. Some say an increase predisposes to knee pain.
         b. Fairbank and coworkers found no relationship between Q angle and knee pain.[8]
      8. Leg length discrepancy.
   C. Knee joint.
      1. Range of motion: if abnormal or locking consider loose bodies, trauma, meniscus, contracture.
      2. Crepitus.
      3. Ligamentus laxity—Lachmann (or anterior cruciate ligament [ACL] instability), McMurray (meniscus) tests.
      4. Effusion.
      5. Pain: location, nature, positional effects.
      6. Palpable bursae.
   D. Patella.
      1. Position (in sitting position) in relation to tibia.
         a. High (patella acta), often associated with subluxation due to pull of the vastus lateralis with resultant lateral patellar shift, predisposes to poor patellar tracking.[21]
         b. Low (patella baja), uncommon: indicates tracking problem due to unusual joint loading, can indicate a quadriceps rupture.[21]
      2. Tracking, especially in terminal extension (30-0 degrees).
      3. Tilting and sliding.
         a. At 90 degrees of knee flexion, patella should be perpendicular to the femoral shaft.
         b. If tilted, patella rotates in horizontal plane so its lateral margin is in a posterior position.

c. Decreased medial slide due to tight lateral retinaculum increasing stress on and instability at the knee.
4. Subluxation.
a. Results from VMO dysplasia.
b. Causes patella to point upward.
c. Lateral subluxation could indicate increased contact at the patellofemoral joint, leading to shear and stress and resulting in cartilage damage.
5. Rotation.
a. Internal (squinting patella).[10]
b. External ("frog's eye patella").[10]

E. Pain.
1. Usually from palpation in the soft tissues in patellofemoral joint pathology.
2. At the lower inferior pole: usually due to insertional tendinitis of patellar tendon.
3. Peripatellar facets: possibly due to plica damage.

F. Muscle function.
1. Tightness.
a. Hip flexors (Thomas test): if tight, can change gait and increase symptoms.
b. Abductors (Ober test).
c. Hamstrings (straight leg raising): if tight, antagonizes quadriceps function and increases patellofemoral joint loading.
d. Knee flexors (modified Thomas test).
2. Weakness: often associated with decreased muscle bulk.
a. Hip flexors: aggravates symptoms in patellofemoral dysfunction.
b. Knee extensors (especially vastus medialis oblique): weakness causes poor patellar tracking.
(1) VMO guides patella in knee extension, displacing it medially and laterally while quadriceps isometrically contract.
(2) Muscle force vectors normally equal (can be measured); in anterior knee pain one may be weak.
(3) The lower the insertion, the greater mechanical advantage for patellar stabilization.[13]

G. Special considerations in young patients: knee pain can be referred from the hip (think Legg-Calvé-Perthes disease or slipped capital femoral epiphysis).

VI. Diagnostic Evaluation (in addition to history and physical examination)
A. Radiographic: no diagnosis based solely on radiographic findings.
1. Plain films: excellent for initial evaluation, especially in acute trauma, of patellar alignment and lateral tilt. Views: anteroposterior (AP), lateral, tunnel/sunrise, and axial projection.[19]
a. AP (to look at patellar position over femoral sulcus).
b. Lateral: at 45 degrees of knee flexion to evaluate patellar height.
c. Tunnel (PA or notch) or sunrise: to evaluate patellofemoral articulation and relative height of the femoral condyles.
d. Axial (at 30 degrees of flexion): to evaluate patellofemoral groove angle; if greater than 130 degrees, may indicate instability.[19]
2. Magnetic resonance imaging to evaluate suspected occult meniscus injury or ACL trauma: rarely appropriate.
3. Computerized tomography.
a. To evaluate for tumor or growth plate injury.[20]
b. For surgical planning.

c. To find and stage patellar subluxation in the last 15 degrees of knee flexion that could be missed on plain film.
4. Radionuclide imaging (bone scan): for judicious use with prolonged symptoms (>3-4 months) with uncertain diagnosis, pain limiting activities of daily living, or history of contact sports.[5]
a. To detect intraarticular processes, meniscal damage, osteochondritis dissecans, altered osseous homeostasis.[5]
b. To rule out tumor or osteomyelitis.[5]

B. Laboratory tests: if systemic, inflammatory, or metabolic disease is suspected.
1. Erythrocyte sedimentation rate.
2. Liver and renal functions.
3. Antibody test: to evaluate for rheumatoid arthritis or ankylosing spondylitis.

VII. Differential Diagnosis
A. Patellofemoral pain/patellar overload syndrome: "runner's knee," "biker's knee."
1. An overuse patellar injury from repeated microtrauma causing peripatellar synovitis.[13]
2. Examination findings: swelling, effusion, crepitus below the patella.
3. Possibly the most common cause of anterior knee pain.
4. In adolescents caused by rapid growth where bone length increases without a balancing increase in hamstring length, reducing hamstring contracture.

B. Plica: redundant fold in synovial lining of the knee joint.
1. Extends from the infrapatellar fat pad medially, around the femoral condyle, under the quadriceps tendon, and above the patella and passes lateral to the lateral retinaculum.[13]
2. Palpable over the medial and lateral retinaculum.
3. Vulnerable to tear as it passes over the femoral condyles.
4. Gradual onset of pain increased with sitting or prolonged knee flexion and aggravated by arising.
5. If fibrosed, can cause popping or snapping with knee extension.[13]
6. If entrapped in the patellofemoral joint between the patella and the medial femoral condyle, the knee may feel as if it will buckle.
7. Associated with tight hamstrings and low tone quadriceps with resulting increase in patellofemoral forces.[18]

C. Patellofemoral malalignment.
1. Patella tends to recenter at 25-30 degrees of knee flexion.[11]
2. Patella tilted and lateralized.
3. Risk of concomitant medial patellar subluxation.

D. Tendinitis.
1. At the patellar tendons.
a. From repeated high quadriceps loading in running, jumping, squatting, kneeling.
b. Can lead to avascular necrosis of poorly vascularized patellar tendon insertion site.[13]
2. At quadriceps tendon: tender to palpation at the superior pole of the patella or at the insertion of the vastus medialis or lateralis.

E. Bursitis.
1. Prepatellar: tenderness and swelling over the anterior patella from repetitive irritation.[13]
2. Retropatellar: pain under the patella, especially at terminal knee extension.[13]

F. Synovial shelf syndrome.
   1. Pain with knee flexion and tenderness of the medial synovial shelf without patellofemoral tenderness.[4]
   2. Increased pain with prolonged sitting.
G. Synovial chorda: perforated synovial shelf results in tight band or "chorda," causing clicking with knee flexion.[4]
H. Trauma.
   1. From direct blow to the knee.
   2. Meniscal tear.
      a. Anterior knee pain.
      b. Locking and clicking.
      c. Decreased range of motion.
      d. Joint line tenderness.
      e. Positive history of injury.
      f. Positive McMurray's test.
   3. Patellar dislocation: often self-evident.
      a. More common if history of trauma, prior dislocation (30% to 50% of all patients), previous lateral release.[12]
      b. Diagnosis based on history of lax patellofemoral ligaments that allow displacement of greater than one third the width of the patella.
      c. Associated with quadriceps weakness or atrophy, medial facet tenderness, or positive apprehension sign.
   4. After ACL reconstruction one third of patients have patellofemoral symptoms 1 year postoperatively, associated with:
      a. Weak quadriceps—due to patellar irritability or flexion contracture.
      b. Knee flexion contracture—causing patellofemoral irritability, leading to quadriceps weakness.
      c. Patellofemoral pain.
I. Osgood-Schlatter disease.
   1. Tibial tubercle apophysitis: due to microfractures.[21]
   2. Tenderness and edema at the tibial tubercle.
   3. Fluffy ossifications over tibial tubercle on plain film.[21]
   4. Usually in growing adolescent males.
J. Slipped capital femoral epiphysis.
   1. In young, growing pubertal patients.
   2. Associated with referred hip pain.
   3. Dull, vague anterior knee pain.
   4. Lower extremity in external rotation with diminished internal rotation of the hip.[10]
   5. Shorter leg on ipsilateral side.
   6. Associated with weak hip abductors.[10]
   7. Evident on AP and lateral plain films of the pelvis.[10]
   8. Consult an orthopedist.
K. Legg-Calvé-Perthes disease.
   1. In prepubertal, short, growing patients with delayed skeletal maturation.[10]
   2. Associated with referred hip pain.
   3. Necrosis of capital femoral epiphysis.
   4. Hip with diminished extension, adduction, and internal rotation.[10]
   5. Can be associated with lumbar radiculopathy.
   6. Consult an orthopedist.

L. Patellofemoral instability.
   1. Subluxation: passive hypermobility of patella with possible abnormal tracking.[13]
   2. Dislocation: visually observed.
M. Neoplasm.
   1. Benign (often must be distinguished from malignant lesions).
      a. Osteochondroma (most common): solitary, sporadic lesions that are the result of misdirected epiphyseal bone growth producing cartilage-capped bony projections from lateral edges of endochondral bones (i.e., femur).[16]
      b. Intraosseous ganglion (cystic lesion found in connective tissue of tendon sheath or joint capsule: the result of softening of connective tissue.
      c. Simple bone cyst: benign cyst on bone.
      d. Giant cell tumor: arises within epiphyses, usually around distal femur or proximal tibia or fibula; must be pathologically differentiated from malignant lesion.
      e. Chondroblastoma: usually in epiphysis; more common in males in the second decade.
   2. Malignant.
      a. Primary osteosarcoma (most common): a malignant tumor of mesenchymal cells; most appear before epiphyseal closure; 2 : 1 male-to-female ratio.[16]
      b. Plasmacytoma: thought to be a precursor to multiple myeloma but can be present for a long time without progression.
      c. Angiosarcoma: neoplasm of vascular origin, usually found in skin, breast, soft tissue, and the liver.
      d. Lymphosarcoma: often associated with leukemia; on radiography appears as metaphyseal bands of radiolucency.
N. Infection: usually primary osteomyelitis.[16]
O. Inflammatory disease.
   1. Rheumatoid arthritis.
   2. Psoriatic arthritis.
   3. Calcium pyrophosphate crystals.[16]
P. Reflex sympathetic dystrophy.
   1. Altered skin color and temperature (skin cold and turns blue, pale, or white), very tender to touch, burning pain, increased sweating.
   2. Vasomotor symptoms in the knee usually less severe than other locations.[3]
   3. Osteoporosis, in late stages, likely secondary to disuse.
   4. Patient often walks without any weight bearing.
   5. Workup: rule out tumor, infection.
   6. Treat with muscle and skin stimulation, contrast baths, medications for neuropathic pain, sympathetic blocks.
Q. Osteochondritis dissecans.[1]
   1. Defect on patellar surface with attached bone fragment.
   2. Separation of subchondral bone and cartilage from another bone.
   3. Usually well circumscribed on imaging studies.
   4. Often at the medial femoral condyle.
R. Chondromalacia patella.
   1. An arthroscopic diagnosis: roughened or fibrillated appearance.[7]
   2. Softening of the patellar articular cartilage.
   3. End stage of cartilage degeneration.

4. The result of trauma or dysplasia.
5. Can be associated with unstable knee with ligamentous or meniscal tear.

S. Hoffa syndrome.
1. Caused by contusive trauma or sprain, repeated microtrauma associated with straining the extended knee, inherently lax ligaments in genu recurvatum.[17]
2. Tenderness anteriorly over the infrapatellar fat pad on each side of the patellar tendon due to impingement of the infrapatellar fat pad between femoropatellar and femoroarticular surfaces.

T. Excessive lateral pressure syndrome.
1. From excessive articular cartilage loading or excessive joint capsule tension.[4]
2. Pain on lateral patellar margin.

VIII. Treatment

A. General principles.
1. Conservative treatment often very successful, even without specific identifiable cause.
2. Surgical treatment should only be done if there is a well-defined specific diagnosis that is not amenable to conservative care alone.[7]
3. Patience, understanding, and support for the patient are important since explanation for pain is not always available.

B. Nonsurgical.
1. Often empiric but successful in 80% of cases.[7]
2. Goal: control symptoms—decrease pain, increase strength, increase range of motion, stretch out contractures.
3. Modify activity.
   a. Decrease climbing, jumping, squatting, kneeling, and other activities that increase patellofemoral pressure.
   b. If the patient is relatively inactive, start with baseline exercises and progress as tolerated.
   c. If patient is very active, moderate the pace of activity.
4. Initial therapy after activity modification.
   a. Acutely, ice (10-15 minutes four to six times per day) not directly on the skin.
   b. If diagnosis pending, splint in 30 degrees of knee flexion to maximize comfort, relax knee ligaments, and remove pressure from cartilage injury.[22]
   c. Pain relief.
      (1) Tylenol (acetaminophen) with or without codeine.
      (2) Nonsteroidal antiinflammatory medications.
5. Therapeutic exercise.
   a. With careful instruction, follow-up, and reinforcement.
   b. To increase muscle strength, especially of the vastus medialis.
   c. To increase flexibility without patellofemoral pain, avoiding heavy patellar loading.
   d. Isometric quadriceps sets.
   e. Isotonic quadriceps exercises in nonpainful range of motion, stretching tight retinacular structures and gradually increasing weight on the quadriceps.
   f. Straight leg raising: to stretch hamstrings.
   g. Stretching for hip adductors.
   h. Increase weight and activity as strength and nonpainful range of motion increase.

i. Proprioceptive exercises: essential in preventing reinjury.
j. Reevaluation if program not successful: consider possibilities of patient noncompliance, inaccurate diagnosis; if these are certain, look for other unusual causes.
k. General principles of patellofemoral dysfunction (PFD) rehab. (See box below.)

6. Patellar taping.
   a. Improves proprioceptive stimuli to change the way the patella tracks.
   b. Evens out the speed and strength of imbalanced contraction forces of the vastus lateralis and medialis.
   c. Useful adjunct in patellar subluxation when done with closed chain exercises to strengthen the vastus medialis.
7. Patellar bracing.
   a. Improves proprioceptive stimuli.
   b. Assists the patient in adhering to activity guidelines.
   c. Very useful in preventing reinjury.
   d. Should be simple in design and easy to don and doff to increase patient compliance.

C. Surgical.
1. Only if nonsurgical treatment fails for over 6 months or obvious surgical lesion.
2. Must have specific diagnosis with clear surgical goals; avoid surgery if physical examination and radiographs are normal.
3. Arthroscopy.
   a. Lateral release of knee capsule and retinaculum.
   b. Proximal or distal realignment.
   c. Cartilage shaving.
   d. Other.
4. Open operation.
   a. Patellar tendon transfer.
   b. Patellectomy.

IX. Summary
A. Careful history and physical.
B. Conservative treatment with emphasis on increasing range of motion, muscle tone, strength (especially the quadriceps), balance, and preventing further injury.

PFD REHABILITATION

1. Relative rest: avoid deep knee bends, stair climbing, etc.
2. Ice: 5-10 minutes before and after activity.
3. VMO strengthening.
   a. Short arc quad sets and knee presses.
   b. Slow, repetitive VMO contractions with eccentric loading.
4. Increase flexibility of hamstrings, vastus lateralis, and iliotibial band.
5. Isometric quadriceps exercise and adductor stretching.
6. Cardiovascular conditioning.
7. Gradual increase of activity when ROM full, good strength (at least 80% of normal), and pain free.
8. Provide athlete with home program.
9. Consider neoprene patellar sleeve to augment proprioception and joint protection during activity.

C. Most resolve with conservative care.
D. Rehabilitation is not over until muscle bulk returns.
E. No return to play or previous activity until 80% of the strength of the uninjured knee by isokinetic testing.

References

1. Bentley G: Anterior knee pain: diagnosis and management, J Roy Coll Surg Edinb 34(Suppl):2-5, 1989.
2. Bose K, Kanagasuntherakm R, Osman MB: Vastus medialis: an anatomic and physiologic study, *Orthopedics* 3:880-883, 1980.
3. Butler-Manuel PA, Justins D, Heatley FW: Sympathetically mediated anterior knee pain, *Acta Orthop Scand* 63(1):90-93, 1992.
4. Dandy DJ: Arthroscopy in the treatment of young patients with anterior knee pain, *Orthop Clin North Am* 17(2):221-229, 1986.
5. Dye SF, Boll DA: Radionuclide imaging of the patellofemoral joint in young adults with anterior knee pain, *Orthop Clin North Am* 17(2):259-261, 1986.
6. Eckhoff DG et al: Femoral morphometry and anterior knee pain, *Clin Orthop Rel Res* 302:64-65, 1994.
7. Eilert RE: Adolescent anterior knee pain. In *Pediatric Orthopedics,* 1991, pp 499, 506, 508-515.
8. Fairbank JC et al: Mechanical factors in the incidence of knee pain in adolescents and young adults, *J Bone Joint Surg* 66B:685-693, 1984.
9. Garrick JG: Anterior knee pain (chondromalacia patella), *Phys Sportsmed* 17:75-84, 1989.
10. Goldberg B: Chronic anterior knee pain in the adolescent, *Ped Ann* 20(4):186, 187, 191-193, 1991.
11. Guzzanti V et al: Patellofemoral malalignment in adolescents, *Am J Sports Med* 22(1):55-60, 1994.
12. Hawkins RJ, Bell RH, Anisette G: Acute patellar dislocations: the natural history, *Am J Sports Med* 14(2):117-120, 1986.
13. Jacobson JE, Flandry FC: Diagnosis of anterior knee pain, *Clin Sports Med* 8(2):179, 181, 184-193, 1989.
14. Jenkins DB: *Hollinshead's Functional Anatomy of the Limbs and Back,* Philadelphia, 1991, WB Saunders, p 234.
15. Kujala UM et al: Scoring of patellofemoral disorders, *Arthroscopy: J Arthroscop Rel Surg* 9(2):159-163, 1993.
16. Lin HH, Gilula LA: A 77 year old man with right anterior knee pain, *Orthop Rev* pp 1333-1339, Dec 1993.
17. Magi M et al: Hoffa disease, *Divisione de chirurgia del Ginocchio e chirurgia Artroscopica* pp 211-216, 1987.
18. Patel D: Plica as a cause of anterior knee pain, *Orthop Clin North Am* 17(2):213-275, 1986.
19. Poole B, Puffer JC, Whipple TL: Knee: watch for the serious problem, *Patient Care* pp 52-53, 57, 61, Feb 29, 1992.
20. Post WR, Fulkerson JP: Anterior knee pain—a symptom not a diagnosis, *Bull Rheum Dis* 42(2):5-6, 1992.
21. Reid DC: Sports injury assessment and rehabilitation, New York, 1992, Churchill Livingstone, pp 347, 349, 357-358, 375, 409-411.
22. Ruffin MT, Kiningham RB: Anterior knee pain: the challenge of the patellofemoral syndrome, *Am Fam Phys* 47(1):185, 192, 1993.
23. Sachs RA et al: Patellofemoral problems after anterior cruciate ligament reconstruction, *Am J Sports Med* 17(6):760, 762-764, 1986.

CHAPTER 56

Rehabilitation of the Injured Knee

David B. Richards, MD

W. Ben Kibler, MD

I. General Overview
  A. Knee injuries extremely common.
    1. Minor sprain → ligament ruptures/fractures.
    2. Key to treatment is timely and accurate diagnosis.
  B. Microtrauma.
    1. Chronic overload injuries.
    2. Develop over long periods of time.
    3. Secondary adaptations may occur.
  C. Macrotrauma.
    1. Single event traumatic injuries.
    2. Can usually define when, where, and how.
  D. Rehabilitation.
    1. Acute phase: resolution of symptoms of injury.
    2. Recovery phase: improve range of motion (ROM), strength, neuromuscular training.
    3. Maintenance phase.
      a. Strengthening, neuromuscular control.
      b. Functional exercises.
  E. Kinetic chain.
    1. Series of connected "links," beginning with ground reactive force and progressing to hand.
    2. Knee an important component in force generation and transfer.
    3. Injured knee may "break the chain" and impair performance (Figs. 56-1 and 56-2).

II. Injuries
  A. Mild sprain → ligament tears/fractures.
  B. Macrotrauma.
    1. Single traumatic event.
    2. Normal anatomy → abnormal.
    3. Instantaneous.

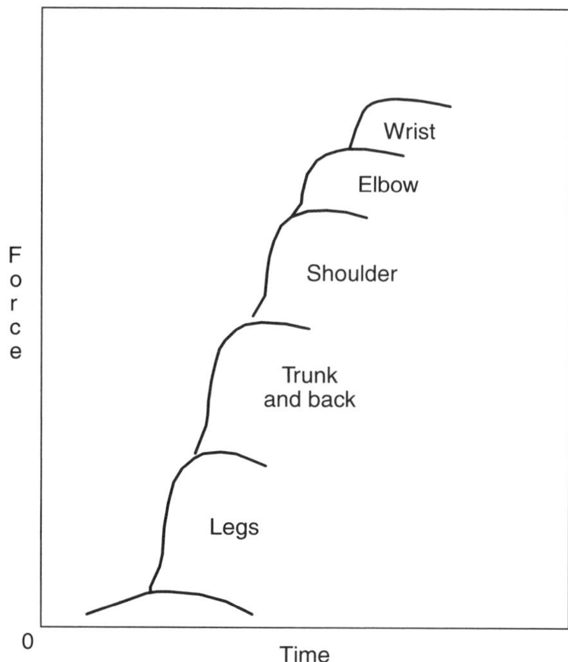

FIGURE 56-1
The kinetic chain for force generation in the tennis serve. The knee serves as an important link in transmitting forces from the calf and allowing generation of forces by the quadriceps and hamstring activation.

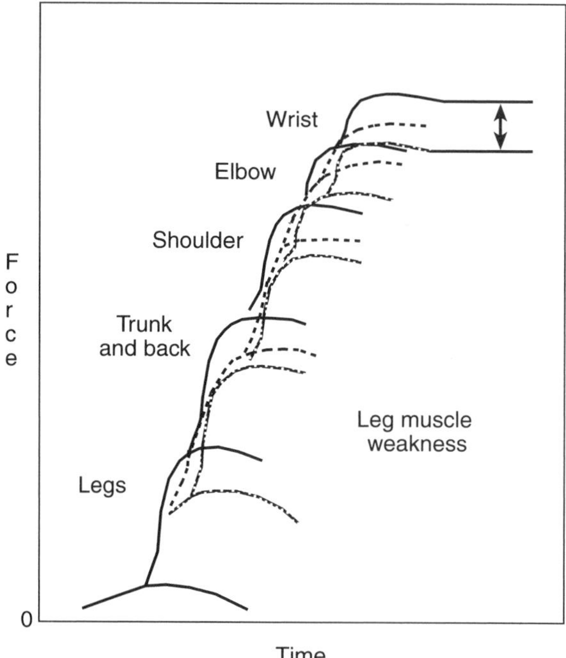

FIGURE 56-2
Kinetic chain of the tennis serve showing the decreased force production due to muscle weakness from incomplete rehabilitation around the knee. The functional result would be decreased service velocity or overuse of the smaller muscles of the shoulder, elbow, or wrist in attempts to make up the force decrement.

C. Microtrauma.
   1. Chronic repetitive tissue overload.
   2. Failure to heal.
   3. Subsequent biomechanical adaptations.
   4. Develops over time.

III. Diagnosis
   A. History.
   B. Physical examination.
   C. Supporting studies.

IV. Goals of Rehabilitation
   A. Resolve symptoms/signs of injury.
   B. Restore ROM and strength.
   C. Restore normal arthrokinematics and neuromuscular firing patterns.
   D. Return to competition.
   E. Prevent reinjury or further injury.

V. Phases of Rehabilitation
   A. Acute (early postinjury or postsurgery).
      1. Goals.
         a. Reduce pain, inflammation, swelling.
         b. Improve ROM.
         c. Minimize muscle atrophy.
         d. Maintain fitness.
      2. Pain, swelling, inflammation.
         a. Nonsteroidal antiinflammatory drugs.
         b. Modalities (ice, heat, electrical stimulation).
         c. Bracing, activity restrictions.
      3. Increase ROM/minimize atrophy.
         a. Isometrics.
         b. Straight leg raises.
         c. Biofeedback: patellar control.
      4. Maintain fitness: aerobic and anaerobic endurance.
      5. Criteria for progression.
         a. Reduce swelling and pain.
         b. Healing of injured tissue.
         c. Begin weight bearing.
   B. Recovery phase.
      1. Goals.
         a. Increase passive/active pain-free ROM.
         b. Improve muscular strength.
         c. Improve neuromuscular control.
         d. Normal single plane joint kinematics.
      2. Increasing ROM.
         a. Patella mobilization.
         b. Cross-friction massage.
         c. Knee flexion/extension.
         d. Stationary bike.
         e. Wall slides.
         f. Stretching quadriceps, hamstrings, iliotibial band, hip flexors, gastrocnemius-soleus.
      3. Improving strength.
         a. Open chain.
            (1) Isotonics (eccentric/concentric).
            (2) Isokinetics.
            (3) Free weights, tubing.

b. Closed chain.
   (1) Stair climber.
   (2) Nautilus.
   (3) Free weights.

4. Neuromuscular control.
   a. Biomechanical ankle platform system (BAPS).
   b. Balance board.
   c. Slide board.
   d. Minitrampoline.
   e. Lifeline.
5. Joint biomechanics: kinetic chain movement patterns.
6. Criteria for progression.
   a. Active/passive ROM equal to opposite side.
   b. Quadricep/hamstring strength ratio 66%, and strength 75% of opposite leg.
   c. One leg squat (10-15 repetitions).
   d. Smooth single plane joint motion.

C. Maintenance phase.
1. Goals.
   a. Increased power and endurance.
   b. Improve multiplane neuromuscular control.
   c. Completion of sport-specific activities.
2. Increased power and endurance.
   a. Isotonics, isokinetics.
   b. Stair climber, stationary bike.
   c. Nautilus.
3. Improved multiplane neuromuscular control.
   a. Multiplane motions.
      (1) Side lunges.
      (2) Slide board.
   b. Plyometrics.
   c. Agility and footwork drills.
4. Sport-specific activities.
5. Criteria for return to play.
   a. Normal ROM/flexibility.
   b. Strength 90% of opposite side.
   c. Normal physical examination.
   d. Normal multiplane kinematics.
6. Following the successful completion of the rehabilitation program, the patient/athlete is encouraged to maintain the level of fitness attained by the rehabilitation program.

Bibliography

Andrews JR, Harrelson GL: *Physical Rehabilitation of the Injured Athlete,* Philadelphia, 1991, WB Saunders.

DeCarlo MS, Sell KE, Klootwyck TE: Faster, better, stronger, *Rehab Management,* pp 66-72, Aug/Sept 1993.

Fu FH et al: *Knee Surgery,* Baltimore, 1994, Williams & Wilkins.

Griffin LY: *Rehabilitation of the Injured Knee,* ed 2, St Louis, 1995, Mosby.

Kibler WB, Chandler TJ: Sport specific conditioning, *Am J Sports Med* 22:3, 1994.

Richardson JK, Iglarsh ZA: *Clinical Orthopedic Physical Therapy,* Philadelphia, 1994, WB Saunders.

Shelborne DK, Nitz P: Accelerated rehabilitation after ACL reconstruction, *J Sports Physical Ther* 15:6, 1992.

CHAPTER 57

Anatomy and Examination of the Hip

Carl Winfield, MD

I. Anatomy of Hip
   A. General.
      1. Ball and socket joint.
      2. Articular surface large and deep, providing substantial mechanical stability, which is adaptive for the high loads it is constantly subjected to.
      3. Capsule extends from femur to acetabulum.
      4. Each part of hemipelvis participates in formation of the acetabulum.
   B. Bony landmarks: anterior superior iliac spine, iliac crest, posterior superior iliac spine, greater tuberosity, lesser tuberosity, pubic symphysis, and ischial tuberosity.
   C. Muscles.
      1. Hip flexors: iliopsoas, rectus femoris, sartorius; pectineus and tensor fasciae latae also function as flexors.
      2. Extensors: gluteus maximus, long head of biceps femoris, semitendinosus, semimembranosus, and posterior portion of adductor magnus.
      3. Abductors: gluteus medius, gluteus minimus, and tensor fasciae latae.
      4. Adductors: adductor longus, adductor brevis, adductor magnus, gracilis, and pectineus.
      5. External rotators: piriformis, superior and inferior gemelli, obturatorius externus and internus, and quadratus femoris.
      6. No pure internal rotators of the hip. A number of muscles provide internal rotation as well as other functions.
   D. Innervation.
      1. Branches of the lumbar and sacral plexus innervate the hip joint. These nerves are derived from the second through the fifth lumbar segments.
      2. Several of the branches originate from the obturator nerve.
   E. Blood supply.
      1. Blood supply to the hip joint in general is generous but to the femoral head itself is tenuous.

2. Femoral head blood supply.
   a. Retinacular arterial system that runs along neck of femur.
   b. Supplied by perforating capsular branches that derive from extracapsular arterial ring formed predominantly by the medial femoral circumflex artery, with contributions from the lateral circumflex vessels.

II. History
   A. Acute.
      1. Mechanism of injury: direct blow, fall, twisting.
      2. Functional disability immediately afterwards.
   B. Chronic: insidious onset of symptoms.
      1. Change in training regimen leading to overuse.
      2. Constitutional symptoms: fever, weight loss.
      3. Biomechanical problems: overpronation, tibial torsion, genu varum.
   C. Age: child or adolescent susceptible to apophysitis, Legg-Calvé-Perthes disease, slipped capital femoral epiphysis, and the like.
   D. Location of pain.
      1. Anterior, lateral, medial, or groin.
      2. May have referred pain to knee.
   E. Timing of pain: pain at rest, first thing in the morning, or lessening with activity is suggestive of inflammatory component.
   F. Review of medications: regular use of corticosteroids may lead to a vascualr necrosis (AVN) of femoral head.

III. Hip Examination
   A. Observation.
      1. Stance.
         a. Anterior superior iliac spine and posterior superior iliac spine should be level with contralateral side.
         b. Increased lordosis of lumbar spine suggests need to evaluate for flexion deformity of the hip.
      2. Gait: should have even distribution of weight bearing as well as pain-free and efficient movement.
   B. Range of motion: pathology involving the true hip joint can best be elicited by testing the passive range of motion. Early abnormalities are best detected by loss of internal rotation and/or abduction. Pain in the groin is very specific for pathology and, when associated with decreased hip range of motion, it is extremely specific for hip joint disease.
      1. Log roll: passive internal and external rotation at hip with patient supine and hip in neutral with knee extended.
      2. Active flexion, extension, abduction, and adduction all tested and compared to the opposite side.
   C. Leg length discrepancy can be evaluated by measuring distance from anterior superior iliac spine to the malleolus.
   D. Muscle strength can be assessed by resisting the patient's movements in the above active ranges of motion.
   E. Special tests.
      1. For sacroiliac joint pathology, Patrick's test (FABERE [flexion, abduction, external rotation, and extension] test): patient lies supine with the foot of the involved side on the opposite knee. The hip joint is now flexed, abducted, and externally rotated. To stress the sacroiliac joint, one hand is placed on the involved knee and the other hand on the opposite anterior superior iliac spine. These are pressed down towards the table. Pain in region of sacroiliac joint indicates a positive test.

2. Trendelenburg test: patient is observed in a standing position from posterior view. Then, while standing on one leg, the patient should maintain level pelvic posture or the contralateral non–weight-bearing side should rise slightly. Pain in the weight-bearing hip joint or weakness of the ipsilateral gluteus medius muscle will result in the pelvis being tilted downward on the contralateral side.
3. Thomas test: detects hip flexion contractures. The unexamined hip and knee are flexed up onto the chest with the patient supine. A flexion contracture in the contralateral examined hip will be demonstrated by the patient's inability to keep the hip fully extended.

Bibliography

Hartzog CW, Boulware DW: A clinical approach to hip pain, *Primary Care Rheumatol* 2(2):1-7, 1992.

Steinberg G, Akins C, Baran D, editors: *Ramamurti's Orthopedics in Primary Care,* ed 2, Baltimore, 1992, Williams & Wilkins.

CHAPTER 58

Common Hip Injuries

Carl Winfield, MD

I. Hip Pointer
  A. History.
    1. Direct blow to iliac crest during collision and contact sports.
    2. Sudden, severe pain in region of iliac crest; commonly with audible pop or snap.
  B. Physical examination: swelling, ecchymosis, and marked tenderness at iliac crest.
  C. Radiographs may be obtained to rule out fracture if clinically indicated.
  D. Treatment.
    1. Ice, compressive dressings, and analgesics.
    2. Progressive supervised stretching program.
    3. May return to contact sports with padding over affected area when pain is tolerable and any limp has disappeared.[7]

II. Hip Adductor Strain ("Groin Pull")
  A. History.
    1. Forced abduction during a fall, twisting injury, or collision.
    2. Pain in the region of the adductors just distal to the origin on the pelvis.
  B. Physical examination.
    1. Pain increased with resisted adduction and at times with resisted hip flexion.
    2. Rarely, ecchymosis is associated. Swelling may be present.
    3. Tenderness at inferior pubic ramus and/or adductor tubercle.
  C. Differential diagnosis: hernia, disorders of bowel, bladder, testicles, kidneys, and other soft tissues.
  D. Treatment.
    1. Rest, ice, nonsteroidal antiinflammatory drugs (NSAIDs).
    2. Strengthening and stretching of adductors.[8]

III. Osteitis Pubis
  A. History.

1. Repetitive overuse of the adductors (e.g., runners with crossover arm swing).
2. Progressive groin pain that may radiate to the thigh.
3. "Popping" sensation with sports participation or walking.

B. Physical examination.
1. Pain with resisted adduction of the thigh.
2. Tenderness at pubic symphysis.
3. One leg stance with hop elicits pain.

C. Studies.
1. Radiographs may show erosions, lytic lesions, sclerosis, or irregularity at the pubic rami adjacent to the syndesmosis.
2. Early diagnosis requires bone scan.

D. Treatment.
1. Rest, NSAIDs, stretching, strengthening of adductors.[11]
2. Severe cases may require corticosteroids or possibly arthrodesis.

IV. Quadriceps Contusion
A. History: direct blow to quadriceps with associated pain and decreased range of motion.
B. Physical examination: thigh with ecchymosis, swelling, and tenderness.
C. Radiographs: may help rule out fracture if suspected.
D. Treatment.
1. Immobilize in full knee flexion for first 24 hours with crutches, rest, and ice.
2. Active and passive gentle flexion, extension exercises, and progressive weight bearing.
3. Stretching, strengthening, proprioception. After patient has 120 degrees of pain-free range of motion, may resume contact sports.[11]

E. Complications: myositis ossificans.
1. History of persistent pain and stiffness.
2. Can be detected by radiography 2-4 weeks following injury.
3. Usually no treatment. Surgical excision is rarely indicated and only after ossification has matured.[5]

V. Posterior Hip Dislocation
A. Most common hip dislocation: 90%.
B. History: forces acting along long axis of femur driving the head posteriorly.
C. Physical examination: hip is flexed, adducted, and internally rotated.
D. Radiographs will demonstrate the dislocation. True lateral of the hip is often necessary to confirm the direction of the dislocation.
E. Treatment.
1. Reduction of the dislocated hip. An orthopedic emergency because of compromise of the blood supply and sciatic nerve.
2. Orthopedic involvement should occur immediately.
3. Reduction occurs with patient supine. As an assistant stabilizes the pelvis, the operator applies traction to the leg from behind the flexed knee along the line of the limb. With continued traction the hip is gently internally and externally rotated (ideally occurs with good pain control and muscle relaxation).[3]
4. Radiographs are obtained to confirm congruous reduction of the hip and to evaluate the presence of any acetabular or femoral head fracture.

VI. Avascular Necrosis of the Femoral Head (Legg-Calvé-Perthes Disease)
A. History.

1. Affects children between the ages of 2-11.
2. Pain usually in groin, anterior thigh, and occasionally in the knee.
3. Onset usually insidious.
4. Some present without pain, but almost all have a limp that increases with activity.

B. Physical examination.
1. Loss of internal and external rotation of hip.
2. Pain with hip motion.
3. Hip flexion produces external rotation.

C. Radiographs.
1. The first bony change may be increased density of the femoral epiphysis.
2. An irregularly mottled appearance of the femoral head and subchondral fracture may appear later.

D. Treatment.
1. Based on the principle that containment of the femoral head within the acetabulum will lead to the best healing and remodeling of the infarcted femoral head.
2. Patients who are young (≤4 years) with involvement of <50% of the head and who lack certain radiographic changes may simply be given symptomatic treatment and observed.
3. For most patients containment of the femoral head within the acetabulum can be achieved with an external brace or cast. For some patients osteotomy of the femur or pelvis is necessary.[10]

VII. Slipped Capital Femoral Epiphysis

A. History.
1. Occurs in children between the ages of 11-16.
2. Insidious onset of groin, hip, thigh, or knee pain associated with a limp.
3. May present with acute hip pain following an injury.
4. More commonly affected are males who are obese with somewhat delayed development of secondary sexual characteristics.

B. Physical examination: in acute phase there is significant muscle spasm and synovitis with restricted range of motion. Because of limitation of internal rotation the extremity tends to externally rotate when the hip is flexed.

C. Studies: radiography demonstrates posterior and medial displacement of the epiphysis.

D. Treatment.
1. Orthopedic referral should be obtained.
2. Treatment is usually surgical and, rarely, immobilization.[10]

VIII. Trochanteric Bursitis

A. History: pain in region of trochanteric bursa, usually when moving hip from full extension to full flexion.

B. Physical examination: with patient lying on unaffected side, the pain is reproduced by the patient actively moving the hip from full extension to 30 degrees of flexion. The examiner's hand may feel a pop or snap when placed over the greater trochanter.

C. Treatment.
1. Remove the athlete from running and place in aerobic activities that do not involve hip flexion and extension.
2. Iliotibial band stretching program and NSAIDs.
3. Corticosteroid injection as a second step.
4. Surgical treatment may be indicated.

IX. Femoral Neck Stress Fracture
   A. History.
      1. Endurance athletes. Thin, amenorrheic females highly susceptible.
      2. Increase in training.
      3. Groin pain with running progressing to pain with activities of daily living.
   B. Physical examination.
      1. May have antalgic gait.
      2. Pain limiting the extremes of internal and external rotation.
   C. Studies.
      1. Radiographs may be negative early or may reveal periosteal new bone formation, endosteal thickening, or radiolucent line formation.
      2. Bone scan typically gives diagnosis 2-8 days after symptoms begin.
   D. Treatment.
      1. If stress fracture is at the tension side, internal fixation is generally performed. Incomplete, nondisplaced fractures may be treated with bedrest, but many recommend open reduction and internal fixation due to high risk of displacement.
      2. If stress fracture occurs on the compression side:
         a. Bedrest until no pain at rest.
         b. Progressive weight bearing within the limits of pain.
         c. If compression fracture progresses from sclerosis to a fracture line, begin strict bedrest and consider immediate internal fixation.
      3. Orthopedic consultation is mandatory. Displaced fractures are an orthopedic emergency!

X. Avulsion Fractures of the Hip
   A. Anterior superior iliac spine (ASIS): sartorius originates here.
      1. History.
         a. Forceful contraction with knee flexed and hip extended.
         b. May have anterolateral thigh paresthesia and pain because of lateral femoral cutaneous nerve entrapment.
         c. Swelling.
      2. Physical examination.
         a. Palpation of ASIS region produces pain.
         b. Pain with resisted hip flexion and knee extension.
      3. Studies: radiography reveals avulsion fracture.
      4. Treatment.
         a. Knee splinted in flexion initially.
         b. Rest, ice, progressive weight bearing, stretching, and strengthening.
         c. Surgery may be required for a displaced apophysis.
   B. Anterior inferior iliac spine: rectus femoris originates here.
      1. History.
         a. Vigorous rectus femoris contractions (e.g., kicking).
         b. Groin pain.
      2. Physical examination.
         a. Resisted quadriceps contraction produces pain.
         b. Hip flexion or extension increases pain.
      3. Studies: radiography reveals avulsion fracture.
      4. Treatment.
         a. Ice, rest, progressive weight bearing. Resistance exercises may begin once full range of motion is obtained.

b. Return to sports may be permitted when full strength and function have returned.
c. Surgery may be necessary for a displaced apophysis.

C. Ischial tuberosity.
1. History.
a. Vigorous hamstring contraction with the hip in flexion and knee extended.
b. Sudden pain in buttock and inability to continue activity.
2. Physical examination.
a. Tenderness to palpation at ischial tuberosity.
b. Pain with straight leg raise and resisted knee flexion.
3. Treatment.
a. Rest, ice, progressive weight bearing.
b. Exercises with resistance can begin once full active range of motion is achieved.
c. May return to sports once full strength and function have returned.
d. Displaced apophysis may require surgery.

D. Iliac crest.
1. History.
a. Direct blow to abdomen or iliac crest.
b. Pain with contraction of abdominal muscles or with resisted hip abduction.
2. Studies: oblique as well as anteroposterior and lateral of pelvis may reveal evidence of avulsion fracture.
3. Treatment.
a. Ice, rest, and crutch ambulation.
b. Stretching and strengthening.
c. Return to sports is not permitted until strength and function have returned.

XI. Hamstring Strain
A. History.
1. Poor flexibility, inadequate warm-up, or fatigue may contribute.
2. Sudden, forceful contraction of hamstrings or forced extension at the knee.
3. Immediate pain in hamstring region and loss of function.
B. Physical examination.
1. Pain with resisted flexion at the knee.
2. Tenderness to palpation at the muscle belly or origin.
C. Treatment.
1. Initially with ice, compression, NSAIDs, and weight bearing as tolerated.
2. Stretching, electrical stimulation.
3. Early functional exercises including jogging, pool running, and stationary biking.
4. Strengthening via curls and isokinetics.[7]

XII. Piriformis Syndrome
A. History.
1. Trauma, prolonged sitting, or overuse.
2. Dull ache in mid-buttock region.
3. Pain walking up stairs or inclines.
B. Physical examination.
1. Tenderness to palpation along course of piriformis muscle from the sacrum to the greater trochanter.

2. Pain with flexing, adducting, and internally rotating the hip with the patient supine.
3. Patient may hold leg in external rotation.
4. May have positive Trendelenburg test.

C. Treatment.
1. NSAIDs and aggressive massage.
2. Stretching by flexing, internally rotating, and adducting at the hip.
3. Ultrasound.
4. Local corticosteroids may occasionally help.
5. Surgical release as a last resort.[9]

XIII. Iliopsoas Bursitis/Tendinitis (Snapping Hip Syndrome)

A. History.
1. Groin pain worse with activity.
2. "Snapping" with hip flexion.

B. Physical examination.
1. Pain with resisted hip flexion.
2. Tenderness to palpation just lateral to the femoral neurovascular bundle over the pubic ramus.

C. Treatment.
1. Activity modification, NSAIDs, ice.
2. Iliopsoas stretching and strengthening.
3. Corticosteroid injection.

References

1. Aronen JG, Chronister RD: Quadriceps contusions: hastening the return to play, *Phys Sportsmed* 20(7):130-136, 1992.
2. Combs JA: Hip and pelvic avulsion fractures in adolescents: proper diagnosis improves compliance, *Phys Sportsmed* 22(7):42-49, 1994.
3. Hartzog CW, Boulware DW: A clinical approach to hip pain, *Primary Care Rheumatol* 2(2):1-7, 1992.
4. Hoppenfeld S: *Physical Examination of the Spine and Extremities,* Syntex Edition, Norwalk, CT, 1976, Appleton-Century-Crofts.
5. Kaeding CC, Sanko WA, Fischer RA: Myositis ossificans: minimizing downtime, *Phys Sportsmed* 23(2):77-82, 1995.
6. Martire JR: Differentiating stress fracture from periostitis: the finer points of bone scans, editor, *Phys Sportsmed* 22(10):71-81, 1994.
7. Mellion MB: *Sports Medicine Secrets,* 1994, Hanley and Belfus.
8. Reider B: *Sports Medicine: The School-Age Athlete,* Philadelphia, 1991, WB Saunders.
9. Rich BS, McKeag D: When sciatica is not disk disease: detecting piriformis syndrome in active patients, *Phys Sportsmed* 20(10):104-115, 1992.
10. Steinberg G, Akins C, Baran D, editors: *Ramamurti's Orthopedics in Primary Care,* ed 2, Baltimore, 1992, Williams & Wilkins.
11. Stewart C: Hip, pelvis and thigh injuries (lecture). Presented at Sports Medicine: An In Depth Review, February 1995, Dallas, Texas. Sponsored by The American Academy of Family Physicians.

CHAPTER 59

Ankle and Foot Anatomy

Aaron Rubin, MD

I. Ankle
   A. Bones.
      1. Calcaneus: the largest and strongest bone in the foot and ankle; transmits energy from foot strike. Has three surfaces that articulate with the talus: large posterior, anterior, and middle. Distally articulates with the cuboid.
      2. Talus: articulates with the tibia and fibula in the mortise. The head articulates with the navicular distally and the calcaneus inferiorly.
      3. Tibia: forms the medial malleolus and medial portion of mortise.
      4. Fibula: a smaller bone that forms the lateral malleolus and the lateral portion of the mortise.
   B. Lateral ligaments.
      1. Anterior talofibular: about 20 mm long, 10 mm wide, and 2 mm thick. Runs parallel to long axis of foot and perpendicular to long axis of leg. Prevents anterior displacement of talus. Most commonly injured ankle ligament. Injured by inversion-plantar flexion.
      2. Calcaneofibular: about 20 mm long, 5 mm wide, and 3 mm thick. Runs vertically and resists inversion of calcaneus. Runs deep to peroneal tendon sheaths.
      3. Posterior talofibular: the smallest of the major lateral ankle ligaments. Acts as a weak restraint against posterior displacement of the talus within the ankle mortise.
   C. Medial ligaments: the deltoid ligament, the largest of the ankle ligaments, is a broad, fanlike, two-layered complex of ligaments. It prevents abduction-eversion of the ankle and subtalar joint.
   D. Muscles (Table 59-1).

II. Foot
   A. Bones: can be thought of in two ways:
      1. By dividing the foot from posterior to anterior into the hindfoot, midfoot, and forefoot.

TABLE 59-1. Muscles of the Ankle

Muscle	Primary Function	Innervation
Anterior Compartment of Leg		
Anterior tibialis	Dorsiflexion and supination of foot	Deep peroneal (L4)
Extensor hallucis longus	Extension and dorsiflexion of great toe	Deep peroneal (L5)
Extensor digitorum longus	Extension and dorsiflexion of toes	Deep peroneal (L5)
Lateral Compartment of Leg		
Peroneus brevis	Eversion and plantarflexion of foot	Superficial peroneal (S1)
Peroneus longus	Eversion plantarflexion and pronation of foot	Superficial peroneal (S1)
Superficial Posterior Compartment		
Gastrocnemius, soleus, plantaris	Plantar flexion, supination of foot	Tibial (S1)
Deep Posterior Compartment		
Flexor hallucis longus	Plantar flexion of great toe	Tibial (S1)
Flexor digitorum longus	Plantar flexion of toes, foot	Tibial (S1, S2)
Tibialis posterior	Supination, adduction of foot	Tibial (L4, L5)

   a. The hindfoot is about one third the length of the foot and is composed of two bones: the calcaneus, which consists of the heel and supports the talus, and the talus itself, which articulates with the lower leg.
   b. The midfoot is about one sixth the length of the foot and is composed of the medial, middle, and lateral cuneiform bones, the cuboid, and the navicular.
   c. The forefoot is composed of the five metatarsal bones and the 14 phalanges.
2. By dividing the foot into columns from medial to lateral.
   a. Medial column: calcaneus, talus, navicular, medial, and middle cuneiform bones, first and second metatarsal bones, and phalanges of first and second toes.
   b. Middle column: lateral cuneiform, third metatarsal, phalanges of third toe.
   c. Lateral column: calcaneus, cuboid, fourth and fifth metatarsal bones, phalanges of fourth and fifth toes.

B. Ligaments: multiple ligaments are present on the plantar and dorsal surface of the foot interconnecting each of the bones.
   1. The medial column is supported by the "spring ligament," which is a fibrocartilaginous, reinforced structure that bridges the gap between the calcaneus and the navicular on the plantar surface, provides a floor to the head of the talus, and prevents excessive midfoot pronation and sag of the talus. The medial arch is further supported by the naviculocuneiform and first tarsometatarsal ligaments.

TABLE 59-2. Muscles of the Foot

Muscle	Primary Function	Innervation
Dorsal Layer		
Extensor digitorum brevis	Extends toe	Deep peroneal
First Plantar Layer		
Abductor hallucis	Abducts great toe	Medial plantar
Flexor digitorum brevis	Flexes toes	Medial plantar
Abductor digiti minimi	Abducts small toe	Medial plantar
Second Plantar Layer		
Lumbricals	Flex metatarsophalangeals/ extend interphalangeals	Medial and lateral plantar
Flexor digitorum and hallucis longus	Flex toes/invert foot	Tibial
Third Plantar Layer		
Flexor hallucis brevis	Flexes great toe	Medial plantar
Adductor hallucis	Adducts great toe	Lateral plantar
Fourth Plantar Layer		
Dorsal interosseous	Abducts toes	Lateral plantar
Plantar interosseous	Adducts toes	Lateral plantar

2. The plantar surface is covered by the plantar aponeurosis and medial and lateral plantar fascia.

C. Muscles (Table 59-2).

III. Biomechanics of the Ankle and Foot

A. Gait cycle: begins at the heel contact of one foot and ends at the next heel strike of the same foot (Table 59-3). The stance phase accounts for 60% of the gait cycle.

TABLE 59-3. Stance Phase of the Gait Cycle

	Contact (25% of stance)	Midstance (40% of stance)	Propulsion (35% of stance)	Swing Phase (40%)
Starts/ends	Heel strike/ forefoot to ground	Foot flat/ heel off	Heel elevation/toe off	Toe off/heel strike
Function	Dissipates energy, adapts to terrain	Foot fully weight bearing for propulsion	Provides force to propel foot forward	Carries extremity from one step to next
Leg motion	Internal rotation	Begins to rotate externally	External rotation	Hip and knee flexion
Subtalar motion	Pronate	Supinate	Supinate	Dorsiflex

1. Stance phase.
   a. Contact phase.
   b. Midstance phase.
   c. Propulsion phase.
2. Swing phase.
   a. During walking, one foot is always in contact with the ground.
   b. During running, a "double-float" phase occurs when both feet are off the ground.

Acknowledgment

The Medical Editing Department, Kaiser Foundation Research Institute, provided editorial assistance.

Bibliography

Fetto JF: Anatomy and physical examination of the foot and ankle. In Nicholas JA, Hershman EB, editors: *The Lower Extremity and Spine in Sports Medicine,* ed 2, St Louis, 1995, Mosby–Year Book, pp 317-334.

Pansky B: *Review of Gross Anatomy,* New York, 1984, Macmillan, pp 532-547.

Reid DC: Selected conditions of the foot, ankle region. In Reid DC, editor: *Sports Injury Assessment and Rehabilitation,* New York, 1992, Churchill Livingstone, pp 129-185, 215-269.

Renstrom PAFH, Kannus P: Injuries of the foot and ankle. In DeLee JC, Drez D, editors: *Orthopaedic Sports Medicine: Principles and Practice,* Philadelphia, 1994, WB Saunders, pp 1705-1767.

CHAPTER **60**

Ankle Ligament Sprains

Aaron Rubin, MD

I. History
  A. Mechanism of injury: ligaments injured.
    1. Plantar flexion with inversion: anterior talofibular (ATFL), calcaneofibular (CFL), posterior talofibular (PTFL), tibiofibular (TFL).
    2. Inversion: CFL (with ATFL or PTFL).
    3. Dorsiflexion: TFL.
    4. Eversion: deltoid, TFL (if severe), interosseous membrane, fibular fracture (proximal or distal).
  B. Presence or absence of "pop."
  C. Ability to continue to play, walk, and so forth.
  D. Swelling and time elapsed before swelling.
  E. Location of swelling.
  F. Previous ankle injury and treatment.
II. Examination
  A. Inspection.
    1. Swelling.
      a. Lateral with ATFL and CFL.
      b. Medial with deltoid.
    2. Ecchymosis.
    3. Palpation.
      a. The ATFL runs from the fibula anteriorly toward the talus.
      b. The CFL arises from the posterior fibula and runs posteriorly and inferiorly to the midportion of the calcaneus.
      c. The PTFL runs from the posteromedial portion of the fibula to the posterior surface of the talus.
      d. The deltoid ligament is a broad collection of ligaments that diverge from the medial malleolus distally and anteriorly to the navicular and posteriorly to the talus.
      e. Syndesmosis injuries cause pain or tenderness at the anterior aspect of the syndesmosis and interosseous membrane.
      f. Check the lateral and medial malleoli, especially the posterior 6 cm and tip (see section on radiographic appearance).
    4. Stress testing: testing the acutely injured ankle may be difficult.
      a. Talar tilt is used to test the lateral ligaments. The heel is grasped in the examiner's hand, the ankle is inverted, and laxity is compared with that of the contralateral side.
      b. The anterior drawer test is used to measure the anterior talofibular ligament and is done by stabilizing the affected leg with one hand and cupping the heel in the opposite hand while placing anterior

force on the heel. Once again, displacement on the affected side is compared with that on the unaffected side.

c. The valgus (eversion) stress test is used to detect instability of the deltoid ligament.

d. The squeeze test is done by compressing the proximal fibula against the tibia. Pain in the distal tibiofibular diastasis indicates syndesmosis injury.

III. Radiographic Appearance

A. Basic views include anteroposterior, lateral, and mortise.

B. Plain radiography: the Ottawa ankle rules.

1. Using these criteria, radiograph films were reduced by 28% and emergency department time and cost were decreased without undiagnosed fractures.

2. Ankle films are required if pain in the malleolar area is accompanied by either

a. Bony tenderness at the posterior medial or lateral malleolus.

b. Inability to bear weight (four steps) immediately after injury and in the emergency department.

3. These rules are valid only in athletes >18 years of age (Stiell et al. 1994).

C. Stress radiography.

1. Talar tilt testing is done as described, the mortise view is obtained, and tilt between the talar dome and the tibial plafond is measured. Consider local anesthetic injection to decrease pain from stressing an injured ankle. Much variability exists in terms of "normal" talar tilt; results range from 0-27 degrees. Cadaveric studies showed much overlap in the amount of talar tilt after sequential sectioning of the ATFL and the CFL. One such study recommended considering the injury an ATFL disruption if talar tilt is 10-20 degrees and considering it an ATFL with a CFL tear if tilt is >20 degrees (and certainly if tilt is >30 degrees). Both must be considered disrupted if the affected ankle's talar tilt is 10 degrees greater than that of the unaffected side.

2. Anterior drawer stress radiography is done by applying posterior force to the distal tibia and by obtaining a lateral view. Displacement of the talus by 4-5 mm with respect to the tibia is probably normal; 8-10 mm displacement is noted with division of the ATFL, and 10-15 mm displacement is noted with division of the ATFL, PTFL, and CFL.

3. Diagnosis of deltoid tears may be aided by using the valgus (eversion) stress test. The heel and midfoot are everted by the examiner as the mortise view is obtained. A tilt >10 degrees is a positive result.

D. Arthrography. Can be used to diagnose acute CFL, ATFL, syndesmotic, and deltoid disruption. Because few false-positive results occur, disruption is improbable if no leakage of contrast is noted. Arthrography is best done 24-48 hours after injury but does not quantitate tear.

1. Superior anterolateral leakage: ATFL rupture.

2. Superior anterolateral and peroneal sheath leakage: ATFL and CFL rupture.

3. Distal tibiofibular space leakage: syndesmosis rupture.

4. Leakage into space above lateral malleolus: deltoid rupture.

E. Bone scanning is useful for evaluating stress fracture, osteochondral fracture, infection, and inflammatory reaction.

F. Computerized tomography localizes osteochondritis dissecans, loose bodies, and subchondral cysts.

G. Magnetic resonance imaging (MRI) shows the soft tissue of the ankle well and can also show osteochondral lesions such as osteochondritis dissecans and talar dome fractures well. Tendons such as the Achilles, peroneal, and posterior tibial are well seen. Usefulness of routine MRI for evaluating ankle ligament injuries is still unknown, although suspected injuries of these structures may be seen.

IV. Treatment
   A. RICE (rest, ice, compression, elevation).
      1. Rest: continued participation in sports with an injured ankle delays healing and may lead to further injury. Crutches are useful for allowing ambulation and partial weight bearing during rehabilitation.
      2. Ice: shown to decrease days required before return to function by about 50% if used within the first 24 hours. Heat should not be applied to an acutely sprained ankle.
      3. Compression: helpful in decreasing pain and swelling. Methods of compression include wrapping with an elastic bandage, stirrup splinting, applying a functional ankle brace, and supporting the ankle with a walking brace, or, in rare cases, with a short leg walking cast. Although it prevents further rehabilitation and icing, a cast may be necessary if early ambulation is required (e.g., because of work demands).
      4. Elevation: raise the ankle above the level of the heart for the first 24 hours.
   B. Rehabilitation.
      1. Decrease swelling
      2. Increase range of motion
      3. Begin muscle strengthening
         a. Isometric
         b. Surgical tubing
         c. Towel slides
      4. Regain proprioception
         a. Spell alphabet with toe
         b. Tilt board, balance board
         c. Place various size balls on floor and move them around with affected foot
   C. Return to sports
      1. Progression: Partial weight bearing→Full weight bearing→Jog→Run half speed→Run full speed→Figure "8's"→Sports specific activities

V. Differential Diagnosis (Causes of the Chronic Sprained Ankle)
   A. Functional instability.
      1. Ligamentous laxity.
      2. Peroneal muscle weakness or subluxating peroneal tendon.
      3. Poor proprioception.
      4. Nerve injury.
   B. Tight, sensitive scar.
   C. Chronic synovitis.
   D. Undiagnosed fracture or osteochondritis dissecans.
   E. Symptomatic os trigonum tarsi.
   F. Reflex sympathetic dystrophy.

Acknowledgment

The Medical Editing Department, Kaiser Foundation Research Institute, provided editorial assistance.

Bibliography

Bennett WF: Lateral ankle sprains. Part I. Anatomy, biomechanics, diagnosis, and natural history, *Orthop Rev* 23:381-387, 1994.

Reid DC: Selected conditions of the foot, ankle region. In Reid DC, editor: *Sports Injury Assessment and Rehabilitation,* New York, 1992, Churchill Livingstone, pp 129-185, 215-269.

Renstrom PAFH, Kannus P: Injuries of the foot and ankle. In DeLee JC, Drez D, editors: *Orthopaedic Sports Medicine: Principles and Practice.* Philadelphia, 1994, WB Saunders.

Singer KM, Jones DC, Taillon MR: Ligament injuries of the ankle and foot. In Nicholas JA, Hershman EB, editors: *The Lower Extremity and Spine in Sports Medicine,* ed 2, St Louis, 1995, Mosby.

Stiell IG et al: Implementation of the Ottawa ankle rules, *JAMA* 271:827-832, 1994.

CHAPTER 61

Ankle Fractures in Athletes

Angus M. McBryde, Jr., MD

I. Introduction and Overview
  A. Incidence and importance.
    1. Ankle injury is generally acute. Foot injury is usually overuse (repetitive stress).
    2. Ankle fracture is relatively rare compared to ankle ligamentous injury (sprain) in the athlete.
    3. Ankle fractures comprise a higher percentage of ankle injuries in nonathletes than in athletes.
    4. Subtle ankle fractures have associated ligamentous injuries. Primary ligamentous injuries often have occult fractures (i.e., grade III ankle sprain with talar dome fracture).
    5. Anatomic reduction of ankle fractures in athletes is necessary due to the functionally high demands. This high demand and need for full functional return to sport require experienced nonsurgical and/or surgical technical competence.
    6. Rehabilitation must be complete (including proprioception) just as with any injury before return to sport.
    7. Results are better and more rewarding in athletes due to:
      a. Excellent bone quality and healing potential.
      b. Compliance with rehabilitation program that permits an aggressive and accelerated approach.
  B. The immature skeleton and ankle fracture.
    1. Ligaments are stronger than bone in the immature athlete, causing the relative incidence of fracture to be higher.
    2. There is a predisposition to physeal injury since the physis has an inherent structural weakness until closing of most of the involved epiphyses (tibia: age 16.4-male, age 14.4-female; fibula: age 16.4-male, age 14.1-female).
      a. Salter-Harris II injury might occur in lieu of an anterior tibiofibular ligament injury with an inversion "sprain."

b. The distal fibular epiphysis (usually Salter-Harris II) is the most common fracture of the ankle in immature athletes.

II. Classification/Mechanism of Injury
   A. General principles.
      1. Low velocity sports (<20 mph) produce more simple fractures (i.e., tennis, volleyball, basketball).
      2. High velocity sports (>20 mph) produce more complex and often open fractures (i.e., skydiving, downhill skiing, ice hockey).
      3. Frank and occult ankle fractures are often an extension of ligamentous injury. The soft tissue injury must be recognized, respected, and included in treatment decisionmaking (i.e., grade III ankle sprain with talar dome or fibula avulsion fracture).
   B. Two classifications are used on a practical basis. The philosophy for ankle fractures in athletes is that the mortise must function normally. Fibular length, fibular position in the tibial groove, and fibular anchoring to the tibia through the syndesmosis are mandatory.
      1. The AO classification system (Danis-Weber) focuses on the fibula and implies that the fibula must be anatomically reduced.
         a. Weber A: fracture of the fibula below the ankle joint level. When displaced, surgery is optional if reduction is not anatomic.
         b. Weber B: fracture at the joint level. Surgery indicated if there is medial tenderness, implying injury to the deltoid ligament and potential instability.
         c. Weber C: higher fibular fracture. Syndesmosis injury requiring surgery and often a syndesmotic screw across the tibia and fibula 2 cm above the ankle joint.
      2. The Lauge-Hansen classification associates specific fracture patterns with the mechanism of the injury.
         a. Foot in supination with adduction force (Weber A).
            (1) Most common mechanism of injury to the ankle.
            (2) Failure first occurs laterally with tibia fracture below the joint.
            (3) Failure then occurs medially with a displaced fracture of the medial malleolus.
         b. Foot in supination with external rotation force (Weber B).
            (1) 40% to 75% of all malleolar fractures.
            (2) Talus rotates, causing fibular torque with spiral oblique fracture of the distal tibia.
         c. Foot in pronation with abduction force (Weber B).
            (1) Medial tension and lateral compression deformity.
            (2) Lateral plafond of tibia can be injured with chondral or osteochondral fracture.
         d. Foot in pronation with external rotation force (Weber C).
            (1) Potential instability.
            (2) Higher fibula fracture.
            (3) Medial failure and then lateral failure.

III. Fractures with Special Considerations
   A. Tillaux fracture.
      1. Occurs in athletes 12-15 years old.
      2. Avulsion of the anterior lateral portion of the distal tibial epiphysis.
      3. Needs open reduction and internal fixation due to joint cartilage disruption. Care must be taken to:
         a. Avoid injury to the distal tibial epiphysis.
         b. Avoid pin or screw transfixion of the distal tibial epiphysis.
      4. Angular or growth-related deformity is rare.

B. Triplane fractures of the distal tibia in the immature skeleton.
   1. Typically a skateboarding injury.
   2. Complicated fracture including distal tibia and its physis.
   3. The foot is supinated with external rotation force.
   4. Growth abnormality can occur.
   5. Surgery is generally necessary.
C. Salter-Harris type II tibia.
   1. Common in football and soccer.
   2. The foot is pronated with external rotation force.
   3. Fibula fracture "compression."
   4. Treatment
      a. Closed reduction (rare ORIF if closed reduction not possible).
      b. 6 weeks in cast; first 3 weeks non–weight bearing.
D. Salter-Harris type III and IV injuries of distal tibia at ankle.
   1. Adduction force with foot in supination.
   2. Surgery necessary if *more than:*
      a. 20-degree angulation.
      b. 2-mm displacement.
E. Stress fractures about the ankle in athletes.
   1. General principles of diagnosis.
      a. Overuse, high use, or repetitive stress. Always an inciting activity. Usually a change in training as etiology.
      b. Gradual or acute onset of symptoms.
      c. Local tenderness and pain are present.
      d. Radiography is negative up to 14-21 days. "Crack" (if cortical) and "blush of callous" often present early.
      e. Bone scan positive after 3-5 days.
      f. Rarely is displacement present or threatened.
   2. Specific stress fractures.
      a. Lateral malleolus ("runner's fracture").
      b. Condensation of bone in distal tibial epiphysis ("trampoline fracture").
      c. Medial malleolus ("adolescent fracture").
      d. Talar neck. Rare but possible.
   3. Principles of treatment.
      a. "Keep the level of pain below the level that hurts." This may require early stopping of the inciting activity or assisted walking with crutches. Casting usually not necessary unless:
         (1) Diagnosis has been delayed.
         (2) Pain uncontrolled with lesser mobilization/support.
      b. Ice, splint, or tape and substitute sport.
F. Often associated fractures.
   1. Tillaux (anterior tibia-fibula ligament avulsion at the tibial attachment).
   2. Volkmann's (posterolateral tibia-fibula ligament avulsion of Volkmann's tubercle).
   3. Posterior malleolar fracture.
      a. Contribution to stability not well documented.
      b. Internally fix if more than 20% articular surface disruption.
   4. Fracture of posterior talar process or os trigonum with primary or secondary impingement.

IV. Imaging
   A. Anteroposterior, lateral, and oblique for initial screening.
   B. Stress radiography is necessary when distal tibia-fibula joint or mortise stability is questionable.

C. Comparison views of the uninjured ankle can help identify abnormal radiographic anatomy.
D. Computerized tomography scan is a clarifying resource for complicated fractures.
E. Occult fractures occasionally require bone scan for localization or confirmation of pathology.
F. Radiographic findings must be correlated with the clinical picture by the clinician. Radiography alone cannot determine diagnosis or indicate treatment for the ankle fracture.

V. Initial Treatment on Court or Field (Immediate Diagnosis)
   A. Determine whether the fracture is open or closed.
   B. Open fracture.
      1. Dress wound or cover sterilely.
      2. Transfer immediately for definitive surgical irrigation and debridement.
      3. "Cover, splint, and transport as soon as possible."
   C. True emergency—gross long bone deformity with:
      1. Loss of ankle pulses.
      2. Loss of motor.
      3. Loss of sensation.
   D. Immediate and long-term morbidity.
      1. Soft tissue.
         a. Skin slough.
         b. Infection.
         c. Neurologic impairment with paralysis.
         d. Compartment syndrome.
      2. Bone.
         a. Avascular necrosis.
         b. Infection.
      3. Bone and soft tissue: vascular embarrassment with possible amputation.

VI. Nonsurgical Treatment of Ankle Fractures
   A. Types.
      1. Minor marginal avulsion fracture of fibula, tibia, talus.
      2. Primary sprain (usually inversion type II-III with fibular avulsion fracture).
      3. Simple fracture configuration (i.e., nondisplaced fibula fractures with no medial pain or tenderness).
   B. Nonsurgical treatment.
      1. Immobilize for comfort and swelling reduction.
         a. Short leg cast (weight bearing/non–weight bearing).
         b. Removable boot type cast.
         c. Air stirrup–type support.
      2. Ice, elevation, taping with primarily sprain injury.
      3. 4-6 weeks of cast immobilization/protected weight bearing for nondisplaced fractures.
      4. "Elevation" implies foot and ankle, one foot above the heart or head.

VII. Criteria for Surgery
   A. Open fracture requires an emergency irrigation and debridement procedure. Procedure prior to open or closed reduction and any internal or external fixation such as:
      1. Intramedullary implant.
      2. Compression or other plate.

   3. Percutaneous skeletal fixation.
   4. External fixator system.
B. >2-3 mm displacement generally unacceptable.
C. Gross instability after reduction.
D. Surgical treatment is chosen in the athlete due to the need for:
   1. Anatomic reduction.
   2. Rigid internal fixation.
      a. Permits early rehabilitation with less early and late loss of motion.
      b. Quicker return to training/competition.
      c. Permits protected early motion rather than cast and immobilization.

CHAPTER 62

Rehabilitation of Ankle Injuries

Stephen M. Simons, MD, FACSM

I. General Goals
   A. Rapid functional recovery; return to sport.
   B. Minimize chronic instability. Etiologies include instability of the talus in the ankle mortise, instability of the subtalar joint, inferior tibiofibular diastasis, peroneal muscle weakness, and motor incoordination following afferent disruption.[16]
      1. Mechanical instability: "motion beyond the physiologic range of motion. Clinically . . . demonstrated by anterior drawer and talar tilt tests."[24]
      2. Functional instability: "the patient's subjective complaints of giving way."[24]
      3. Chronic symptoms incidence following acute ankle injuries: 10% to 30%.[1,3,18]

II. Phase 1 (Acute Phase)[2,6,9,11,16]
   A. Goals: decrease edema, pain, and spasm and reduce chance for further injury.
   B. Cryotherapy: ice bath, ice bags. Apply 15-20 minutes three to four times daily.
   C. Compression: Ace wrap, commercial compression, cooling devices (i.e., Cryo-Cuff (Aircast), Jobst Cryo/Temp System[21] (Fig. 62-1).
   D. Weight bearing: non–weightbearing to touchdown as tolerated.
   E. Elevation alone can significantly reduce ankle edema.[19]
   F. Rehabilitation exercises: limited to pain-free mobilization, isometric open kinetic chain and no closed kinetic chain exercises, heel cord stretches.

III. Phase 2 (Subacute Phase)
   A. Goals: maintain mobility, minimize muscle contracture, restrengthen, and reeducate proprioception.
   B. Cryotherapy continues. Contrast baths.

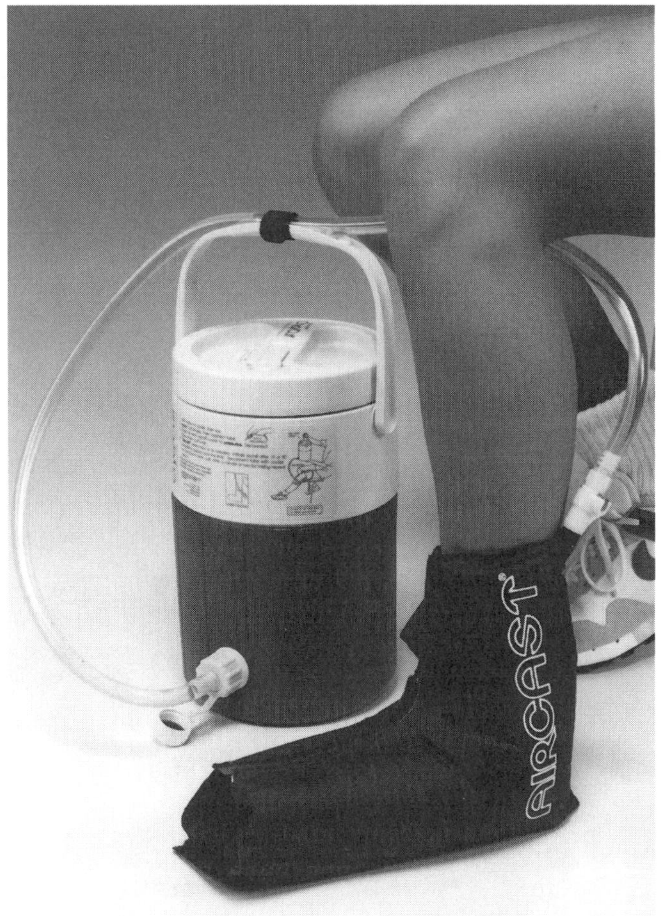

FIGURE 62-1
Commercial compression cooling devices such as the Cryo-Cuff (Aircast) can hasten swelling reduction and early mobilization.

- C. Compression with pneumatic compression brace (Fig. 62-2). Provides inversion/eversion protection and compression.
- D. Weight bearing: partial to full weight bearing.
- E. Rehabilitation exercises: alphabet range of motion, Achilles stretching, heel raises (non–weight bearing progression to weight bearing), body weight transfers with bilateral stance, biomechanical ankle platform system (BAPS) board exercises in partial weight bearing.

IV. Phase 3 (Return to Activity)
- A. Goals: functional progression, proprioceptive retraining, mechanical control, preparation for return to sport.
- B. Cryotherapy postexercise.
- C. Support with splints, taping, orthotics.
- D. Weightbearing: full
- E. Rehabilitation exercises
  1. Achilles stretching, heel raises: begin flat and progress to step raises. Begin bilateral and progress to unilateral injured side.
  2. Open kinetic chain strengthening. Weights applied to the foot. Resistance exercises in all planes using flexible elastic tubing.
  3. Body weight transfers with resistance. Running.

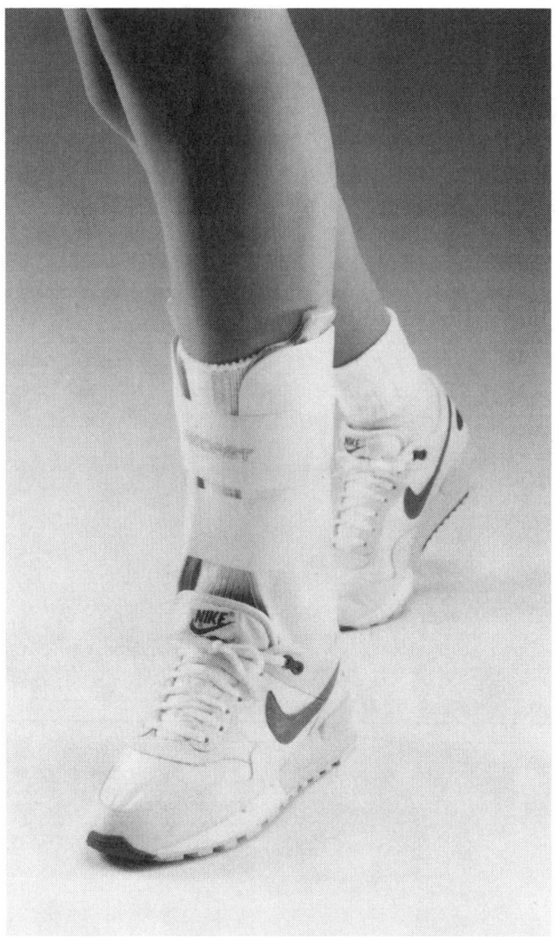

FIGURE 62-2
A pneumatic compression brace can be used for early protection and effusion management. It can also be used for reinjury prophylaxis upon return to sport.

4. BAPS board, four-square hopping, backpedaling, figure eights with progressively smaller circles, cariocas.

V. Rehabilitation Timing
   A. Progression through the above outline depends on severity of ankle injury. Each step should be monitored by a qualified therapist, trainer, or physician.
   B. Return to sport is determined by assessing the sport demands, risk of further injury, and performing the above rehabilitation activities pain-free.

VI. Early Mobilization
   A. Early mobilization while protecting the ankle with some support yields earlier return to routine activity and sport.[7]
   B. Early mobilization can be used for mild to moderate ankle sprains without instability as well as for more severe ankle sprains that demonstrate instability.[15]
   C. Long-term residual functional instability is equivalent for ankles treated with early mobilization or initial immobilization.[7,15]

VII. Ankle Injury Prevention
   A. Taping.[8,10,25,26]
      1. Laboratory evidence that taping reduces talar tilt and ankle inversion when compared to no taping.

2. Clinical ankle injury reduction when using taping prophylaxis for previously injured ankles. Probable mechanism: improved proprioception.
3. Tape loses considerable ability to control inversion after 10-20 minutes of exercise.
4. Tape requires a skilled person to apply daily. Very costly when used on daily basis.

B. Ankle bracing.[14,20,22,23]
1. Several braces available (i.e., Swede-o-Universal ankle support and Aircast Sport-Stirrup).
2. Laboratory evidence that bracing reduces talar tilt and ankle inversion when compared to no bracing.
3. Clinical field studies demonstrating reduced incidence of ankle injuries for both first-time trauma–type (collision) injury and recurrent injury. Improved proprioception as proposed mechanism.
4. Bracing provides inversion protection for a longer exercise time than taping.
5. Bracing, although initially more costly, is less expensive than daily taping.
6. Insufficient studies comparing effectiveness of various braces.[4,12,13,17]
7. Small performance decrements (1.6% to 3.5%) for vertical jump, shuttle run, and sprint when using ankle taping or bracing.[5]

References

1. Anderson ME: Reconstruction of the lateral ligaments of the ankle using the plantaris tendon, *J Bone Joint Surg* 67A:930-934, 1985.
2. Balduini FC et al: Management and rehabilitation of ligamentous injuries to the ankle, *Sports Med* 4:364-380, 1987.
3. Brostrom L, Sundelin P: Sprained ankles: histological changes in recent and chronic ligament ruptures, *Acta Chir Scand* 132:248-253, 1966.
4. Bunch RP et al: Ankle joint support: a comparison of reusable lace-on braces with taping and wrapping, *Phys Sportmed* 13(5), 1985.
5. Burks RT et al: Analysis of athletic performance with prophylactic ankle devices, *Am J Sports Med* 19:104-106, 1991.
6. Diamond JE: Rehabilitation of ankle sprains, *Clin Sports Med* 8:877-891, 1989.
7. Eiff MP, Smith AT, Smith GE: Early mobilization versus immobilization in the treatment of lateral ankle sprains, *Am J Sports Med* 22:83-88, 1994.
8. Fumich RM et al: The measured effect of taping on combined foot and ankle motion before and after exercise, *Am J Sports Med* 9:165-170, 1981.
9. Garrick JG: When can . . . ? A practical approach to rehabilitation illustrated by treatment of ankle injury, *Am J Sports Med* 9:67-68, 1981.
10. Glick JM, Gordon RB, Nishimoto D: The prevention and treatment of ankle injuries, *Am J Sports Med* 4:136-141, 1976.
11. Gould JA: *Orthopedic and Sports Physical Therapy,* ed 2, St Louis, 1990, CV Mosby.
12. Gross MT et al: Comparison of support provided by ankle taping and semirigid orthosis, *J Orthop Sports Physical Ther* 9(1):33-39, 1987.
13. Gross MT, Lapp AK, Davis JM: Comparison of Swede-o-Universal® ankle support and Aircast® Sport-Stirrup® orthoses and ankle tape in restricting eversion-inversion before and after exercise, *J Orthop Sports Physical Ther* 13(1):11-19, 1991.
14. Kimura IF et al: Effect of the AirStirrup® in controlling ankle inversion stress, *J Orthop Sports Physical Ther* 9(5):190-193, 1987.
15. Konradson L, Holmer P, Sondergaard L: Early mobilizing treatment for grade III ankle ligament injuries, *Foot Ankle* 12(2):69-73, 1991.
16. Mulligan E: Lower leg, ankle and foot rehabilitation. In Andrews JR, Harrelson GL, editors: *Physical Rehabilitation of the Injured Athlete,* ed 1, Philadelphia, 1991, WB Saunders.
17. Rovere GD et al: Retrospective comparison of taping and ankle stabilizers in preventing ankle injuries, *Am J Sports Med* 16:228-233, 1988.
18. Sammarco GJ, DiRaimondo CV: Surgical treatment of lateral ankle instability syndrome, *Am J Sports Med* 16:501-511, 1988.
19. Sims D: Effects of positioning on ankle edema, *J Orthop Sports Med Phys Ther* 8:30-33, 1986.

20. Sitler M et al: The efficacy of a semirigid ankle stabilizer to reduce acute ankle injuries in basketball, *Am J Sports Med* 22:454-461, 1994.
21. Sloan JP, Giddings P, Hain R: Effects of cold and compression on edema, *Physician Sportsmed* 16:116-120, 1988.
22. Stover CN: Air stirrup management of ankle injuries in the athlete, *Am J Sports Med* 8:360-365, 1980.
23. Surve I et al: A fivefold reduction in the incidence of recurrent ankle sprains in soccer players using the sport-stirrup orthosis, *Am J Sports Med* 22:601-605, 1994.
24. Trevino SG, Davis P, Hecht PJ: Management of acute and chronic lateral ligament injuries of the ankle, *Orthop Clin North Am* 25:1-16, 1994.
25. Tropp H, Askling C, Gillquist J: Prevention of ankle sprains, *Am J Sports Med* 13:259-262, 1985.
26. Vaes P et al: Comparative radiological study of the influence of ankle joint bandages on ankle stability, *Acta Orthop Belgica* 50:636-644, 1984.

CHAPTER 63

Common Foot Injuries

Craig Wargon, DPM

I. Introduction
  A. Scope of the problem.
    1. Foot and ankle injuries are endemic to the running, jumping, and kicking sports. When combined with cutting and sliding maneuvers, the incidence increases greatly.
    2. Studies of sports-related injuries have suggested an overall injury rate of between 10% and 15% for the foot and ankle.
    3. Football alone is estimated to cause between a low of 186,000 and a high of 2,480,000 injuries of the foot and ankle in the United States each year.
  B. Nature of the problem.
    1. Pain is the most common reason athletes seek medical attention for their feet, followed by foot deformity and lastly, instability.
    2. Without treatment, even minor foot ailments can lead to protracted pain due to the constant forces of weight bearing.
    3. Painful conditions can frequently be treated effectively by relatively simple measures with a basic working knowledge of foot anatomy, function and common foot pathology.

II. Selected Clinical Anatomy of the Foot
  A. Rearfoot
    1. Subtalar joint (talocalcaneal): a complex joint that permits inversion and eversion (triplane motion). At initial ground contact the subtalar joint undergoes rapid eversion, which is a passive energy-absorbing mechanism. Active inversion follows, which reaches a maximum at toe-off.
    2. Tarsal tunnel: a canal that lies posterior and inferior to the medial malleolus. Tendons of the deep posterior compartment of the leg (flexor hallucis longus [FHL], flexor digitorum longus [FDL], and posterior tibial) pass through this canal as well as the posterior tibial nerve.

3. Posterior tibialis.
   a. A muscle of the deep posterior compartment of the leg.
   b. The tendon runs behind the medial malleolus; it has a primary insertion into the navicular and then has separate attachments to the cuneiforms and bases of the lesser metatarsals.
   c. It functions to maintain the longitudinal arch and provides active inversion and plantarflexion of the foot.

B. Midfoot.
1. Midtarsal joint (transverse tarsal joint or Chopart's joint): consists of the talonavicular and calcaneal cuboid joints. Motion of this joint allows rotation, abduction, and adduction. This joint is "locked" when the subtalar joint is supinated and "unlocked" when the subtalar joint is everted. This is the key mechanism that allows the foot to adapt to uneven surfaces yet function as a stable platform from which to propel.
2. Spring ligament.
   a. Lies between the sustentaculum tali of the calcaneus and the navicular; cradles and supports the head of the talus.
   b. Rupture of this ligament leads to collapse of the medial longitudinal arch.
3. Peroneal longus and brevis.
   a. Muscle of the lateral compartment of the leg.
   b. The peroneal brevis tendon runs behind the lateral malleolus and inserts into the base of the fifth metatarsal. A powerful everter of the foot.
   c. The peroneal longus runs with the brevis; at the cuboid it sharply changes directions and inserts into the base of the first metatarsal. It acts as a sling to stabilize the transverse arch and first metatarsal. It also counterbalances the strong inversion of the posterior tibial muscle.
4. Tibialis anterior.
   a. This is a muscle of the anterior compartment of the leg.
   b. The tendon functions to dorsiflex the ankle and invert the foot.
5. Plantar fascia: an aponeurosis that originates at the medial plantar border of the calcaneus, it divides distally into several slips and inserts into the proximal phalanges. This fascia helps maintain the medial longitudinal arch. The fascia is under tension, which plays a role in coordination of muscular activity from the great toe to the gastrocnemius-soleus complex ("windless effect").
6. Sinus tarsis (Fig. 63-1): a funnel-shaped tunnel with a large opening on the lateral side of the foot and a very narrow opening on the medial side. The talar neck defines the roof of the tunnel, and the floor is the distal superior portion of the calcaneus.
   a. Several ligaments occupy the tunnel including the interosseous talocalcaneal.
   b. The sinus tarsis area contains abundant synovial tissue that is prone to synovitis and inflammation when injured.
7. Lisfranc's joint.
   a. The articulation of the cuneiforms and cuboid with the metatarsals.
   b. The second metatarsal cuneiform joint recesses between the medial and lateral cuneiforms, providing stability to the Lisfranc's joint and the second metatarsal.

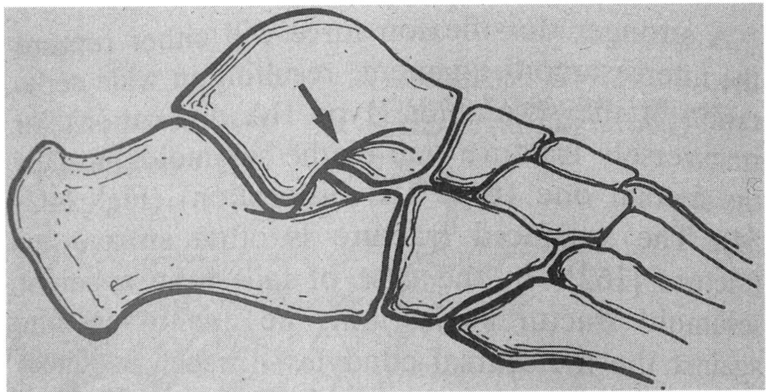

FIGURE 63-1
Lateral opening of the sinus tarsi (arrow).

C. Forefoot.
  1. First metatarsophalangeal joint.
    a. This joint is differentiated from the lesser toes by the sesamoid mechanism.
    b. There is a high degree of variability of the shape and stability of this joint.
      i. A round, more mobile joint may have a tendency toward development of hallux valgus (bunions).
      ii. A square, more rigid joint has more of a tendency toward development of hallux limitus and arthritis.
  2. Sesamoids.
    a. Accessory bones contained within the double tendon of the flexor hallucis brevis that articulate dorsally with the first metatarsal head (Fig. 63-2).
    b. The sesamoids provide an increased mechanical advantage for the flexor hallucis brevis to plantarflex the first metatarsal phalangeal joint (MTP).
    c. Multipartisim can be a normal variation of these bones; the medial sesamoid is more commonly bipartite than the lateral.
  3. Posterior Tibial Nerve
    a. Divides into two major branches in the sole of the foot.
      (1) Medial plantar nerve: It also divides into two branches, a medial branch that provides sensations to the plantar aspect of the medial hallux and the first, second, and third common digital branches that provides sensation to all the toes except the fifth toe.
        (a) The second and third common digital branches are the most frequent location for the development of interdigital neuromas.
      (2) Lateral plantar nerve: Innervates interossei muscles as well as sensation to the lateral foot and fourth and fifth toes via communication with branches of the medial plantar nerve.

III. Injuries to the rearfoot
  A. Sever's disease (calcaneal apophysitis).
    1. An extremely common traction apophysitis occurring in athletes age 7-15.

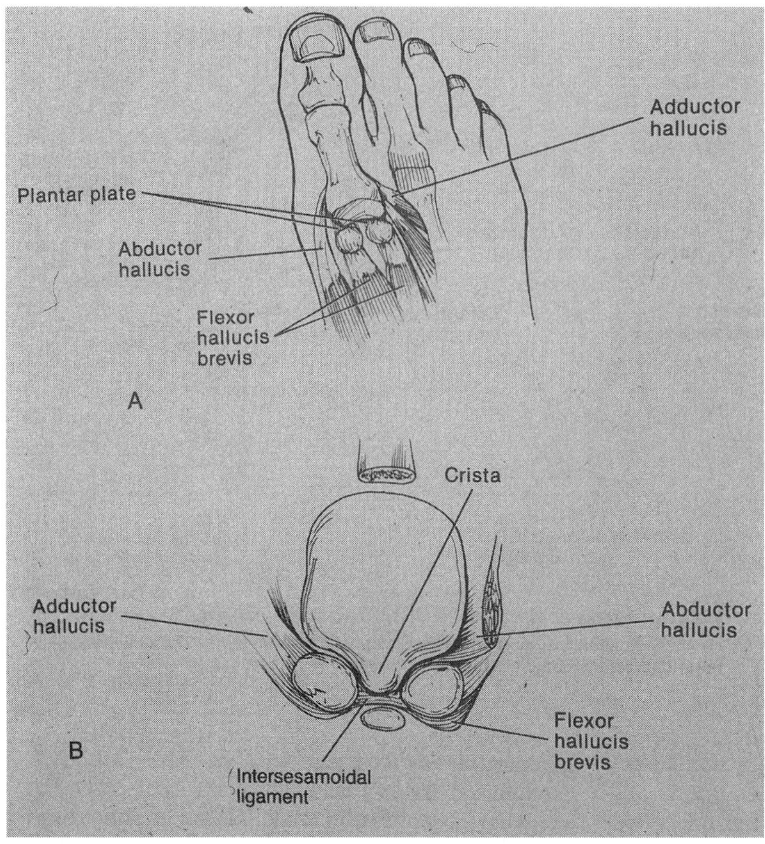

FIGURE 63-2
A, The sesamoids are contained within the double tendon of the flexor hallucis brevis. **B,** Cross-section through the metatarsophalangeal joint demonstrating relationship of sesamoids and extrinsic muscles.

2. Examination: tenderness to palpation of the posterior calcaneus at insertion of Achilles' tendon.
3. Children with cavus (high arch) rigid feet may be predisposed.
4. Radiographs generally are not indicated; typically shows fragmentation and sclerosis even in asymptomatic children.
5. Treatment.
   a. Heel lifts; effectively shortens distance to insertion, thus less force to the apophysis.
   b. Rest, activity as tolerated with heel lifts.
   c. Cryotherapy.
   d. Crutches or cast if necessary.
   e. Reassurance that once growth plate is closed (at about 12-15), the symptoms will resolve.

B. Achilles' tendinitis: may represent several pathological conditions concerning the Achilles' tendon or structures adjacent to it.
   1. Paratenonitis: symptoms—diffuse swelling, focal tenderness (usually medially more than laterally) to the midportion of the tendon, and crepitus may be present. Athletes complain of pain in the morning, which may improve later in the day.
   2. Partial rupture.
      a. Usually occurs as the result of a distinct episode or series of episodes. The tendon trauma can result from shear stresses or cu-

mulative microtrauma in an area of degeneration within the tendon.
   b. There can be local fusiform thickening or a palpable nodule with the tendon. Pain is exacerbated by dorsiflexion of the foot.
3. Tendinosis: tendon degeneration unassociated with an inflammatory reaction. Degenerative changes are related to the aging process and/or vascular change within the tendon. Most common area is the midthird section of tendon (relative avascular zone). This may represent so called mucinoid degeneration histologically.
4. Retrocalcaneal bursitis: a distinct entity denoted by pain that is anterior to the tendon, just superior to its insertion on the os calcis. Positive two-finger squeeze test.
5. Insertional tendinitis (enthesitis): true inflammatory reaction within the tendon. Patients have direct tenderness over the Achilles' tendon insertion. May be associated with a calcification on the superior calcaneus within the tendon insertion.
6. Treatment: nonsurgical management is usually successful in alleviating most symptoms; however, progress can be extremely slow in many cases. In cases of true mucinoid tendon degeneration or chronic inflammation, surgery may be indicated. Nonoperative treatment consists of:
   a. Ice massage.
   b. Deep friction massage.
   c. Dorsiflexed night splint.
   d. Physical therapy ultrasound treatment.
   e. Rest and cross-training.
   f. Gentle stretching once acute symptoms have resolved.
   g. Heel lifts and/or functional foot orthoses.
   h. Injections are rarely used; if an injection is employed, care must be taken not to inject steroid directly into the tendon or tendon insertion.

C. Haglund's deformity ("pump bump").
   1. An exostosis over the lateral posterior aspect of the calcaneus caused by recurrent friction. Often an adventitious bursa may develop.
   2. Etiology.
      a. Abnormal mechanics leading to excessive motion of the calcaneus.
      b. Structural congenital deformity of the calcaneus.
      c. Shoe gear irritation (pumps).
   3. Treatment.
      a. Open heel shoes or shoe with a lower heel and softer heel counter.
      b. Accommodative padding (e.g., moleskin to protect the skin).
      c. Orthotics to control the excessive motion.
      d. Cryotherapy.
      e. If all else fails, surgical excision of the offending bone (this generally requires 6 weeks of cast immobilization to protect the Achilles' tendon).

D. Heel pain syndrome (plantar fasciitis).
   1. Symptoms: pain in the plantar or plantar-medial aspect of the calcaneus where the plantar fascia and intrinsic muscles of the foot insert into the calcaneus. The pain is usually worse upon arising in the morning and gradually gets better with the first few steps. The onset of the pain is typically insidious in nature, though a relative increase in activity can be a precipitating factor. Commonly, the pain is of several months duration.

2. An exceptionally cavus or planus foot type can be an exacerbating factor. Frequently, people with this condition are overweight.
3. Mechanical etiology: as the foot pronates, the medial arch lowers. This lengthens the foot. When the foot is lengthened, the plantar structures are on stretch. Consequently, the plantar fascia pulls excessively at its origin on the calcaneus. This pull leads to inflammation of the periosteum on the calcaneus and hence pain. When the periosteum is irritated, it will often cause the formation of new bone, resulting in a plantar heel spur. Thus the spur is the result of this condition, not a cause of the inflammation.
4. Successful treatment of this condition involves addressing the mechanical issues and decreasing the inflammation that is present.
   a. Local injections of steroid.
   b. Arch supports or orthotics to limit pronation (in the vast majority of cases quality over-the-counter arch supports are used).
   c. Shoe modification: I recommend shoes with a thicker midsole or slightly higher heel. This effectively raises the arch and transfers weight anteriorly.
   d. Ice massage.
   e. Gastrocnemius-soleus stretching.
   f. Antipronation taping or strapping can be effective.
   g. Night splints can be beneficial; compliance is often low.
   h. Physical therapy modalities may be helpful.
   i. Oral antiinflammatory medications can be used as an adjunctive therapy.
   j. Surgery is rarely indicated due to the success of conservative treatment. Surgery consists of release of the plantar fascia.
5. For persistent cases one needs to rule out stress fracture, entrapment of the medial calcaneal branch of the posterior tibial nerve, or inflammatory arthropathies. Generally radiographs are not ordered unless other etiologies are suspected.

E. Heel bruise/heel fat pad syndrome.
1. Symptoms: unlike plantar fasciitis, heel bruise pain is located directly under the weight-bearing portion of the calcaneus. Periostitis may be responsible for the protracted pain.
2. The precipitating cause may be one traumatic incident or the repetitive microtrauma of running or walking. This leads to disruption of the fibrous septae and fat pad. Predisposing factors include obesity, age, or atrophic fat pad.
3. Treatment.
   a. The heel cup (Fig. 63-3): acts as a containment device into which the heel sits. The heel pad is not allowed to displace laterally and medially; the fat pad remains plantar to the bone and serves as a cushion for which it was designed. (I find that heel cups do not work well for plantar fasciitis.)
   b. "Donut" accommodative padding or padded insoles (e.g., Spenco).
   c. Rest and antiinflammatory medications.
   d. Ice early, later heat.

IV. Injuries to the Midfoot

A. Tarsal tunnel syndrome.
1. Tarsal tunnel syndrome represents an entrapment neuropathy of the posterior tibial nerve as it passes through the fibroosseous tunnel created by the laciniate ligament. This may be due to mechanical factors such as overpronation.

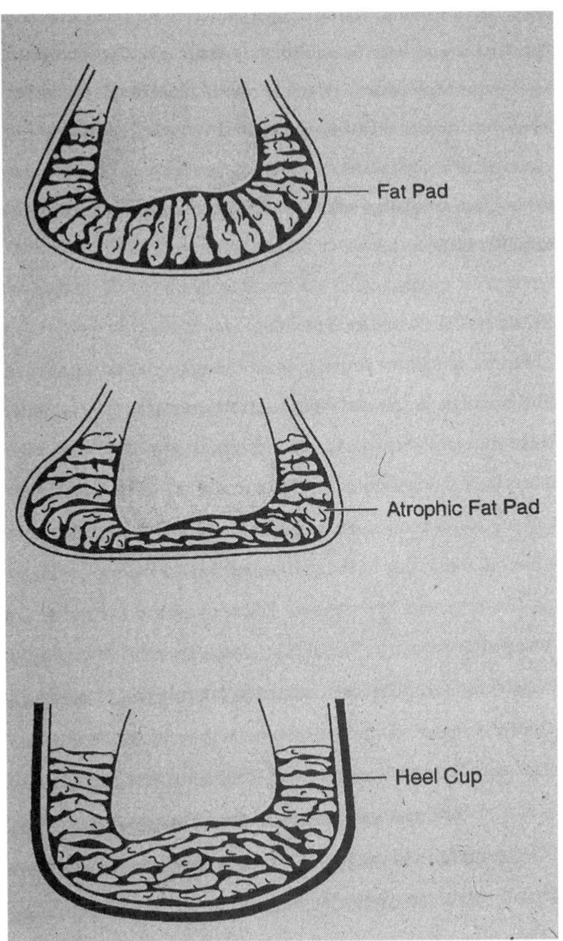

FIGURE 63-3
Heel cup acts as a containment device, not allowing heel pad to displace laterally or medially with weight bearing.

2. Symptoms usually occur in the forefoot and may include shooting, burning, and radiating pain from the medial plantar aspect of the foot to the toes.
3. Tendinitis of the tendons in this region (FHL, FDL, PT) may be a precipitating factor. Effective treatment of this may reduce neurogenic symptoms.
4. Examination: often a positive Tinel's sign is present. Nerve conduction velocity (NCV) studies may confirm physical findings.
5. Systemic etiologies such as diabetes or alcoholism should be ruled out. Varicosities can also put pressure on this nerve.
6. Treatment.
   a. Rest: casting of foot in plantarflexed and inverted position.
   b. Antiinflammatory medications.
   c. Orthotics to control foot motion.
   d. Surgery if conservative treatment fails.
7. It should be noted that tarsal tunnel syndrome is far less common than carpal tunnel syndrome.

B. Posterior tibial tendinitis.
   1. This tendon is responsible for inversion and plantar flexion. It functions to stabilize the arch. The muscle tendon unit undergoes eccen-

tric contraction during the stance phase of gait to limit the normal flattening of the arch (pronation). Arch collapse places excessive burden on the muscle tendon unit. Overuse can also be a significant factor in the etiology of injury to this tendon. People with flexible planus foot type are more susceptible to posterior tibial tendinitis.

2. Diagnosis is made by eliciting tenderness to palpation along the course of the posterior tibial tendon as it courses posterior and distal to the medial malleolus. Tenderness may also be present at the medial portion of the navicular. Pain will also be elicited by stressing the tendon.
   a. Stressing the tendon is accomplished by placing the foot in a position of inversion and plantarflexion. The patient is then asked to maintain this position while the opposite force is applied by the examiner.
   b. The tendon can also be stressed by asking the patient to do a single limb toe raise. In the case of tendinitis this will elicit pain and may be difficult to do. In the case of posterior tibial tendon insufficiency or rupture the patient will not be able to do this or the heel will not reinvert.
3. Treatment consists of rest and often immobilization. In the acute phase it is not uncommon to place the patient in a below-the-knee slightly inverted and plantarflexed cast for several weeks to take the tendon off of stretch. Rest may also be accomplished by maintaining the arch of the foot with orthotics, thus lessening the load on this tendon. Walking barefoot or in flat, nonsupportive shoes should be avoided.
4. Complete tears or severe attenuation of the tendon are accompanied by loss of the medial longitudinal arch (unilateral flat foot) and progressive forefoot abduction. These cases are difficult to manage and probably should be referred to a specialist.

C. Köhler's disease (aseptic necrosis of the tarsal navicular).
   1. Usually affects males between the ages of 5 and 10.
   2. The patient usually presents with a painful limp. Pain and swelling are localized to the medial navicular.
   3. Radiographs show a poorly developed ossification center with condensation and fragmentation. It may take several years for the radiographic appearance to change.
   4. Treatment consists of rest and a below-the-knee cast if necessary. An arch support and a stiff-soled shoe may also be helpful. The pain will resolve when the growth plate closes.

D. Navicular stress fracture.
   1. This is a rare injury. An index of suspicion is raised when there is a dull ache over the dorsum of the medial arch combined with a history of overuse.
   2. Radiographs are rarely positive. A bone scan will help make the diagnosis. A positive bone scan should be followed by a computerized tomography scan to detail the extent of injury.
   3. Treatment consist of 6-8 weeks of non–weight bearing below-the-knee casting. Inadequate treatment may lead to nonunion or avascular necrosis.

E. Fifth metatarsal injuries.
   1. The base of the fifth metatarsal serves as the attachment site of the peroneal brevis. Forceful inversion often leads to an avulsion fracture of the base of this bone.

2. Treatment consists of either a short leg cast for 2-3 weeks or a post-surgical wooden-soled shoe for 3-4 weeks. Nonunions are rare, and surgical reduction is almost never indicated.
3. Jones fracture occurs at the juncture of the base of the fifth metatarsal and the proximal diaphysis (1.5 cm distal to the base). This fracture heals much less readily than the former, and at least 6-8 weeks of non–weight-bearing casting is required. Many authors prefer Open Reduction Internal Fixation (ORIF) with bone graft due to reported high nonunion rates.

V. Injuries to the Forefoot
   A. Metatarsal stress fractures (Fig. 63-4).
      1. Most people complain of dull, aching pain in the forefoot to varying degrees. The forefoot may demonstrate edema. Moving the affected metatarsal or direct palpation will be painful.
      2. Radiographs will not be positive for 2-3 weeks after the injury. Displaced fractures are rare. Radiographs will demonstrate callus formation at the fracture site; this is a sign of bone healing.
      3. Treatment consists of use of a postsurgical wooden shoe for 4-6 weeks, rest, and elevation. A below-the-knee walking cast can be used if the symptoms warrant this.

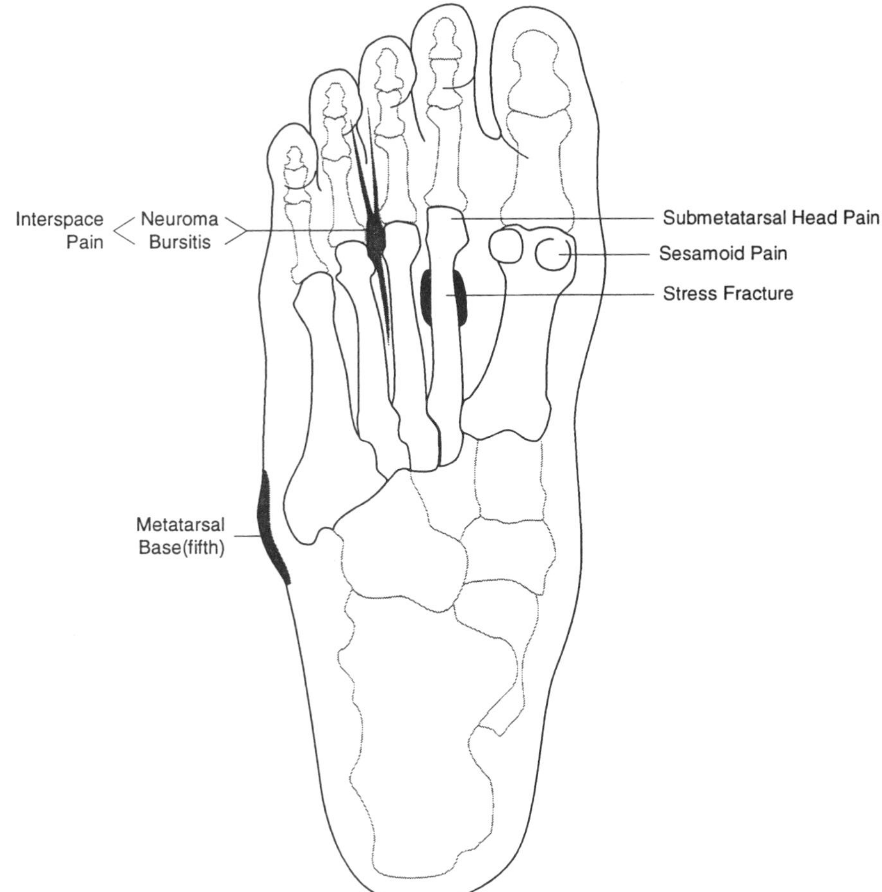

FIGURE 63-4
Metatarsal stress fractures. Intermetatarsal neuroma.

4. The second metatarsal takes more stress and is the most commonly injured. The third and fourth metatarsals follow in frequency.
5. Athletic activity can be resumed when the patient has no swelling, pain, or limp.

B. Submetatarsal head pain (anterior metatarsalgia).
1. This is defined as pain with direct palpation of the plantar aspect of the metatarsal head. It is sometimes difficult to determine if the pain is coming from the metatarsal head, a nearby neuroma, or an intermetatarsal bursitis. Dorsiflexing the corresponding toe can sometimes help to localize the metatarsal head.
2. Pain under the metatarsal head is usually the result of increased pressure there. Common structural causes leading to excessive pressure under a metatarsal head are:
   a. Depressed metatarsal.
   b. Elongated metatarsal with abnormal metatarsal parabola.
   c. Decreased plantar fat pad.
   d. Accessory sesamoids or hypertrophied metatarsal condyles.
   e. Overpronation with hypermobile first ray.
3. Treatment: relief is generally obtained by decreasing pressure under the affected metatarsal head. This can generally be accomplished by a number of conservative measures.
   a. Shoes with thick, curved midsoles (rocker bottom style) can serve to decrease force under all the metatarsals.
   b. Metatarsal pads to unload one of the lesser metatarsals (Fig. 63-5).
   c. Arch supports or orthotics with or without a metatarsal pad incorporated.
   d. Spenco-style insoles can reduce shear forces and provide padding.
   e. It is not unreasonable to immobilize the foot with a walking boot or short leg cast to allow the injured area to recover.

C. Sesamoiditis.
1. The first metatarsal head is unique in that it has two sesamoid bones, which are accessory bones that function to provide a mechanical advantage for the flexor hallucis longus tendon in much the same way the patella does for the quadriceps tendon.
2. Disorders of the sesamoids are usually the result of direct trauma or repeated microtrauma, as in running. This trauma commonly leads to sesamoiditis (inflammation of the sesamoid and its surrounding structure). The tibial sesamoid is most commonly involved.
3. Certain individuals are predisposed to sesamoiditis due to anatomical factors.
   a. Forefoot valgus.
   b. Rigid pes cavus.
   c. Multipartite sesamoid.
4. Symptoms consist of pain in the area of the metatarsal head and pain with palpation of the affected sesamoid. There may be associated swelling in the area and limitation of dorsiflexion.
5. With a history of significant trauma or severe persistent pain, a fractured sesamoid should be ruled out.
   a. Anteroposterior, oblique, lateral, and axial radiographs should be ordered.
   b. One must try to determine if the sesamoid is partite or fractured. Partite sesamoids are usually in two pieces and have smooth borders, with little separation. Fractures can have rough borders, be comminuted, and have more separation.

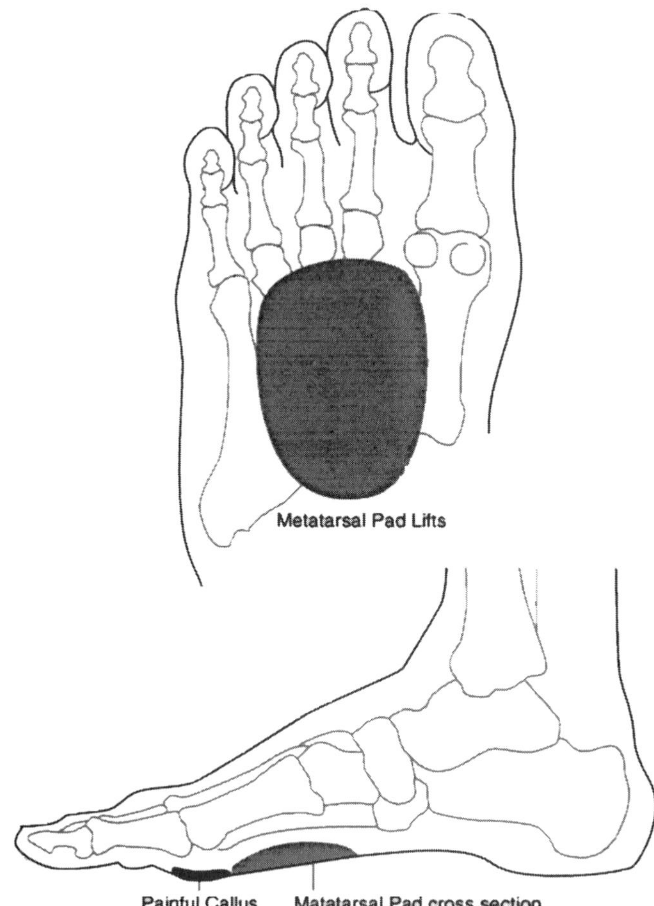

FIGURE 63-5
Metatarsal pads.

c. Fractures require cast immobilization and can have a high non-union rate.

6. Treatment involves means to unload the area. This can be accomplished with aperture padding (I often use an easily removable felt accommodative padding sandwiched between two layers of Elastoplast tape; Fig. 63-6). Resting the area by having the patient use crutches is commonly done. Thick-soled rocker bottom style shoes can be helpful.
7. In cases of persistent pain custom orthotics employing accommodative padding are prescribed. Local injections with steroid may also be indicated.

D. Intermetatarsal neuroma (Fig. 63-7).
1. The intermetatarsal nerve becomes pinched by adjacent metatarsal heads. This leads to scarring and nerve damage (perineural fibrosis).
2. Symptoms consist of neuritic-type pain, burning, radiating pain, numbness, and paresthesias in the interspace and to the associated toes. The symptoms tend to be sporadic in nature.
3. Physical examination is done by pushing up on the plantar aspect of the interspace between the involved metatarsal heads while at the same time with the other hand squeezing the metatarsal heads together from medial to lateral. Occasionally, the thickened nerve can

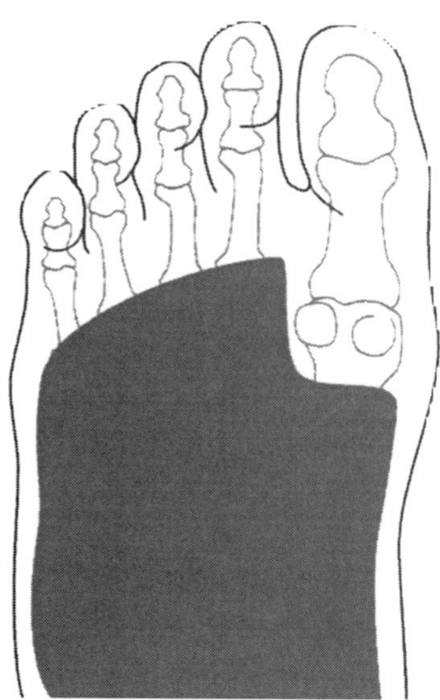

FIGURE 63-6
Treatment of sesamoiditis using easily removable felt accommodative padding sandwiched between two layers of Elastoplast tape.

be felt as a pop between the metatarsal heads. This maneuver should reproduce the symptoms the patient experiences during walking.

4. Treatment.
   a. Injections consist of a long-acting local anesthetic combined with an intermediate-acting steroid. The injections are given in a series, if necessary (I generally will give up to three injections at 2-month intervals). When giving the injection, one must deposit the solu-

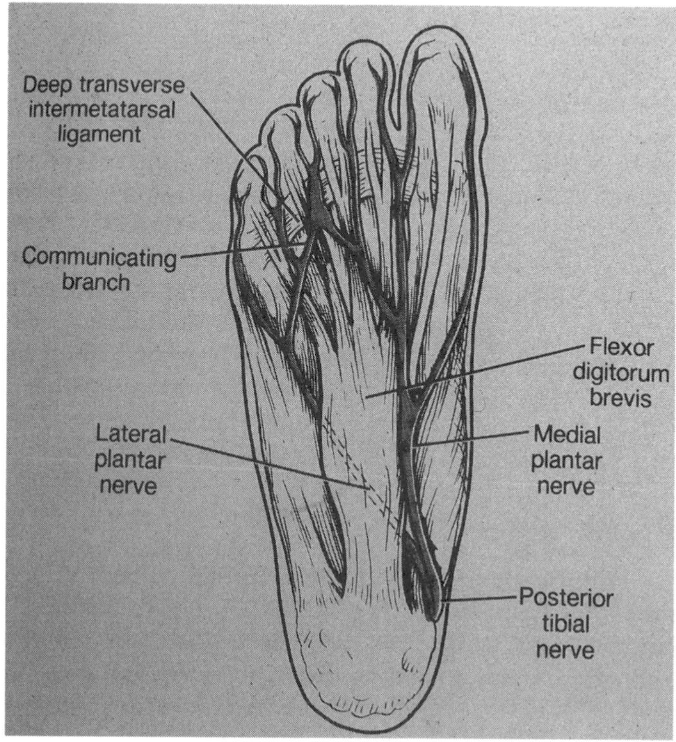

FIGURE 63-7
Anatomy of plantar aspect of foot showing location of neuroma and relationship of lateral plantar nerve to flexor digitorum brevis muscle belly that forms "brevis sling".

tion deep in the region between the metatarsal heads. Care should be taken not to inject the solution superficially near the dorsal skin.

b. Metatarsal pads can be helpful in that they act to lift and separate the metatarsal heads.

c. The patient should be advised to use shoe gear with plenty of room in the toe box (ski boots, bicycle shoes, and women's fashion shoes can be particularly offending).

5. An intermetatarsal bursitis is often difficult to distinguish from an intermetatarsal neuroma, and, not uncommonly, the condition occurs in tandem.
   a. Most commonly found in the second and third interspace as are intermetatarsal neuromas.
   b. The patient may describe a sense of fullness in the area in addition to symptoms commonly encountered with neuromas.
   c. Treatment is similar to that for neuromas, though injections of steroid may provide more long-lasting and reliable relief for this condition.
6. If conservative treatment fails, surgical excision may be indicated. It should be noted that failure rates have been reported to be as high as 20%.

E. Turf toe is a ligamentous sprain following hyperextension of the great toe.
   1. The mechanism generally involves aggressive pushoff and pivoting.
   2. Symptoms include edema and tenderness with range of motion, especially in extension.
   3. Treatment includes immobilization taping combined with the use of a rigid postsurgical shoe and control of inflammation. Stiff-soled shoes will help to deter recurrence.

F. Hallux valgus (bunions).
   1. This is a common condition with a strong hereditary component, which can be exacerbated by shoe gear and activity.
   2. The main structural abnormalities are:
      a. A prominent metatarsal head dorsomedially.
      b. An increase in the intermetatarsal angle.
      c. Abduction and valgus rotation of the great toe.
   3. Most patients complain of increased pressure and pain over the prominent first metatarsal head. It is not uncommon for patients to describe sharp shooting pain at night when they are not weight bearing.
   4. Conservative treatment consists of orthotics to control overpronation, accommodative padding, wide shoes, shoe modification, cryotherapy, nonsteroidal antiinflammatories, and, occasionally, an injection of short-acting steroid with local anesthetic (this should be injected extra-articularly).

G. Toenail problems.
   1. Onychocryptosis (ingrown toenails).
      a. Common causes of ingrown toenails are congenitally curved nails, fungal infection, and trauma.
      b. The nail border may be hypertrophied from chronic inflammation or it may be acutely infected.
      c. If infected, the nail border needs to be removed as it acts as a foreign body. Antibiotics are *rarely* indicated in a non-compromised host; it is not appropriate to put the patient on oral antibiotics and

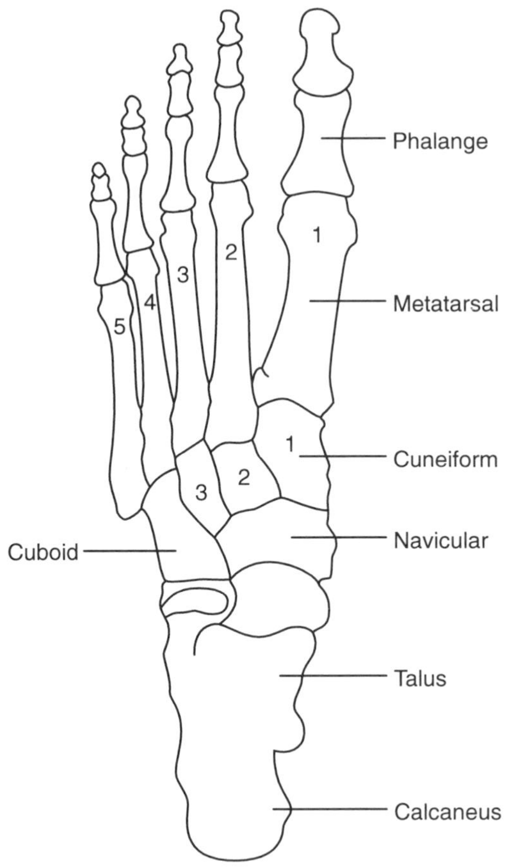

FIGURE 63-8
Bones of the foot.

not remove the ingrown portion of the nail. Partial or total nail avulsion is followed by warm water soaks with Epsom salts.

d. If ingrown toenails are a recurrent problem, partial or total nail matricectomy can offer a long-lasting solution.

2. Onychomycosis (fungal infection of toenails).
   a. Thick, discolored toenails are commonly the result of fungal infection. This can be caused by previous repeated microtrauma to the nail or a single traumatic episode.
   b. Total eradication is almost impossible; treatment involves teaching the patient how to keep the nail debrided using pliers-like nail shears. Topical antifungal application will not lead to a cure but may in some cases provide some aesthetic benefit (I rarely advocate systemic antifungal medication).
   c. Permanent removal of the nail, if painful or infected, may be the best solution.

Bibliography

Bossley CJ, Cairney PC: The intermetarsal-phalangeal bursa—its significance in Mortori's metatarsalgia, *J Bone Joint Surg* 62B:184-191, 1980.

Dockery GL: *Nails: Fundamental Conditions and Procedures. Comprehensive Textbook of Foot Surgery,* Baltimore, 1992, Williams & Wilkins, pp 277-303.

Gage JR: *An Overview of Normal Walking. American Academy of Orthopaedic Surgeons Instructional Course Lecture No 39,* Taunton, MA, 1990, Rand McNally.

Garrick JG, Requa R: The epidemiology of foot and ankle injuries in sports, *Clin Sports Med* 7:29-36, 1988.

Heckman JD: *Fractures and Dislocations of the Foot,* Philadelphia, 1991, JB Lippincott, pp 2041-2182.

Holmes GB, Mann RA: Possible epidemiological factors associated with rupture of the posterior tibial tendon, *Foot Ankle* 13:70-78, 1992.

Hunter SC et al: Foot problems. In: The *Team Physician's Handbook,* Philadelphia, 1990, Hanley & Belfus, pp 452-463.

Karr S: Subcalcaneal heel pain, *Orthop Clin North Am* 25(1):161-175, 1994.

Mann RA, Reynolds JC: Interdigital neuroma: a critical clinical analysis, *Foot Ankle* 3:328-234, 1983.

Schepsis AA, Wagner C, Leach RE: Surgical management of Achilles tendon overuse injuries, a long term follow-up study, *Am J Sports Med* 22:611-619, 1994.

CHAPTER 64

Biomechanics of Running and Gait

Karl B. Fields, MD

Mitch Craib, PhD

I. Introduction
   A. Definition of biomechanics: effects of external and internal forces on a biological system.
   B. Biomechanics is an offshoot of classical mechanics; classical mechanics is based on Newton's three laws: inertia, action, and reaction.[14]
   C. Three essential areas of biomechanics include study of anatomical factors, neurophysiological factors, and external forces that affect movement of a biological system.
   D. Running involves all three areas.
   E. Biomechanical analysis may be directed toward performance or understanding injury.
   F. Mechanics is subdivided into *statics* and *dynamics,* with biomechanics primarily related to dynamics.
   G. Two commonly used terms related to dynamics are kinematics and kinetics. *Kinematics* describes position, displacement, velocity, and acceleration; *kinetics* relates force applied to a body to its mass and motion.[14]

II. Key Aspects of Biomechanics Related to Running
   A. Force.
      1. Force is basically a push or pull of one body on another, and in running both external and internal forces affect the individual.
      2. Examples of *external force* include the force of gravity, ground impact forces, friction, and wind resistance.
      3. *Internal forces* relate to joints, muscles, tendons, ligaments, and body structures.
   B. Movement related to force.
      1. Force results in movement unless balanced by an equal and opposite force.
      2. Force results in either translational (movement along a straight line) or rotational movement.
      3. Force about a joint is least when motion is purely translational.

4. Logically, a force resulting in almost a pure translational movement would lead to more efficient running.
5. Torque (moment of force) is a measure of rotational movement.
6. Rotational force at a joint increases stress and the likelihood of injury.
7. Excess rotational force (primarily pronation) hinders running efficiency.[14]

C. Kinematics.
   1. Running primarily involves translational movement, and this movement is defined by a combination of position, displacement, acceleration, and velocity.
   2. Average speed = distance/time and this is a product of stride length × stride frequency.
   3. Logically, running speed increases with increasing stride length or increasing stride frequency until an optimal balance is achieved above which any further increase in one leads to a concomitantly greater decrease in the other.
   4. Efficient running involves moving the center of mass forward (translational movement) while minimizing the vertical displacement of this center of mass.
      a. Problems occur with excess motion outside the plane of primary movement.
      b. For example, overstriding may allow the center of mass to fall too low, requiring additional force in a vertical direction to return the center of mass to the normal level of its translational displacement. This becomes an inefficient expenditure of energy.
   5. In running, rotational movement always occurs in certain anatomical areas to allow translation to occur along a single straight vector.
   6. This differs from walking, during which two parallel vectors result from strides in which one foot always makes ground contact.
   7. Running also differs significantly from walking in that an airborne phase is present.
   8. A third key difference between walking and running is that foot strike and stance occur in approximately one third the time that they take for walking.[12]
   9. In running, contraction of adductor muscles and hip flexion help pull the foot strike onto the same vertical plane during forward movement. Some degree of pelvic/internal hip rotation is required for this to occur.
   10. Foot strike involves rotation in that most runners strike in some supination and accommodate with pronation to move the foot into position for toe off.
      a. Neutral position of the ankle leaves the foot in slight supination.
      b. Subtalar joint motion facilitates rotation along the longitudinal axis of the foot to transfer weight to the medial aspect of the foot for more efficient pushoff.
      c. Excessive pronation does not promote efficient pushoff, increases stresses on various joints, and leads to more frequent injury.

D. Kinetics.
   1. Force is transferred to the lower extremity from the impact of the foot with the ground. In running, the stance phase is markedly shorter than in walking so that there is less time for shock absorption; therefore shock is of greater magnitude.[12]
   2. Ground reaction forces occur in three planes: vertical, mediolateral, and anteroposterior.

3. Force platforms allow us to understand the relative contribution of force vectors in each of these planes to the movement of the runner and to the stress transferred to the foot and lower extremity.
4. Force platforms demonstrate that runners with different forms have differing patterns of impact force.
    a. The typical heel striker has a first peak of impact force shortly after heel strike.
    b. A second distinct force peak comes from active pressure applied to the forefoot at pushoff.
    c. A runner who lands on the forefoot will have a different pattern in that the force peaks from impact and from active pushoff are closer together and may merge into one peak.
    d. With increasing running speed both heel strikers and forefoot strikers will show movement toward one peak because of the compressed time for impact and toe off.[12]
    e. This implies that the force transmitted to the foot and lower extremity differs in runners based on form. The demands placed on lower extremity muscles for cushioning vary.[13]
5. Impact forces vary with multiple factors including running speed, running style, shoe shape, and shoe material construction.
6. The magnitude and timing of the impact force on the runner also vary directly with the type of surface so that an absolutely rigid surface shows an almost immediate, high impact peak whereas running in soft sand shows virtually no impact peak.
7. This means that muscle must become more active as a shock absorber the harder the surface or the shoe.
8. Force is measured by external impact via the force plate, but the internal force experienced at a joint can only be calculated mathematically.
9. Internal forces are called active forces since they are largely determined by muscle action.
10. External forces average 2-3 times body weight for easy running and probably peak at about 4 times body weight with sprinting.
11. Internal or active impact forces reach 6 times body weight for running calculated at the ankle and knee.
12. Maximal active force from the effect of muscle contraction for sprinting (pushoff) may reach 10-13 times body weight at the ankle.[14]

E. Concept of a kinetic chain.
1. Force is dissipated over a linked connection of anatomical structures from the foot to the lower extremity to the trunk.
2. When the foot is in contact with the ground the kinetic chain is considered closed.[11]
3. At early foot strike shock absorption, stabilization of the knee, hip and ankle joints, and accommodative flexibility of the foot are required for normal function.
4. Each joint from the subtalar to the hip in the lower extremity helps absorb the force.
5. Soft tissues, particularly muscle, are primary shock absorbers.
6. Injury or dysfunction at any level of this shock-absorbing chain results in a transfer of excessive load to other areas of the chain.
7. Normal motion within the kinetic chain is also important when the chain is open (foot off the ground) during the swing phase of gait.
8. Rotational forces acting over greater distance magnify stress.

a. For example, an equal rotational force starting from a valgus alignment of the knee increases stress at the Achilles' tendon more than a rotational stress originating at the subtalar joint.
b. This is explained by the equation T = dF, where *T* is torque (moment of force), *d* is distance from a line of action, and *F* is force acting on the body.
c. Torque is always present as a part of the normal gait cycle of running as internal rotation takes place at foot strike followed by external rotation at toe off.
d. A second example is that standing places ½ body weight on each hip joint, but standing on one leg multiplies the torque at the weight-bearing hip joint to 3 to 5 times body weight.[14]

9. Anything that affects the ability of the kinetic chain to function alters the runner's ability to dissipate force.
   a. Injury.
   b. Specific muscle weakness.
   c. Limited range of motion at any joint.
   d. Damage to soft tissue structures: bone, cartilage, tendon, or ligament.
   e. Fatigue.
   f. Shoe characteristics.[11]
10. Persistent kinetic chain dysfunction from whatever cause is postulated as a major cause of running injury.

F. Gait cycle.
   1. Key phases include the swing phase and the stance phase.
   2. Stance phase is divided into foot strike (usually on the heel), midstance, and toe off.
   3. Swing phase is divided into early, mid, and late cycle.
   4. Part of the running gait cycle is a "float" phase during which the athlete is airborne with neither foot in contact with the ground.[12]
   5. Excess pronation is generally defined by an Achilles' tendon angle in excess of 10 degrees[4]; during walking normal arches show pronation of about 6-8 degrees and flat feet show pronation of 10-12 degrees.[12]
   6. Pronation of 0 degrees or less identifies a runner who would be classified as displaying excessive supination.
   7. The laboratory measurement of angles to define pronation or supination gives a guideline only, as the clinical manifestations of pronation or supination vary with fatigue, running speed, and other dynamic factors.

G. Muscular activity during gait cycle (Table 64-1).[15]
   1. General: muscle activity during gait cycle has been determined by electrical activity. The specific role of each function is extrapolated based on these physiological data plus the understanding of anatomical principles.
   2. Stretch-shortening cycle: a key concept of muscular activity in locomotion is that a stretch triggers an eccentric contraction of a particular group followed by a rapid concentric contraction. This activity forms a natural type of muscle action that results in a more powerful final action.[10]
      a. Hamstrings: stabilize the knee at initial ground contact; function synergistically with gluteus maximus to bring about rapid hip extension during stance phase.[12]
      b. Gluteus maximus: helps decelerate forward swing of the thigh in late swing phase and is primary initiator of rapid hip extension.

TABLE 64-1. Muscle Activity During Running

	Stance Phase			Swing Phase		
Muscles	**Foot Strike**	**Mid Stance**	**Toe Off**	**Early**	**Mid**	**Late**
Rectus femoris	×	×	×	×		×
Hamstrings	×	×	×			×
Anterior tibialis	×		×	×	×	×
Gastrocnemius	×	×				×
Soleus	×	×				×

Modified from Reference 15. × indicates muscle activity.

c. Quadriceps: brief phase of stabilization of the knee at initial ground contact; bring about knee extension in swing phase.
d. Hip abductors: stabilize the stance leg and hemipelvis during stance phase and prevent sagging of hemipelvis during swing phase.
e. Hip adductors: active throughout gait cycle and specific role less clear; probably assist in positioning thigh for more efficient toe off and help position the leg for initial ground contact.
f. Anterior compartment: tibialis anterior, extensor hallucis longus, and extensor digitorum longus; stabilize the foot and ankle during stance phase and probably help accelerate the tibia forward during toe off.
g. Peroneal muscles: during late swing phase and early stance phase stabilize the ankle joint; initiate the first 50% of plantar flexion for toe off.
h. Gastrocnemius and soleus: pushoff for the acceleration phase of running.
i. Posterior tibialis: plantar flexion and stabilization of the ankle joint to prevent excess pronation.

III. Biomechanics and injury.
A. Clinical assessment of gait is essential in detecting dysfunction of the kinetic chain.
B. Some asymmetry of weight bearing, foot strike, or form is not unusual and is often balanced by compensatory adjustments.
C. Significant asymmetry of gait or true limp points toward injury or limitation of motion that may be subtle on static examination.
D. Excess pronation is measured by the Achilles' tendon angle (the angle formed by the Achilles' tendon and a line bisecting the calcaneus).[14]
1. Clinically, pronation has been associated with numerous running injuries including the most common (patellofemoral stress syndrome [PFSS], iliotibial band syndrome [ITB], medial tibial stress syndrome, and plantar fasciitis).[7]
2. Prospective association of running injury with excessive pronation has been reported.[14]
E. Eccentric muscle contraction is related to injuries to the musculotendinous unit.
1. Eccentric means that the muscle is lengthened while muscle units are active.

2. Muscles undergoing eccentric contraction experience greater forces and would place more stress on the weak point in the anatomical system, which is the musculotendinous attachment.[6]
3. Clinically this is confirmed by the occurrence of hamstring,[16] calf, and Achilles' tendon tears during eccentric contraction; rarely in concentric contraction.

F. Leg length inequality is associated with an increase in running injuries.[7]
1. Clinical observation shows that the long leg is the more commonly injured extremity.
2. Perhaps this has some relationship to the mathematical formula for torque in that force is multipled by distance. In this case the long leg may be subject to greater stress although the biomechanical causes for this have not been established.

G. Cavus feet, particularly when inflexible, show a high peak impact on force plate studies. Clinically, cavus feet have been shown prospectively to have a relative risk of 6.1 for injury, with flat feet showing a relative risk of 1.[2]

H. Increased torque adds stress to joints, and joint injury is much more common in running than in walking.
1. Observed motion changes in degrees comparing running versus walking for various joints[12]:

Hip flexion-extension	50 vs. 40
Knee flexion-extension	80 vs. 40
Plantar flexion-extension	45 vs. 25

I. Summary.
1. Biomechanics ties the static principles of anatomy and physics to dynamic stresses associated with running.
2. Biomechanical studies and mathematical calculations predict the stresses that will occur at joints and in soft tissues of the lower extremity.
3. Limited clinical trials confirm increased injury risk associated with biomechanical stress.
4. Clinical observations conform to predicted stresses derived from the biomechanical model.
5. Relating biomechanical stresses to running injury is an area of intense study at present with few proven associations.
6. A knowledge of biomechanics does help the clinician postulate probable causes of injury.

IV. Orthotics for Running

A. Orthotics.
1. An orthosis is basically a mechanical device that exerts a counterforce.
2. In the most basic sense any arch pad or metatarsal pad is a form of orthosis.
3. Current use of orthotics in runners includes variably sophisticated shoe inserts that range from a rigid to semirigid to soft construction.
4. Generic orthotic devices are formed from orthopedic felt, variable density rubber compounds, graphite-rubber mixtures, sorbothane, and any of the various materials employed in orthotic preparation.
5. Prescribed orthotics have a core blank of a memory plastic, an outer cover, a padded support layer, and a base.

6. Orthotic materials include rigid and moldable plastics for a core.
   a. Support materials including ethyl vinyl acetate, polyvinyls, poron, and various forms of rubber.
   b. Coverings of nylon, felt, suede, or leather.
   c. Base materials ranging from firm plastics to vinyl acetate derivatives to styrofoam.
7. Orthotic preparation can be done by developing inserts from non–weight-bearing casts or weight-bearing casts or by molding malleable blanks with partial or full weight bearing.

B. Clinical use of orthotics.
   1. Orthotic use gained credibility in medical circles after James and coworkers reported using orthotics for treatment of 46% of 180 injured runners in a 1978 study.[7]
   2. They reported a 78% "beneficial" result from this treatment.
   3. The basic principle that underscored their approach was that the subtalar neutral position was best for runners.
   4. They defined three keys to successful orthotic preparation.
      a. Correct analysis of alignment.
      b. Correct casting.
      c. Precise fabrication.
   5. Clinical observations included[7]:
      a. Orthotics were most effective for controlling excess compensatory pronation.
      b. They were useful for short-term acute injury treatment as well as long-term treatment of form or alignment problems.
      c. A slight undercorrection of measured abnormalities worked best.
      d. Soft, flexible orthotics worked best for cavus feet.
   6. Clement and associates also recommended orthotic use in their 1981 report of treatment of 1650 runners.[1]
      a. Soft orthotics with a medial wedge were used for most runners with varus alignment (who were presumably suspected of showing excess compensatory pronation).
      b. Dr. Scholl's and Spenco over-the-counter orthotics were also helpful.
      c. Rigid orthotics were reserved for extreme biomechanical problems.
   7. Vixie observed that 60% to 80% of patients could use a soft orthotic.[17]
   8. Overcontrol of pronation by an orthotic can render the foot too rigid and actually worsen shock absorption.[4]
   9. D'Ambrosia and Douglas looked at a series of 50 runners and found a 72% improvement rate.[4]
      a. Flat or pronated feet (81%) did much better than cavus feet (62%).
      b. Cavus feet responded best to soft materials.
      c. Materials used were fairly rigid.
      d. Gender and age made little difference.
      e. Mileage run made some difference; unimproved averaged 30 miles per week versus 23.6 for the improved group.
      f. Running surface may be a factor as well, as 72% of improved limited running on paved surface whereas 71% of unimproved group ran only on paved surfaces.
   10. D'Ambrosia tracked runners for 5 years and found the following results[3]:
      a. 17% needed orthotics.

TABLE 64-2. Response of Injuries to Orthotics

Percent Improved by Diagnosis	Males	Females
Medial tibial stress syndrome	70	83
Pes planus	90	*
Metatarsalgia	84	89
Plantar fasciitis	85	76
Iliotibial band	66	*
Cavus foot	25	*

*number of women too small to evaluate.
†n = 200.

b. MTSS (posterior tibial syndrome) was the leading diagnosis.
c. Results varied by diagnosis (Table 64-2).

11. Newer orthotic materials have probably improved compliance and pain relief with orthotic use.
    a. Survey of 53 orthotic users.
    b. 96% pain relief when coupled with other therapy.
    c. 94% continued usage.
    d. 52% would not do anything without orthotics in shoes.[5]

C. Summary.
1. Orthotic use for runners gained clinical popularity after limited clinical trials reported improvement in 72% to 78% of runners.
2. The rationale for their use and the one condition they seem most clearly to help is excessive pronation. While biomechanical studies show reduction of pronation with the use of orthotics, effect on the knee function has not been clearly demonstrated.[9]
3. Clinical use has become widespread and includes other conditions that lead to running injury such as leg length inequality, cavus feet, bunions, and the like, although causal relationship of malalignments with running injury remains to be determined.[8]
4. Overall success may have a strong relationship to the clinician's skill in assessing the correction needed and the patient who might benefit.
5. Cavus feet, particularly when rigid, pose an increased injury risk, and their response to treatment with orthotics is less predictable.
6. Improved materials and more clinical experience with these suggest that products made today may be superior to those used in the early trials.
7. A movement away from heavier, more rigid orthotics has made their use by runners more acceptable.
8. Orthotics are a classic example of applying biomechanical principles to the direct treatment of running injuries.

References

1. Clement DB, et al: A survey of overuse running injuries, *Phys Sportsmed* 9(5):47-58, 1981.
2. Cowan D, Jones BH, Robinson JR: Foot morphologic characteristics and risk of exercise-related injury, *Arch Fam Med* 2(7):773-777, 1993.
3. D'Ambrosia R: Orthotic devices in running injuries, *Clin Sports Med* 4(4):611-618, 1985.
4. D'Ambrosia R, Douglas D: Orthotics. In D'Ambrosia R, Drez D, editors: *Prevention and Treatment of Running Injuries,* Thorofare, NJ, 1982, Charles B. Slack publishers, pp 55-64.
5. Donatelli R et al: Biomechanical foot orthotics: A retrospective study, *JOSPT* 10(6):205-212, 1988.

6. Jacobs R, Bobbert MF, Schenau GJ: Function of mono- and biarticular muscles in running, *Med Sci Sports Exerc* 25(10):1163-1173, 1993.
7. James SL, Bates BT, Osternig LR: Injuries to runners, *Am J Sports Med* 6(2):40-50, 1978.
8. Kannus V: Evaluation of abnormal biomechanics of the foot and ankle in athletes, *Br J Sports Med* 26(2):83-89, 1992.
9. Kilmartin TE, Wallace WA: The scientific basis for the use of biomechanical foot orthoses in the treatment of lower limb sports injuries—a review of the literature, *Br J Sports Med* 28(3):180-184, 1994.
10. Komi PV: The musculoskeletal system. In Dirix A, Knuttgen HG, Tittel K, editors: *The Olympic Book of Sports Medicine,* vol 1, London, 1988, Oxford, pp 15-39.
11. MacIntyre J, Lloyd-Smith R: Overuse running injuries. In Renstrom PAFH, editor: *Sports Injuries, Basic Principles of Prevention and Care,* Cambridge, MA, Blackwell Scientific Publications, 1994, pp 139-160.
12. Mann RA: Running sports: biomechanics of running. In Mack R, editor: *American Academy of Orthopaedic Surgeons Symposium on The Foot and Leg in Running Sports,* Chicago, 1982, Year Book Medical Publishers, pp 1-29.
13. Martin PE, Morgan DW: Biomechanical considerations for economical walking and running, *Med Sci Sports Exerc* 24(4):467-473, 1992.
14. Nigg BM: Biomechanics as applied to sports. In Harries M, Williams C, Stanish WD, Micheli LJ, editors: *The Oxford Textbook of Sports Medicine,* New York, 1994, Oxford Medical Publications, pp 94-111.
15. Ounpuu S: The biomechanics of walking and running, *Clin Sports Med* 13(4):843-863, 1994.
16. Stanton P, Purdam C: Hamstring injuries in sprinting—the role of eccentric exercise, *J Orthop Sports Phys Ther,* pp 343-349, March 1989.
17. Vixie DE: Orthotics and shoe corrections. In Mack R, editor: *American Academy of Orthopaedic Surgeons Symposium on The Foot and Leg in Running Sports,* Chicago, 1982, Year Book Medical Publishers, pp 76-79.

CHAPTER **65**

Athletic Taping and Bracing

Kirk Jones, MD

ANKLE TAPING AND BRACING

I. Introduction
   A. Ankle sprains are among the most common musculoskeletal injuries affecting both sedentary individuals as well as all types of athletes. Of these, approximately 80% are inversion injuries.[28]
   B. Valuable practice and game time is lost during the recovery process and the chance of recurrence is high.
   C. In an attempt to prevent or lessen the possibility of reinjury various forms of prophylactic ankle taping and/or bracing have been employed.
   D. It is believed that providing an external source of stability to the ligamentous structures without compromising normal joint mechanics will aid in prevention as well as joint protection once injury has occurred.

II. Ankle Taping
   A. The traditional and most commonly used form of stabilization is adhesive ankle taping.
   B. A variety of taping techniques are utilized in the field, although for the most part the same components are present: anchors, stirrups (vertical), horseshoe strips (horizontal), heel locks, and figure eights.
   C. Ankle taping methods.
      1. A tape adherent usually precedes the strips.
      2. Tape may be applied directly to the skin or underwrap may be utilized.
      3. The number of layers of strips and the sequence in which they are applied vary between trainers and are also determined by the size and shape of the ankle.
   D. Types of ankle taping.
      1. Open basketweave: alternating stirrup and horseshoe strips application whereby the strips do not come together anteriorly along the shin or dorsum of the foot. This tape job is beneficial immediately

postinjury because it provides support without excessive constriction, which may hinder circulation.[5]

2. Closed basketweave: similar to the open; however, the layers overlap and encircle the ankle and foot.

III. Ankle Bracing
   A. Ready-made stabilizers.
      1. Included within this category are elastic-type sleeves and lace-up ankle supports.
      2. The benefits as a group are that they are easy to apply, cost effective, and reusable.
      3. Common brand lace-up ankle supports include Cramer, McDavid, Swede-O.
      4. Variations between the braces are heel lock straps, plastic or steel stays for extra support, and Velcro closures.
      5. In treatment of acute injuries, these are not recommended because they do not provide uniform pressure; however, lace-up stabilizers may be worn over a tape job.[5]
   B. Semirigid orthosis.
      1. A semirigid orthosis consists of a prefabricated plastic or thermoplastic shell.
      2. The Air-Cast is a leading example, which consists of medial and lateral shells that are lined with air bags and are connected at the heel. It is held onto the leg with Velcro straps.
      3. It is recommended following acute injury in conjunction with taping as an immobilizer for stable malleolar fractures and in subacute stages.[5]
      4. There are additional brands available but there is a lack of research comparing their effectiveness.
      5. It must also be recognized that comfort will have a strong influence in dictating compliance.

IV. Effectiveness of Ankle Taping
   A. There is disagreement within the literature in regards to the effectiveness and therefore efficacy of ankle taping.
   B. Support is provided by the following.
      1. It is generally believed that the effectiveness of taping is due to improvement in ankle stability by reducing ankle motion, thereby preventing ankle injury.
      2. The effectiveness of ankle taping has been demonstrated by a significant reduction of ankle sprains when compared with nontaped ankles.[10,25]
      3. Additional benefits included the following:
         a. The severity of ligamentous injury was reduced.
         b. Reduction of injury risk was as great as 50% and was even further lowered with the combined use of high-top shoes.
         c. The incidence of recurrence was reduced by as much as two thirds.[10]
      4. Enhanced proprioceptive recruitment has been demonstrated in athletes with significant talar tilt when taping was utilized.[11]
      5. The closed basketweave has been utilized in most studies and appears to be beneficial in minimizing ankle injuries.[10,18,26]
   C. Disadvantages were demonstrated by the following:
      1. It has been shown that taping loses its ability to restrict motion within minutes into the exercise.[9,12,16,18,19]

2. Postexercise motion restriction has been reported to have decreased to 10% to 15% from initial values, ranging from 30% to 41% following various sporting activities.[9,12,19]
3. These differences may be due to the variety of activity levels, modes of measurement, as well as the taping methods that were used.

V. Ankle Taping Versus Bracing
   A. Advantages of bracing.
      1. Taping is costly and requires trained personnel to apply.
      2. Bracing provides motion restriction over a longer period of time.
         a. A semirigid brace lost only 12% of its initial motion restriction of 42% after exercise.[12]
         b. This loss could easily be accounted for by retightening during exercise.
         c. The ability to keep a stabilizing device at adequate levels of restriction is a consideration, especially once fatigue occurs.
      3. Bracing can reduce the incidence of injury, especially when combined with low-top shoes as demonstrated in a retrospective study analysis.[26]
   B. Advantages of taping.
      1. Ability to conform to any ankle, thus providing a custom fit.
      2. It has not been demonstrated whether bracing can provide proprioceptive influences as has been demonstrated with taping.
      3. Mechanism of taping effectiveness may be due to other factors yet to be determined.

VI. Effect of Taping and Bracing on Athletic Performance
   A. An important issue raised with ankle stabilization is whether athletic performance will be hindered.
   B. Research has documented that motor skills have and have not been significantly affected with the use of both taping and certain types of braces.
   C. Prior to drawing any conclusions, the types of taping methods and braced used, time of testing (i.e., immediately after application versus after warm-up), and the types of motor skills being tested must be considered.
   D. There has been no indication that taping or bracing will result in an increase of injuries to other joints.

VII. Summary
   A. It appears that taping and bracing have a worthwhile role in the stabilization of both sound and unstable ankles for the purpose of prevention, management, and rehabilitation.
   B. Their method of effectiveness may be different.
      1. Taping appears to provide less mechanical stability over time but may increase proprioceptive stimulation.
      2. Bracing appears to provide more mechanical stability.
   C. The superiority of one method over the other has been debated as has their effect on athletic performance.
   D. Taping or bracing should not be used as a substitute for a sound rehabilitation program but rather used in conjunction with it.

KNEE BRACING

I. Introduction
   A. The high occurrence and severity of injuries to the knee in sports represent a significant problem.

B. Given that the knee is located in the middle of a long lever arm, is a relatively shallow joint, and lacks soft tissue protection, it is vulnerable to injury.
C. Injuries may range from mild sprains to complete ruptures of one or more soft tissue structures, which may necessitate surgical intervention. The medial collateral ligament (MCL) and anterior cruciate ligament (ACL) are the most commonly injured.
D. In an attempt to prevent injuries and protect and provide support to acute and postsurgical knee conditions, a variety of knee braces have emerged. However, clinical research as to their efficacy is controversial.

II. Instabilities
   A. Instabilities as the result of ligamentous injury are classified by tibial movement in relationship to the femur. The two classifications are:
      1. Straight—defined as abnormal motion in one plane around a single axis with medial, lateral, anterior, and posterior movements as possibilities.
      2. Rotational—defined as abnormal motion in two or more planes around two or more axes, resulting in anteromedial, anterolateral, posterolateral, or combinations of these movements.

III. Types of Braces
   A. In 1984 the American Academy of Orthopaedic Surgeons classified knee braces into three basic categories.
      1. Prophylactic: designed to prevent or decrease the likelihood of serious injury in a normal knee.
      2. Rehabilitative: designed to allow for protective motion in an acutely injured knee on which surgery may or may not have been performed.
      3. Functional: designed to provide joint stability to an unstable or postsurgical knee in performance of activities of daily living or sports.[1]

IV. Prophylactic Knee Braces
   A. It has been reported that a football player with a 4-year career has a 64% chance of sustaining a knee injury, 73% of which involves the MCL.[14]
   B. The development of this type of brace was based on the premise that most forces that cause injury to the MCL are delivered laterally. Such a device would theoretically help disperse force away from the medial structures.
   C. There are two basic types of prophylactic knee braces (PKBs).
      1. A lateral bar with a single, dual, or polycentric hinge, which is applied to the lateral aspect of the knee joint. Examples include Stromgen, McDavid, Anderson-Omni.
      2. A hinged medial and lateral bar encased in a plastic shell, which is fitted around the knee and held in place by straps or cuffs. Examples include Am Pro, Iowa.
   D. Research studies have found positive effects concerning the use of certain PKBs.
      1. PKBs significantly reduced anteroposterior (AP) translation and internal/external (IE) rotation at low loads in cadavers.[2]
      2. With the use of a mechanical knee model, PKBs provide a beneficial effect in protection of both MCL and ACL against lateral blows.[22]
   E. In contrast, some research studies conducted on cadavers have concluded the following.
      1. At angles other than 0 degrees, PKBs did not alter medial joint line opening or ACL loading. At 0 degrees a reduction of strain was observed along the posterior portion of the MCL.[3]

2. No significant protection was concluded in another study, which also found four adverse effects which included[23]:
   a. Preload force on MCL.
   b. Center of axis shift.
   c. Premature joint line contact.
   d. Brace slippage.
3. Another study refuted the preload effect as tested in vivo and found that PKBs tested did not enhance proprioceptive responses. In vitro PKBs tested at flexion angles of 30 degrees or greater did not provide any benefit.[24]

F. Epidemiological studies conducted primarily on football players over a number of years have also been controversial in determining the efficacy of PKBs.[27,29,30]
   1. There have been studies that have concluded a significant increase in number of knee injuries in those athletes with braces as compared to those without of which the severity was not decreased.[27,30] The possibility of a reduction in a player's agility was attributed to this finding.[27]
   2. Other studies have indicated the reduction of incidences of ACL and MCL injuries; however, the severity was not reduced.[29] This reduction appeared to be dependent on player position, whereby braced defensive players benefited more than nonbraced defensive players. This benefit was not observed with offensive players.

G. Problems associated with the various studies. It is difficult to replicate real-life situations leading to injury.
   1. Cadavers used for the most part ranged in age from 50 to 75 years of age. They do not provide the dynamic stability provided by muscular contractions. Lack of soft tissue compliance does not allow for proper brace application.
   2. Low load forces applied in the research studies are not representative of the higher load forces found in athletics.
   3. The environment—consisting of playing surface, weather, and type of shoes—varies greatly.
   4. Player characteristics such as height, weight, position, prior knee injuries, level of experience, and conditioning are also variables that must be considered.
   5. Rule changes that have occurred during the epidemiological studies may have accounted for some of the injury reductions noted.
   6. Definition and degree of injury vary within the medical community.

H. Summary.
   1. Researchers generally agree that continued work and improvement in brace design are needed.[4,23,24]
   2. Athletes should be made aware of the availability of PKBs; however, their use should be voluntary. Information regarding the possibility that injury and/or its severity may not be prevented should be provided.
   3. Until further clinical studies are conducted, the recommendation for wearing a brace cannot be made.
   4. If a brace is to be worn, it (1) should not slip, (2) should not contact the joint line, and (3) should be properly maintained.

V. Rehabilitative Knee Braces

A. Historically, casts or cast braces were utilized to provide protection to injured, unstable knees for postsurgical situations.

B. Rehabilitative knee braces (RKBs) have replaced casting secondary to their light weight and ability to compensate for changes in girth as the result of swelling, atrophy, and eventual hypertrophy. An additional advantage is the ability to inspect the surgical incision easily.
C. The purpose of RKBs is to provide protection to healing structures while allowing for a progressive increase in controlled range of motion over time.
D. RKBs are composed of medial and lateral sidebars, which provide long leverage protection and which are held in place with Velcro straps that surround both the thigh and calf. Hinges located about the joint lines can be set for a desired amount of range of motion. These characteristics lead to versatility in application to a variety of patients.
E. Research has not focused as much attention on these types of braces even though they are used more often than both prophylactic and functional braces. Some of the studies available have indicated the following.
   1. An investigation of eight different RKBs revealed that significant reduction in translation and rotational forces at low loads in mechanical knee models can be achieved.[6] The characteristics of those braces that led to increased stability included:
      a. The necessity for medial and lateral joint line contact.
      b. The greater number of straps, which in essence increases the total contact surface area.
      c. The ability of the brace to function as a single unit regardless of the individual makeup of the individual components.
   2. Braces that include medial and lateral supports along with sidebar rigidity increase stability about the knee in cadavers.[15]
F. Problems associated with the use of RKBs.
   1. Pressure sores and skin irritation, excessive heat retention, and vertical brace migration.
   2. Circulatory impedance if strapping is too tight.
   3. Patient non-compliance.
   4. Psychological dependency as well as risk taking.
G. Summary.
   1. Patients require education regarding the use of RKBs to minimize problems.
   2. Further research is necessary, especially since rehabilitation programs are utilizing a more aggressive approach requiring RKBs to act more as functional braces.[22]
   3. Research investigating effect on specific sports skills such as jumping, running, cutting drills, and endurance is lacking.

VI. Functional Braces
A. During the 1970s the first functional brace designed for an athletic population was created as the result of recognition of rotational instability.[20]
B. Since then, a variety of functional knee braces (FKBs) have emerged, which can be classified into two general types.
   1. Hinge/post/strap: a few examples include Lenox Hill, Don Joy Defiance, Omni Scientific Elite.
   2. Hinge/post/shell: examples include CTi, Generation II, Bledsoe.
C. These braces can either be custom-fitted or bought off the shelf and range in price from $145 to $570.
D. The purpose of FKBs is to augment stability in an unstable or post-surgical knee in performance of activities of daily living and sports.

E. Numerous studies have been conducted; even so, the literature does not adequately support or negate the efficacy of FKBs in controlling knee instabilities in ACL-deficient knees.
F. Similar problems as noted in research involving PKBs in regards to low load testing levels and use of cadavers complicate applicability towards in vivo situations (see p. 491).
G. Research studies have generally concluded that an increase in stability with the use of FKBs can occur under low load situations. It should be noted that loads were not representative of those loads produced in activities as of daily living as demonstrated by Noyes.[21]
H. Subjectively, however, at least 90% of participants in one study felt that they performed better with FKBs and noted less incidences of the knee giving way.[8] Instability was not totally eliminated.
I. Summary.
   1. The use of FKBs may provide some benefit in activities, especially at low loads in an ACL-deficient knee.
   2. Even though objective biomechanical support has not substantiated the efficacy of FKBs, subjective improvements are a consideration.
   3. Patients should be informed that FKBs may not prevent subluxation.
   4. FKBs must not substitute for a rehabilitative program designed to improve range of motion, strength, and functional activities.
   5. Further research is required, especially in light of continuing advances in surgical and rehabilitative techniques.

References

1. American Academy of Orthopaedic Surgeons: *Knee Braces Seminar Report.* Chicago, 1985, American Academy of Orthopaedic Surgeons.
2. Anderson K et al: A biomechanical evaluation of taping and bracing in reducing knee joint translation and rotation, *Am J Sports Med* 20(4):416-421, 1992.
3. Beynnon BD, Renstrom PA: The effect of bracing and taping in sports, *Ann Chir Gynaecol* 80:230-238, 1991.
4. Brown TD, VanHoeck JE, Brand RA: Laboratory evaluation of prophylactic knee brace performance under dynamic valgus loading using a surrogate leg model, *Clin Sports Med* 9:751-762, 1990.
5. Buschbacher RM: Ankle sprain evaluation and bracing. In Buschbacher RM, editor: *Sports Medicine and Rehabilitation: A Sport-Specific Approach,* St Louis, 1994, Mosby–Year Book.
6. Cawley PW: Postoperative knee bracing, *Clin Sports Med* 9:(4)763-769, 1990.
7. Cawley PW, France EP, Paulos LE: Comparison of rehabilitative knee braces, *Am J Sports Med* 17:141-146, 1989.
8. Colville MR, Lee CL, Ciullo JV: The Lenox Hill brace. An evaluation of effectiveness in treating knee instabilities, *Am J Sports Med* 14:257-261, 1986.
9. Fumich RM et al: The measured effect of taping on combined foot and ankle motion before and after exercise, *Am J Sports Med* 9(3):165-169, 1981.
10. Garrick JG, Requa RK: Role of external support in the prevention of ankle sprains, *Med Sci Sports* (3):200-203, 1993.
11. Glick JM, Gordon RB, Mishimoto D: The prevention and treatment of ankle injuries, *Am J Sports Med* 4:136-141, 1976.
12. Green TA, Hillman SK: Comparison of support provided by a semirigid orthosis and adhesive ankle taping before, during, and after exercise, *Am J Sports Med* 18(5):498-506, 1990.
13. Green TA, Wight CR: A comparative support evaluation of three ankle orthoses before, during and after exercise, *J Orthop Phys Ther* 11:453-466, 1990.
14. Hewson GF, Mendini RA, Wand JB: Prophylactic knee bracing in college football, *Am J Sports Med* 14:262-265, 1986.
15. Hofmann AA et al: Knee stability in orthotic knee braces, *Am J Sports Med* 12:371-374, 1984.
16. Larsen E: Taping the ankle for chronic instability, *Acta Orthop Scand* 55:551-553, 1984.
17. Miyasaka K et al: The incidence of knee ligament injuries in the general population, *Am J Knee Surg* 4:3-8, 1991.
18. Morris HH, Musnicki W: The effect of taping on ankle mobility following moderate exercise, *J Sports Med* 23:422-426, 1983.

19. Myburgh KH, Vaughan CL, Isaacs SK: The effects of ankle guards and taping on joint motion before, during and after a squash match, *Am J Sports Med* 12(6):441-445, 1984.
20. Nicholas JA: Bracing the anterior cruciate ligament deficient knee using the Lenox Hill derotation brace, *Clin Orthop* 172:137-142, 1983.
21. Noyes FR et al: Biomechanical analysis of human ligament grafts used in knee ligament repairs and reconstruction, *J Bone Joint Surg* 66A:344-352, 1984.
22. Paulos LE, Cawley PW, France PE: Impact biomechanics of lateral knee bracing, *J Sports Med* 19(4):337-342, 1991.
23. Paulos LE et al: The biomechanics of lateral knee bracing. Part I: Response of the valgus restraints to loading, *Am J Sports Med* 15(5):419-429, 1987.
24. Paulos LE et al: The biomechanics of lateral knee bracing. Part II: Impact response of the braced knee, *Am J Sports Med* 15(5):430-438, 1987.
25. Quigley TB, Cox J, Murphy J: A protective wrapping for the ankle, *JAMA* 132:924, 1946.
26. Rovere GD et al: Retrospective comparison of taping and ankle stabilizers in preventing ankle injuries, 16(3):228-233, 1988.
27. Rovere GD, Haupt HA, Yates CS: Prophylactic knee bracing in college football, *Am J Sports Med* 15(2):111-116, 1987.
28. Roy S, Irvin R: *Sports Medicine Prevention, Evaluation, Management and Rehabilitation,* Englewood Cliffs, 1983, Prentice-Hall.
29. Sitler MR et al: The efficacy of a prophylactic knee brace to reduce knee injuries in football, *Am J Sports Med* 18(3):310-315, 1990.
30. Teitz CC et al: Evaluation of the use of braces to prevent injury to the knee in collegiate football players, *J Bone Joint Surg* 69A:2-9, 1987.
31. Zuelzer, WA: Knee Bracing. In Buschbacher RM, editor: *Sports Medicine and Rehabilitation: A Sport-Specific Approach,* St Louis, 1994, Mosby–Year Book.

PEDIATRIC CONCERNS

CHAPTER 66

Musculoskeletal Injuries Unique to Growing Children And Adolescents

Angela D. Smith, MD

I. Ways the Immature Musculoskeletal System Differs from the Mature
   A. Open growth plates.
      1. Provide longitudinal and appositional growth (Fig. 66-1).
      2. Lead to relative disproportion between lengths of the long bones and their adjacent musculature.
      3. Some evidence of increased fracture rate at time of peak height velocity.
   B. Thicker periosteum.
      1. Stabilizes the bone whether it is intact or fractured.
      2. In the event of fracture, periosteum may act as a deforming force as it contracts over time.
      3. Takes more force to disrupt than adult periosteum.
      4. Highly vascular, so aids in the more rapid healing observed in younger individuals.
   C. Long bones more porous.
      1. Especially at the metaphysis.
      2. Torus (buckle) fractures common among children.
   D. Long bones absorb more energy before fracture than do adult's long bones.
      1. In the very young may spring back or bend rather than break.
      2. Look for plastic deformation if fracture is suspected but no fracture line is observed.
   E. Different injury patterns at different ages: pattern probably depends on relative strengths of adjacent structures at the particular skeletal age.
   F. Thicker articular cartilage.
      1. Articular cartilage also growing.
      2. For reasons not known (possibly related to the differences of articular cartilage between the mature and immature states) children and adolescents develop chondral or osteochondral fragmentation from

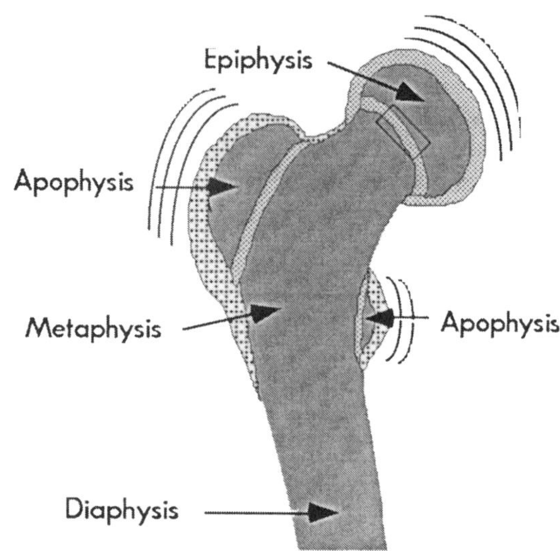

FIGURE 66-1
The parts of a growing bone. Growth occurs in all the stippled areas.

overuse—at the distal femoral condyle, capitellum, radial head, and (more rarely) humeral head.

G. Greater vascularity of menisci of the knee: better potential for healing of more types of meniscal tears than in adult.

II. Growth plate (physis)
   A. Growing cartilaginous physis resists less force than the bone surrounding it.
      1. Epiphysis: at end of a long bone.
      2. Apophysis: attachment of musculotendinous unit.
   B. In certain types of acute injuries, the weakest link is at the physis.
      1. Traction: fibula physeal fracture from ankle inversion injury instead of ankle sprain.
      2. Shear, bending: medial collateral ligament sprain vs. femur fracture.
      3. Compression: Salter V fracture of distal radius from fall onto outstretched hand.
   C. Overuse injuries of physis.
      1. Traction: Osgood-Schlatter disorder.
      2. Compression: growth arrest of distal radial physis of gymnasts.
      3. Possibly shear: may be part of reason for gymnasts' distal radial growth arrest.
   D. Spinal growth overload disorders: Scheuermann's disease (ring apophyses of vertebral bodies), spondylolisthesis (progression of vertebral slippage from defect in pars interarticularis).
   E. Slipped capital femoral epiphysis disruption of physeal structure, loss of columnation of dividing chondrocytes.

III. Physeal Fractures (Fig. 66-2)
   A. Salter-Harris classification often aids in prognosis and is important for determining specific treatment.
      1. Type 1: through physis only; radiographs may be normal except for soft tissue swelling over physis; growth arrest rare.
      2. Type 2: through physis, with corner of metaphysis; growth arrest may occur, especially in certain locations, at certain ages.
      3. Type 3: through physis and epiphysis, into joint; growth arrest rare, but concern about articular congruity.

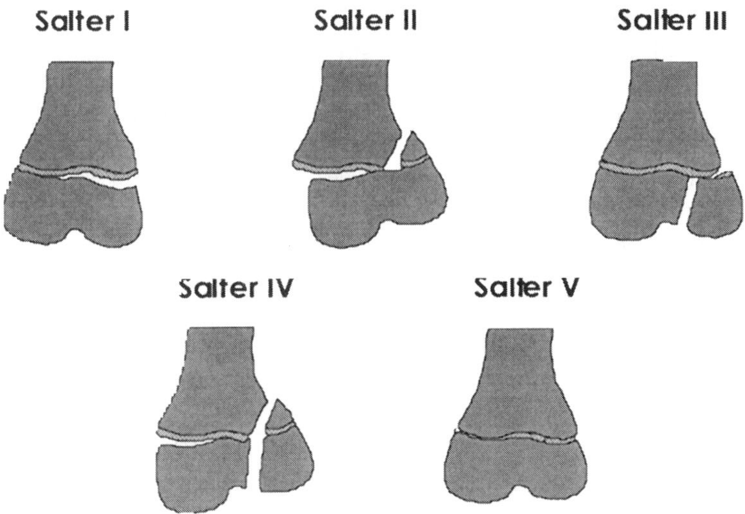

FIGURE 66-2
The Salter-Harris classification of physeal fractures.

4. Type 4: through metaphysis, across physis, through epiphysis, into joint; bony bridge from epiphysis to metaphysis may occur and cause growth arrest; also concerns about articular congruity.
5. Type 5: compression of physis; radiographs may appear normal.

B. Alter the on-field examination from the usual for adults.
   1. Injury may be a fracture rather than a sprain.
   2. Before doing *any* stress test to a joint of a skeletally immature individual, ascertain that there is almost no chance of a fracture being present.

C. Know the anatomy of epiphyseal regions well.
   1. Thoroughly palpate physes that might be involved in the injury
   2. *Strongly* consider obtaining radiographs before doing any stress testing of the knee, ankle, elbow, wrist, shoulder, or digit of a skeletally immature athlete.

D. Initial treatment for most significant extremity injuries in athletes with open physes.
   1. Splint and elevate the limb.
   2. Apply ice.
   3. Send the athlete for further evaluation (radiography, etc.) before allowing return to play.

E. Initial treatment for obvious severe deformity.
   1. With significant threat to viability of the limb, consider closed reduction.
   2. For most young athletes in North America, appropriate emergency room and radiography facilities are usually nearby, so reduction on site is rarely warranted unless limb has loss of circulation or injury is recurrent (i.e., recurrent shoulder dislocation).

IV. Additional injury factors not directly related to musculoskeletal system

A. Temporary changes in coordination: with growth spurts and weight gain.

B. Inadequate matching in contact sports: matched by age, rather than by height, weight, or Tanner stage, for most contact sports.

C. Motivational differences.
   1. May be pushed by parent or coach (or self), so afraid to stop when pain occurs, leading to increased incidence or severity of injury.
   2. More likely to have less qualified coaches.

D. Other psychological considerations.
   1. Perceived needs for athletic success (or needs to retain attention of coaches and parents) may lead to disordered eating, which may in turn cause increased injury due to physical or mental fatigue or weakness.
   2. Athlete may perceive (sometimes correctly) that his or her worth to a parent is as a successful athlete rather than as a unique individual; therefore, may be afraid to admit injury until it is so severe that major or prolonged treatment is needed.

Bibliography

Bak K: Separation of the proximal tibial epiphysis in a gymnast, *Acta Orthop Scand* 62:293-294, 1991.

Barnett LS: Little League shoulder syndrome: proximal humeral epiphyseolysis in adolescent baseball pitchers, a case report, *J Bone Joint Surg* 67A:495-496, 1985.

Caine D et al: Stress changes of the distal radial growth plate. A radiographic survey and review of the literature, *Am J Sports Med* 20:290-298, 1992.

Currey JD, Butler G: The mechanical properties of bone tissue in children. *J Bone Joint Surg* 57:810-814, 1975.

Goldstein JD et al: Spine injuries in gymnasts and swimmers. An epidemiologic investigation, *Am J Sports Med* 19:463-468, 1991.

Mubarak SJ, Carroll NC: Juvenile osteochondritis dissecans of the knee: etiology, *Clin Orthop Rel Res* 157:200-211, 1981.

Ogden JA: Skeletal growth mechanism injury patterns, *J Pediatr Orthop* 2:371-377, 1982.

Stanitski CL, Harvell JC, Fu F: Observations on acute knee hemarthrosis in children and adolescents, *J Pediatr Orthop* 13:506-510, 1993.

CHAPTER **67**

Rehabilitation for Children and Adolescents

Angela D. Smith, MD

I. Concepts of Rehabilitation
   A. Following injury, rehabilitation essential to prevent recurrent injury or related injury.
   B. Return muscle strength to full power, strength, and endurance.
   C. Regain flexibility and coordination.
   D. Restore full performance capability.
   E. *Pre*habilitation: identify deficits in muscle strength, flexibility, and coordination and correct them preseason.

II. Principles of Rehabilitation for Children and Adolescents
   A. Rationale.
      1. Similar exercises for youth and adult, but different ways of increasing compliance.
      2. Problems to work with.
         a. Shorter attention span.
         b. Don't care to understand purpose of rehabilitation program or why it's important.
         c. Teenagers feel invulnerable.
         d. Don't wish to be different from peers.
      3. Possible solutions.
         a. Teach program in the most concise, entertaining manner possible.
         b. Organize exercise program to be brief but effective.
         c. For teenagers, use improvement of performance as motivator.
         d. Allow patient to do any part of sport/practice that is safe to optimize psychological status (maintain social contacts, improve motivation to rehabilitate).
      4. Specific principles for this age group.
         a. Defined period of time to meet goals.
         b. Short exercise bouts.
         c. Small number of exercises—do these regularly and correctly.
         d. Make evidence of progress obvious.

e. Build in incentives.
f. Integrate the rehabilitation program into the patient's schedule.

B. Defined rehabilitation period.
1. Set a period of time to meet goals, preferably not more than 2 months.
2. Gain young person's interest and cooperation when pain and physical limitations still present.
3. Limit doing things *to* patient—have patient be active participant, beginning as rapidly as possible.
4. Control pain and swelling as rapidly as possible, to begin therapeutic exercise as soon as possible.

C. Short rehabilitation exercise bouts.
1. Preferably only 15 minutes.
2. Recognize that the "ideal" program is often (usually) unrealistic.
3. Treat critical regions first.
4. Children unlikely to perform *any* portion of program that takes too long to complete.

D. Small number of exercises.
1. Limited number of exercises, specific to the particular injury.
2. Let young person feel accomplished at finishing entire group of only three or four different exercises.
3. If more prescribed, realize that the easiest exercises to perform (and the ones preferentially selected by most children) tend to be the least useful for improving the condition being treated.
4. Emphasize the most critical exercises: written handouts with stars, stickers, bright underlining; should do critical exercises *first.*

E. Visible progress.
1. Goal-oriented progression, with many intermediate levels on the ladder of goals.
2. Indicate progress by:
a. Changing colors of elastic bands.
b. Increasing numbers of repetitions.
c. Increasing pounds of resistance.

F. Interesting and entertaining therapeutic exercise programs.
1. Entertain while instructing.
2. Concise and interesting instructions, including
a. Cartoon characters
b. Sports stars
c. "Gimmicks"
3. Enticing equipment—bright colored, decorated

G. Integration into regular schedule with incentives.
1. Six days per week.
2. Once a day.
3. One day off "for good behavior."
4. Do short exercises any time waiting for something.
5. Do while watching television or talking on the telephone; do exercises during first phone call, reward is to make a second call.
6. "Personal treat" on day off from exercises.

III. Components of the Rehabilitation Program
A. Similar to those for adults.
B. Includes injured area, adjacent regions, and remote muscles and joints.
C. Anaerobic power.
D. Aerobic endurance.

E. Realistically, only the most motivated or elite young athletes pursue a rehabilitation program to endpoint of full return of all the above.
F. Special considerations for children.
    1. Flexibility and strengthening.
    2. Muscles may be relatively short compared with the bones.
    3. Have little concept of nonballistic methods for stretching.
    4. Exercise programs should be supervised carefully.
    5. Machines must be adjusted carefully to fit child's frame; child must be instructed appropriately and supervised.
G. Modalities.
    1. Ice, compression, elevation.
    2. Ultrasound therapy and phonopheresis: some evidence suggests need for caution when using therapeutic ultrasound near open growth plates.
    3. Electrical stimulation for controlling muscle spasms and for controlling pain, especially in ankle or knee.
H. Medications.
    1. *Acute injury:* pain management may include low dose of narcotic, but usually nonsteroidal antiinflammatory drugs (NSAIDs) are appropriate; probable NSAID effect of slightly speeding soft tissue healing in addition to pain relief.
    2. *Overuse injury:* with significant pain or swelling, may need antiinflammatory medication to control symptoms sufficiently to allow rehabilitation.
    3. Sometimes difficult to convince adolescent to take NSAID on a regular basis.
    4. *Milder overuse injury:* use medication only when in a situation with no risk of further injury to the structure that is being rehabilitated.
    5. If pain is masked before an activity, the healing process may be disrupted or a different injury may result.
    6. Elite athlete may choose to take risk but should be informed of risk.
I. Instructions regarding athletic activity during rehabilitation (see box below).
    1. *First rule:* amount of tissue healing that occurs over a 24-hour period must exceed the amount of tissue destruction that occurs during that period, so must be pain-free the following morning.

ATHLETE'S FOUR RULES FOR PLAYING WHILE INJURED

Pain may be present at the end of activity, but must be gone by the next morning, indicating that the amount of tissue injury is probably not exceeding tissue healing.

Limping, or favoring the injured limb, means it's too risky to participate in activities where you are not in control of the situation. If you continue in an activity where collision or slipping is likely—and the muscles about the knee are not firing in a normal, coordinated manner—then serious, permanent injury could occur.

Ability to complete the prescribed exercise program effectively, 6 days a week, is necessary. If you have so much discomfort following the sport activities that you cannot do the strengthening exercises properly, then you should either decrease the amount of sport activity or perform the strengthening exercises in the morning.

You should not use pain-masking drugs or ice application *before* sport activity, so that you can monitor your body's signals of pain.

2. *Second rule:* activities must be avoided if they cause pain that interferes with the patient's ability to do the therapeutic exercises correctly and efficiently.
3. *Third rule:* athlete cannot compete if the weakened region is likely to lead to further injury.
4. *Fourth rule:* cannot use modalities or medications that mask pain before "at risk" activity.

IV. Specific Example: Patellofemoral Pain Syndrome
   A. One of the most frequent sports injuries for children and adolescents.
   B. Primary or secondary to muscular imbalance from another injury.
   C. Type of Program.
      1. For mild to moderate pain, home program.
      2. For severe symptoms, must relieve inflammation and begin therapeutic exercise program slowly; may need NSAID, ice, patellar brace, McConnell taping.
      3. Program below has been effective in returning greater than 95% of my patients to their former activity levels without any surgery (including many initially diagnosed with mild or moderate lateral patellar compression syndrome); the only known failures all had recurrent dislocations of one or both patellae before starting this program.
   D. Defined rehabilitation period.
      1. For typical adolescent patellofemoral pain syndrome, takes 2 months to decrease pain by half.
      2. Additional 1 to 2 months to resolve entirely (patient usually quits program before then).
   E. Small number of exercises.
      1. Concentrate on strengthening quadriceps and stretching hamstrings and quadriceps; correct other flexibility deficits such as in calf muscles.
      2. Straight leg raise progressive resistance exercises, three sets each leg (Fig. 67-1), alternating right and left sides (even if symptoms are unilateral).
      3. Increase amount of exercise by increasing repetitions or by adding 1 lb of weight.
      4. May add terminal short arc knee extensions.
   F. Visible progress.
      1. Do exercises once daily, 6 days per week.
      2. Several times each week, should be able to increase either repetitions or weight; increase incrementally from 8 to 12 repetitions, then increase weight by 1 lb and decrease repetitions to 8 again.

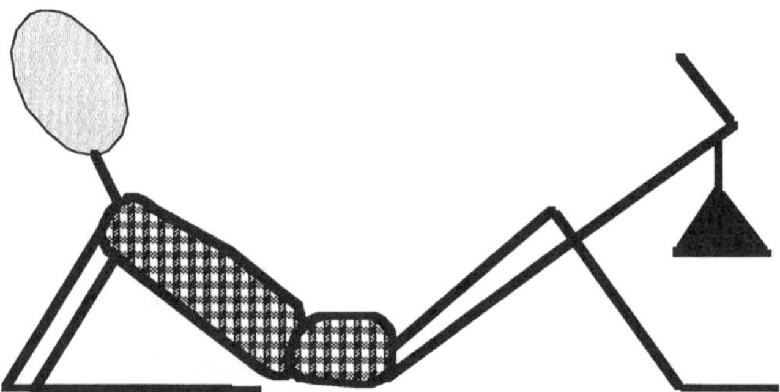

FIGURE 67-1
Straight leg raise strengthening exercise.

3. For 120-lb teenager, half of symptoms gone when able to complete straight leg raises with 12 lb of weight, entirely gone with about 20 lb.
4. Maintenance program three or four times per week, for 1 month.
5. Next 2 months, test strength with maintenance weight weekly.
6. Finally, check for maintenance of strength gains monthly for a final 6 months.

G. Interesting and entertaining therapeutic exercise programs and integration into the daily schedule.
1. Explain etiologic factors. Usually succeed in boring patient with this, but it helps parent understand need for compliance with program.
2. Then ask, "do you ever watch TV or talk on the phone?" Usually get laughter or smiling nods from parent and patient; now that patient's attention is regained, teach principles of exercise program.
3. Use weights. Most respond more positively (in compliance) and more rapidly, as compared to using elastic bands or needing to leave home to use machines.
4. Many centers utilize elastic bands as resistance for quadriceps strengthening.
5. Incentives: complete exercises during the first 15 minutes of a television show, get to watch the rest of the show.

Bibliography

Cahill BR, Griffith EH: Effect of preseason conditioning on the incidence and severity of high school football knee injuries, *Am J Sports Med* 6:180-183, 1978.

Danish S: Psychological aspects in the care and treatment of athletic injuries. In Vinger PE, Hoerner E (eds): *Sports Injuries—The Unthwarted Epidemic,* ed 2, Littleton, MA, 1984, PSG Publishing.

Gann N: Ultrasound: current concepts, *Clin Management* 11(4):64-69, 1996.

Heil J: *Psychology of sport injury,* Champaign, IL, 1993, Human Kinetics Publishers.

Kibler WB, Chandler TJ, Stracener ES: Musculoskeletal adaptations and injuries due to overtraining, *Exerc Sports Sci Rev* 20:99-126, 1992.

Lysens RJ et al: The accident-prone and overuse-prone profiles of the young athlete, *Am J Sports Med* 17:612-619, 1989.

Murphy S: Behavioral considerations. In Canten RC, Micheli LJ (eds): *ACSM's guidelines for the team physician,* Philadelphia, 1991, Lea & Febiger.

Sewall I, Micheli LJ: Strength training for children, *J Pediatr Orthop* 6:143-146, 1986.

Smith AD: A four-year longitudinal study of injuries of elite figure skaters, *Med Sci Sports Exerc* 23:S151, 1991.

Smith AD: Rehabilitation of children's sports injuries. In Bar-Or O, editor: *International Olympic Committee Encyclopedia of Sports Medicine: The Child Athlete,* London, Blackwell, 1996.

Smith AD, Stroud L, McQueen C: Flexibility and anterior knee pain in adolescent elite figure skaters, *J Pediatr Orthop* 11:77-82, 1991.

Smith AM et al: Emotional responses of athletes to injury, *Mayo Clin Proc* 65:38-50, 1990.

CHAPTER **68**

Strength Training for Children and Adolescents

Sally S. Harris, MD, MPH

I. Introduction
   A. Strength training is an increasingly popular activity for children and particularly adolescents, both as an independent recreational or fitness activity and as a conditioning activity in association with other sports.
   B. This chapter address the benefits and risks of strength training and what kinds of strength training activities are appropriate for this age group.
II. Definitions
   A. Strength training (resistance training).
      1. Strength training is the use of a variety of training methods to improve muscle strength, endurance, and/or power for sports participation or fitness enhancement.
      2. Strength training methods include exercises such as push-ups and pull-ups, which use body weight as the resistive load, exercises that use spring or rubber tubing to provide resistance, weight training using free weights or weight machines to provide resistance, isometric training against immovable resistance, and training with various devices (isokinetic, pneumatic, and hydraulic machines) that provide accommodating resistance.
   B. Weight lifting (Olympic lifting). Competition in:
      1. Clean and jerk.
      2. Snatch.
   C. Power lifting. Competition in:
      1. Squat.
      2. Dead lift.
      3. Bench press.
   D. Body building. Competition in muscle size, symmetry, and definition achieved through various resistance training methods.
III. Recommendations for Children and Adolescents
   A. Strength training is thought to be the safest and therefore most appro-

GUIDELINES: STRENGTH TRAINING FOR CHILDREN AND ADOLESCENTS

1. Preparticipation evaluation by physician knowledgeable in sports medicine.
2. Good quality equipment suitable to the size and age of the athletes.
3. Strength training should be part of an overall conditioning and fitness program.
4. Supervision by a well-trained adult.
5. Appropriate warm-up and cool-down period before and after strength training.
6. Selection of sports-specific exercises appropriate to the level of physical and emotional maturity of the participant.
7. Attention to proper technique: avoid Valsalva maneuver, hyperventilation, back hyperextension.
8. Emphasis on dynamic concentric contractions as opposed to eccentric overload exercises.
9. Emphasis on sets of high repetitions at low resistance.
10. Each exercise should be taken through the full range of motion for maximum muscle development and maintenance of flexibility.
11. Competition (weight lifting, power lifting, body building) should be prohibited.
12. Maximal lifts should not be performed until skeletal maturity (Tanner stage 5).
13. Program design should be based on the principle of progressive resistance.

priate of the above activities for children and adolescents because it involves training methods utilizing several sets of multiple repetitions of submaximal resistance.

B. Weight lifting, power lifting, and body building, which typically involve lifts with maximal amounts of weight and/or ballistic maneuvers, are not recommended for children prior to skeletal maturity (Tanner stage 5) due to potential for injury associated with extremely high loads or physical stress on the immature skeleton.

IV. Development of Muscle Strength During Childhood

A. Physiology of strength development.
  1. Muscle strength is closely related to the number and cross-sectional area of the contracting muscle fibers.
  2. Muscle fiber number is fixed shortly after birth.
  3. Muscle growth is accompanied by increased fiber diameter (hypertrophy).
  4. Strength improves linearly with growth during childhood.

B. Gender differences.
  1. Prior to puberty girls and boys have similar strength (boys are slightly stronger by 1-2 kg).
  2. Boys show marked acceleration in development to strength at puberty (due to dramatic increase in muscle mass), peaking at ages 20-30.
  3. Girls do not show appreciable increases in strength at puberty (due to the fact that most of the increase in body mass is a result of increase in body fat rather than muscle mass).
  4. In boys peak isometric strength occurs 6-12 months after peak height velocity (PHV), while in girls peak strength occurs at the same time as PHV.
  5. Girls may be temporarily somewhat stronger than boys 1-2 years during early puberty due to:
     a. Initiation of their growth spurt 1-2 years sooner than boys.
     b. Earlier relationship of peak strength to PHV.

V. Efficacy of Strength Training
   A. Both boys and girls demonstrate significant gains in strength after an appropriate program of resistance training. As for adults, strength increases depend on providing an adequate training stimulus in terms of the intensity, volume, and duration of the training program.
   B. Prepubescent children make similar relative strength gains compared to later stages of pubertal development and adulthood but demonstrate smaller absolute strength increases.
   C. It is unknown whether a critical stage of development exists during which the response to strength training is greatest.

VI. Mechanisms of Strength Gains
   A. Lack of changes in muscle size. Strength training prior to adolescence has little if any effect on muscle size (hypertrophy); training-induced strength gains are largely independent of changes in muscle size.
   B. Neurological adaptations are important for strength gains.
      1. Increased neural drive (increased % motor unit activation, increased integrated electromyographic activity).
      2. Changes in intrinsic contractile muscle function (increased twitch torque).
      3. Improved motor skill coordination.

VII. Musculoskeletal Injury Patterns
   A. National Electronic Injury Surveillance Survey.
      1. Statistics: weight-training injuries requiring emergency treatment for all ages.
         a. 19% of weight-training injuries occurred in children aged 0-14.
         b. 49% occurred in children aged 15-24.
         c. 39% occurred in the home setting.
      2. Most common type of injury (by prevalence).
         a. Sprains/strains.
         b. Contusions/abrasions.
         c. Lacerations.
         d. Fractures.
      3. Most common site of injury (by prevalence).
         a. Lower trunk.
         b. Finger.
         c. Toe.
         d. Foot.
   B. There is no evidence that strength training during childhood places an individual at greater risk for musculoskeletal injury than participation in other sports and recreational activities.
   C. There is no evidence that prepubertal children are more prone to strength training–related injury than older children or adults.
   D. There is no evidence of subclinical injury based on markers of repetitive stress to bone (bone scan), collagen (urinary hydroxyproline), cartilage (keratin sulfate), or muscle (creatinine phosphokinase).

VIII. Epiphyseal Injury
   A. There are numerous case reports of epiphyseal fracture due to weight training in children.
   B. The majority of these injuries occurred in pubescents and adolescents (none less than age 12).
   C. The majority of these injuries appear preventable by avoiding improper technique, excessive loading, ballistic movements, and lack of supervision.

SAMPLE PROGRAM PRESCRIPTION

One to three sets of 6-10 exercises per session
Frequency of two to three sessions per week with rest day in between
Duration of 20-60 minutes per session
Progressive resistance:
  Start at no resistance/weights until proper form is achieved.
  Then initiate resistance at the 6 repetition level; advance to 15 repetitions.
  Weight then added in increments of 1-3 lb until child can do just 6 repetitions.
  Advance again to 15 repetitions before increasing weights.

D. There are no reports of epiphyseal injury in supervised prospective strength training studies. Epiphyseal fracture is a relatively rare occurrence in sports in general and is associated with low risk of long-term consequences when treated properly.

IX. Injury Prevention
  A. Two studies in adolescents show decreased number and severity of injuries and shorter rehabilitation time following injury in adolescent high school athletes as a result of strength training.
  B. No studies in prepubescents.

X. Flexibility
  A. Prospective studies show that strength training programs have no detrimental effect on flexibility.
  B. If stretching exercises are included, these programs can result in moderate improvements in flexibility.

XI. Effects of Strength Training on Performance
  A. Motor fitness tests.
    1. Strength training appears to improve performance on selected motor fitness tests (vertical jump, standing long jump).
    2. Knee extension program improved vertical jump performance (12%) but not as much as training for the vertical jump per se (19%).
    3. Correlation with improvements on motor fitness tests with sports performance is unclear.
  B. Sports performance.
    1. Sports with a substantial strength and power component theoretically might be improved.
    2. One study in swimmers showed improved 100-yard swim times after strength training; however, another study showed no change.
    3. There is no compelling evidence that sports performance is enhanced; however, few studies have addressed this question.

Bibliography

American Academy of Pediatrics: Strength training, weight and power lifting, and body building by children and adolescents, *Pediatrics* 86:801-803, 1990.

Blimkie CJR: Resistance training during preadolescence: issues and controversies, *Sports Med* 15(6):389-407, 1993.

Blimkie CJR: Benefits and risks of resistance training in children. In Cahill BR, Pearl AJ, editors: *Intensive Participation in Children's Sports,* Champaign, Il, 1993, Human Kinetics Publishers.

Cahill BR, editor: *Proceedings of the Conference on Strength in the Prepubescent,* Chicago, 1988, American Orthopedic Society for Sports Medicine.

How to Build a Strength and Conditioning Program in Your High School, Lincoln, NE, 1986, National Strength and Conditioning Association.

Mazur LJ, Yetman RJ, Risser WL: Weight-training injuries: common injuries and preventative methods, *Sports Med* 16(1):57-63, 1993.

National Injury Clearinghouse: 1987 data summary on injuries caused by weight lifting. Washington, DC, National Electronic Injury Surveillance System, US Consumer Product Safety Commission.

Rowland TW: Muscle strength and endurance. In Rowland TW, editor: *Exercise and Children's Health,* Champaign, Il, 1990, Human Kinetics Publishers.

CHAPTER 69

Fracture Diagnosis and Management of Common Injuries

Michael E. Robinson, MD

I. Introduction
  A. The primary care practitioner treating active individuals or serving as team physician should have a basic knowledge of fracture diagnosis and management.
  B. Many fractures (including the closed reduction of some fractures) can be successfully managed by the primary physician, although individual practice may vary depending on level of training and experience.
  C. Other factors influencing the decision to manage fractures include the availability of casting materials and radiography equipment as well as medicolegal concerns.
  D. A good working relationship with an orthopedic consultant should be developed.
  E. Exhaustive textbooks of fracture management have been published. This chapter addresses a limited number of common injuries.

II. Field Management
  A. Consider diagnosis of fracture after any musculoskeletal trauma, especially when the patient has local deformity, edema, ecchymosis, or pain.
  B. Splint possible fractures in the field to facilitate transporting the patient, obtaining radiographs, and relieving the patient's pain.
  C. Traditional splinting of the injury where it lies is an acceptable method of treatment. Some authors believe that gentle longitudinal traction improves outcome and has little risk of further soft tissue damage.
  D. Keep brace supplies on hand.
    1. Formal: rigid or air splints.
    2. Improvised: wood slats, moldable aluminum, foam padding.

III. Fracture Nomenclature
  A. Goal: Learn to accurately describe a fracture.
  B. Fracture pattern (Fig. 69-1): transverse, oblique, spiral, comminuted.
  C. Fracture site (Fig. 69-2).

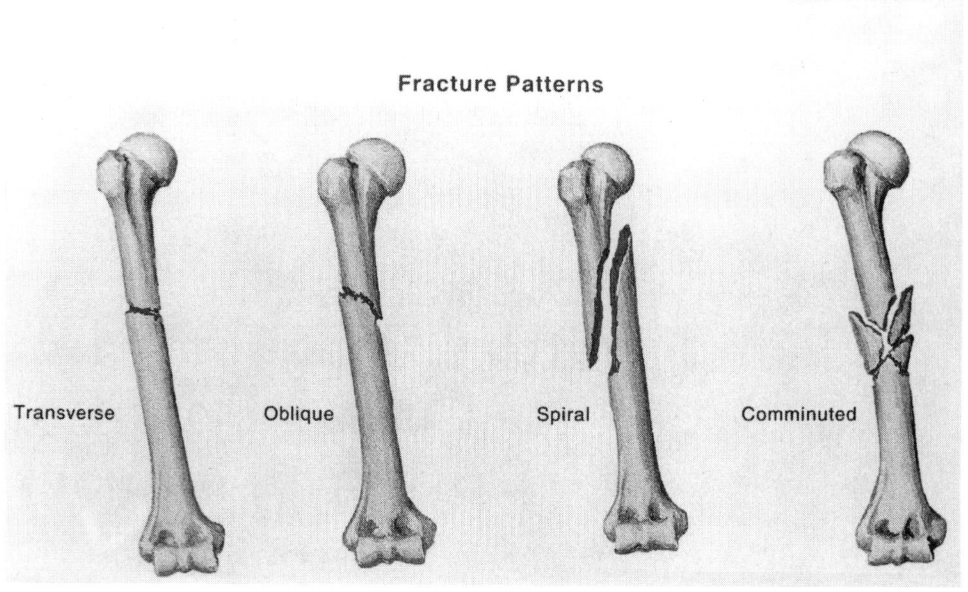

FIGURE 69-1
Fracture patterns. (Reproduced by permission of the author and publisher from Heckman JD: Fractures: emergency care and complications, *Clin Symp* 43(3):7, 1991.)

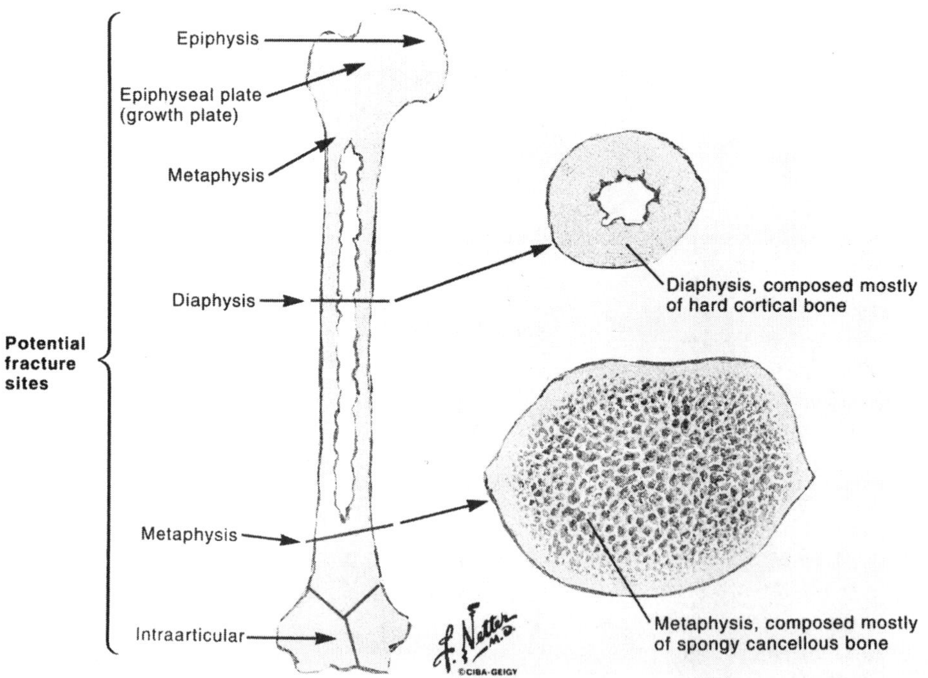

FIGURE 69-2
Characteristics of long bone at various fracture sites. (Reproduced by permission of the author and publisher from Heckman JD: Fractures: emergency care and complications, *Clin Symp* 43(3):4, 1991.)

1. Diaphyseal: cortical bone. Small cross-sectional area may decrease fracture stability.
2. Metaphyseal: cancellous bone. Larger contact area exists.
3. Epiphyseal: extends to articular surface.

D. Angulation: defined as direction of the apex of the angle that the fracture creates (Fig. 69-3).

E. Displacement: location of distal fragment in relation to proximal fragment.

F. Rotation: position of distal fragment in relation to anatomical position (external or internal).

G. Compression fracture: loss of volume, height, or both, usually in region of cancellous bone.

H. Avulsion fractures: occur at the sites of ligament and tendon insertion on bone.

I. Open or closed fractures: skin over fracture site may be either broken or unbroken.

IV. Pediatric Fracture Principles

A. Understand epiphyseal plate fracture classification of Salter (Fig. 69-4).

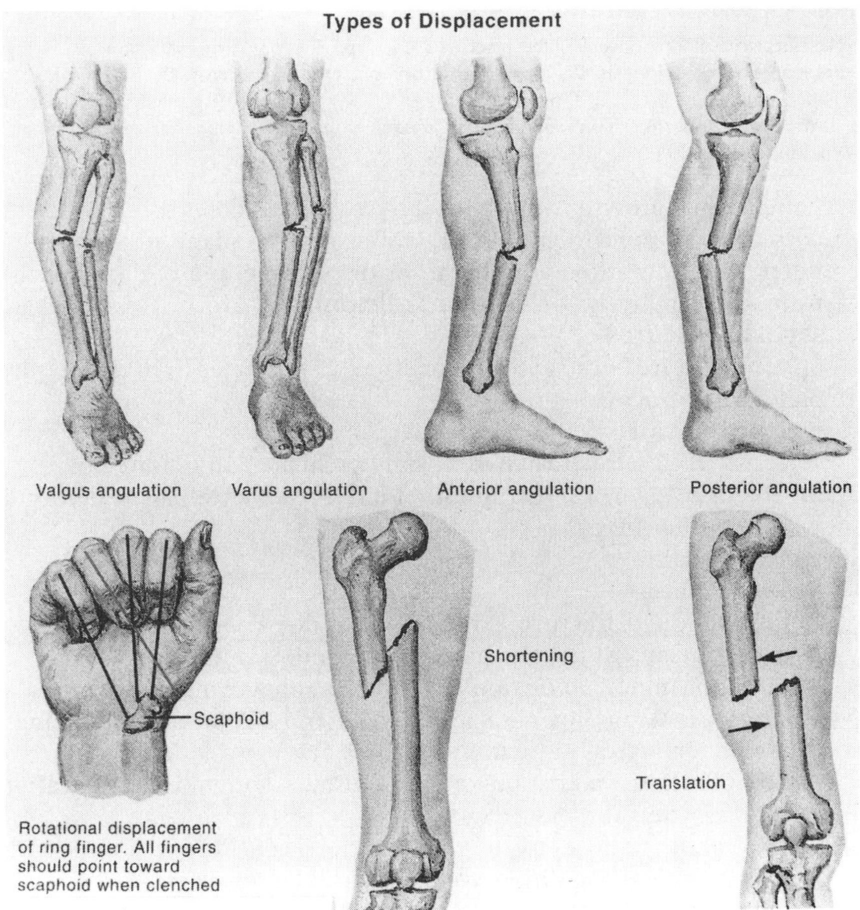

FIGURE 69-3
Types of displacement. (Reproduced by permission of the author and publisher from Heckman JD: Fractures: emergency care and complications, *Clin Symp* 43(3):5, 1991.)

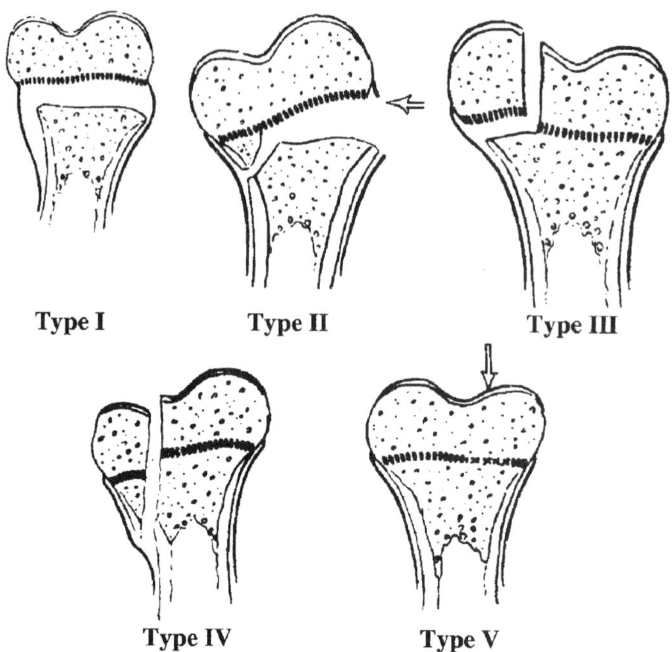

FIGURE 69-4
Salter classification of epiphyseal plate fractures. **A,** Type I: separation of epiphysis. **B,** Type II: fracture-separation of epiphysis. **C,** Type III: fracture of part of epiphysis. **D,** Type IV: fracture of epiphysis and epiphyseal plate. **E,** Type V: crushing of epiphyseal plate. (Reproduced by permission of the author and publisher from Gartland JJ: *Fundamentals of Orthopaedics,* ed 3, Philadelphia, 1987, WB Saunders, p. 90.)

B. Longitudinal growth from the epiphyseal plate allows some spontaneous correction of mild fracture angulation in same plane of motion as the nearest joint. Marked angulation or displacement, angulation removed from the epiphysis, or rotational deformities are not acceptable and should be reduced.
C. Sprains are rare because ligament strength is greater than the epiphyseal plate (think fracture).
D. Fracture patterns.
   1. Torus: buckle fracture in metadiaphyseal portion of long bone.
   2. Greenstick: cortical disruption of one cortex with plastic deformation of opposite cortex.

V. Specific Fractures
   A. Mallet fracture.
      1. Description: a fracture extending into dorsal articular surface of the distal phalanx at the site of extensor tendon insertion.
      2. Mechanism: forced flexion of distal interphalangeal (DIP) joint.
      3. Diagnosis: drop finger—inability to extend DIP joint. Assess congruity of joint on lateral radiograph (Fig. 69-5).
      4. Complication: volar subluxation of distal fragment is an indication for surgical referral.
      5. Treatment (same as for tendon injuries): continuous splinting of DIP joint in extension for 6 weeks. Dorsal or volar padded aluminum splint, Stax™ (Stax Link™ America, New Jersey) splint.
   B. Middle phalanx fracture.
      1. Description: jammed finger—fracture involving the volar articular base of the middle phalanx at attachment of volar plate. Usually stable if less than 30% to 40% of joint surface is affected.

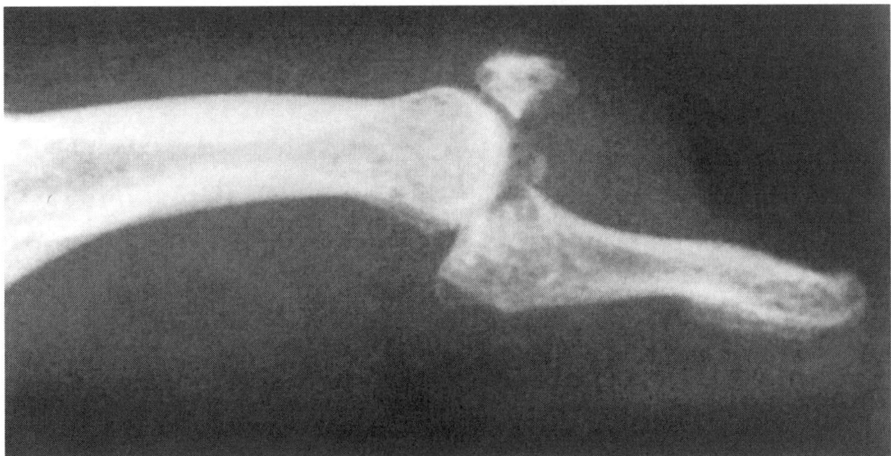

FIGURE 69-5
Mallet finger of bony origin with volar subluxation of the distal phalanx. (Reproduced by permission of the author, editor, and publisher from Rockwood CA Jr, Green DP, Bucholz RW, editors: *Rockwood and Green's Fractures in Adults,* ed 3, Philadelphia, 1991, JB Lippincott, p. 452.)

2. Mechanism: direct axial load, also after dorsal dislocation of proximal interphalangeal (PIP) joint.
3. Diagnosis: local edema and pain at PIP joint but able to demonstrate intact tendon function. Confirm by radiography.
4. Complications: the stability of any phalangeal fracture must be assessed. Treatment is influenced by possibility of displacement or rotation.
5. Treatment.
   a. Mild injury: buddy tape fractured finger to adjoining fingers for 2 to 4 weeks, and start early range-of-motion exercises.
   b. Formal: dorsal padded aluminum extension block splint with PIP in 30 degrees of flexion for 2 weeks, then buddy tape and initiate range-of-motion exercises.

C. Metacarpal neck fractures.
   1. Description: fracture at level of the metacarpal neck. Boxer's fracture of the fifth metacarpal neck. Metacarpal bone is usually impacted and has dorsal angulation. This fracture is inherently unstable; however, good functional results can be expected with up to 40 degrees of angulation in fifth and 20 degrees in fourth metacarpal bone due to carpal-metacarpal flexibility. Little angulation is acceptable in second and third metacarpal bones.
   2. Mechanism: direct impact on metacarpal head while hand is in clenched fist position.
   3. Diagnosis: local pain, edema, deformity. Assess angulation on lateral radiography. Check finger rotation.
   4. Complications: excessive palmar tilt of metacarpal head may result in tendon imbalance and claw deformity. Cosmetic loss of knuckle is a common feature.
   5. Treatment: gutter splint or short arm spica cast with metacarpophalangeal joint flexed 60 degrees for 2 to 4 weeks, then initiate range-of-motion and grip-strengthening exercises. If reduction is done, a well-molded cast is important to maintain position and should be left on for 4 weeks.

D. Scaphoid fractures.
   1. Description: common fracture at wrist and a commonly missed diagnosis.

2. Mechanism: dorsiflexion load on wrist—fall on palm.
3. Diagnosis: typical history. High index of suspicion. Pain over scaphoid bone on floor of anatomical snuffbox. Initial radiographs may not show fracture.
4. Complications: nonunion in 5% to 10% of fractures. Scapholunate dissociation (ligamentous disruption). Normal scapholunate angle = 45 to 60 ±15 degrees.
5. Treatment.
   a. Equivocal fracture: apply short arm thumb spica cast for 2 weeks, then do a second examination and obtain radiographs.
   b. Nondisplaced fracture: apply long arm thumb spica cast for 6 weeks, then apply a short arm spica cast until clinical and radiographic healing has occurred. Average healing time is 12 weeks.

E. Distal radius fracture
1. Description: many eponyms and classification schemes exist. Colles' fracture of the distal metaphysis of the radius within 2 cm of articular surface, which is often dorsally displaced and angulated. The fracture may extend into the joint.
2. Anatomy: recognize normal radiocarpal joint alignment (Fig. 69-6).
3. Mechanism: fall onto outstretched hand.
4. Diagnosis: local pain, edema. Fracture identified on radiographs.
5. Complications: alteration of the normal radiocarpal alignment through intraarticular extension, angulation, or displacement of fracture fragments can lead to functional impairment and degenerative changes.
6. Treatment: for stable, undisplaced extraarticular fractures (and nonangulated greenstick fractures in children) use a short arm cast for 6 weeks. Consider applying a removable splint during the last 2 weeks for early range-of-motion exercise and rehabilitation in reliable patients. Torus fracture requires 4 weeks to heal. Marked alteration of normal wrist alignment is not acceptable, and anatomical reduction should be carried out through appropriate closed (or open) methods.

F. Radial head fractures.
1. Description: nondisplaced or minimally displaced fractures involving <30% of the surface of the radial head with little or no separation or impaction. Nondisplaced neck fractures.
2. Mechanism: fall onto outstretched hand with axial loading of elbow.
3. Diagnosis: elbow effusion; pain over radial head and with forearm rotation; no mechanical block to elbow motion. If equivocal, aspirate joint and instill local anesthesia for a second examination. Assess elbow stability (collateral ligaments). Palpate interosseous membrane and distal radioulnar joint to rule out radial-ulnar dissociation.
4. Radiographic appearance: typical wedge-shaped pattern (Fig. 69-7) or transverse neck. Occasionally, no definite fracture but increase in fat pad/joint effusion.
5. Complications: displaced fractures or those with mechanical block to range of motion should be referred.
6. Treatment: sling and/or removable splint with early range-of-motion exercises for 2 weeks followed by protected return to functional activities.

G. Clavicle fractures.
1. Description: about 80% occur in middle third of clavicle bone.
2. Mechanism: fall onto outstretched hand or lateral shoulder.
3. Diagnosis: clinical deformity, pain, or edema over midclavicle bone. Bone crepitus and motion. Check skin for tenting. Obtain anteroposterior and 45-degree cephalic tilt radiographs.

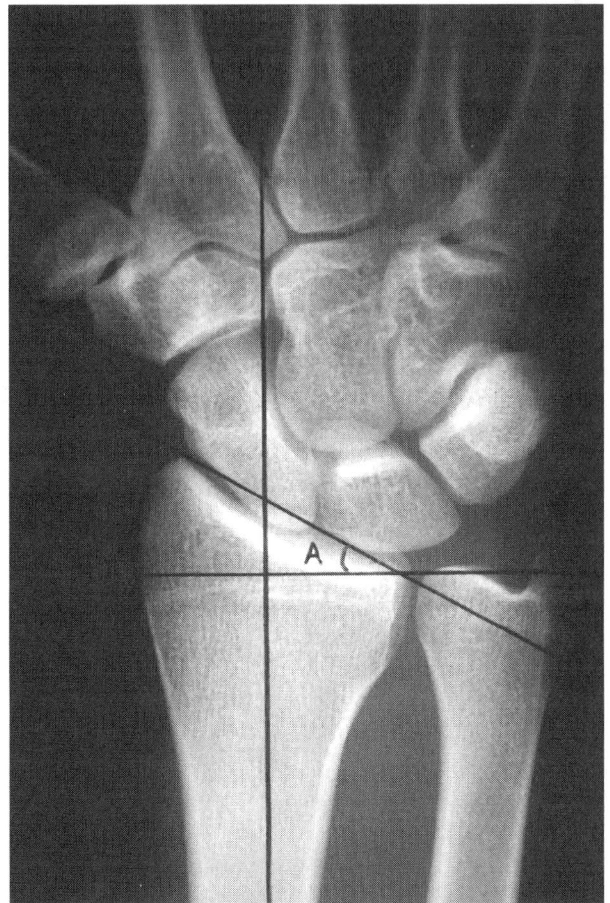

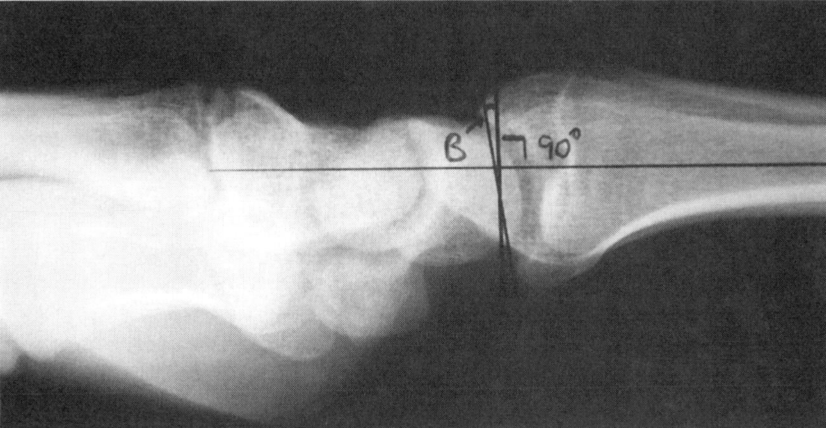

FIGURE 69-6
On anteroposterior radiography, normal radial inclination at the wrist (angle A) is 22-24 degrees. On lateral radiography, volar inclination (angle B) is 10-12 degrees.

4. Complications: markedly displaced fractures and fractures of proximal and distal thirds of clavicle warrant consultation and may have higher nonunion rates.
5. Treatment: use an arm sling and swathe, or apply a figure-8 bandage until pain subsides (usually 4 weeks in adults). Initiate mobilization exercises as pain allows. Clinical and radiographic healing typically occurs in 8 weeks.

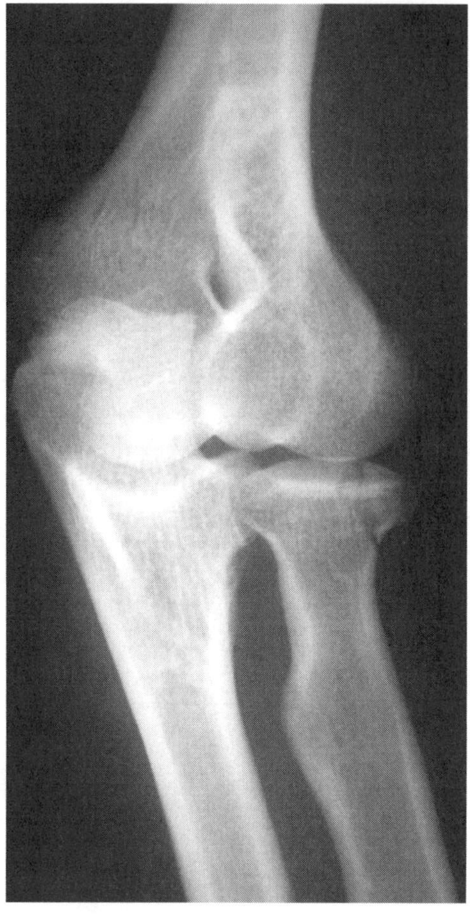

FIGURE 69-7
Nondisplaced radial head fracture affecting 25% of joint surface.

Acknowledgment

The Medical Editing Department, Kaiser Foundation Research Institute, provided editorial assistance.

Bibliography

Browner BD et al, editors: *Skeletal Trauma: Fractures, Dislocations, Ligamentous Injuries,* Philadelphia, 1992, WB Saunders.

DeLee JC, Drez D Jr, editors: *Orthopaedic Sports Medicine: Principles and Practice,* Philadelphia, 1994, WB Saunders.

Gartland JJ: *Fundamentals of Orthopaedics,* ed 3, Philadelphia, 1987, WB Saunders.

Heckman JD: Fractures: emergency care and complications, *Clin Symp* 43(3):2-32, 1991.

Medley ES, Shirley SM, Brilliant HL: Fracture management by family physicians and guidelines for referral, *J Family Pract* 8:701-710, 1979.

Rockwood CA Jr, Green DP, Bucholz RW, editors: *Rockwood and Green's Fractures in Adults,* ed 3, Philadelphia, 1991, JB Lippincott.

Wiesel SW, Delahay JN, Connell MC: *Essentials of Orthopaedic Surgery,* Philadelphia, 1993, WB Saunders.

CHAPTER **70**

Overuse Injuries

Warren A. Scott, MD

I. Introduction to Overuse Injuries
   A. Progressive overload training is sought by athletes to stimulate muscle growth, strength, speed, agility, flexibility, power, and accuracy.
   B. Athletes need to strike a balance in their training programs between stress overload and rest-recovery-adaptation. (See box on page 518.)
   C. Repetitive microtrauma that overwhelms the tissue's ability to repair itself will produce an overuse injury.
   D. Injury severity can progress from microdamage (pain) to macrodamage (swelling, redness, warmth). (See Table 70-1.)
   E. High velocity cyclic overloading can produce an "overuse" injury in seconds. An example would be a 100-m runner, who sprints for 8 seconds and then suffers a hamstring muscle pull. (See Tables 70-2 and 70-3.)
   F. Low velocity cyclic overloading, combined with increasing training volumes, can lead to an overuse injury after weeks or months of continuous overload. An example would be a marathon runner with a 2-year history of progressively worsening Achilles' tendinitis. (See Tables 70-2 and 70-3.)

II. Tissue Response to Injury (see Table 70-4)
   A. There is a continuous progression from microtrauma (pain) to macrotrauma (pain, swelling, warmth, redness) and decreased function.
   B. This is mirrored and influenced by the inflammatory response.
      1. Cell mobilization (1-2 weeks).
      2. Ground substance proliferation (2-4 weeks).
      3. Collagen protein formation (1-2 months).
      4. Final organization (2-12 months).
   C. Time frame for full healing can extend from 1-18 months.
   D. Tissue types vary in their response to overload stress. Injuries vary according to how much macrotrauma has developed over time and how much scar tissue is present. ***Think of the muscle-tendon-bone unit.***
      1. Different stress patterns will produce different injuries.

SIGNS OF OVERTRAINING

- Increase in morning resting heart rate (approximately 10 beats)
- Positive orthostatic pulse test (approximately 10 beats)
- Poor sleep
- Inadequate caloric intake, with subsequent weight loss
- Increased thirst
- Increased work effort during submaximal testing
- Muscle soreness
- Mood swings (decreased libido, decreased vigor, increased fatigue, depression, anger)
- "Heavy legs," susceptible to injuries
- Depressed immune function
- Loss of menstruation (amenorrhea) in females

2. A good example is medial tibial stress syndrome. The mechanism of injury is torsion and compression. The exact site of tissue damage can vary between tendinitis, periostitis, and tibial stress fracture. The pattern of injury can vary among different athletes.

III. Approach to the Patient

A. Introduction

1. Strive to establish a positive relationship. Many athletes experience depression, anger, fear, and relief when they become injured. Encourage their active participation in the rehabilitation process. Engage patient in goals they can quickly accomplish. The treatment programs for chronic severe overuse injuries can require up to 18 months to complete. Time until recovery should be clearly established so the athlete can develop realistic expectations.
2. Determine their interests and goals concerning sports play.
3. Determine their motivation and commitment to the rehabilitation process.
4. Take a leadership role, and organize and coordinate the care of your patient. Depending on circumstances the rehabilitation team may include the physician, patient, parent, coach, physical therapist, and athletic trainer. Strive to customize the rehabilitation program so as to maximize compliance/completion.

TABLE 70-1. Functional rating of injury severity

Level	Healing Time	Description of Pain and Activity Level
Grade I	2-4 weeks	Injury produces discomfort during play. Onset usually with hard exertion. Pain relief at cessation of play. Activities of daily living are not affected. Competitive level unaffected.
Grade II	1-3 months	Increasingly painful during sport, decreased ability to play competitively. Activities of daily living can produce pain.
Grade III	3-6 months	Cannot compete in sports. Activities of daily living are compromised.
Grade IV	9-18 months	Activities of daily living are significantly compromised. Major injury. Significant macrodamage. Cannot play sports; out for season.

TABLE 70-2. Common overuse injuries by sport

Sport	Injury
Running	Patellar tendinitis, iliotibial band tendinitis, chondromalacia patellae, metatarsal stress fractures, medial tibial stress syndrome, Achilles' tendinitis, plantar fasciitis
Swimming	Breast stroker's knee (medial collateral ligament sprain and/or medial patellar shelf synovitis, long head biceps brachii tendinitis, supraspinatus tendinitis, subacromial bursitis
Dancing	Lumbosacral strains, Achilles' tendinitis, plantar fasciitis, metatarsalgia, stress fractures of tibia, fibula, or metatarsals, pars interarticularis, medial tibial stress syndrome, patellofemoral syndromes
Weight lifting	Nontraumatic acromioclavicular joint osteolysis, carpal tunnel syndrome, supraspinatus and long head biceps brachii tendinitis
Tennis, baseball, volleyball, javelin	Subacromial bursitis, supraspinatus and biceps brachii tendinitis
Gymnastics	Medial tibial stress syndrome, radiocarpal joint stress reaction, stress fractures of lumbar spine, tibia, fibula, or metatarsals
Basketball/Volleyball	Achilles' tendinitis, patellar tendinitis, stress fractures of metatarsals, distal tibia, or fibula

TABLE 70-3. Common overuse injuries grouped by injury site

Site	Injury
Knee	Medial shelf plica, patellar and iliotibial band tendinitis, biceps femoris tendinitis, chondromalacia patellae, pes anserinus and prepatellar bursitis
Foot	Plantar fasciitis, metatarsalgia, interdigital neuroma, metatarsal stress fractures, sesamoiditis
Shoulder	Biceps and supraspinatus tendinitis, subacromial and subscapular bursitis, acromioclavicular osteolysis
Elbow	Medial and lateral epicondylitis
Wrist/Hand	Thumb extensor tenosynovitis, finger flexor tendon ganglion cysts, dorsal wrist ganglion cysts
Hip/Gluteal	Piriformis tendinitis, gluteus tendinitis, ischiogluteal bursitis, greater trochanteric bursitis, iliotibial band tendinitis (at hip), proximal hamstring tendinitis
Lower leg	Exertional compartment syndrome, medial tibial stress syndrome, stress fracture of distal tibia-fibula
Ankle	Achilles' tendinitis, pre- and post-Achilles' bursitis, dorsolateral ankle ganglion cysts, posterior tibial tendinitis
Lumbar spine	Pars interarticularis stress fracture, extension-facet overload, erector spinae and quadratus lumbar muscle spasms
Cervical-thoracic spine	Trapezius muscle spasms

TABLE 70-4. Common overuse injuries by tissue type

Tissue Type	Injury
Tendon	
• Bone-tendon interface	Medial and lateral epicondylitis, Achilles' tendon, patellar tendon
• Midtendon	Achilles' tendon, supraspinatus, biceps brachii
• Muscle-tendon junction	Achilles' tendon, medial and lateral epicondylitis
Muscle	Delayed onset muscle soreness, acute overuse muscle injury ("muscle pull"; medial head gastrocnemius, long head biceps brachii, hamstring complex)
Bone	Adolescent apophyseal injuries, osteochondritis dissecans, stress reaction—fracture (compression [tarsal navicular], traction [humerus], periostitis [medial tibial stress syndrome])
Nerve	Compressive (metatarsal interdigital, suprascapular, ulnar, median, radial, digital) Taction (ulnar, peroneal nerve, posterior tibial, axillary)
Cartilage	Chondromalacia (grade I through IV)
Bursae/Ganglion	Cysts (pre- and post-Achilles, olecranon, prepatellar, iliopectineal, ischiogluteal, dorsal lateral ankle, dorsal wrist, finger flexor tendons)
Miscellaneous types	Compartment syndromes (forearm, lower leg), plantar fasciitis

5. The main reasons athletes drop out of a rehabilitation program include:
   a. Inconvenient setting.
   b. Inaccessible.
   c. Lack of time.
   d. Work/school conflict.
   e. Poor spousal-family support.

IV. Approach to the Injured Athlete
   A. A careful, thorough history can usually reveal the diagnosis.
   B. Athletes usually have a good reason why they are injured.
   C. Common periods of injury vulnerability include:
      1. Adding training volume.
      2. Adding training intensity.
      3. New movement pattern (skill).
      4. Return from absence (seasonal, illness, injury).
   D. Find out what they were doing and what changes they made.
      1. Training progressions produce injuries according to their intensity and duration. "Too much, too hard, too soon, too frequent" translates into:
         a. A training increase of 10% per week will begin to produce tissue overload and injury in approximately 6-8 weeks.
         b. A training increase of 50% per week will produce injuries in 2-3 weeks.
         c. A training increase of 100% per week will produce injuries in 1 week.

d. A training increase of greater than 100% will produce an injury in several days.
2. New skills: Check with athlete; have him or her obtain information from coach. Question about road surfaces (hills, slanted/uneven, asphalt trails, concrete).
3. Equipment variables: new shoes, tennis racquets, weight machines, bikes, golf clubs. Forcing a rapid adaptation to new equipment can produce an injury.
4. Attempt to learn the exact mechanism of injury.

E. The physical examination in overuse injury cases.
1. Observe athlete doing sport, and look for possible linkage effects. For example, patellofemoral pain and medial tibial stress syndrome can be secondary to excessive foot pronation.
2. Watch patient perform sport and pinpoint exact moment when pain occurs.
3. Perform a vigorous examination. Most athletes will not experience much pain during a "low stress" physical examination.
4. Sometimes it is necessary to intentionally aggravate injury (temporarily) by having the patient perform sport until it produces pain. Immediately perform physical examination to uncover source of pain.
5. Check:
   a. Leg length.
   b. Standing and lying.
   c. True bone length with radiographic measurements.
   d. Femoral neck angle.
   e. Knee alignment.
   f. Tibial alignment.
   g. Foot type (neutral, flat, cavus).
   h. Muscle size/strength imbalances.
   i. Muscle flexibility deficiencies.
   j. Muscle weakness.
6. Carefully observe injury site for inflammatory changes.
   a. Warmth, swelling, redness.
   b. Tender to touch, tender with passive and/or active movement.
   c. Palpate for scar tissue formation (especially in muscle-tendon injuries).
   d. Test injury with progressive loading. (Hop on one leg, deep squats, push-ups). Use this to assess reinjury vulnerability.

V. Phase I

A. Antiinflammatory phase
1. Basic first aid should be applied to all injuries. Grade I injuries (see Table 70-1) rarely require much except ice. Grade II-IV injuries can benefit from a variety of interventions. The goal of this phase is to arrest further tissue damage and promote healing.
2. Pain control.
   a. Ice is one of the best interventions that can be applied.
   b. Sequential icing technique is very effective.
      i. Cover skin with two layers of plastic wrap.
      ii. Apply a bag of crushed ice. (Gel packs, frozen vegetables are substitutes.)
      iii. Secure with an Ace wrap.
      iv. Massage and mold ice pack over injury site.
      v. Time: 20 minutes. Remove ice (refreeze). Let skin warm up for 10 minutes. Perform two more cycles of 20 minutes on, 10 minutes off.

vi. Repeat this entire sequence several times a day for several days.

c. Medications.

i. Nonsteroidal antiinflammatory drugs (NSAIDs) are frequently prescribed for overuse injuries. NSAIDs are most helpful during the initial treatment process. Encourage proper compliance with regular usage for several weeks to produce antiinflammatory changes (as opposed to analgesic effect). Avoid long-term use to minimize possible side effects. Some patients will need to try several different NSAIDs before finding one that is helpful and tolerable.

d. Other therapeutic modalities.

i. Helpful for pain control and decreasing inflammation.

ii. A variety of other therapeutic measures are available and can be applied by physical therapists and athletic trainers.

iii. Therapeutic ultrasound, transcutaneous nerve stimulation (TENS), and functional electrical stimulators are a few examples.

iv. The use of modalities is dependent on availability (cost) to athlete, accessibility to athlete, time commitment, and positive therapeutic response.

3. Protective bracing.
   a. Protective bracing should be applied to the injury site immediately to prevent further tissue damage.
   b. Allow the maximal joint movement that is below pain threshold.
   c. Sometimes it is necessary to begin with rigid splinting materials and progress to flexible/supportive braces as injury improves.
   d. A variety of splints can be made from fiberglass casting and other moldable thermoplastics.
   e. Additionally, many prefabricated, custom-designed, and injury-specific braces are available.
   f. See Table 70-5 for types of braces used in overuse injuries.
4. Review with athlete.
   a. Injuries can vary regarding the inflammatory response.
   b. If inflammation is minimal, proceed to phase II program.
   c. If tolerated, it is helpful to initiate stretching, strengthening, and cross-training at the beginning of the rehabilitation process. (See Phase II.)
   d. Review return to play criteria with athlete at the onset. This will provide the athlete with realistic expectations.

VI. Phase II

A. Once the inflammation is under control and the injured part adequately protected from further injury, we can focus on the rehabilitation process.

B. During phase II:

1. Keep up (or increase) cross-training program below soreness threshold.
2. Review return to play criteria.
3. Start a regular stretching program, making sure to work all muscle groups used in the athlete's primary sport.
4. If weakness or imbalances are detected at the injury site, begin a strengthening program.
5. Review REST concept (see below).
6. Use of corticosteroid and anesthetic injections.

TABLE 70-5. Braces for overuse injuries

Types	Injury	Materials
Counterforce	Long head biceps brachii, medial and lateral epicondylitis, thumb extensor tendinitis, patellar and Achilles' tendinitis, chondromalacia patella	Materials include fiberglass splints, canvas, moldable plastics, cloth tape
Supportive	Medial tibial stress syndrome, metatarsalgia, lumbar corsette, plantar fasciitis. Compression can vary with different materials.	Usually neoprene or elastic material sleeve-type brace, goes over joints or long bone. Felt pads. Ace wraps, Coban, flexible orthotics
Tension-producing night splint	Achilles' tendinitis, plantar fasciitis, gastrocnemius-soleus tendinitis/muscle strain, medial and lateral epicondylitis, hamstring strains and tendinitis	Made from fiberglass casting or moldable plastics
Rigid	Necessary for all injuries that are aggravated by activities of daily living and when all other types of braces are not satisfactory	Polypropylene orthotics, fiberglass casting materials, prefabricated joint-specific braces
Semirigid	Any injured joint	Prefabricated joint-specific braces. Plastic polymers and neoprene are common.

C. Corticosteroid injections.
   1. Very helpful in chronic problems with bursitis, tenosynovitis, tendinitis, periostitis, intraarticular synovitis.
   2. Typically inject 5-10 ml (one-third corticosteroid, two-thirds anesthetic).
   3. Experience with over 1000 injections is excellent using 0.5% bupivacaine and betamethasone.
   4. Bupivacaine provides 8-12 hours of anesthesia and can "break" a muscle spasm cycle.
   5. Betamethasone is very potent and long-acting ($t_{1/2}$ = 3 weeks).
   6. Avoid hard exercise for 2-3 weeks after an injection.
   7. Combine injection with stretching, cross-training, strengthening, and icing to achieve best results.

D. Trigger point injections.
   1. Muscle bellies can develop hard knots secondary to an overuse injury.
   2. Stretching, strengthening, massage, and ice are the best first aid measures for a muscle knot.
   3. Triggerpoint injections are easy, safe, and very effective.
   4. Palpate for sensitive trigger points in muscles.
   5. Using 27-gauge 1½-inch needle, inject 5-10 ml of 0.25% to 0.5% of

bupivacaine in a fan-like distribution. A 25-gauge 3½-inch spinal needle can be used for the large back and leg muscles.
6. Follow up injections with combined therapy measures listed above.
7. In the office setting, following an anesthetic block it is helpful to move the joints through a full range of motion.
8. The proprioceptive neuromuscular facilitation (PNF) technique "contract-relax" also works well in this setting.

E. REST = resume exercise below soreness threshold.
   1. Most overuse injuries are secondary to repetitive motion overload. The tissues cannot adapt quickly enough.
   2. The primary sport that caused the injury will need to be modified or temporarily stopped to prevent reinjury and overall worsening.
   3. Protective bracing (see Table 70-5) is very effective in allowing the athlete to continue play while the injury is healing.
   4. Modification of play should include:
      a. Reduced volume (25% to 50%).
      b. Reduced intensity (10% to 20%).
      c. Reduced frequency (25% to 50%).
      d. Reduce or eliminate painful maneuvers. (For example, a tennis player with supraspinatus tendinitis can usually perform the forehand and backhand but has pain during the service motion. Simply eliminating the offending forces [the serve] may be all that is necessary.)
      e. Try to keep some training in the primary sport as long as injury is not aggravated.
      f. Competitions are sometimes easier than training and may not aggravate the injury. (For example, a swimmer with biceps tendinitis incurred by swimming 8,000 m per day may be able to perform 100- and 200-m races relatively pain-free.)
   5. The ***R***esume ***E***xercise below ***S***oreness ***T***hreshold serves as a reminder to continue play in a reduced, *careful* fashion.
      a. Determine injury threshold prior to the institution of NSAIDs and corticosteroid injections.
      b. Both medications will provide a "false confidence" in measuring tolerable levels of exercise.
      c. Retest each week, and increase volume and intensity of exercise load, as tolerated.

F. Cross-training program.
   1. Usually injury is aggravated by the athlete's primary sport. Athletes need to find a substitute sport that uses the same muscle groups as their primary sport.
   2. For example, most athletes with knee and ankle injuries that occur from running/jumping sports can usually cross-train via:
      a. Pool running in deep water.
      b. Bicycle riding.
      c. Cross-country ski machine.
      d. Rowing machine.
      e. Stair climber.
      f. Weight training.
   3. Athletes should perform both aerobic and interval type training in the secondary sports. This will help preserve overall fitness.
      a. Be creative and try cross-training in several sports; see which one most closely resembles the primary sport and does not aggravate the injury.

   b. Studies have shown that a very high fitness level in the primary sport can be maintained by cross-training in alternative sports, lasting for several months.
   c. Cross-training also keeps volume of exercise per week at a constant, preventing weight gain.
4. Flexibility: stretching.
   a. Most injuries cause a component of muscle spasm. This can be as subtle as asymmetrical "tightness" or as severe as a maximal cramping muscle.
   b. Stretching exercises are essential in all phases of the rehabilitation process.
   c. Overuse injuries are commonly associated with loss of flexibility in the injured extremity.
   d. Maximal muscle power is proportional to the length of the muscle fibrils. Stretching exercises restore natural resting length of muscle-tendon unit.
   e. Stretching is best carried out when the body is warmed up.
   f. Any aerobic activity for 10-20 minutes will warm up the muscles and enhance flexibility.
   g. Teach athletes to feel the stretch in the muscle belly. This *should not* produce tension at the injury site. Modify the stretch to avoid aggravating the injury site.
   h. Hold stretching positions for up to 30 seconds. Add stretching tension to take up the slack as the muscle relaxes.
   i. Repeat stretch twice.
   j. Some athletes may want to stretch 5-10 times a day to prevent tightening of muscle-tendon unit.
   k. Stretching without a warm-up can be safe, given a gradual approach.
5. Strengthening.
   a. Usually injured area is inherently weaker.
   b. Weight training conducted in a progressive format can stimulate muscle growth and development.
   c. Weight training is very controlled and can be performed relatively early in the rehabilitation process.
   d. Resistance training can be carried out with weights, machines, resistance tubing (Thera-Band, "bungee cords," surgical tubing are all good substitutes).
      i. Closed chain kinetic exercises can be performed using body weight for resistance (push-ups, pull-ups, one-third knee bends, and side board are examples).
      ii. Water can also be used for resistance exercises.
      iii. Water allows an infinite variety of patterns. The resistance is proportional to the velocity at which you perform the exercise.
      iv. Slow movements yield low resistance.
      v. Fast movements yield high resistance.
      vi. Move continuously, exercising large muscle groups that mimic primary sport for 1-2 minutes. Build to 5-10 minutes. Vary movement patterns. Avoid positions that aggravate injury.
      vii. There are products commercially available to vary the amount of water resistance. Such products include foot/ankle/hand flotation resistance devices, and flotation jackets, water-compatible radios/tape players can make water rehabilitation more fun.

e. Whatever method you choose the DAPRE (daily adjusted progressive resistance exercise) protocol can be used with all.
   i. Essentially, the injured tissues require stimulation/stress to promote healing and remodeling of scar tissue.
   ii. Small, incremental stresses applied longitudinally to the muscle tendon unit provide the proper stimulus to aid healing.
   iii. The exercises are well controlled and can be advanced rapidly with careful attention.
   iv. The DAPRE program can be illustrated with the example in the box below.

VII. Phase III of Program: Return to Play Criteria
   A. Progress from pain-free level with increasingly more difficult skills, all below pain threshold.
   B. Compare right vs. left.
      1. Vertical jump.
      2. Diagonal jump.
      3. Horizontal jump.
      4. Timed one-third knee bends.
      5. Jump rope one leg.
   C. Sport-specific functional progressive-type programs.
      1. For example, a football player will lift weights and bike ride during the general rehabilitation phase and then change to run, jump, cut, and pivot during the sports-specific phase.

USING THE DAPRE PROGRAM: EXAMPLE USING WEIGHTS

Pick Starting Weight

As a test: You should be able to lift "starting weight" 10 times comfortably. Trial and error will reveal a starting weight.

Too easy—Add 20% more weight and retest. 10 repetition test should *not* be a maximal effort.

Encourage athlete to push the 80% to 90% level. Avoid maximal effort. You risk injury, and it is not necessary for the rehabilitation process.

Avoid pain during testing process. Pain takes priority over rapid advancement. Simply drop weight below pain threshold.

Set 1—Perform 10 repetitions of exercise with half of starting weight.

Set 2—Perform 10 repetitions of exercise with three-quarters of starting weight.

Set 3—Perform as many repetitions as possible.

If set 3 was greater than 15 repetitions, add 10% to 20% more weight for set 4.

If set 3 was less than 5 repetitions, subtract 10% to 20% weight for set 4.

If set 3 was approximately 10 repetitions, keep weight the same for set 4.

Perform maximum number of reps on set 4. Trial and error will yield the correct weight to work with.

Adjust weights so that sets 3 and 4 are about 10 repetitions.

Some weeks progress will be more pronounced than other weeks.

Perform resistance exercises, 3-4 days per week.

Every other day routine works well.

Athletes can usually expect to increase strength approximately three- to fourfold during their rehabilitation program.

Complement resistance exercises with *before, during,* and *afterward* stretching. Stretch whenever muscle tension seems to be progressing.

2. The complex skill of football can be broken down into smaller, simpler steps that can be practiced and progressed to more difficult maneuvers.
3. The final phase of all rehabilitation programs should include sport-specific drills.
4. Test progressively in sport-specific play.
   a. Jumping maneuvers.
   b. Lateral maneuvers.
   c. Backward maneuvers.
   d. Cutting-pivot maneuvers.
   e. Running maneuvers.

D. Special advice to athletes when they are 90% healed.
   1. Athletes tend to back off on their rehabilitation exercises before completion of healing. Allow adequate time for full recovery. Controlled and progressive overload is necessary to stimulate full tissue healing and sport-specific adaptation. Progress at a rate of approximately 10% per week.
   2. Reinjury rate is high during this period. Athletes experience minimal pain at injury site. During sports play they suddenly experience pain. Sudden tissue overload causes reinjury. The athlete is usually surprised at the level of exertion that produced the reinjury. Continue protective bracing (see Table 70-5) for as long as necessary to prevent reinjury.
   3. Minimal pain is experienced at this phase. Pain is important. It tells the athlete how hard to push. We modulate the activity to stay below pain level (REST). At this phase pain is only produced during strenuous activity. Greatly overshooting the soreness threshold will set the athlete back.

Bibliography

The articles below are from *Clinics in Sports Medicine,* WB Saunders.

The Athletic Elbow and Wrist, Part I; April 1995, Vol. 14 No. 2
Basic Science and Clinical Application in the Athlete's Shoulder; October 1991, Vol. 10:4
Basketball Injuries; April 1993, Vol. 12 No. 2
Bicycling Injuries; January 1994, Vol. 13 No. 1
The Exercise Prescription; January 1991, Vol. 10 No. 1
Foot and Ankle Injuries; October 1994, Vol. 13 No 4
Gymnastics; January 1985, Vol. 4 No. 1
Neurovascular Injuries; April 1990, Vol. 9 No. 2
New Trends and Developments in Sports Medicine; January 1993, Vol. 12 No. 1
Patellofemoral Problems; April 1989, Vol. 8 No. 2
Racquet Sports; January 1995, Vol. 14 No. 1
Rehabilitation; October 1989, Vol. 8 No 4
Rehabilitation of the Injured Athlete; July 1985, Vol. 4 No. 3
Spine Problems in the Athlete; July 1993, Vol. 12 No. 3
Tendinitis I; July 1992, Vol. 11 No. 3

CHAPTER 71

Physiology of Musculoskeletal Growth

Mimi D. Johnson, MD

I. Introduction
  A. Although the initiation of pubertal growth and development may vary, all children undergo the same sequence of maturational and skeletal changes.
  B. Once the process has begun, the chronology is quite predictable.

II. Height and Weight
  A. Height.
    1. Growth velocity is similar in boys and girls from ages 1-10 years.
    2. Pubertal growth spurt begins 2 years earlier in girls than in boys.
    3. The growth spurt covers 24-36 months and accounts for 20% to 25% of final adult height.
    4. In girls the average age of peak height velocity (PHV) is 12.1 years.
      a. The growth spurt begins as early as 9.5 years and as late as 14.5 years.
      b. Maximal growth rate is reached 6-12 months prior to menarche.
      c. Most girls have reached 90% to 95% of adult height by menarche. After menarche median height gain is 7.4 cm.
      d. The median age when adult stature is reached is 17.3 years; 10% of girls grow until 21.1 years of age.
    5. In boys the average age for PHV is 14.1 years.
      a. The growth spurt begins as early as 10.5 years and as late as 16 years.
      b. The median age of reaching adult stature is 21.2 years; 10% of boys grow until 23.5 years of age.
  B. Weight.
    1. The pubertal growth spurt accounts for 50% of ideal adult body weight.
    2. In girls peak weight velocity occurs 6 months after peak height velocity.
    3. In boys peak weight velocity and peak height velocity are simultaneous.

TABLE 71-1. Classification of pubertal staging in girls

Stage	Pubic Hair	Breasts
1	None	Prepubertal; no glandular tissue
2	Sparse, long, straight, lightly pigmented on labia majora	Breast bud; small amount of glandular tissue
3	Darker, beginning to curl, extend laterally	Breast mound and areola enlarge; no contour separation
4	Coarse, curly, abundant, less than adult	Breast enlarged; areola and papilla form mound projecting from breast contour
5	Adult type and quantity, extending to medial thigh	Mature; areola part of breast contour

Adapted from Tanner JM: *Growth at Adolescence,* ed 2, Oxford, England, 1962, Blackwell Scientific Publications.

III. Pubertal Development
   A. Pubertal stages (i.e., Tanner stages) provide fairly reliable guidelines about growth and growth potential (Tables 71-1 and 71-2).
      1. Prepubescence: Tanner I.
      2. Early pubescence: Tanner II and III. Pubertal development begins in Tanner II. Growth spurt begins in Tanner II for females and Tanner III for males. PHV in females occurs during Tanner III.
      3. Midpubescence: Tanner III (late), Tanner IV. PHV in males occurs during Tanner IV. In females menarche begins in Tanner IV.
      4. Late pubescence: Tanner V. Growth rate decreases, epiphysiodesis (physeal closure) occurs, articular cartilage is that of an adult, apophyses close.

IV. Axial and Appendicular Skeletal Growth
   A. Growing bone is in a constant state of change where fibrous, cartilaginous, and osseous morphological patterns are controlled microscopically

TABLE 71-2. Classification of pubertal staging in boys

Stage	Pubic Hair	Genitalia
1	None	Penis, testes, and scrotum are prepubertal
2	Sparse, long, straight, lightly pigmented at base of penis	Enlargement of scrotum and testes; penis is not enlarged
3	Darker, beginning to curl, extend laterally	Enlargement of penis in length; further growth of testes and scrotum
4	Coarse, curly, abundant, does not extend to thigh	Further growth of testes and scrotum; increased size of penis, especially in breadth
5	Adult type and quantity, extending to medial thigh	Genitalia are adult in size and shape

Adapted from Tanner JM: *Growth at Adolescence,* ed 2, Oxford, England, 1962, Blackwell Scientific Publications.

and macroscopically by genetic programming, changing hormonal activity, and variably applied mechanical loads.

B. Physiological control of growth.
   1. Testosterone.
      a. Stimulates the physis to undergo rapid cell division and widening during the growth spurt.
      b. Eventually manifests a slow-down of growth and consolidation of cartilage.
   2. Estrogen.
      a. Appears to stimulate growth of already differentiated osseous tissue.
      b. May slow down cartilage growth by affecting the subchondral plates on either side of the physis.
      c. Suppresses growth plate activity by suppressing sulfation factor and increasing calcification of the matrix.
      d. The effect of estrogen in the female is stronger than the similar effect of testosterone in the male.
   3. Other hormonal influences.
      a. Growth hormone: has no significant direct effect on bone or cartilage growth; however, it causes the liver to produce somatomedin C, which does promote growth (causes secretion of chondroitin sulfate and collagen by the chondrocytes).
      b. Thyroxin.
      c. Sulfation factor.
   4. Mechanical factors.
      a. Intrinsic tension due to muscle force across the joints.
      b. Repetitively applied external forces.
   5. Other factors affecting relative rate of growth.
      a. Vascular changes.
      b. Direct trauma.
      c. Neurological factors.
      d. Nutritional deprivation.

C. Longitudinal and latitudinal bone growth. The appendicular and axial skeleton are derived from initial transformation of the mesenchymal model to a cartilaginous model, with subsequent transformation to an ossified structure; this is called endochondral ossification.
   1. Longitudinal growth: the physis (growth plate).
      a. The physis is the primary site of longitudinal bone growth.
      b. In the physis, a longitudinal column of cells may be divided on the basis of physiological function and histiological appearance into zones of growth, maturation, transformation, and remodeling.
         i. The layer of resting cells in the zone of growth, closest to the epiphysis, contains immature chondrocytes. As cells mature, enlarge, and migrate toward the metaphysis, progressive ossification and then calcification occur.
         ii. Cells may be added peripherally through the zone of Ranvier, a specialized region surrounding the physis. This zone contains fibrovascular tissue, mesenchymal tissue, differentiated epiphyseal and physeal cartilage, and the osseous ring of Lacroix.
         iii. Contribution of growth plates to growth of individual bones.

Humerus	Distal humeral physis	20%
	Proximal humeral physis	80%
Radius	Distal radial physis	75% to 80%
	Proximal radial physis	20% to 25%

Femur	Proximal femoral physis	30%
	Distal femoral physis	70%
Tibia/Fibula	Proximal physes	55%
	Distal physes	45%

2. Latitudinal bone growth takes place in the diaphysis and metaphysis by means of appositional growth through the combined mechanisms of periosteal osteogenesis and endosteal remodeling. In the physis latitudinal growth occurs by cell division and matrix expansion within the physis and by cellular addition peripherally at the zone of Ranvier.
3. Interstitial expansion occurs within the epiphysis and physis as a result of the enlargement of the secondary center of ossification.

D. Coordination of skeletal and muscle growth. With few exceptions, the periosteum serves as the origin for most muscular fibers along the metaphysis and diaphysis. This allows growth of bone and muscle units to be coordinated.

E. Stage of growth may affect injury patterns.
1. Macrotrauma.
   a. A child's bone fails differently than an adult's bone.
      i. Greenstick fracture.
      ii. Torus fracture.
   b. Differences in the interrelationships between soft tissue and bone/cartilage result in the tendency toward avulsion of soft tissue-bone interface in an adult and intraosseous failure in a child (tibial spine avulsion in child vs. cruciate ligament tear or avulsion in adult).
   c. During prepubescence, the physis and its attachment to the zone of Ranvier are stronger than ligamentous structures around the joint. The opposite is true in midpubescence. A lateral blow to the knee produces different injuries in differing stages of growth.
      i. Tanner I-II: injury to medial collateral ligament (MCL), not physis.
      ii. Tanner III-IV: injury to physis.
      iii. Tanner V: injury to MCL.
   d. Apophyseal avulsion fractures may occur in child/adolescent.
2. Microtrauma.
   a. Repetitive microtrauma may result in variable secondary injury depending on stage of growth.
      i. Traction apophysitis can result from microtrauma at the apophysis.
      ii. Osteochondritis dissecans may be a result of repetitive microtrauma at the articular cartilage.
      iii. Irregularity, widening, and premature closure of the distal radial physis in gymnasts are more likely to occur from repetitive stress during midpubescence, as opposed to prepubescence.
   b. There may be an increased incidence of soft tissue injury due to muscle-tendon imbalance during the growth spurt.
      1. Decreased flexibility of muscle groups.
      2. Inconsistencies in the strength of muscle groups around a joint.

V. Body Composition

A. Fat.
1. In girls there is a modest decrease in fat accumulation 3 years prior to PHV. Once PHV is reached, there is an increase in fat accumulation. At 18-22 years old the standard female has 22% to 26% body fat.

2. In boys there is usually loss of fat at PHV. At 18-22 years old the standard male has 12% to 16% body fat.

B. Muscle.
   1. Muscle mass increases steadily from the onset of puberty until its completion.
   2. Muscle fiber and total cross-sectional area of muscle in females averages 60% to 85% of those areas in males.
   3. The proportion of slow and fast twitch fibers in males and females are similar.

C. Bone density.
   1. There is a gradual acquisition of bone mass in early childhood, which accelerates during adolescence until sexual maturity is reached.
   2. 50% of adult bone mass is formed during the second decade.
   3. Peak bone mineral density (BMD) is attained by 20 years of age and perhaps by 16 years.
   4. Pubertal stage and weight are the greatest predictors of axial and peripheral bone density, respectively, during growth.
   5. Physical activity and dietary calcium are positively associated with increased BMD in children and adolescents.
   6. Females with delayed menarche or secondary amenorrhea lose BMD and experience a decreased rate of bone accretion when compared with their eumenorrheic counterparts.

Bibliography

Bachrach LK et al: Decreased bone density in adolescent girls with anorexia nervosa, *Pediatrics* 86:440-447, 1990.

Barnes HV: Physical growth and development during puberty, *Med Clin North Am* 59:1305-1317, 1975.

Copeland KC: Variations in normal sexual development, *Pediatr Rev* 8:18-26, 1986.

Gilsanz V et al: Vertebral bone density in children: effect of puberty, *Radiology* 166:847-850, 1988.

Guyton AC: *Human Physiology and Mechanisms of Disease,* ed 5, Philadelphia, 1992, WB Saunders.

Katzman DK et al: Clinical and anthropometric correlates of bone mineral acquisition in healthy adolescent girls, *J Clin Endocrinol Metab* 73:1332-1339, 1991.

Matkovic V: Calcium metabolism and calcium requirements during skeletal modeling and consolidation of bone mass, *Am J Clin Nutr* 54(Suppl):245S-260S, 1991.

Micheli LJ: Overuse injuries in children's sports: the growth factor, *Orthop Clin North Am* 14:337-360, 1983.

Ogden JA: *Skeletal Injury in the Child,* ed 2, Philadelphia, 1990, WB Saunders.

O'Neill DB, Micheli LJ: Overuse injuries in the young athlete, *Clin Sports Med* 7:591-610, 1988.

Roche AF, Davila GH: Late adolescent growth in stature, *Pediatrics* 50:874-880, 1972.

Rockwood CA, Wilkins KE, King RE, editors: *Fractures in Children,* ed 3, Philadelphia, 1991, JB Lippincott.

Roy S et al: Stress changes of the distal radial epiphysis in young gymnasts, *Am J Sports Med* 13:301-308, 1985.

Rubin K et al: Predictors of axial and peripheral bone mineral density in healthy children and adolescents, with special attention to the role of puberty, *J Pediatr* 123:863-870, 1993.

Slemenda CW et al: Role of physical activity in the development of skeletal mass in children, *J Bone Mineral Res* 6:1227-1233, 1991.

Tanner JM: *Growth at Adolescence,* ed 2, Oxford, 1962, Blackwell Scientific Publications.

Warren MP: The effects of exercise on pubertal progression and reproductive function in girls, *J Clin Endocrinol Metab* 51:1150-1157, 1980.

CHAPTER 72

Finding and Correcting Flexibility Deficits for Injury Prevention and Rehabilitation

Angela D. Smith, MD

I. Are Inflexibility and Injury Related?
   A. Evidence of relationship between relatively inflexible muscles and injury at or near sites of attachment.
   B. No careful scientific studies to support causation, but good information concerning relationship.
   C. Resolution of flexibility deficit (without any other treatment) rapidly leads to resolution of pain for some injuries in clinical practice.

II. Scientific Evidence for Relationship
   A. Profile of individual prone to overuse injuries: lax ligaments, weak muscles, and inflexible muscles.[2]
   B. Quadriceps inflexibility and anterior knee pain.[4]
   C. Hamstrings inflexibility and patellofemoral pain.[5]
   D. Triceps surae inflexibility and calcaneal apophysitis.[3]
   E. Loss of shoulder internal rotation and impingement.[1]

III. Clinical Evidence for Relationship
   A. Inflexible muscle associated with specific injury.
   B. Iliopsoas inflexibility.
      1. Avulsion fracture of lesser trochanter.
      2. Increased lumbar lordosis.
   C. Sartorius inflexibility: avulsion fracture of anterior superior iliac spine (ASIS).
   D. Hamstring inflexibility.
      1. Avulsion fracture of ischial tuberosity.
      2. Muscle strain.
      3. Low back pain.
      4. Increased swayback and roundback posture.
   E. Rectus femoris inflexibility.
      1. Avulsion fracture of anterior inferior iliac spine.
      2. Muscle strain.

F. Tensor fascia lata tight.
   1. Iliotibial band friction syndrome.
   2. Greater trochanter bursitis
G. Gastrocnemius inflexibility.
   1. Partial avulsion of one head of muscle.
   2. Achilles' tendinitis.
   3. Plantar fasciitis.
H. Tight shoulder external rotators and posterior capsule: impingement syndrome.

IV. Principles Regarding Flexibility Deficits of Adolescence
   A. Dynamically changing relationship between bone length and muscle length with growth.
   B. Muscles related to overuse injuries generally cross two joints.
   C. Preferable to warm up muscles first; however, better for growing children and adolescents to stretch "cold" than not to stretch at all.
   D. Stretch in nonballistic manner; instead, perform slow and gradual stretches.
   E. Hold each stretch for about 30 seconds.
   F. Relax into the stretch; should feel muscle stretching, but should not hurt.
   G. Repeat each stretch three times (get most stretch first and second time; still get enough increase third time to make it worthwhile, but by fourth and fifth time get little increment and beyond fifth get none).[6]
   H. Compliance tip: may do some stretching exercises whenever waiting for someone.

V. Reproducible Flexibility Tests
   A. Hip flexors.
      1. Thomas test (Figure 72-1).
      2. Adolescents should have no contracture.
   B. Iliotibial band (tensor fascia lata) (Figure 72-2).
      1. Ober or modified Ober test.
      2. Abduct and extend hip, while flexing ipsilateral knee; then observe how close to midline the knee returns as the hip adducts (by gravity

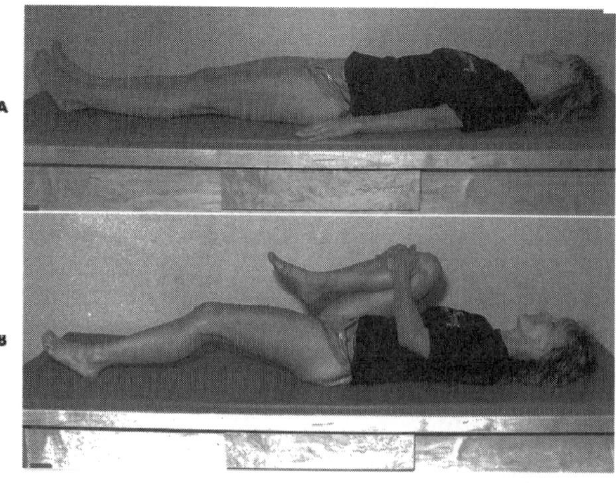

FIGURE 72-1
Positive Thomas test

in the Ober test, by gently swinging the knee toward midline in the modified test).

3. The extended hip should adduct to neutral (knee at midline).

C. Rectus femoris (quadricep) (Figure 72-3).

1. Examinee lies prone, ASIS on firm surface, knees together.
2. Examiner records angle of maximal knee flexion.
3 Maximal knee flexion with hip extended − Maximal knee flexion with hip flexed = Amount of contracture of rectus femoris
4 Adolescents should be able to touch heel to buttock except unusually mature males.

D. Hamstrings (Figure 72-4).

1. Straight leg raise less reliable than popliteal angle.
2. For popliteal angle, examiner passively flexes examinee's hip and ipsilateral knee 90 degrees, then (maintaining the hip flexion at 90 degrees) extends the knee until tension is noted in the hamstrings; the angle between the tibia and true vertical is generally the one used clinically.
3. Adolescents should be able to straight leg raise to 85 degrees and have popliteal angle of 10 degrees or less.

E. Gastrocnemius (Figure 72-5).

1. Align the heel with the tibia by supinating the foot.
2. Knee fully extended.
3. Passively dorsiflex the ankle as far as possible with examiner's body weight leaning against examinee's foot; do not allow examinee to "help" by contracting ankle dorsiflexors (this often pulls hindfoot out of alignment with tibia and gives inflated measurement).

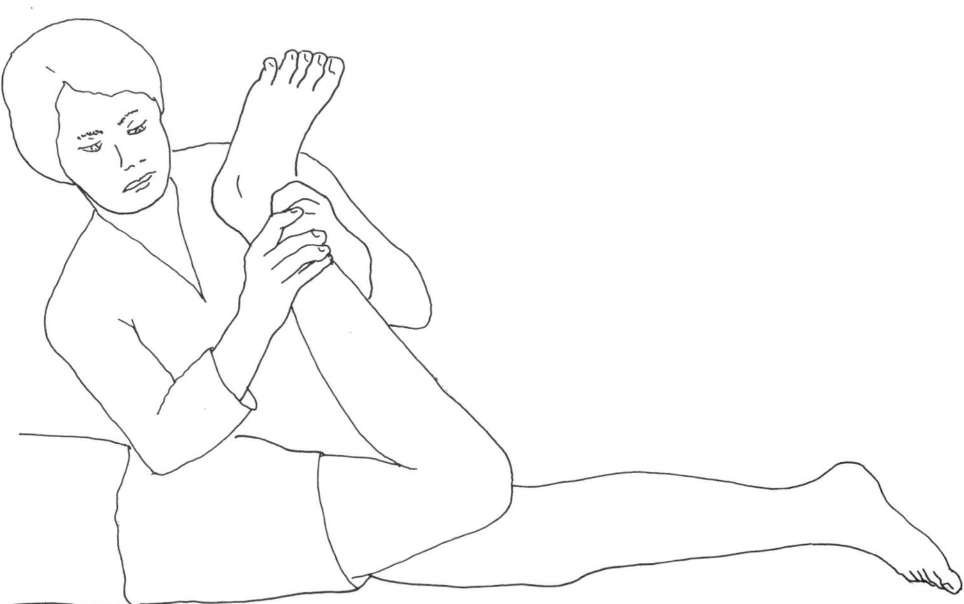

FIGURE 72-2
Modified Ober test

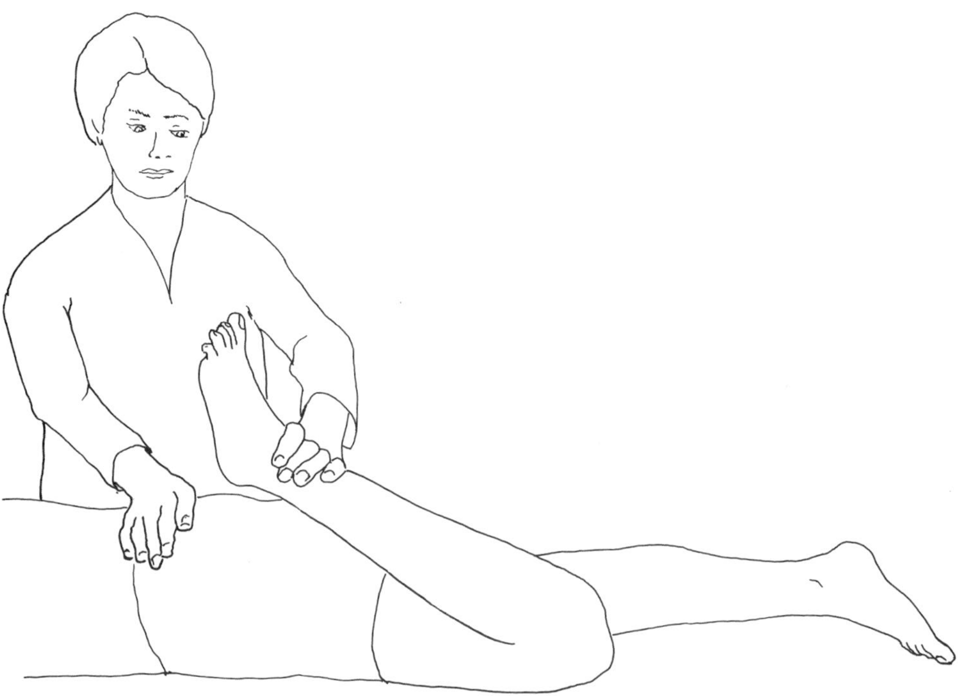

FIGURE 72-3
Rectus femoris flexibility test

4. Adolescents should have 10 degrees or more of ankle dorsiflexion with the knee extended.

F. Shoulder rotators.
   1. Here, comparison with the opposite side is important.
   2. With scapula firmly on examination table and shoulder abducted 90 degrees, flex elbow 90 degrees to be able to use forearm as a goniometer arm.
   3. For most average adolescents, medial and lateral rotation are about 90 degrees each; dominant arm of throwers and tennis players and both shoulders of swimmers often have excessive lateral rotation and diminished medial rotation.

VI. Simple Stretches That Work

A. Triceps surae (Figure 72-6).
   1. Wall stretch: both feet should be perpendicular to the wall.
   2. To stretch right gastrocnemius, right foot back, right knee straight, lean forward as if doing push-up against the wall.
   3. To stretch right soleus, do not change position of feet but simply sit back a bit, flexing right knee slightly; should feel a deeper muscle than for gastrocnemius.

B. Hamstrings (Figure 72-7).
   1. Sit on a firm surface, chest on thighs, knees bent, hands gently grasping lateral borders of feet.
   2. "Walk" heels away from buttocks until slight stretch is felt.
   3. Hold position for 30 seconds.
   4. Then lift chest up to release stretch, walk heels further away, lean chest down onto thighs again, keeping shoulders and upper back relaxed.
   5. Repeat several times.

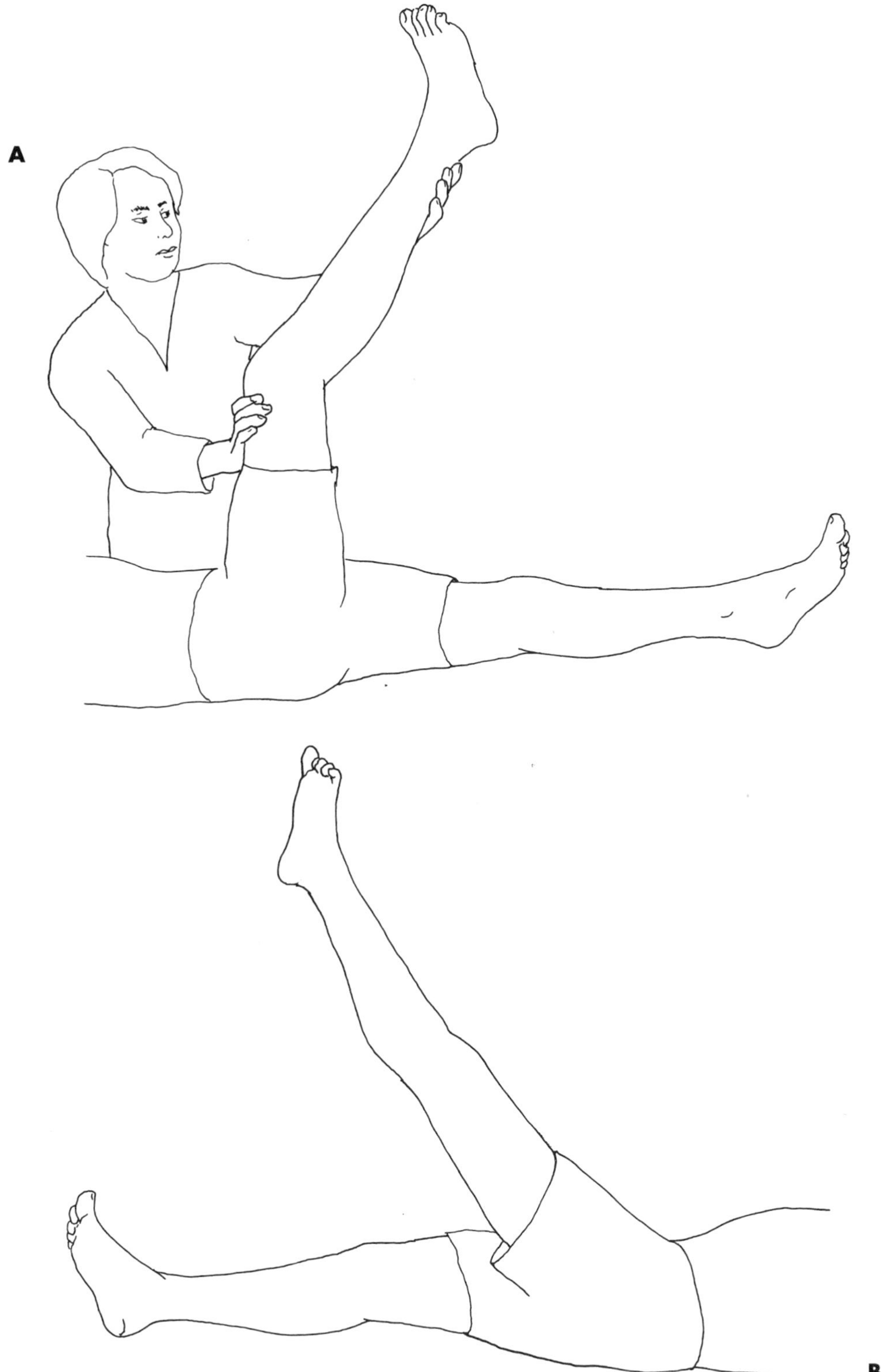

FIGURE 72-4
A, Popliteal angle flexibility test. **B**, Straight leg raise

6. This can also be done standing up if no place available to sit, but impossible to relax into the stretch as well when standing.
7. For additional exercise, see Adductors below.

C. Quadriceps (Figure 72-8).
1. Lie prone, ASIS firmly on table or floor, knees together.

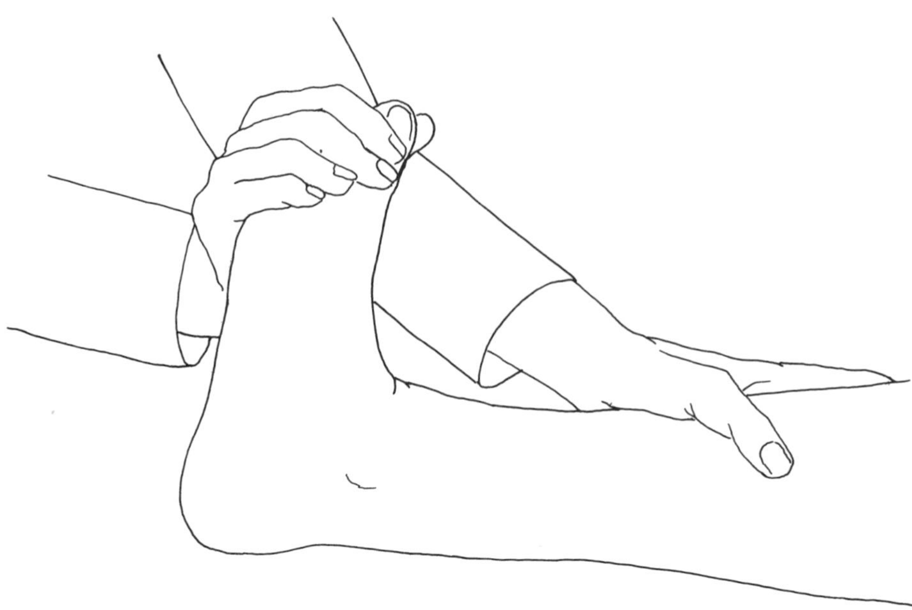

FIGURE 72-5
Gastrocnemius flexibility test

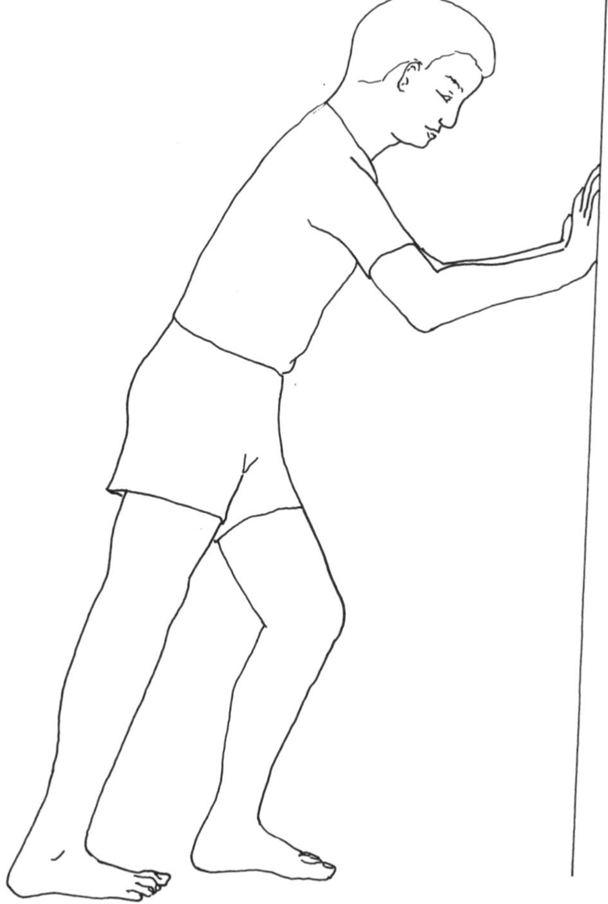

FIGURE 72-6
Triceps surae stretches

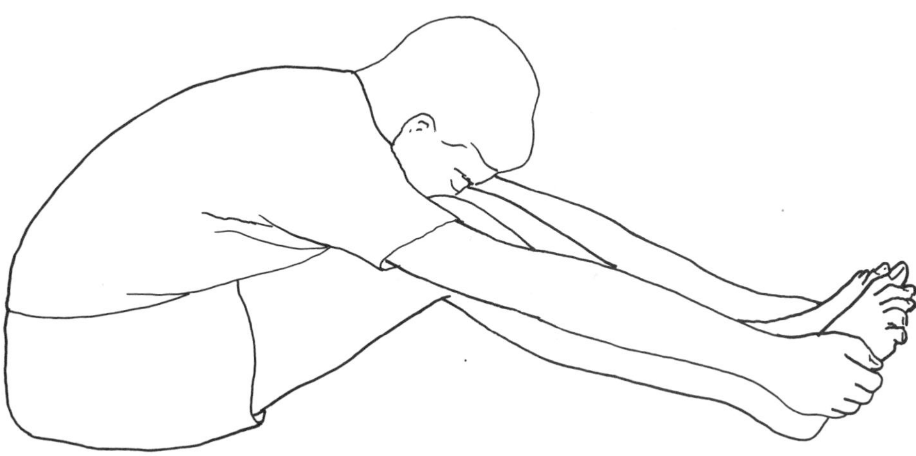

FIGURE 72-7
Hamstring stretch

2. Bend one knee, and grasp that foot or ankle with the opposite hand.
3. Bring foot toward buttock, try to touch buttock with foot.
4. To increase the stretch, extend the hip.
5. If doing this exercise standing, make certain that hip remains extended and adducted to neutral.

D. Adductors.

1. Straddle stretch: easy way for teenagers to do this (while talking on phone, reading, etc.) is to lie supine, perpendicular to a wall, with feet up on the wall and buttocks as close to the wall as possible; allow feet to slide outward on the wall (abducting hips).
2. As flexibility increases, move buttocks closer to the wall, and let feet slide farther apart.
3. May also be done seated on the floor; then add to stretch by leaning trunk towards one leg or straight between the legs.
4. These exercises stretch adductors and hamstrings; the specific muscle stretched is dependent on relative positions of trunk and hips.

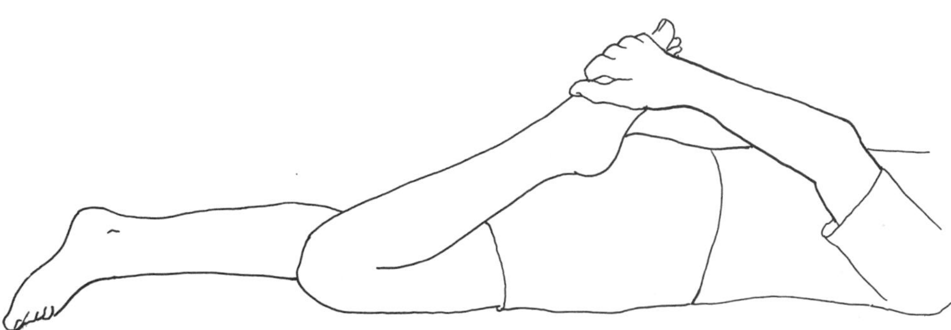

FIGURE 72-8
Quadriceps stretch

E. Iliopsoas and/or rectus femoris (hip flexors).
    1. Perform Thomas test maneuver.
    2. Increase stretch by letting limb that is to be stretched hang off table.
F. Iliotibial band.
    1. Hip in neutral position, feet pointing forward, no trunk rotation; adduct hip to be stretched.
    2. To stretch right iliotibial band, cross left foot in front of right, push right greater trochanter into iliotibial band.
    3. Alternatively, stand on platform on right foot, let left hip drop a few inches lower than right, not twisting or rotating at all (Figure 72-9).
G. Lumbodorsal muscular and fascial structures.
    1. Seated hamstring stretch as above.
    2. Curl up.
H. Lateral rotators of the shoulder (patient lacks internal rotation).
    1. Lie supine, shoulder abducted 90 degrees, elbow flexed 90 degrees.
    2. With upper arm supported on table, weight in hand or on wrist, allow passive medial rotation of shoulder.

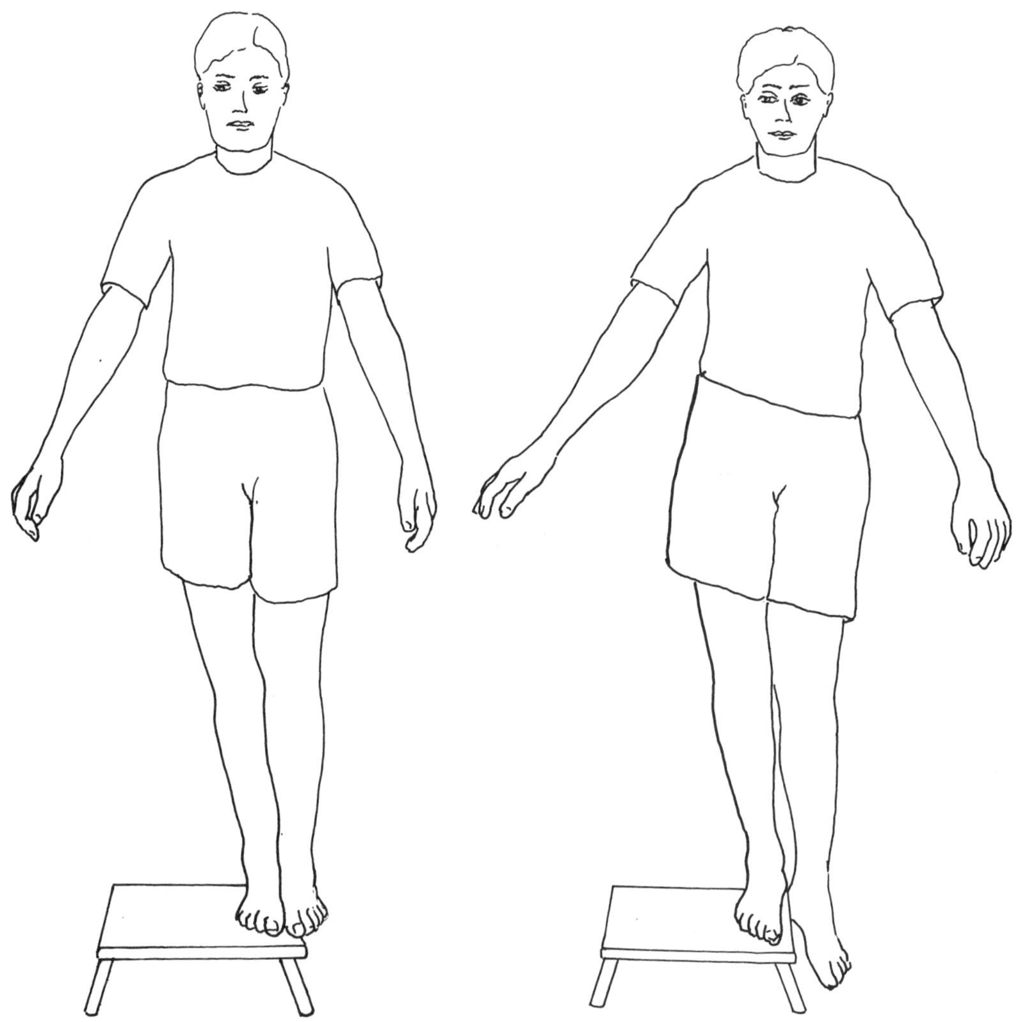

FIGURE 72-9
Iliotibial band stretch

References

1. Kibler WB, Chandler TJ, Stracener ES: Musculoskeletal adaptations and injuries due to overtraining, *Exerc Sports Sci Rev* 20:99-126, 1992.
2. Lysens RJ et al: The accident-prone and overuse-prone profiles of the young athlete, *Am J Sports Med* 17:612-619, 1989.
3. Micheli LJ, Ireland ML: Prevention and management of calcaneal apophysitis in children: an overuse syndrome, *J Pediatr Orthop* 7:34-38, 1987.
4. Smith AD, Stroud L, McQueen C: Flexibility and anterior knee pain in adolescent elite figure skaters, *J Pediatr Orthop* 11:77-82, 1996.
5. Stroud L, Smith AD, Kruse R: The relationship between femoral anteversion and patellofemoral pain, *Orthop Trans*
6. Taylor CC, Seaber AB, Garrett WE Jr: Response of muscle-tendon units to cyclic repetitive stretching, *Trans Orthop Res Soc* 10:84, 1985.

CHAPTER 73

Epidemiology of Injuries

James G. Garrick, MD

I. Historical
  A. First used to study skiing injuries.
    1. Used techniques from highway safety.
    2. Major innovation was the use of matched controls.
  B. Ankle injuries and cleat configuration in football.
  C. Synthetic turf and football injuries.
  D. Catastrophic cervical spine injuries in football.
  E. Prophylactic knee braces.
  F. Sliding injuries in baseball/softball.

II. Types of Studies
  A. Descriptive.
    1. Most common.
    2. A tally of injuries arising from a particular activity.
    3. A precise definition of injury is essential.
      a. Injuries reported to insurance carriers will tend to oversample more severe injuries (fractures and dislocations) and injuries requiring immediate medical attention (lacerations).
      b. Injuries reported to coaches will oversample injuries precluding participation and obvious acute injuries.
      c. Injuries reported to athletic trainers will include all of the above as well as chronic and overuse (gradual onset) injuries and injuries not resulting in time lost to participation.
      d. Injuries reported in personal interviews of players will include all of the above plus even more "minor" injuries.
    4. Injuries should be classified by:
      a. Anatomy (knee, leg, ankle, foot, etc.).
      b. Pathology (fracture, sprain, strain, etc.).
      c. Onset (acute or gradual).
      d. History (recurrent).

5. A denominator is essential for the creation of injury rates.
   a. Group studied should be precisely identified (e.g., a team of 67 high school football players).
   b. Some measure of exposure should be noted (e.g., participating in 10 games and 67 practices).
6. General observations.
   a. The more sensitive the definition of injury (e.g., those collected by athletic trainers or personal interviews):
      i. The higher the injury rates.
      ii. More gradual onset, overuse injuries.
      iii. Lower proportion of fractures and dislocations.
      iv. Lower proportion of acute injuries.
   b. "Causes" of injuries can be suggested but not "proven" due to the lack of controls.

III. Case-Control Studies
   A. Data collected from both injured and uninjured.
   B. Permits documentation of causes (synthetic turf) and effects (use of breakaway bases).
   C. The use of simultaneous controls, while ideal, may be impossible. (A new field is installed on which everyone plays, or everyone is required to wear knee braces.)
   D. Historical controls (commonly used [e.g., comparing current data with those gathered in the years before the synthetic field was installed]) may introduce additional biases.
      1. New coach and/or techniques.
      2. Addition of new protective equipment.
      3. Different weather conditions.
      4. Different win/loss records.
      5. New diagnostic and treatment methods.
   E. Must be hypothesis generated. "Data dredging" (testing many/all combinations of variables looking for "significance") often rampant and always inappropriate.
   F. Require comprehensive planning, trained personnel, appreciable additional effort, and skilled analyst.

Bibliography

Garrick JG, Requa R; Medical care and injury surveillance in the high school setting, *Phys Sportsmed* 9(8):46-50, 1981.

Lenaway DD, Ambler AG, Beaudoin DE: The epidemiology of school-related injuries: new perspectives, *Am J Preventive Med* 8(3):193-198, 1992.

Pinkham JR, Kohn DW: Epidemiology and prediction of sports-related traumatic injuries, *Dental Clin North Am* 35(4):609-626, 1991.

Shirely RA, Grana WA, Ellis D: High School Sports Injuries, *Phys Sportsmed* 9(8):46-50, 1981.

Van Mechelen W, Hlobil H, Kemper HC: Incidence, severity, etiology, and prevention of sports injuries: a review of concepts, *Sports Med* 14(2):82-99, 1992.

CHAPTER 74

Injuries in Football and Soccer

James M. Moriarity, MD

I. Scope of Participation
   A. Soccer.
      1. 40 million registered participants worldwide.
      2. United States has seen a meteoric rise in the number of participants.
      3. Has introduced women to contact sport.
   B. Football: 1.5 million high school participants.
   C. National Collegiate Athletic Association (NCAA) injury rates[13] per 1000 athletic exposures (practice or game).
      1. Spring football: 9.59.
      2. Fall football: 6.57.
      3. Men's soccer: 7.87.
      4. Women's soccer: 7.90.

II. Head Injuries/Concussion
   A. 1 in 5 football athletes will suffer head injury.[4]
   B. Soccer athletes report a similar injury rate of 4% to 22%.
   C. Grading concussion: Colorado Guidelines.[9]
      1. Grade I: No loss of consciousness (LOC), confusion without amnesia. May return to competition if observed for 20 minutes and examination is normal.
      2. Grade II: No LOC, confusion with amnesia. Remove from contest, minimum return 1 week after symptoms gone.
      3. Grade III: LOC, transport to hospital with neck precautions if necessary, full neurological evaluation, minimum return 2 weeks.
   D. Head injury and soccer.
      1. There has been recent concern about long-term neurological sequelae from cumulative head trauma in soccer.
      2. An increased incidence of cerebral atrophy found on computed tomography (CT) scan, abnormal electroencephalography (EEG), and abnormal psychometric tests were found in former and current soccer athletes.

3. None of these athletes were felt to be clinically or socially impaired.[24]

E. Nontraumatic head injury.
   1. Weightlifter's headache: a condition of uncertain etiology described as a sudden onset of intense head and neck pain sometimes associated with minor neurological symptoms occurring during maximal lifting effort. Many times seen with inexperienced lifters who incorrectly lift with Valsalva's maneuver.
   2. Exertional headache: an intense vascular reproducible type of headache brought on by exertion. Effectively treated with indomethacin.
   3. Footballer's migraine: first described in soccer athletes who experienced typical migraine symptoms initiated by heading the ball. Athlete experiences headache in absence of other concussive symptoms.[10]

F. Second impact syndrome.
   1. A condition in which a player who has sustained minor head trauma in the recent past develops sudden, massive brain swelling in response to a relatively minor second impact.
   2. The precise cause is unknown but is thought to involve loss of autoregulation of the cerebral vasculature with resultant increase in cerebral blood flow and subsequent increase in cerebrospinal fluid (CSF).
   3. Underscores need to restrict contact in individuals diagnosed with concussion syndrome until symptoms have resolved.[9]

III. Neck Injuries

A. Strong neck musculature is a prerequisite for football and soccer play.
   1. Helps prevent rotational/shear injury to the brain.
   2. Helps protect spinal cord.
   3. Neck serves as attachment for shoulder/scapular muscles.

B. Persistent pain or limited motion in the neck of an injured athlete is a fracture until proven otherwise. An unconscious athlete should be assumed to have a cervical spine injury and treated with neck immobilization.

C. Neck conditions that preclude soccer and football participation.[23]
   1. Spear tackler's spine.
   2. Unstable cervical spine.
   3. Klippel-Feil anomaly type I (fusion of cervical vertebrae).
   4. Odontoid anomalies.
   5. Atlantooccipital fusion.
   6. Acute cervical disc.
   7. Chronic cervical disc with neurological impairment.

D. Spinal stenoses: defined as a spinal canal to vertebral body ratio of <0.8. An alternative definition is loss of CSF cushion around the spinal cord as demonstrated by magnetic resonance imaging (MRI).
   1. Associated with transient quadriparesis lasting less than 24 hours.
   2. 92% of cases of transient quadriparesis have occurred in athletes with ratios <0.8.
   3. However, the presence of ratios <0.8 in asymptomatic individuals should not exclude them from competition.
   4. In nonathletic populations the incidence of spinal stenoses is roughly 12%. In professional and college ranks the incidence increases to roughly 33%. This disparity reflects the larger vertebral bodies found in larger individuals.[16]

5. Routine screening of athletes for cervical spine stenoses not recommended.

IV. Brachial Plexus Injuries[7]

A. Are one of the most common injuries seen in contact sports. Also known as "stingers" or "burners" because of the character of pain felt radiating down the arm. Are caused by one of several mechanisms but all involve compression or traction on the nerves of the brachial plexus. Common presentation occurs after a tackle or collision. Player exits the field with affected arm dangling at side.

B. Most common nerve root affected is C5-C6.
   1. After the stinging has subsided, muscle strength of the deltoid, spinati, biceps, brachioradialis, and wrist extensors/flexors should be tested.
   2. The athlete should have full range of motion (ROM) of the neck and no spasm.
   3. Bilateral arm, hand, or leg symptoms signal neurapraxia of the spinal cord, and the athlete should be evaluated for possible cervical instability or spinal stenoses.

C. Grading of brachial plexus injury.[18]
   1. Neurapraxia: interruption of physiological function without anatomical damage. Symptoms transient or lasting up to a few hours. Full recovery.
   2. Axonotmesis: interruption of function with axonal damage and wallerian degeneration. Neurolemma spared. Function returns as myelin regenerates. Symptoms of paresthesia and weakness may last from weeks to months. Recovery generally complete. Electromyogram (EMG) positive 3-4 weeks postinjury.
   3. Neurotmesis: loss of function with damage to neurolemma. Poor prognosis for return (0-30%). EMG reflects neuronal damage and muscle denervation.

D. Profile of football athletes with burners.[11]
   1. The average time missed by an athlete with axonotmesis is 10 days.
   2. Burners secondary to extension/compression of the neck are three times more common in athletes with spinal stenoses.
   3. Risk by position (greatest to least):
      a. Defensive end and linebackers.
      b. Defensive lineman.
      c. Offensive lineman.
      d. Defensive back.
      e. Offensive backs.

E. Return to play/prevention.
   1. Players suffering from a burner should not be allowed to resume competition until all symptoms have subsided, strength has completely recovered, and full, painless ROM of the neck is demonstrated.
   2. Bilateral symptoms, prolonged symptoms for more than a few days, or recurrent burners merit more complete neurological evaluation for spinal stenoses, cervical instability and injury, and possible disc disease.
   3. Athletes with recurrent unilateral neurapraxic burners without evidence of cervical instability and complete recovery between episodes may return to play.
   4. These athletes may benefit from neck strengthening exercises to facilitate shoulder retraction, and devices such as the "cowboy collar"

to prevent neck hyperflexion and deflect traction forces during tackling.

V. Shoulder Injuries
   A. Sternoclavicular joint.
      1. Is the only bony attachment of the shoulder to the trunk.
      2. Mechanism of injury is fall on the lateral shoulder.
      3. Anterior subluxation is more common than posterior and often associated with a proximal clavicular fracture.
      4. Posterior subluxation may dangerously compress the trachea or brachial vessels and in the event of respiratory embarrassment requires immediate reduction. This is best accomplished by lateral traction on the abducted arm and, if necessary, anterior elevation of the clavicle.
   B. Clavicular fractures.
      1. The most common fracture of the shoulder.
      2. Mechanism of injury is fall on the lateral shoulder or in rare cases secondary to pull of the pectoralis major muscle.
      3. Treated with shoulder retraction in a clavicle strap. No throwing rehabilitation for 6-8 weeks and no contact till bony healing has occurred.
   C. Acromioclavicular (AC) separation.
      1. Is one of the most common shoulder injuries in soccer and football.
      2. Mechanism of injury is depression of the lateral shoulder.
      3. The two ligaments supporting the AC joint are the weak AC and the strong coracoclavicular (CC).
      4. Injuries can be divided into three grades.
         a. Grade 1: sprain or tear of the AC ligament. Painful joint, painful abduction. Minimal loss of time from competition.
         b. Grade 2: sprain or partial tear of both the AC and CC ligaments. Painful joint, limited shoulder motion, residual depression of the joint.
         c. Grade 3: tear of both ligaments with significant residual depression of the joint. Marked pain and limited ROM.
      5. AC separations of the shoulder with significant displacement of the clavicle have been described and classified. These may require closed or open manipulation to restore function.
      6. Treatment of AC separations is slinging and progressive rehabilitation. All grades of AC separations may result in degenerative changes in the AC joint with continued pain and tenderness, especially on adduction of the shoulder.
      7. Importantly, the same mechanism of injury that causes AC separations can also inflict damage to the Sternoclavicular (SC) joint, the rotator cuff, and glenohumeral ligaments. Do not overlook associated pathology.
   D. Shoulder instability: a common condition found in football and soccer athletes.
      1. The primary pathology in shoulder instability is derangement or insufficient function of the glenohumeral ligaments due to congenital laxity, acute traumatic injury, chronic overload, or associated failure of the rotator cuff.
      2. The net result is a humeral head that dislocates, subluxes, slips, or impinges adjacent structures during activities that stress the glenohumeral joint.
      3. Instability may be quiescent until unmasked as a "shoulder slippage" felt in the weight room, progressive as seen in recurrent subluxers, or chronic following shoulder dislocation.

4. Secondary manifestations of shoulder instability include rotator cuff tendinitis due to cuff impingement or overload, "dead arm" syndrome from brachial plexus stretch, and bony changes of the glenohumeral complex (Hill-Sachs lesion of the humerus and Bankart lesion of the glenoid).

E. Treatment depends greatly on the pathology, playing position, and training requirements.
   1. Rotator cuff strengthening: will provide musculotendinous support to the glenohumeral joint
   2. Scapular stabilizers: strengthening the rhomboids, serratus, latissimus, levator scapulae, and trapezius will stabilize the "origin end" of the rotator cuff muscles.
   3. Mechanical devices: such as harnesses that prevent arm abduction and external rotation.
   4. Surgery: stabilization procedures such as capsular shifts and rotator cuff repair.

VI. Hand and Wrist Injury
   A. Common in contact sports.
   B. The diagnoses and treatment of injuries to the hand and wrist are well outlined in accompanying chapters.
   C. Unique to a discussion of these injuries in football and soccer are the techniques used to permit athletes to compete and practice.
   D. Rules governing casts and splints
      1. The NCAA rules regarding protective equipment in football state that "hard, abrasive or unyielding substances of the hand, wrist, forearm or elbow of any player is not allowed unless covered on all sides with closed-cell, slow recovery foam padding no less than 1/2 inch thick."
      2. "Casts are permitted only to protect a fracture or dislocation and must similarly be covered." Athletes requiring casts should have a protected cast for practice and games and a regular cast for normal wear. This can be accomplished by fashioning a fiberglass cast, bivalving it, and gluing foam padding to its surface.
   E. Protective splinting.
      1. Orthoplast splinting material custom-molded for dislocated or sprained fingers provides the athlete with strong, lightweight support.
      2. Off-the-shelf splinting is available for a variety of hand injuries including gamekeeper's splints, thumb spica splints, wrist braces, finger splints, and custom-made molded splints.

VII. Muscle Injury
   A. Muscles may be subjected to cramps, bruises, strains, or tears. Since soccer and football depend on speed for success, injuries to running muscles can markedly impair performance.
   B. Quadriceps muscle injury is the most muscle common injury in soccer, hamstrings the most common in football.[8]
   C. Muscle injury can be classified into six phases of healing (Table 74-1).[17]
   D. Experimental data[22] suggest that the musculotendinous unit is the most susceptible to injury in the muscle strain-stretch model.
      1. The injured muscle's ability to withstand tensile force is markedly diminished but not lost.
      2. Clinical implications are that early, limited ROM exercises are possible, but functional, high intensity loads place the muscle at increased risk of further damage.

TABLE 74-1. Muscle injury and healing

Time	Histological Findings	Treatment
0-6 hours	Peritrauma	Ice, elevation, compression
6-24 hours	Intense inflammation	Nonsteroidal antiinflammatory drugs, ice, protection
24-36 hours	Phagocytosis	Active ROM, ultrasound, no resistance work
3-6 days	Early healing	Ultrasound, heat, minimal resistance work
7-14 days	Established healing	Full ROM, heat, increased resistance
15-60 days	Restoration of function	Full resistance, normal and athletic movement

3. Techniques that anesthetize the muscle or otherwise reduce pain so a high degree of use can be maintained are not advisable.

E. Hamstring injury.
1. The three hamstring muscles are the semitendinosus, semimembranosus, and biceps femoris (long and short head). All three muscles have origins from the ischial tuberosity except for the short head of the biceps with origins on the femur.
2. The hamstrings span the hip and knee joint and exert force across both.
3. The biceps femoris is unique in having dual innervation of its long head (tibial portion of sciatic nerve) and short head (peroneal portion of sciatic nerve).
4. Hamstring injury commonly occurs in the swing phase of running when the hamstring is acting as a decelerator to the strong quadriceps contraction.
5. Rehabilitation of hamstring injuries should include stretching, spanning both hip and knee joints and emphasizing eccentric strengthening.
6. Hamstring contractile strength is dynamic: it changes with position and speed of contraction.
7. Time to recovery is highly variable (2-12 weeks).

F. Quadricep injury.
1. The quadricep muscle is composed of the rectus femoris, vastus lateralis, vastus intermedius, and vastus medialis. All four muscles converge to form the quadriceps tendon. Of the four, only the rectus femoris has an origin not on the femur (anterior-inferior iliac spine), and it, like the hamstrings, crosses two joints.
2. Injuries occur from forceful contractions, from excessive stretch, or from direct blows to an unprotected thigh.
3. The rectus femoris is the most common muscle injured.
4. Treatment goals are the same as for hamstrings: compression, icing, passive stretching, early mobilization, regain of ROM, and strengthening.
5. Quadriceps contusions and hemorrhage can be especially disabling. An innovative treatment utilizing 120 degrees of knee flexion applied immediately at time of injury and lasting 12-24 hours was found to markedly reduce swelling and time lost from competition.[3]

G Hip flexors.
1. The major hip flexors are the powerful iliopsoas and the rectus femoris, which function to bend the trunk, raise the leg, and stabilize the pelvis.
2. These injuries are seen in soccer athletes who are hit as they attempt to strike the ball, placing a hyperextension force on the hip flexors. Offensive linemen exploding from their stance or pass blocking also present with these injuries.
3. Isolated rectus femoris injury can be established by having the patient extend a dangling knee while lying flat on the examination table and palpating the proximal muscle.

H. Groin Injury: can encompass many diagnoses.
1. Specifically, the muscles most commonly involved in groin injury include the adductor longus, adductor brevis, and gracilis.
2. Adduction of the hip and stabilization of the pelvis during cutting maneuvers are their primary function. The strength of the adductors is remarkable and is comparable to that of the quadriceps.
3. The mechanism of injury is usually an eccentric stretch during a cutting maneuver. The location of the injury may be proximal at the adductor tendon insertion of the pubic tubercle and superior pubic ramus or in the body of the muscle belly.
4. Often, identification of the cause of groin pain is difficult owing to the large number of anatomical structures coursing through this area. The differential list includes inguinal hernia, adductor tendinitis, osteitis pubis, entrapment of the ilioinguinal, iliohypogastric, or genitofemoral nerves, rectus abdominis insertional tendinitis, or strain of the transversalis or external oblique fascia.
5. Treatment is similar to that for other muscle injuries and return to competition is allowed when nonpainful cutting and acceleration can take place.
6. Surgical treatment for chronic groin pain has been proposed, including adductor tenotomy with reinsertion distal to the pubic tubercle and herniorrhaphy.[1,19]

VIII. Knee Injury

A. Injuries to the knee in football and soccer can result from both trauma and training. No attempt will be made to describe all the specific injuries, their diagnoses, and rehabilitation.
1. Physicians caring for football and soccer athletes should be thoroughly familiar with knee examination, diagnoses, rehabilitation, and the surgical options available to athletes with injured knees.
2. The concept of "career-ending injury" is less applicable with the advent of reconstructive knee surgery and advanced rehabilitative techniques. A few general comments may be stated.
   a. An acutely swollen injured knee with hemarthroses has approximately a 75% statistical chance of anterior cruciate ligament (ACL) injury.[14]
   b. There is approximately a 50% chance of associated meniscus injury with ACL disruptions.
   c. ACL reconstruction appears to prevent subsequent development of meniscal injury.[6]
   d. The sensitivity of clinical examination by experienced orthopedists to diagnose arthroscopically proven ACL injury is approximately 60%.[15]

B. Bracing knees in football and soccer.
   1. Each year, millions of dollars are spent by school systems in hope of preventing serious knee injury. Even though many investigations on the possible benefits of prophylactic knee bracing have been undertaken, there is no clear consensus of opinion regarding its efficacy.
   2. One of the tendencies found in a recent collaborative study by the Big Ten was an increase in the "survival" time of athletes wearing braces to serious knee injury. Currently, there are no recommendations regarding the advisability of prophylactic knee bracing.

IX. Ankle Injury
   A. One of the most frequently encountered injuries in all sport and the most common injury in soccer.
   B. There are three types of ankle sprains.
      1. Lateral sprains from an inversion/plantar-flexed stress.
      2. Medial or deltoid from an eversion stress.
      3. High ankle sprain from a dorsiflexed/rotational stress.
   C. Ankle injuries can be classified into I, II, and III degree injuries based on the extent of injury of the ligaments involved.
   D. Treatment is best accomplished with immediate compression with horseshoe-shaped pads and elastic wraps or off-the-shelf compressive stirrups combined with icing, rest, and antiinflammatories.
   E. Functional rehabilitation with orthotic support allows for more prompt return to activity. Emphasis is placed on reacquisition of full ROM and proprioceptive awareness. Return to competition is allowed when high speed running, cutting, and jumping can be accomplished without impairment and pain.
   F. Conditions that predispose to ankle injury include tight gastrocnemius muscles with associated Achilles' tendon inflexibility, rearfoot supination, loss of prioprioception from previous injuries, incompetent supporting ligaments, peroneal nerve or muscle injury, and traditional cleated shoes versus soccer style shoes.

X. Syndesmotic Ankle Sprains
   A. Although injury to the lateral ankle ligaments accounts for 85% of all ankle sprains in sport, the high ankle or syndesmotic tibia-fibula sprain is especially troublesome in football and soccer athletes.[21]
   B. Whereas the lateral and medial ankle ligaments span the ankle (talocrural) joint, the high ankle ligaments are confined to the tibia-fibula interface and function to maintain the integrity of the ankle mortise and fibular motion. During ankle dorsiflexion the anterior tibia-fibula ligament resists the normal posterior displacement and external rotation of the fibula.
   C. Injuries to these ligaments can be isolated or associated with medial deltoid sprains and fibular fractures.
      1. The mechanism of injury is that of an externally or internally directed rotational force applied to a dorsiflexed and axially loaded ankle as demonstrated in the posture of a pass blocking lineman or a soccer athlete planting a foot in preparation for a kick.
      2. The pain of high ankle sprains is worse in a weight-bearing position and during take-off from a stance position. Recovery is prolonged in comparison to lateral sprains.

XI. Prophylactic Taping and Bracing[20]
   A. Taping ankles in athletics is a time-honored ritual. Studies evaluating taped ankles demonstrate enhanced resistance to inversion that quickly

dissipates during competition. Interest in reducing time and cost of taping ankles has spawned the development of off-the-shelf prophylactic braces.

B. In a study of South African soccer athletes, prophylactic bracing was found to significantly reduce the incidence of recurrent sprain in a previously injured ankle. No benefit from bracing was demonstrated in ankles not previously injured. The study suggests that only athletes with previous ankle injuries should be braced or taped.

XII. Turf Toe[5]

A. Turf toe is a hyperextension injury to the first metatarsal-phalangeal joint. Its occurrence parallels the development of artificial surfaces and more flexible soccer-type footwear.

B. Athletes with less than 60 degrees of extension at the metatarsal-phalangeal joint are more susceptible to this injury.

C. Stiff-soled shoes that resist forefoot extension help in the treatment and prevention of this painful injury.

D. The extent of the injury ranges from a mild capsular sprain to frank subluxation. Return to competition is hampered by the athlete's inability to push off.

XIII. Stress Injuries

A. Football and soccer athletes are subjected to the same rigors of year-round training as many other sports participants and as a consequence suffer from overuse phenomena.

1. Stress fractures of the spine, pelvis, hip, femur, tibia, fibula, tarsal navicular, metatarsals, and sesamoids have all been described.
2. Tendinitis of the shoulder rotators, iliopsoas, iliotibial band, adductors, quadriceps, patella, peroneals, and Achilles' tendon are common occurrence.

B. Bone stress and training.

1. Bone stress appears to peak 3 weeks after the initiation of a more intense training regimen, suggesting that a decrease in training intensity may be appropriate at that time.
2. Athletes should not attempt to train through bone pain. The early recognition of bone stress injury and institution of non–weight-bearing training may substantially shorten the recovery phase of stress injury.[2]

C. The female athlete triad and training.

1. Amenorrhea, disordered eating, and osteoporosis are an interrelated triad of medical problems prevalent in athletic women who are predisposed to overuse injury.
2. With increasing participation of young women in soccer, attention to frequency of menstrual periods, calorie intake, and bone health is necessary.[12]

D. Training and the kinetic chain.

1. The term kinetic chain implies a functional connection between all the working parts of an exercising extremity. A breakdown in one link of the chain influences the action of an adjacent link.
2. Accordingly, evaluation of an overuse injury merits a search for other potential causative factors along the chain. Likewise, rehabilitation must proceed in the same manner.
3. With the advent of resistance training in soccer and especially football, imbalances in muscle strength may inadvertently occur that disrupt the kinetic chain. An example is hamstring/quadricep strength

and its effect on hamstring injury. If concentric muscle development is overemphasized, eccentric injury is likely to occur.

References

1. Akermark C, Johansson C: Tenotomy of the adductor longus tendon in the treatment of chronic groin pain in athletes, *AMJ Sports Med* 20(11):640-644, 1992.
2. Arendt E: Stress injuries to bone, AMSSM Annual Meeting, Palm Springs, CA, June 1994.
3. Aronen J: Quad contusion: minimizing the length of time before return to full activity, AMSSM Annual Meeting, Palm Springs, CA, June 1994.
4. Cantu R: Cerebral concussion in sport, *Sports Med* 14(1):64-74, 1992.
5. Coughlin M: Conditions of the forefoot in DeLee J, Drez D, editors: *Orthopedic Sports Medicine,* Philadelphia, 1994, WB Saunders, pp 1859-1865.
6. Daniel D et al: Fate of the ACL injured patient: a prospective outcome study, *Am J Sports Med* 22(5):632-645, 1994.
7. Garth W: Evaluating and treating brachial plexus injuries, *J Musculoskeletal Med* pp 55-67, Oct 1994.
8. Gordon D: Physiotherapy of muscle injuries of the lower limb, *J Chartered Soc Physiother* 61(4): 102, 1975.
9. Kelly J et al: Concussion in sports, *JAMA* 266(20):2867-2869, 1991.
10. Matthews WB: Footballer's migraine, *Br Med J* (2):326-327, 1972.
11. Meyer S et al: Cervical spine stenoses and stingers in collegiate football players, *Am J Sports Med* 22(3):158-167, 1994.
12. Nattiv A et al: The female athlete triad: the interrelatedness of disordered eating, amenorrhea, and osteoporosis in the athletic woman, *Clin Sports Med,* pp 405-418, April 1994.
13. *1993-94 NCAASports Medicine Handbook,* ed. 7 Publications Ed, Overland Park, KS.
14. Noyes Frank, Bassett W: Arthroscopy in acute traumatic hemarthroses of the knee, *J Bone Joint Surg* 62a:678, 1980.
15. Oberlander M, Shalvoy R, Hughston J: The accuracy of the clinical knee examination documented by arthroscopy: a prospective study, *Am J Sports Med* 21(6):773-778, 1993.
16. Oder J et al: Incidence of cervical spine stenoses in professional and rookie football players, *Am J Sports Med* 18:507-509, 1990.
17. Reid D: *Sports Injury: Assessment and Rehabilitation,* New York, 1992, Churchill Livingstone, pp 85-103.
18. Sedden H: *Surgical Disorders of the Peripheral Nerves,* Baltimore, 1972, Williams & Wilkins, pp 174-198.
19. Smedberg S et al: Herniography in athletes with groin pain, *Am J Surg* 149:378, 1985.
20. Surve I et al: A fivefold reduction in the incidence of recurrent ankle sprains in soccer players using the sports stirrup orthoses, *Am J Sports Med* 22(5):601-607, 1994.
21. Taylor D, Bassett F: Syndesmotic ankle sprains, *Phys Sports Med* 21(12):39-51, 1993.
22. Taylor D et al: Experimental muscle strain injury: early functional and structural deficits and the increased risk of reinjury, *Am J Sports Med* 21(2):190-195, 1993.
23. Torg J: *Athletic Injuries to the Head, Neck, and Face,* ed 2, St Louis, 1991, Mosby–Year Book.
24. Tysvaer A: Head and neck injuries in soccer: impact of minor trauma, *Sports Med* 14(3):200-213, 1992.

CHAPTER 75

Track and Field

Carol L. Otis, MD

I. Introduction
  A. Many diverse sports.
  B. Historically, some of the oldest athletic events.
    1. Outgrowth of training for soldiers.
    2. Male dominated.
  C. Emphasis on the *individual.*
  D. Winning judged by competition against others and against standards.

II. Sport Specificity of Training, Competition and Injury: Know Each Sport Individually
  A. Understand what is involved in training, competing, and being successful for each sport.
  B. What types of injuries are seen in training.
  C. What injuries in competition.
  D. What environmental factors affect the event.

III. Specific Events
  A. Throwing events involve the greatest risk to injury for spectators/others: shot put, discus, javelin, hammer.
    1. Sports involve technique.
    2. Training injuries.
      a. Upper extremity.
        i. Acromioclavicular (AC) joint.
        ii. Shoulder.
        iii. Upper arm.
        iv. Elbow.
        v. Wrist.
        vi. Fingers.
      b. Back: imbalance of throwing side.
      c. Lower extremity.
    3. Competition injuries/illness.
      a. Injuries to competitors.

- b. Medical concerns: hydration
- c. Injuries to noncompetitors from thrown item.

B. Jumping Events.
1. Long jump.
   a. Technical: four phases.
      i. Approach.
      ii. Take-off.
      iii. Aerial.
      iv. Landing.
   b. Injuries in each phase.
      i. Approach: muscle strains, strains, falls.
      ii. Takeoff: knee injuries, ankle injuries, impact deceleration.
      iii. Aerial.
      iv. Landing impact.
2. High jump.
   a. Three styles.
      i. Eastern-scissor kick.
      ii. Western roll.
      iii. Fosbury flop.
   b. Four phases.
      i. Run-up.
      ii. Planting.
      iii. Aerial over bar.
      iv. Landing.
3. Triple jump.

C. Pole vault.
1. Technically difficult.
2. Requires speed, strength, timing, balance.
3. Narrow margin of error. Catastrophic if injury occurs.
4. Equipment: fiberglass poles. May snap at take-off.
5. Four phases.
   a. Run-up.
   b. Plant pole: complex motion.
   c. Aerial over bar.
   d. Landing.

D. Sprint events.
1. Block starts.
2. Anaerobic activity.
3. Three phases of run.
   a. Start.
   b. Middle.
   c. Finish.
4. Training injuries.
   a. Muscle balance: hamstrings/quadriceps strains, tears.
   b. Toe running: imbalance to gastrocnemius and toe flexors.

E. Hurdles.
1. Timing critical in running (not jumping) over hurdle.
2. Flexibility important.
3. Overuse injuries to lower extremities, pelvis.
4. Contusions to medial aspect of trailing leg.

F. Endurance events 1500 m and up.
1. Aerobic training with distance, time, intensity, and surface as cofactors to injury.
2. Injuries usually due to overuse.
   a. Tendinitis.

b. Bursitis.
c. Stress fractures.
3. Surface: pavement (concrete) three times more likely to cause injury.
4. Experience.
5. Equipment.
a. Shoe wear loses shock absorption after 250-400 miles.
b. Spikes for racing.
6. Environmental factors more important.

IV. Coverage of Events
A. Track meets.
B. Road races.
C. Triathlons.
D. Endurance events.

V. Coverage of Traveling Teams: Pretrip Organization
A. Review athlete's history.
B. Advise on jet lag, weather, food, customs, dress.
1. Vaccinations, other health precautions.
2. see International Amateur Athletic Federation (IAAF) medical manual or USA Track and Field Team Physician manual for further information.

VI. Environmental Hazards
A. Hypothermia.
B. Hyperthermia.
C. Surface.

VII. Special Concerns for Track Athletes
A. Drug Testing.
1. USA Track and Field: random year-round.
2. NCAA: at events.
3. IAAF: at events
4. Call U.S. Olympic Committee (USOC) Drug Info Hotline: 1-800-233-0393.
B. B_{12} and other requests.
C. Psychology.
D. Sport massage.
E. Female athlete triad.
1. Amenorrhea.
2. Disordered eating.
3. Osteoporosis.
4. A concern for all female athletes. May be more prevalent in distance runners.
a. Myth of "thinner is faster."
b. Myth that amenorrhea is a marker of training adequacy.
F. Medical problems.
1. Asthma.
a. May present as exercise-induced asthma only.
b. Variable symptoms.
c. Multiple effective drug regimens. Begin with pretraining inhalers.
d. Clear all medications with USOC Drug Info Hotline 1-800-233-0393.
2. Gastrointestinal disturbance.
a. Reflux.
b. Gastritis: look for use of nonsteroidal antiinflammatory drugs.
c. Diarrhea: common.
i. Try diet modifications.
ii. Use nonsedating antimotility drugs (Imodium).

3. Incontinence: Kegel exercises.
4. Screen for anemia.
   a. Common in runners.
   b. Pseudoanemia vs. iron deficiency.
5. Hematuria.
   a. May be due to bladder contusions (male) or renal ischemia.
   b. If hematuria does not clear with stopping sports activity for 1-2 days, do work-up.

CHAPTER 76

Basketball Injuries

Michael D. Jackson, MD

James L. Moeller, MD

David O. Hough, MD

I. General Overview
   A. The sport of basketball predisposes the athlete to significant injury as a result of the running, jumping, cutting, pivoting, and explosive movements required for sudden acceleration and deceleration.
   B. With the ever increasing popularity of the sport, injury management and prevention have become important. This is especially true for the nonelite athlete as studies have shown that the majority of injuries occur among the nonprofessional population.[4]
   C. Epidemiological data also suggest that the injury risk is greatest in female basketball players.[9,22,28]
   D. Studies on injury rates have demonstrated that the most common injuries in basketball players involve the ankle, followed by the knee and foot.[2,10,28]

II. Lower Extremity
   A. Ankle injuries.
      1. Lateral (inversion) ankle sprains.
         a. The mechanism of injury typically involves landing of the body weight on the foot while it is plantar flexed and internally rotated. This may occur as a result of stepping on another player's foot and rolling the ankle inward or landing on the foot as it rolls inward.
         b. Physical examination typically reveals:
            (1) Tenderness over the lateral ankle ligaments. Anterior talofibular ligament (ATFL) is most commonly injured followed by the calcaneofibular (CFL) ligament.
            (2) Edema and bruising over the lateral aspect of the ankle.
            (3) Decreased range of motion with dorsiflexion and plantar flexion.
            (4) Positive anterior drawer if ATFL is disrupted.
            (5) Positive talar tilt if CFL is disrupted.

(6) Pain with syndesmosis compression test if the tibiofibular syndesmosis is disrupted. Tenderness over the distal tibiofibular syndesmosis is also typically present.

c. Lateral ankle sprains are classified by the degree of ligamentous damage.
   (1) Grade I indicates stretching of the ATFL with some of the fibers torn but without significant ligamentous disruption.
   (2) Grade II indicates significant disruption of the ATFL, typically with a partial tear of the CFL.
   (3) Grade III indicates complete tear of the ATFL and CFL with possible disruption of the posterior talofibular ligament.

d. Treatment of lateral ankle sprains is based primarily on classification of the injury.
   (1) All sprains should be treated with the rest, ice, compression, and elevation (RICE) principle.
   (2) Immobilization.
      (a) With grade I and grade II sprains this may be accomplished with taping or an orthotic ankle brace.
      (b) Grade III sprains may require casting, but rarely indicated.
   (3) Rehabilitation.
      (a) Begin with early range of motion (ROM) exercises to restore normal mechanics.
      (b) Strengthening of the lower extremity musculature is added when ROM is pain-free.
      (c) Proprioceptive training should be started early to help prevent recurrent sprains.
      (d) Finally, sport-specific training should be added (i.e., running, jumping, cutting, and pivoting).
      (e) When the athlete is ready to return to competition, he or she may benefit from prophylactic ankle bracing and/or taping.

2. Medial (eversion) ankle sprain.
   a. Mechanism of injury is typically dorsiflexion combined with eversion, or external rotation of the foot, particularly when cutting to the opposite side. This type of sprain is less common than the inversion sprain but has the potential to be more severe.
   b. Eversion sprain typically results in tear of the medial deltoid ligament. There may also be injury to the anterior inferior tibiofibular ligament, the interosseous membrane, and if severe, avulsion fracture of the medial malleolus.
   c. Physical examination is similar to that for inversion sprain but should also include eversion stress of the deltoid ligament and palpation of the distal fibula for tenderness and possible fracture.
   d. Treatment consists of general ankle rehabilitation principles as previously described.

3. Peroneal tendons.
   a. Basketball requires a significant amount of lateral movement and as a result requires adequate stability of the peroneal tendons (both longus and brevis).
   b. The primary functions of the peroneus longus and peroneus brevis muscles are eversion and plantar flexion of the foot. These muscles are therefore very important in lateral push-off.
   c. Peroneal tendon rupture is rare, whereas tendinitis or strain is frequently associated with other injuries of the foot or ankle.

(1) Peroneal tendon strain is commonly associated with inversion ankle sprains.
(2) Peroneal tendinitis is often an overuse injury occurring after injury to the opposite foot or ankle.

d. Symptoms are generally localized to the lateral ankle or over the peroneal muscle bellies with tendinitis.
e. Tear of the peroneal longus tendon typically occurs at the sesamoid (os peroneum) adjacent to the cuboid tunnel where the tendon turns from the lateral aspect of the foot medially.
    (1) This is typically elicited by pain and weakness in the area of the cuboid.
    (2) Tendon integrity can be assessed by placing the foot in dorsiflexion and inversion, and asking the patient to return the foot to neutral while resisting this motion.
f. Treatment is variable.
    (1) Tendinitis responds to stretching and strengthening of the peroneal muscles.
        (a) Physical therapy and the use of modalities may also be beneficial in speeding recovery.
        (b) Nonsteroidal antiinflammatories (NSAIDs) are helpful in decreasing inflammation and symptoms.
    (2) Tendon strains respond to the general principles of ankle rehabilitation.
    (3) Tendon rupture is best treated by surgical repair.

4. Anterior ankle impingement.
    a. This results from repetitive forced dorsiflexion of the foot as a result of frequent jumping.
    b. The repetitive dorsiflexion results in osteophyte formation on the contact points of the tibia and talus.
    c. As the osteophytes increase in size, dorsiflexion of the ankle becomes restricted.
    d. Physical examination reveals pain with forced dorsiflexion of the ankle and tenderness to palpation over the osteophyte.
    e. Diagnosis is made by lateral radiographs with the ankle in a dorsiflexed position. This will reveal osteophyte formation with abutment of the tibia and talus.
    f. Treatment may consist of heel elevation, the use of a negative heel, or both.[16] Surgical removal of the osteophyte may be necessary if size increases and range of dorsiflexion decreases.
    g. This pathology is felt to be the result of lateral ankle ligamentous instability in most cases. When present, the patient benefits from stabilization of the ligamentous laxity.

B. Knee injuries.
    1. Anterior cruciate ligament.
        a. As a result of the running, jumping, pivoting, cutting, and deceleration required, basketball places the anterior cruciate ligament (ACL) at significant risk of injury.
        b. The mechanism most commonly causing ACL injury in basketball is deceleration and change of direction when the tibia is externally or internally rotated. The athlete typically feels a sudden pain in the knee associated with a pop or tearing sensation usually followed shortly by effusion and the inability to continue competition.

c. Physical examination reveals anterior laxity of the knee. This is best demonstrated by Lachman's and the pivot-shift test.
d. Magnetic resonance imaging (MRI) of the knee is a useful tool in the diagnosis of ACL injury, especially in cases where the physical examination is equivocal.
e. Surgical reconstruction is clearly the trend in management of the ACL injuries. In adolescent athletes with open growth plates, conservative treatment of rehabilitation focusing on preferential strengthening of the hamstrings combined with custom-fitted braces may be the treatment of choice.

2. Meniscal injuries.
   a. Meniscal tears typically result from internally rotating (lateral meniscus) or externally rotating (medial meniscus) the axially loaded, partially flexed knee.
   b. The athlete will usually report gradually increasing pain and, possibly, swelling of the knee.
      (1) In most cases the athlete is able to continue competition for a short period after the injury.
      (2) History typically reveals decreased ROM, locking, and give-way of the knee.
   c. Physical examination is often positive for joint line tenderness. Specific meniscal tests include:
      (1) McMurray's test.
      (2) Apley compression test.
   d. MRI is often beneficial in the diagnosis of meniscal injury.
   e. Most meniscal tears require some form of surgical intervention. Options include:
      (1) Surgical repair (usually peripheral tears).
      (2) Partial meniscectomy.
      (3) Total meniscectomy.
3. Medial and lateral collateral ligament sprains.
   a. Medial collateral ligament (MCL) and lateral collateral ligament (LCL) sprains result from direct valgus and varus forces, respectively, to the stationary knee.
   b. Physical examination.
      (1) Tenderness may be elicited anywhere along the course of the ligament.
      (2) Laxity may be present with varus (LCL) or valgus (MCL) stress.
   c. These injuries respond well to conservative treatment.
      (1) Active and passive ROM exercises.
      (2) Quadriceps and hamstring strengthening.
      (3) Orthotic knee bracing at 30-40 degrees of flexion, for variable periods depending on severity.
      (4) Progressive functional exercise.
4. Patellar tendinitis.
   a. Patellar tendinitis is often referred to as "jumper's knee."
   b. The jumping, sprinting, sudden acceleration, and deceleration required in basketball predispose the athlete to tendinitis around the knee.
      (1) The repetitive forces generated across the knee with these activities may result in microscopic tears and inflammation of the patellar tendon.

   (2) These pathological changes usually occur at the distal pole of the patella or just proximal to the tibial tubercle.
  c. Symptoms are typically insidious in onset and associated with exercise, especially jumping and landing.
  d. Physical examination reveals tenderness to palpation of the patellar tendon, typically at the inferior pole. The "wet leather sign" may also be present on palpation.
  e. In adolescents, "jumper's knee" often refers to Osgood-Schlatter disease.
   (1) This is patellar tendinitis combined with inflammation of the apophysis of the tibial tubercle.
   (2) Symptoms are similar to patellar tendinitis.
   (3) Physical examination will reveal tenderness to palpation of the tibial tubercle as well as the patellar tendon. After symptoms have been present for a long period the tibial tubercle will become prominent.
  f. Treatment for these two conditions is conservative.
   (1) Activity is limited by the patient's symptoms.
   (2) Hamstring and quadriceps stretching and strengthening are initiated. Strengthening should include an eccentric program with partial squats.
   (3) Physical therapy and modalities to include ice, ultrasound, and, occasionally, phonophoresis or iontophoresis may be beneficial. Physical therapy should include sport-specific activities such as jumping.
   (4) NSAIDs are helpful.
   (5) Patellar tendon taping may help decrease forces across the patella during activity.[17]
  g. Chronic patellar tendinitis may result in tendon rupture. This requires surgical repair.
5. Patellofemoral dysfunction.
  a. Forces generated across the patella in basketball place the patellofemoral joint at significant risk for tracking problems. This occurs more commonly in women as a result of increased Q angles.
  b. Symptoms include:
   (1) Anterior knee pain with activity, especially with ambulating stairs.
   (2) Anterior knee pain when sitting with the knee flexed for long periods.
   (3) Grinding sensation with knee flexion.
  c. Physical examination may reveal:
   (1) Patella crepitance.
   (2) Increased Q angle.
   (3) Patella alta.
   (4) Squinting patella.
   (5) Vastus medialis obliquis (VMO) atrophy.
  d. Treatment should concentrate on quadriceps strengthening.
   (1) VMO exercises.
    (a) Leg extensions from 30 to 0 degrees.
    (b) Straight leg raises.
   (2) McConnell taping and orthotic knee bracing may also be beneficial.

(3) Surgical intervention is reserved for patients who fail conservative therapy, depending on age and level of activity.

6. Semimembranosus tendinitis.
   a. Presents as vague medial knee pain. May mimic meniscal tear.
   b. Treatment includes rest, icing, NSAIDs, ultrasound, and stretching.

C. Lower leg injuries.

1. Shin splints.
   a. The term *shin splints* commonly refers to posterior tibial muscle tendinitis and periosteal irritation. Also referred to as *medial tibial stress syndrome.*
   b. Symptoms are typically insidious in onset. Presents as pain and swelling over the posteromedial crest of the tibia diffusely that become worse with activity.
   c. Physical examination.
      (1) Diffuse tenderness over the muscles attachment to the tibia.
      (2) Small hematomas may be palpated over the posteromedial aspect of the tibia.
      (3) Pain and weakness with testing of the posterior tibial and flexor hallucis longus muscles.
      (4) Localized tenderness over the tibia may indicate stress fracture.
   d. Treatment is most often conservative.
      (1) Ice massage to the painful area.
      (2) NSAIDs.
      (3) Decrease running and jumping.
      (4) Arch taping and shoe orthotics may be beneficial.
      (5) Physical therapy directed at strengthening the posterior tibial, flexor digitorum longus, flexor hallucis longus, and foot intrinsic muscles.
2. Achilles' tendinitis.
   a. Occurs frequently in athletes who jump repetitively.
   b. Symptoms may occur gradually or after an acute event. Tenderness at the insertion to the calcaneus or over the distal Achilles' tendon.
   c. Physical examination.
      (1) Tenderness to palpation of the tendinous area.
      (2) Palpation may reveal nodules, palpable defect, or crepitation ("wet leather" sign).
   d. Treatment initially should be conservative.
      (1) Ice massage after activity.
      (2) Relative rest.
      (3) Stretching and strengthening of the posterior leg musculature (eccentric program).
      (4) NSAIDs.
      (5) Physical therapy to include iontophoresis or phonophoresis.
      (6) Heel lifts and orthotics.
      (7) Surgical intervention is reserved for patients who fail to respond to conservative therapy.
3. Achilles' tendon rupture.
   a. Occurs in sports associated with forceful push-off of the foot.
   b. Patient experiences acute onset of pain in the posterior aspect of the lower leg.
      (1) Feels like a shot in the back of the leg.
      (2) Athlete will have difficulty or be unable to ambulate.

c. Physical examination reveals markedly decreased or absent foot plantar flexion when the calf is squeezed while the patient lies prone.
d. Treatment commonly is surgical repair. Casting is also an option.

D. Foot injuries.
 1. Plantar fasciitis.
  a. Presents as arch pain of gradual onset. Pain is worse in the morning with the first steps and with activity.
  b. Physical examination typically reveals tenderness on the sole of the foot in the area of the plantar fascia's insertion to the calcaneus and tight heel cords.
  c. Treatment options include icing, arch taping, heel lifts, orthotics, NSAIDs, and tension night splints.
  d. Activity is limited by the athlete's symptoms.
 2. Sesamoiditis.
  a. Inflammation of the tissues around the sesamoids commonly affects the medial (tibial) sesamoid more than the lateral (fibular) sesamoid.
  b. Cavus feet with a rigid, plantar-flexed first ray, a high arch, and a tight Achilles' tendon are more commonly affected.
  c. Physical examination typically reveals localized tenderness, swelling occasionally, and discomfort with passive dorsiflexion of the foot.
  d. Treatment options include ice, massage, iontophoresis, ultrasound, NSAIDs, and orthotics. Surgical removal frequently is not beneficial and may result in a biomechanical muscle imbalance and subsequent deformity.
  e. Stress fractures or acute fractures of the sesamoids may occur. These can be differentiated from bipartite bone by appearance on plain radiographs or, more commonly, by bone scan.
 3. Calcaneal beak fractures.
  a. Adduction and plantar flexion of the foot predispose the athlete to fracture of the beak of the os calcis.
  b. The chief complaint is pain and point tenderness in the area of the os calcis. This is located one fingerbreadth anterior to the area halfway between the lateral malleolus and the base of the fifth metatarsal.
  c. Treatment typically involves a non–weight-bearing cast for 4 weeks followed by a walking cast for 4 weeks.
 4. Navicular avulsion fracture.
  a. Mechanism of injury is acute eversion of the foot.
  b. The athlete complains of pain in the area of the navicular bone.
  c. Nonunion is possible after conservative treatment with casting.
 5. Os trigonum fractures.
  a. The os trigonum is an accessory bone on the lateral tubercle of the posterior talus. Found in approximately 10% of the population.
  b. In basketball, fracture of the os trigonum typically occurs when one player steps on the foot of another player, forcing the second player to fall posteriorly, causing hyperplantar flexion of the foot.
  c. The athlete, acutely, presents with pain in the posterolateral ankle and decreased range of motion in both the ankle and subtalar joints.

d. Physical examination will reveal pain with passive hyperextension or active flexion of the great toe.
e. Diagnosis is confirmed by plain radiographs.
f. Treatment is typically casting and non–weight-bearing for 4-6 weeks. Surgical excision is occasionally necessary.

6. Avulsion fracture of the base of the fifth metatarsal.
   a. Mechanism of injury is similar to that of an inversion ankle sprain.
   b. The athlete commonly presents with an inversion ankle sprain and point tenderness at the base of the fifth metatarsal.
   c. Diagnosis is confirmed by plain radiographs.
   d. Treatment consists of either casting or surgical pinning.
7. Cuboid subluxation.
   a. Cuboid subluxation is rare.
   b. This results in midfoot pain on the lateral plantar aspect of the foot.
   c. Diagnosis may be confirmed radiographically. The cuboid may be displaced plantarly with increased joint space dorsally and decreased joint space plantarly.
   d. Treatment consists of manipulation of the cuboid. This may be accomplished by the cuboid thrust or the cuboid squeeze.

III. Upper Extremity Injuries
   A. Finger injuries; the distal interphalangeal joint (DIP).
      1. Mallet finger: the most common DIP injury.
         a. Extensor tendon injury that occurs when a sudden flexion force is applied to an actively extended DIP: this usually occurs when the ball strikes the tip of the digit.
         b. Physical examination reveals distal phalanx droop and inability to actively extend the DIP fully.
         c. Radiography should be performed to rule out fracture or subluxation.
         d. Treatment.
            (1) Splint DIP in full extension continuously for 4-6 weeks. Proximal interphalangeal joint (PIP) may be left free.
            (2) Wean from splint over next 2-4 weeks.
            (3) Splint for athletics over the next 2-3 months.
      2. Jersey finger.
         a. Flexor digitorum profundus tendon avulsion occurs when DIP is forcefully extended while being actively flexed. Fourth digit is most commonly involved.
         b. Physical examination reveals swelling and tenderness over the flexor sheath and lack of active DIP flexion.
         c. Radiographs may reveal an avulsion fracture.
         d. Surgical treatment is required.
   B. Finger injuries; the PIP.
      1. Boutonnière deformity.
         a. Due to disruption of the central extensor tendon slip at its insertion into the middle phalanx. Mechanism: sudden forceful flexion of actively extended PIP.
         b. Four grades are described, with each sequential step being more difficult to treat and having a worse prognosis.
            (1) Grade I: the deformity is passively correctable.
               (a) Swollen PIP.
               (b) Dorsal PIP tenderness to palpation.
               (c) Dorsal pain and weakness on resisted PIP extension.

(d) Active extension may be possible.
(2) Grade II: PIP flexion contracture <30 degrees, not passively correctable.
(3) Grade III: PIP flexion contracture > 30 degrees and loss of flexion of the DIP.
(4) Grade IV: fixed PIP flexion contracture and degenerative change in the joint.

c. Treatment.
(1) Grade I and II injuries.
(a) Splint PIP in full extension, leave DIP free for 6 weeks continuously.
(b) Active and passive ROM exercises of DIP to remobilize the lateral bands and allow the central slip to heal at its proper length.
(c) Night splinting and protection during play should be continued for an additional 4 weeks.
(2) Grade III: treatment involves surgery, but splinting or casting should be used prior to surgery in an attempt to correct the flexion contracture.
(3) Grade IV: treatment is operative. Surgery may yield little active motion gain. Arthrodesis is often necessary.

C. Wrist injuries.
1. Scaphoid fractures.
a. The scaphoid bone is unique in that it bridges the two rows of carpal bones, which makes it more susceptible to injury.
b. Mechanism of injury is usually a fall onto the outstretched hand.
c. Physical examination findings.
(1) Tenderness and swelling in the anatomical snuff box.
(2) Pain with active wrist dorsiflexion and radial deviation.
d. Radiographs are often negative (5% to 15%).
(1) Follow-up films should be obtained in 2 weeks if initial films are negative.
(2) Bone scan should be considered if diagnosis is required sooner.
e. Treatment. Long arm thumb spica cast for 6 weeks followed by short arm thumb spica cast until fracture is healed.
(1) Average healing time for scaphoid waist fractures is 9-12 weeks.
(2) Proximal pole fractures may take up to 24 weeks to heal due to the distal blood supply of the scaphoid.
f. Complications.
(1) Nonunion: this is reported at 3% to 10%.
(2) Avascular necrosis: occurs in 30% of wrist fractures.
2. Hamate fractures.
a. Usually results from a fall onto the hypothenar eminence.
b. Physical examination findings.
(1) Palmar ulnar wrist pain.
(2) Neurovascular symptoms in the ulnar nerve/artery distribution may be present.
c. Radiographs are often negative, and this leads to a delay in diagnosis.
(1) Oblique and carpal tunnel views may be helpful.
(2) Bone scan or computerized tomography (CT) may be useful.
d. Treatment of choice is excision of the fracture fragment. If diagnosis is made early, a period of immobilization prior to surgical referral may be attempted.
3. Scapholunate dissociation: the most common wrist ligament injury.

a. Mechanism is usually a fall on an outstretched hand. The scaphoid rotates from a longitudinal to a horizontal position and the lunate angulates in the opposite direction.
b. Physical examination findings.
(1) Pain over the dorsoradial wrist.
(2) Pain over the scapholunate joint.
(3) Positive Watson test. Subluxation of the proximal scaphoid when pressure on the distal pole is combined with radial wrist deviation.
c. Radiographs.
(1) Anterior-posterior views (AP): will reveal a >2-mm gap between the scaphoid and lunate if the ligament is totally disrupted (the "Terry Thomas" sign).
(2) Posterior-anterior (PA) clenched fist view may accentuate any instability.
(3) Arthrograms may be needed for definitive diagnosis.
d. Treatment is generally by closed reduction and K wire stabilization.
(1) Open reduction may be necessary.
(2) Partial ligament injuries with no radiographic changes may be treated by thumb spica cast for 6 weeks.

D. Shoulder injuries: rotator cuff injuries.
1. Due to repetitive overhead activities such as shooting the basketball.
a. Supraspinatus tendon is where most problems arise because it passes in such close proximity to the coracoacromial ligament, the acromioclavicular joint, and the bony roof of the acromion.
b. Hand dominance seems to contribute to the occurrence of shoulder symptoms as most patients feel symptoms on the dominant side.
2. Physical examination findings.
a. Rotator cuff muscle weakness.
b. Tenderness over anterior and superior aspects of the glenohumeral joint.
c. Impingement signs may be present.
3. Treatment.
a. Regular icing.
b. Physical therapy modalities to decrease pain and inflammation.
c. NSAIDs.
d. Relative rest: especially a decrease in the amount of overhead activity.
e. Rotator cuff strengthening.

IV. Back Injuries
A. In older populations, muscular injuries are the most common type of back injury encountered. Other possible etiologies include intervertebral disc disease and degenerative changes, among others. In younger populations, muscular injuries are still the most common cause of back pain; however, back pain in younger athletes requires thorough evaluation.
B. Pars interarticularis injuries are due to repeated stresses on the posterior elements of the spine.
1. The patient presents with back pain that is usually worse during activity, especially running and jumping. The pain is often relieved by rest.
2. Physical examination may reveal tenderness to palpation of the back just lateral to the spinous processes in the lower lumbar region. Pain may be exacerbated by hyperextension.

3. Radiographic examination should be performed if pars interarticularis lesions are suspected.
    a. Oblique radiographs may show sclerosis or fracture in the area of the pars (a collar on the "Scottie dog" or a broken neck of the "dog").
    b. If radiographic findings are negative and suspicion is high, bone scan should be performed.
4. Treatment includes rest from the inciting activities. Bracing may be needed, especially in cases where bilateral pars lesions and subsequent forward slippage of one vertebral body on another has occurred (spondylolisthesis). Conditioning of the back is an important part of the treatment of this type of back injury. Conditioning includes flexibility, strength, and endurance training.

V. Facial and Head Injuries

A. In the United States, basketball is second only to baseball in the number and severity of eye injuries and oral trauma sustained while playing organized sports.
1. Organized basketball only accounts for 20% of basketball injuries.
2. No regulations for prevention of facial injuries currently exist for basketball (i.e., mandatory mouthguards or eye protection).

B. Facial lacerations.
1. As for any laceration, thorough cleansing, irrigation, and debridement are essential before closing the wound.
2. Closure under sterile conditions should be performed as soon as possible to ensure the best possible outcome.

C. Nasal bone fractures.
1. Nasal bone fractures occur most commonly due to a lateral force that may lead to significant dislocation of the fracture fragments. Other injuries should be ruled out by examination.
    a. Septal hematoma: a collection of blood between the cartilage and mucoperichondrium that may lead to collapse of the nasal dorsum through the loss of septal cartilage support due to abscess or pressure necrosis.
    b. Septal fracture.
2. Treatment includes realignment of the fracture fragments. Septal fracture requires realignment and possibly splinting.
3. Many feel that it takes a minimum of 6 weeks for proper healing to occur. Protective devices may allow players to return to action earlier.

D. Concussions. Basketball is a contact sport and any grade of concussion may occur during competition.
1. Many different systems for classifying concussions exist. In most of these systems the most important factors to consider while grading concussions are loss of consciousness (LOC) and its duration and the presence/absence of posttraumatic and/or retrograde amnesia.
2. There are many different views on when an athlete who has suffered a concussion should return to play. It is generally accepted that play should not be resumed so long as postconsussive symptoms (e.g., headache, confusion, poor concentration, etc.) are present at rest or during light activity.

E. Eye injuries. In the United States, basketball accounts for approximately 7500 eye injuries annually, primarily in younger age groups. Basketball players are considered to be in a "high risk" category for eye injury.
1. Corneal abrasions are the most commonly encountered eye injuries; the mechanism is usually a finger in the eye.

a. Symptoms include pain, photophobia, foreign body sensation, and tearing.
b. Diagnosis is confirmed by epithelial staining defect with fluorescein.
c. Treatment includes antibiotic eye drops or ointment.
   (1) Individuals who do not wear contact lenses should have a pressure patch applied for 24 hours. Contact lens wearers do not require a pressure patch.
   (2) Individuals with small lesions who do not wear contact lenses do not require follow-up unless symptoms persist or worsen. Contact lens wearers should be followed up daily until the epithelial defect resolves. Contact lenses should not be worn during treatment.

2. Hyphema is the collection of blood in the anterior chamber and may lead to marked visual deficits and even permanent loss of vision.
   a. Symptoms include pain and blurred vision, and there is a history of trauma.
   b. Blood in the anterior chamber is usually readily visible. Complete ocular examination should be performed.
   c. Treatment includes bed rest with the head of the bed elevated, eye shield (no eye patch), no aspirin products, atropine 1% drops three or four times daily, and mild analgesics.
      (1) Some patients may require hospitalization.
      (2) Follow-up should be daily for at least the first 5 days.
3. Protective eyewear should be considered for patients with a history of eye injury. Some feel that eyewear should be mandatory in high risk sports such as basketball.

F. Dental injuries occasionally occur. The most important aspects of care of the patient who has suffered a dental injury are careful handling of the avulsed tooth and rapid referral to the proper health care professional.
   1. An avulsed tooth should be rinsed in tap water and placed back in the socket for transport to the dentist. Other ways to transport the tooth include the patient holding the tooth in his or her mouth, in saline, in milk, or, as a last resort, in a cup of water.
   2. Mouthguards should be considered for any basketball participant at any level of competition. Mouthguards not only protect the teeth but may guard against lacerations to the tongue and lips, absorb shock that could cause mandibular fracture, and absorb shock that may cause concussion.

Bibliography

Barrett JR et al: High versus low-top shoes for the prevention of ankle sprains in basketball players. A prospective randomized study, *Am J Sports Med* 21(4):582-585, 1993.

Colliander E et al: Injuries in Swedish elite basketball, *Orthopedics* 9(2):225-227, 1986.

Cooney WP: Sports injuries to the upper extremity, *Postgrad Med* 76(4):45-50, 1984.

Emerson RJ: Basketball knee injuries and the anterior cruciate ligament, *Clin Sports Med* 12(2):317-328, 1993.

Everson LI et al: Radiologic case study. Cuboid subluxation, *Orthopedics* 14:1004, 1991.

Ferretti A: Epidemiology of jumper's knee, *Sports Med* 3(4):289-295, 1986.

Friedberg MA, Rapuano CJ eds. In: *Wills Eye Hospital Office and Emergency Room Diagnosis and Treatment of Eye Disease,* Philadelphia, 1990, JB Lippincott, pp 20-32.

Goyette RF: Facial injuries in basketball players, *Clin Sports Med* 12(2):247-263, 1993.

Gray J et al: A survey of injuries of the anterior cruciate ligament of the knee in female basketball players, *Int J Sports Med* 6(6):314-316, 1985.

Henry JH et al: The injury rate in professional basketball, *Am J Sports Med* 10(1):16-18, 1982.

Howse C: Wrist injuries in sport, *Sports Med* 17(3):163-175, 1994.

Johnson KA, Teasdall RD: Sprained ankles as they relate to the basketball player, *Clin Sports Med* 2(2):363-371, 1993.

Liu SH, Jason WJ: Lateral ankle sprains and instability problems, *Clin Sports Med* 13(4):793-809, 1994.

Lo YPC, Hsu YCS, Chan KM: Epidemiology of shoulder impingement in upper arm sports events, *Br J Sports Med* 24(3):173-177, 1990.

MacAfee KA: Immediate care of facial trauma, *Phys Sports Med* 20(7):78-91, 1992.

McDermott EP: Basketball injuries of the foot and ankle, *Clin Sports Med* 12(2):373-393, 1993.Molnar TJ, Fox JM: Overuse injuries of the knee in basketball, *Clin Sports Med* 12(2):39-62, 1993.

Noyes FR et al: Partial tears of the anterior cruciate ligament. Progression to complete ligament deficiency, *J Bone Joint Surg* 71-B(5):825-833, 1989.

Rosenberg JM, Whitaker JH: Bilateral infrapatellar tendon rupture in a patient with jumper's knee, *Am J Sports Med* 19(1):94-95, 1991.

Roy S, Irvin R: *Sports Medicine. Prevention, Evaluation, Management, and Rehabilitation,* Englewood Cliffs, NJ, 1983, Prentice-Hall.

Shambaugh JP et al: Structural measures as predictors of injury in basketball players, *Med Sci Sports Exerc* 23(5):522-527, 1991.

Sickles RT, Lombardo JA: The adolescent basketball player, *Int J Sports Med* 12(2):207-219, 1993.

Sitler M et al: The efficacy of a semirigid ankle stabilizer to reduce acute ankle injuries in basketball. A randomized clinical study at West Point, *Am J Sports Med* 22(4):454-461, 1994.

Vegso JJ, Harmon LE: Nonoperative management of athletic ankle injuries, *Clin Sports Med* 1(1):85-98, 1982.

Weisman G et al: Cyclic loading in knee ligament injuries, *Am J Sports Med* 8(1):24-30, 1980.

Wilson RL, McGinty LD: Common hand and wrist injuries in basketball players, *Clin Sports Med* 12(2):265-291, 1993.

Wirtz PD: High school basketball knee ligament injuries, *J Iowa Med Soc* 72(3):105-106, 1982.

Zelisko JA et al: A comparison of men's and women's professional basketball injuries, *Am J Sports Med* 10(5):297-299, 1982.

CHAPTER 77

Bicycling Injuries

Robert Kronisch, MD

I. Scope of Participation
  A. Recreational bicycling.
    1. There are currently more than 100 million bicyclists in the United States, with over 30 million adults cycling regularly.
    2. The number of U.S. adults cycling regularly has more than doubled in the last 10 years.
    3. The majority of this increase is due to the rapid growth in popularity of off-road bicycling (mountain biking).
  B. Competitive bicycling.
    1. Membership in the United States Cycling Federation (USCF), the national governing body for road and track bicycle racing, has remained relatively stable at around 35,000 for the last several years.
    2. Membership in the National Off-Road Bicycle Association (NORBA), the governing body for off-road bicycle racing, is currently in excess of 34,000 and continues to rise steadily.

II. Fitting the Bicycle to the Rider.
  A. General considerations.
    1. Select a frame style that will meet the rider's needs and intended use (e.g., road bike, mountain bike, or hybrid model; Figure 77-1).
    2. Rider comfort is the most important consideration in frame selection.
    3. Overuse injuries may result from improper fit.
  B. Frame size. Proper frame size is determined by having the cyclist stand with the legs straddling the bike and measuring the distance between the top tube and the cyclist's crotch.
    1. For a road bike the distance should be 1-2 inches.
    2. For a mountain bike the distance should be 3-6 inches.
    3. For hybrid bikes select a size based on the rider's intended use of the bike (i.e., primarily road or off-road use).
  C. Saddle height.
    1. Proper saddle height is determined by having the cyclist sit on the bike while it is stationary and measuring the angle of the knee

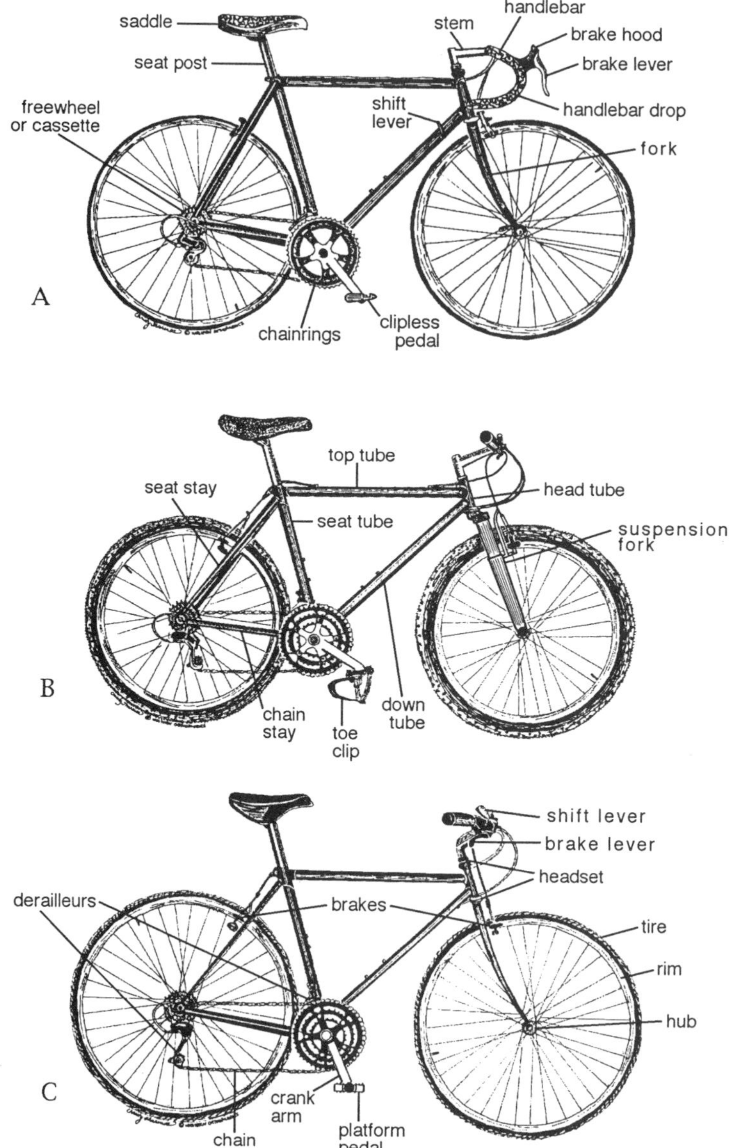

FIGURE 77-1
Bicycle anatomy. (**A**) Road bicycle. (**B**) Mountain bicycle. (**C**) Hybrid bicycle. (Adapted from Holmes JC, Pruitt AL, Whalen NJ: Cycling injuries. In Nichols JA, Hershman EB, editors: *The Lower Extremity and Spine in Sports Medicine,* ed 2, St Louis, 1995, Mosby–Year Book, used with permission.)

(greater trochanter to lateral femoral condyle to lateral malleolus). The saddle height is adjusted so that there is 25-30 degrees of knee flexion with the pedal at bottom dead center (6:00 position).

2. Off-road cyclists may want the seat slightly lower to improve stability and maneuverability while riding off-road.
3. Individuals may fine-tune seat height adjustments with changes of ¼ inch every few rides.

D. Saddle fore and aft position.
  1. Use a plumbline or yardstick to adjust the saddle so that the front of the patella is directly over the axle of the front pedal when the pedals are horizontal (3:00 and 9:00 positions).

2. Off-road cyclists may want the seat slightly further aft (½ inch) to increase rear wheel traction while climbing.

E. Saddle tilt.
   1. Use a carpenter's level to ensure that the saddle is level or tilted slightly upward in front.
   2. Men may get urological or neuropathic symptoms if the front is tilted up too much.
   3. Women may want the front tilted down slightly to decrease pressure on the perineum.

F. Reach.
   1. Reach is determined by the combination of saddle fore and aft position, top tube length, and handlebar stem length. Changes are generally made by replacing the stem.
   2. This is a less exact measurement than lower body positioning and may be influenced by experience and flexibility.
      a. Competitive cyclists generally prefer a longer reach.
      b. Rider comfort is the most important factor.
      c. Finding the ideal position may take time.

G. Handlebar height.
   1. Bars should be 1-2 inches below the top of the saddle for short cyclists and up to 4 inches for tall cyclists.
   2. Off-road and novice cyclists may want the bars slightly higher.
   3. Bars should be raised slightly in the early part of the season or if upper body or lower back syndromes develop.

H. Pedal selection. Several types of pedals are available and should be selected based on the rider's level of experience as well as the presence or absence of lower extremity overuse syndromes.
   1. Platform pedals are primarily for low intensity recreational riding or commuting.
   2. Toe clips and straps enable a more secure attachment to the pedal for improved power transmission from the legs to the bike.
   3. Clipless pedals use a cleat on the rider's shoe to firmly attach the foot to the pedal and have become standard equipment for competitive cyclists and many bicycle enthusiasts.
      a. Fixed clipless pedals do not allow any movement at the shoe-pedal interface.
      b. Floating clipless pedals allow some internal and external rotation at the shoe-pedal interface during the pedaling motion.

I. Foot position.
   1. The widest part of the foot (first MTP joint) should be directly over the pedal axle.
   2. Cleats should be adjusted so that the cyclist's neutral foot position is maintained on the bicycle. The rotational adjustment device (available for a fee at some bicycle shops) is the most efficient way to accomplish this.

III. Traumatic Injuries.

A. Epidemiology.
   1. There are over 500,000 emergency room visits per year in the United States from bicycling accidents.
   2. Around 1000 deaths per year, half in children and adolescents.
   3. Most injuries are superficial (abrasions, contusions, lacerations) and minor in nature.
   4. Body regions most commonly injured: upper extremity > head and face > lower extremity > trunk.

5. Factors associated with injury.
    a. Road bicycling.
        (1) Road surface irregularities, gravel, turning, riding downhill, mechanical problems with the bicycle.
        (2) A motor vehicle is usually involved in cases of severe or fatal trauma.
    b. Off-road bicycling.
        (1) Excessive speed, riding downhill, turning, obstacle in the trail, sand or gravel, inattentiveness, riding beyond one's ability, competition.
        (2) Off-road cyclists are often thrown from their bicycles, which may increase the severity of injury.

B. Extremity injuries.
1. Upper Extremity.
    a. Usually injured in trying to break a fall. Scaphoid, distal radius, and radial head or neck fractures may result.
    b. Shoulder injuries are common.
        (1) Clavicle fractures and AC separations are common.
        (2) Some shoulder dislocations are seen in off-road cyclists.
2. Lower extremity.
    a. Spoke injuries occur when the foot is caught between the wheel and the frame and may range from abrasion to amputation; usually seen in barefooted bicycle passengers.
    b. Fractures of the lower extremity are uncommon in cyclists.

C. Head and face injuries.
1. Head injuries account for the majority of bicycling deaths and are usually due to a collision between a motor vehicle and an unhelmeted cyclist.
2. Bicycle accidents are the most common cause of serious head injuries in children.
3. Helmet use decreases the risk of head injury by 85%.
4. Concussions are relatively common, particularly in mountain biking, even with proper helmet use.
5. Facial injuries are common.
    a. May be associated with underlying head injury.
    b. Most bicycle helmets provide little or no facial protection.

D. Abdominal and chest injuries.
1. Abdominal injuries are uncommon and are usually seen in children.
    a. Usually caused by blunt trauma from handlebars; a motor vehicle is usually involved in the accident.
    b. Diagnosis may be delayed due to insidious symptoms.
2. Chest injuries other than rib fractures are uncommon.

IV. Overuse Injuries

A. General considerations.
1. Overuse injuries in cyclists result from the interaction between the cyclist's anatomy and the mechanical restraints of the bicycle.
    a. Anatomical variations may produce excessive loads on muscles, joints, and tendons during the pedaling motion.
    b. Modern pedal systems firmly attach the cyclist's shoes to the pedals and require perfect individualized adjustment to avoid generating forces that can lead to overuse injuries.
    c. Cycling involves a very high number of repetitions of lower extremity movements, which can magnify the effects of small errors in bicycle fit.

2. Treatment of overuse injuries in cyclists involves the same standard therapeutic measures used in other athletes (not discussed here) but may also involve adjustment of bicycle fit, compensation for anatomical variations, and modification of the cyclist's training habits.
3. Competitive cyclists should build a training base early in the season by cycling 1000 miles over a 6-week period on relatively flat terrain using a high cadence (80-100 rpm) and avoiding their large chainrings. Touring cyclists should do the same for 500-600 miles. Hill work and training for power and intensity should be added only after this training base has been established.

B. Lower extremity.
   1. General considerations.
      a. Lower extremity overuse injuries often develop early in the season from training increases without an adequate training base or following sudden increases in hill work, mileage, or intensity.
      b. In addition to the specific measures mentioned below, treatment usually involves temporary avoidance of hills and limiting cycling to pain-free, high-cadence, easy spinning using small chainrings on flat terrain.
   2. Knee extensor mechanism problems.
      a. Patellofemoral pain and quadriceps and patellar tendinitis are common in cyclists and are treated similarly.
      b. Question the cyclist regarding training base, hill climbing, and use of the large chainring and about weight training or other extensor mechanism–loading activities.
      c. Look for anatomical variants such as patellofemoral malalignment, internal tibial rotation, overpronation, or valgus or varus alignment.
         (1) Anatomical variants, particularly rotational variations, should be compensated for with cleat position adjustments. Limit floating pedals to 5 degrees of rotation.
         (2) Encourage quadriceps strengthening for patellofemoral malalignment.
         (3) Active pronation (while cycling) is treated with cycling orthotics, which are longer and more rigid than running orthotics.
         (4) Valgus alignments are accommodated with lifts or shims between the pedal and the shoe or with orthotics
         (5) Varus alignments are accommodated with spacers between the crankarm and the pedal
      d. The saddle may be too low or too far forward, leading to excess knee flexion. Correct the saddle to neutral fore-aft position with 25-30 degrees of knee flexion at bottom dead center (BDC).
   3. Iliotibial band (ITB) friction syndrome.
      a. The ITB moves over the lateral femoral condyle with each pedaling stroke; contact is greatest at about 30 degrees of knee flexion and is accentuated by internal tibial rotation.
      b. Question the cyclist regarding excessive hill work or inadequate training base.
      c. Look for varus alignment, active pronation with internal tibial rotation, prominent lateral femoral condyle, or tight ITB.
         (1) Consider using spacers for varus alignment.
         (2) Consider orthotics for active pronators.
         (3) Floating pedals with fixed endpoint may limit active internal tibial rotation.

d. The cleats may be too internally rotated, or the saddle may be too high or too far aft.
   (1) Adjust the cleats to reflect the cyclist's lower extremity alignment or place them in slight external rotation.
   (2) Switch to floating pedals if fixed clipless pedals are used.
   (3) Lower the saddle to 30-35 degrees of knee flexion at BDC or even lower.
   (4) Spacers between the crankarm and pedal may improve hip-foot alignment and decrease stress on the ITB.

4. Medial synovial plica irritation.
   a. The medial synovial plica and/or medial patellofemoral ligament may become irritated from cycling, especially following sudden increases in mileage or intensity.
   b. Valgus alignment, active pronation, and internal tibial rotation may increase medial knee stress; correct for these as described above.
   c. Ensure that the saddle is properly positioned and that cleat position reflects the cyclist's anatomical alignment.
5. Pes anserine tendinitis/bursitis.
   a. Overpronation, valgus alignment, or external tibial rotation may produce excessive stress on the pes anserinus; correct for these as described above.
   b. Saddle may be too high or leg length discrepancy (LLD) may be present.
   c. Treatment of LLD:
      (1) Fit the bike to the long leg and correct the short leg.
      (2) Corrections should slightly undercompensate the discrepancy.
      (3) Tibial LLD is corrected with orthotics and/or a lift between the pedal and the shoe.
      (4) Femoral LLD requires a lift and cleat adjustment; move the foot of the short leg slightly back on the pedal and the foot of the long leg forward.
6. Hamstring tendinitis.
   a. Less common than other knee complaints.
   b. Question the cyclist regarding training base and excessive use of the large chainring.
   c. Look for varus or valgus alignment or LLD; correct for these as described above.
   d. Saddle may be too high or too far aft; cleats may be incorrectly placed.
      (1) Ensure neutral fore-aft position and temporarily decrease seat height to 30-35 degrees of knee flexion at BDC.
      (2) Adjust cleats to reflect lower extremity alignment.
7. Achilles tendinitis.
   a. May be due to flexion/extension or angular stress on tendon.
   b. Look for pes planus, overpronation, LLD; treat as described above.
   c. Observe the cyclist for excessive ankling (dorsiflexion plantar flexion while pedaling).
   d. The foot may be too far behind the pedal axle, leading to excessive flexion/extension, or the foot may be excessively rotated, leading to angular stress on the tendon.
      (1) Make sure the foot is correctly placed on the pedal.
      (2) Consider temporarily moving the foot 1-3 mm forward on the pedal.

C. Upper extremity.
 1. Ulnar nerve compression.
  a. The ulnar nerve is susceptible to external compression at Guyon's canal due to its superficial location.
  b. Motor, sensory, or mixed motor and sensory loss may occur.
  c. Onset may be progressive or acute.
  d. Conservative treatment is almost always effective.
   (1) Relative or complete rest with avoidance of pressure to the ulnar palmar area; may take up to 3-6 months.
   (2) Advise the cyclist to change hand position frequently while cycling.
   (3) Changes to the bicycle may be needed.
    (a) Ensure proper frame size.
    (b) Padded gloves and handlebar grips may help limit microtrauma to the hand and wrist.
    (c) Consider adjusting the handlebar height and/or reach so that less of the rider's weight is on the handlebars (raise or change to a shorter stem).
    (d) Consider drop handlebars with a deeper drop for road cyclists; occasionally may need to change to upright or aero-style bars.
    (e) Consider front suspension for off-road cyclists (adjust if already present).
 2. Median nerve compression.
  a. Much less common in cyclists than ulnar nerve compression (consider other possible causes).
  b. May coexist with ulnar neuropathy.
  c. Same recommendations as for ulnar nerve compression.

D. Neck and back pain.
 1. Neck pain.
  a. Very common, usually due to prolonged neck extension or to shock and vibrations transmitted to the neck via the upper extremities.
  b. Treatment may involve changes to the bicycle.
   (1) Reduce neck extension by raising the handlebars, changing to a shorter stem, or moving the seat forward; consider upright bars.
   (2) Reduce shock by using wider tires and/or lower inflation pressure, padded gloves, and handlebar grips or tape; consider front suspension (adjust if already present).
  c. Ensure proper riding position.
   (1) Avoid riding with the elbows fully extended.
   (2) Change hand and head/neck position frequently.
   (3) Decrease the amount of time spent cycling with the hands in the handlebar drops.
   (4) Avoid riding in a hunched position.
  d. Stretching before, during, and after riding is helpful for prevention and treatment.
 2. Low back pain.
  a. Very common, especially early in the season and in novice cyclists (often resolves as conditioning improves).
  b. Off-road cyclists may develop low back pain from the repetitive jolting and stress associated with off-road riding conditions.
  c. Changes to the bicycle may be needed.

(1) Proper fit of the bicycle is essential to allow the spine to remain in neutral position.
(a) Ensure proper saddle height and fore/aft position.
(b) Consider decreasing the reach for cyclists with pain arising from the posterior spinal elements.
(c) Consider increasing the reach for cyclists with pain arising from the intervertebral disks.
(2) Consider larger tires and/or lower inflation pressure.
(3) Consider front suspension system for off-road bicycles. Some concern exists as to whether certain rear suspension systems may actually increase the shock transmitted to the lower back.

d. Ensure proper riding technique.
(1) Encourage high cadence, low resistance pedaling, especially early in the season.
(2) Discourage sudden increases in mileage and intensity.
(3) Change hand position and position on the seat frequently while riding.
(4) Stand and stretch on the bike while cycling.

e. A dynamic lumbar stabilization program may be needed for definitive treatment.

E. Saddle-related problems.

1. Skin problems.

a. Saddle sores may develop from overuse or improper saddle positioning and may range from mild chafing and pain to ulceration and secondary infection.

b. Treatment is generally symptomatic for mild cases.
(1) Ensure good hygiene.
(2) Clean, padded cycling shorts that wick moisture away from the skin.
(3) Padded saddle that is wide enough to support the ischial tuberosities.
(4) Consider repositioning or changing the saddle.

c. More severe cases may require temporary cessation of cycling.

2. Neuropathic problems.

a. Pudendal neuropathy is very common in male cyclists.
(1) Numbness of the penile shaft from compression of the dorsal branch of the pudendal nerve between the symphysis pubis and the saddle.
(2) Almost always is transient and resolves after cycling.
(3) Ensure proper saddle position and use of padded cycling shorts.
(4) Consider changing to a different saddle.

Bibliography

Holmes JC, Pruitt AL, Whalen NJ: Cycling injuries, In Nichols JA, Hershman EB, editors: *The Lower Extremity and Spine in Sports Medicine*, ed 2. St Louis, 1995, Mosby–Year Book.

Mellion MB, Burke ER, editors: Bicycling injuries, *Clin Sports Med* 13(1):1-262, 1994.

Pfeiffer RP, Kronisch RL: Off-road cycling injuries, an overview, *Sports Med* 19(5):311-325, 1995.

CHAPTER **78**

Running

Karl B. Fields, MD

I. Overview
  A. Running is the fitness sport of choice for 40 to 50 million Americans.
  B. Runners score high on overall assessments of general health.
  C. Nevertheless, the sport of running is associated with a high injury risk.
    1. Various studies, depending on the definition of injury employed, find that 40% to 60% of runners have at least one significant injury each year.
    2. Women's and men's cross-country have high injury rates among high school athletes, with as many as 50% to 60% injured for more than 5 days during a season.[10]
    3. Injury patterns differ greatly among competitive track and field athletes, recreational road racers, and joggers.
  D. Studies of runners indicate that they have lower overall musculoskeletal disability[9] and do not appear to have an increased risk of degenerative joint disease.[19]
  E. Fitness has prospectively been associated with longevity, and unfit individuals who improve their fitness lessen their health risks.[1] Running appears to be one of the best ways for people to reach a very good or excellent fitness level.

II. Training
  A. General.
    1. In studies of running injury, training error is listed as the most common cause.
    2. To determine whether an injury is due to a training error, the clinician needs a basic understanding of training theory.
    3. The physician must establish credibility with a runner before suggesting that he or she modify a regimen that has led the individual to run faster.
    4. In all training schedules the athlete must progressively stress the biological system without causing tissue breakdown and injury.

5. There is a thin line between overtraining and maximal training.
6. Most runners seen for injury are adults participating in road races of distances from the 5000 m to the marathon.
   a. Youth and adolescent participation in track and field has actually declined in the past two decades.
   b. Approximately 50% of runners are now over age 40.
   c. Master's athletics (women > 35 and men > 40) is increasing in popularity.

B. Principles of training.[11]
   1. Periodization: the division of training into different phases to achieve a desired outcome.
      a. For example, one 3-month cycle may emphasize endurance; another strength and speed; another shorter phase might be for rest and sharpening form; etc.
      b. Advantages include lessening boredom and reducing fatigue.
   2. Progressive overload: once the body becomes accustomed to a specific level, the training load must be increased to stimulate new musculoskeletal adaptation.
   3. Specificity: training must resemble the requirements of the sport activity.
      a. Example one: The training pace for a 1500-m race and marathon race is dramatically different.
      b. Example two: Variable terrain is more important for cross-country training than for track racing.

C. Types of training for distance runners.[6]
   1. Interval training: runners complete a specific distance repetitively at an approximate pace with a fixed period of rest with the goal of increasing VO2 max. These can be designed to stress aerobic recovery, mixed aerobic-anaerobic stress, or pure anaerobic (speed) stress.
   2. Distance training: longer runs stress slow twitch muscle fibers with the ultimate outcome of increasing enzyme induction and other muscle cell adaptations.
   3. Tempo runs: a workout of 18 to 20 minutes at 15 to 20 seconds per mile slower than 10-km race pace with the intent of accustoming the runner to the stress of race pace and extending the "lactate threshold."
   4. Maximum pace workouts: a low number of repeats with full rest in between at maximal speed.
   5. Recovery runs: easy efforts at about 50% of maximum and no longer than 10% to 15% of weekly mileage; usually follow hard workouts.

III. Studies That Have Examined Running Injuries

A. Early classic studies were based on case series of patients who came to physician offices for running injury.
   1. Brubaker and James[2]: review of 109 runners who visited an orthopedic clinic for care between 1955 and 1972 (collegiate and high school runners averaging 49 miles per week; Table 78-1).
   2. Clement and associates[3]: review of 1650 patients with 1819 injuries seen in a primary care sports medicine clinic between 1978 and 1980 (all classes of runners; Table 78-2).
   3. Selection bias is inherent in each of these studies as they reflect the particular patient population of each clinic.
   4. Nevertheless, each study added substantially to the clinical understanding of running injuries.

TABLE 78-1. Running injuries as seen by Brubaker and James[2]

Injury Categories	%	Stress Fracture Type	%
Strains	33.1	Tibia	41.2
Stress fractures	15.6	Metatarsal	29.4
Sprains	11	Fibula	17.6
Tendinitis	11.6	Cuneiform	5.9
Patellar problems	14.7	Navicular	5.9

5. Brubaker and James[2] cared for a more competitive group of runners, and the injury distribution is different than that in studies that include recreational runners and less competitive road racers. They were the first to point out that tibial stress fractures were the most common among runners.
6. Clement and associates[3] cared for a population more typical of primary care practices.
   a. They were among the first to emphasize that the knee was the most commonly injured anatomical area among runners.
   b. Their data identified the six injuries still felt to be most common in runners.
7. Marti and coworkers[4] completed a study based on survey data from 4358 male runners in a road race.
   a. Injury pattern: knee, 27.9%; lower leg including Achilles', 29.9%; and foot and ankle, 28.5%.
   b. Achilles' tendon and calf symptoms were the two most common specific overuse symptoms and were more common among older runners.

IV. Prospective Studies of Running Injury are Limited
   A. Lysholm and Wiklander[12] prospectively studied competitive runners in a track club.
      1. Injuries more closely resembled Brubaker and James[2] study.
      2. Study confirmed high injury rate as 65% of runners were injured during 1 year.
   B. The Ontario Cohort Study[23] provides the best prospective data that reflect patients typical of a primary care practice. Authors enrolled 1680 runners at two road races for a prospective survey of running injuries

TABLE 78-2. Running injuries seen by Clement et al.[3]

Injury Categories	%	Anatomical Location	%
Patellofemoral stress syndrome	25.8	Knee	41.7
Tibial stress syndrome	13.2	Leg and ankle	27.9
Tendinitis	14.9	Foot	18.1
Plantar fasciitis	4.7	Hip	5
Iliotibial band syndrome	4.3	Lower back	3.7
Tibial stress fracture	2.6	Thigh	3.6

over 12 months. Of these 1288 had complete follow-up data and 1000 had a physical assessment. During the year 48% were injured (Table 78-3).

V. Summary of Prospective and Retrospective Studies
   A. Prospective and retrospective studies generally agree on the anatomical locations and the most common injuries seen in runners.
   B. In general, competitive runners show more strains and stress fractures compared to recreational runners and local road racers.
   C. Knee injury, particularly PFSS, is the most common injury of road racers.
   D. Older runners may have an increased risk of Achilles' tendon and calf problems.
   E. Most common locations of running injury in order are the knee, leg and ankle, and foot.
   F. Most common specific injuries are[13]:
      1. Patellofemoral stress syndrome (PFSSO).
      2. Iliotibial band (ITB).
      3. Medial tibial stress syndrome (MTSS).
      4. Achilles' tendinitis.
      5. Plantar fasciitis.
      6. Patellar tendinitis.
   G. More recent surveys indicate that stress fractures comprise about 10% of running injuries.

VI. Causes of Running Injury Overview
   A. No studies have definitively identified the causes of running injury, suggesting that multiple factors are involved.
   B. Problems in defining causality relate to selection bias: studies chose either runners who came to a particular office for injury or who attended a given race.
   C. In no study has data collection been comprehensive: for example, injuries are often self-defined and determined by survey, and injury definitions are not uniform.
   D. The true denominator of the number of runners in the general population is not known; thus extrapolations of injury rates are from the selected population samples.
   E. In most studies investigators did not confirm the diagnosis for the injured runners.
   F. Examination for anatomical factors was not standardized among studies.
   G. Factors identified in studies must be considered associated rather than causal.

TABLE 78-3. Running injuries: The Ontario Cohort Study[23]

Anatomical Location	%
Knee	27
Leg and ankle	27
Foot	16
Hip	9
Back	11 (only 5% new injuries)
Thigh	7

VII. Specific Factors Related to Running Injury
  A. Training error
    1. Brubaker and James[2] found training error to be the most common factor by clinical history.
    2. Clement and associates[3] noted specific aspects of training including:
      a. High intensity without rest days.
      b. Sudden increases in mileage or intensity.
      c. A single severe training session or competition.
    3. Marti and coworkers[4] noted an increased association of injuries with running mileage (highest >50 km/week). Competitive orientation of the runner was also significant.
    4. Prospective association was found by in two studies.
      a. Lysholm and Wiklander noted training error as a cause in 23 of 55 injuries.
      b. The Ontario Cohort study[23] found an association with running > 40 miles per week. Lesser association was noted with:
        i. Running more miles per day on training runs.
        ii. Length of long run.
        iii. Running more days per week (biggest jump is for 7 days/week).
  B. Anatomical factors.
    1. Brubaker and James[2] found certain anatomical factors on clinical examination.
    2. Clement and associates[3] listed numerous anatomical factors that they felt related to the injuries they examined, including:
      a. Leg length discrepancy.
      b. Femoral neck anteversion.
      c. Weakness or inflexibility of the quadriceps or hamstrings.
      d. Genu valgum, varum, or recurvatum.
      e. Q angle >15 degrees.
      f. Patella alta.
      g. Tibial torsion.
      h. Tibia varum.
      i. Gastrocnemius soleus insufficiency.
      j. Leg-heel or heel-forefoot malalignment.
      k. Pes cavus or pes planus.
      l. Structural irregularities of the toes.
    3. Lysholm and Wiklander[12] found anatomical factors in 19 of 55 injuries.
    4. Marti and coworkers[4] and the Ontario Cohort study[23] did not find an association, but limited physical evaluation was done each study.
    5. Cowan[4] found a strong prospective association with arch height and injury in soldiers.
      a. Cavus feet with a soft tissue arch height >3.14 cm were associated with a relative risk of 6.1.
      b. Flat feet had the lowest RR.
  C. Functional errors.
    1. Pronation has been identified by most clinicians as the most common functional error leading to running injury.
    2. Limited prospective study relates pronation to injury,[18] but most orthotic studies designed at controlling excess pronation resulted in good clinical resolution of injury.

3. Supination without compensatory pronation has been postulated as the functional factor that contributes to the increased injury rate in cavus feet.
4. Excess supination has also been related to occurrence of ITB syndrome.
5. Cross-over striding; overstriding, "toeing out," body lean, and other form errors have been postulated as causing running injury, but no documentation exists.

D. Extrinsic factors.
   1. Shoe problems.[3]
      a. Inadequate heel wedge.
      b. Poor heel counters.
      c. Inflexible soles.
      d. Narrow toe boxes.
      e. Lateral heel wear.
      f. Removal or breakdown of orthotics.
   2. Running surface.[3]
      a. Uneven.
      b. Hardness.
      c. Road camber.
      d. Soft surfaces do not require the muscles to provide as much shock absorption.
   3. Clement and associates[3] and James and Brubaker[2] implicated extrinsic factors as causes of injury.
   4. Lysholm and Wiklander[12] in their prospective study found shoes or surface to play a role in 13 of 55 injuries.
   5. The Ontario Cohort study[23] did not find shoe characteristics or running surface to be predictors of injury.

E. Kinetic chain dysfunction.
   1. Limited agreement about what constitutes a significant problem hinders studies of causality.
   2. Robbins and Hanna[20] looked at barefoot running and how this led to better function of the medial longitudinal arch. They concluded that running shoes led to "pseudoneuropathic" function of the arch.
   3. Runners who had sustained an injury showed more limited range of motion at the hip on both the injured and uninjured side.[22]
   4. Strengthening of the posterior tibialis muscle reduces the degree of pronation.[7]

F. Psychological factors.
   1. In a small prospective trial, type A behavior appeared to be related to running injury.[8]
   2. McKelvie and colleagues[17] did not find that a particular personality type in marathoners was associated with increased risk of injury.
   3. Schafer and McKenna[21] in a survey noted an association between stress and running injury.

G. Summary of injury causes.
   1. Multiple factors probably contribute to running injury, and causality is difficult to determine.
   2. Strongest evidence exists for excessive running mileage.
   3. Strong evidence also exists for an association with previous injury.
   4. Of the anatomical factors, cavus feet, leg length inequality, and enlarged Q angle for PFSS are most likely to be causally related to injury.

5. Of the functional problems, only pronation is felt to be strongly related to injury.
6. Kinetic chain dysfunction and psychological factors are areas where additional research may identify probable causes of running injury.
7. Extrinsic factors need further study.

VIII. Review of the Most Common Running Injuries

A. Patellofemoral stress syndrome.

1. Generally referred to as PFSS, "runner's knee," or chondromalacia patella, this is the most common running injury.
2. A syndrome of anterior knee pain from any of a variety of causes, although true chondromalacia findings on arthroscopy are present in a minority of cases.
3. Symptoms include pain and sometimes swelling of the anterior knee exacerbated by downhill running and speed work.
4. "Theater sign" or increased pain when sitting with knees bent are classic symptoms.
5. Anatomical associations include vastus medialis obliquus (VMO) weakness, abnormal patellar shape, shallow patellofemoral groove, increased Q angle, abnormal patellar tracking.
6. Examination may reveal puffiness, "double hump sign," positive pain on patellar contraction against resistance or on patellar compression, unilateral crepitus, VMO atrophy, and increased patellar mobility.
7. Running gait may show excessive pronation.
8. Radiological evaluation is rarely helpful.
9. Treatment centers on reduction of inflammation, quadriceps strengthening, hamstring stretches, and either patellar tendon straps or patellar braces with a lateral horseshoe and open patella.
10. McConnell taping technique has been helpful.
11. In runners who pronate, an antipronation pad or formal orthotic may be tried.
12. Modification of training includes reduction of speed work, avoidance of hill workouts and particularly downhill running, and reduction of total mileage.
13. Runners who cannot train without limping should be placed on substituted activity.
14. Quadriceps strengthening should avoid excessive loading of the patellofemoral joint, particularly with the knee bent greater than 45 degrees.

B. Iliotibial band syndrome.

1. This is the second most common knee problem of runners and causes sharp lateral knee pain that occurs during knee flexion, usually during the late swing phase of gait.
2. Pain is variable at different running paces; pain may worsen on sloped running surfaces. Stairmaster, biking, and nonimpact activity causes minimal if any discomfort.
3. Anatomical factors may include varus alignment and unequal leg lengths. An excessively pronated foot with increased internal tibial rotation.
4. Form changes include supination or "cross-over" during running gait and sometimes an excessive compensatory pronation.
5. Physical examination reveals point tenderness over lateral femoral epicondyle and pain reproduced at a certain phase of knee flexion with a varus stress (usually about 30 degrees).

6. Positive Ober's test suggests ITB tightness.
7. Differential diagnosis includes plica, popliteus tendinitis, and meniscus injury.
8. Treatment includes a combination of the following factors depending on the individual situation:
   a. Stretches.
   b. Lateral strengthening.
   c. Orthotics when biomechanical problem exists.
   d. Ice.
   e. Transverse friction massage.
   f. Nonsteroidal antiinflammatory drugs (NSAIDs) for 5 to 10 days.
   g. Injection can occasionally be helpful in severe cases (often a small bursa below ITB).
   h. Phonophoresis or iontophoresis.
9. Training modification includes flat, nonbanked surfaces, variable paced workouts, stopping for sharp or persistent pain and alleviating with stretches and ice, correction of any excessive lateral shoewear.

C. Plantar fasciitis.
1. Painful overuse syndrome in which a hallmark is pain on the first step out of bed in the morning.
2. Pain pattern is severe on the first steps into a run and may lessen after 5 to 10 minutes.
3. Dull, toothache-like pain may persist during the day and be exacerbated by standing in hard shoes on hard floors.
4. Physical examination shows point tenderness at the medial insertion of the plantar fascia onto the calcaneus. Extension of the great toe may cause symptoms. Squeeze of the calcaneus is nonpainful. Examination often is otherwise unremarkable.
5. Cavus feet or pronation on gait may predispose runners to problems.
6. Differential diagnosis includes calcaneal stress fracture and neuropathy.
7. Treatment is often frustrating and slow and includes a variable combination of:
   a. Ice massage.
   b. Arch exercises and stretches.
   c. Heel cups or special strapping with moleskin and tape.
   d. NSAIDs.
   e. Flexible shoes and barefoot running, which may restore arch function.
   f. Injection.
   g. Orthotics or arch pads.
   h. Night splints.
   i. Physical therapy with modalities.
8. In general when symptoms are greatest most runners will be unable to train. Rest alleviates the most painful symptoms; training can resume on soft surfaces with a reduction in intensity and distance.
9. Careful attention to altered biomechanics after return is important to avoid a compensatory injury.

D. Achilles' tendinitis
1. The Achilles' tendon is the "thermometer" of the runner. When a light squeeze of the Achilles' tendon produces pain, the runner is almost certainly overtraining.

2. The Achilles'-calf complex plays a crucial role in the push-off that allows runners to have an airborne "float" phase of gait.
3. Any weakness or excessive pain leads to an uneven gait.
4. Tendinitis or partial tear is characterized by pain over the major chord of the tendon or anywhere along the broad-based musculotendinous connections to the gastrocnemius-soleus complex.
5. Swelling or crepitation in the tendon sheath indicates a more severe tendinitis.
6. Nodules suggest the possibility of partial tears.
7. Mild tendinitis may be treated with antiinflammatory measures including ice massage and NSAIDs along with heel cups or heel pads.
8. In a mild tendinitis the runner may continue to train on a reduced schedule as long as symptoms continue to lessen.
9. More severe tendinitis cases require rest, substitute activity, and the same treatment as above.
10. Strengthening exercises for both gastrocnemius and soleus.
11. Stretching must be gentle so as not to worsen the injury.
12. Ultrasound, massage, and formal physical therapy may be needed in difficult cases.
13. Steroid injection is to be avoided.

E. Medial tibial stress syndrome and tibial stress fracture.
    1. Medial tibial pain is the condition most commonly labeled "shin splints."
    2. Symptoms include persistent aching and pain along the medial border of the shin.
    3. Pain may variably seem muscular or bony in origin.
    4. Physical findings include pain on palpation of the distal third of the tibial border; occasionally, swelling, thickening, or elevation of the periosteum and warmth can be detected on palpation.
    5. Positive pain on tuning fork vibration or on a simple "hop test" suggests the possibility of tibial stress fracture as does an extremely focal area of pain. (Ultrasound at 2.5-3 W/cm^2 produces pain as well.)
    6. Early season hill training and increased mileage for inexperienced runners are leading causes of MTSS. In established runners this symptom more commonly suggests tibial stress fracture.
    7. Running gait may reveal excessive pronation or increased internal rotation of the tibia.
    8. Some runners appear to have "miserable malalignment" syndrome with a combination of anatomical changes.
    9. Nocturnal pain is more common with stress fracture.
    10. Weakness or numbness suggests compartment syndrome.
    11. Etiology remains controversial: repeated torque on lower tibia, traction microfractures from pull of interosseous membrane, a compartment syndrome involving the posterior tibialis muscle and fascia, etc.
    12. Treatment varies by the intensity of symptoms.
        a. Mild MTSS: ice massage; exercises including heel, toe, and backwards walking as a part of the warm-up for running; antipronation pads or orthotics if warranted by running form; NSAIDs; reduce training and avoid hills; cross training and gentle stretches of calf, posterior tibialis, and anterior tibialis.
        b. Moderate MTSS: all of the above are indicated but usually substituted activity must replace running until tenderness lessens.

If tenderness is persistent, further work-up to exclude stress fracture or even compartment syndrome may be warranted. When retraining starts, surface should be soft.

c. Severe MTSS: this is a tibial stress fracture until proven otherwise; bone scans will usually show focal uptake of stress fracture or more diffuse uptake characteristic of periostitis. Above measures plus no weight-bearing sports activity for a minimum of 2 weeks or until "hop test" is negative; long air cast, very gradual retraining program.
d. Tibial stress fractures other than the posterior shaft of the lower third of the medial tibia: these may not respond as predictably as MTSS. Anterior midtibial shaft stress fractures have more commonly been seen in dancers and jumping athletes. Radiographs show a horizontal lucency ("dreaded black line"), which is often an area of nonunion. Healing is slow.[15]
e. When exercise compartment pressures are high in the deep posterior compartment, these patients will respond to limited fasciotomy.[5] This has been a very common condition of world class middle distance runners.

IX. Symptoms That May Indicate a High Risk Running Injury

A. Groin pain: the differential diagnosis varies considerably depending on the age of the patient; femoral neck stress fractures are particularly worrisome as they can displace with serious complications. Malignancy must always be a consideration as a mimicker of joint symptoms.[16]
   1. Pediatric (below age 10): Legg-Calvé-Perthes and infectious causes are considerations as is injury.
   2. Adolescents: slipped capital femoral epiphysis (may present as knee pain), snapping hip syndrome, adductor strains.
   3. Adults: femoral stress fracture, osteoarthritis, avascular necrosis, osteitis pubis.

B. Medial arch pain: the primary concern is navicular stress fracture since this may be difficult to detect on plain films.
   1. Bone scan and/or computerized tomography may be needed if pain is persistent.
   2. Navicular fractures need conservative treatment with non–weight-bearing casts for 6-8 weeks.[5]
   3. Nonunion and avascular necrosis are problems.

C. Recurrent knee effusion: this suggests intraarticular pathology.
   1. Osteochondritis dissecans of the medial femoral condyle has been noted in runners and is a particularly difficult entity to treat.
   2. Severe PFSS or true chondromalacia patellae can cause recurrent effusion but needs definitive diagnosis.
   3. Degenerative meniscus tear or new injury to a previously injured anterior cruciate ligament is a problem that can occur with overuse in runners, although each is more typical of traumatic injury.
   4. Intraarticular stress fracture of the tibial plateau.

D. Joint swelling: this is not typical of overuse problems of runners so must trigger a thought of intraarticular stress fracture, arthritic change, or other significant problems whether this involves tarsal joints, metacarpophalangeals, or ankle.

E. Chronic metatarsalgia in an adolescent: look for avascular necrosis of the second metatarsal head (Freiberg's infarction).

F. Sciatica in a runner: consider piriformis syndrome or other causes of extrinsic compression of the sciatic nerve as well as disk injury.

X. General Approach to Running Injury

A. Principle 1: Special treatments may be helpful for specific injuries. For example, patellar tendon straps may relieve symptoms in PFSS and sometimes in Osgood-Schlatter syndrome but have a limited role in other conditions. Similarly, a heel lift may help in Achilles' tendinitis or a second insole or orthotics may reduce injury risk in athletes with problems secondary to a leg length inequality.

B. Principle 2: Ice helps in most running injuries. For example, icing after activity for the duration of symptoms may be the key to resolution of problems like plantar fasciitis and metatarsalgia, when padding, NSAIDs, and other treatments seem to offer limited relief. For most joint problems ice is a cornerstone. The role of heat is more limited and probably works best as an adjunct to treatment in chronic muscular strains.

C. Principle 3: Use NSAIDs short term. Runners normally should respond to 1-2 weeks of NSAID therapy. Rarely do they have chronic inflammatory conditions such as arthritis that require prolonged therapy. When 1-2 weeks of NSAIDs have not helped, consider other aspects of treatment or reconsider the original diagnosis.

D. Principle 4: Modification of the training schedule is an essential part of treatment.

1. Specific changes to consider include reduction of stressful activity. For example, a runner with PFSS will usually experience most pronounced symptoms on downhill running and to a lesser extent on uphill. For this reason eliminating hill workouts may remove a key trigger for symptoms.
2. Reduce speed. Achilles' tendinitis or a hamstring strain is stressed maximally in eccentric contraction, usually during speed workouts. Removal of these workouts may allow the athlete to continue training at a lower level while rehabilitating the injury.
3. Determine if running curves aggravates the condition. For example, hip rotators such as the piriformis muscle undergo maximal stress (particularly on the outside leg) in speed runs around a turn. For this reason a similar quality effort may be tolerable for an athlete with piriformis syndrome if run on a straight-away.
4. Reduce mileage. The soleus muscle is essentially composed of slow twitch fibers. Overwork such as long runs in preparation for a marathon is often the key factor in developing "soleus syndrome." Runners may be able to train with this injury if distance and total mileage are reduced enough so as not to overstress the injured muscle group.
5. Add rest days. Few runners can consistently run 7 days weekly without rest days. This was one factor identified as a cause of injury in the Ontario Cohort study.[23] Similarly, few runners can do more than three quality workout sessions per week and adequately recover. Staleness and overtraining syndromes often follow excessive quality work.

E. Principle 5: Consider a change in training surface for frequently injured runners. Tracks, roads, trails, and grass have markedly different characteristics as surfaces. Impact of running on these surfaces varies with the resistance of the surface. For this reason runners who have recurrent conditions thought related to impact (e.g., MTSS or certain stress fractures) should try moving to a softer training surface.

F. Principle 6: Substitute to supplement aerobic condition. Using a wet vest, biking, swimming, Stair stepper, Nordic tracks, and the like are all good methods of cross-training that can help maintain basic aerobic fitness during times of injury. Not all runners are equally able to gain benefit from each of these, so the specific cross-training should be determined by individual preference.

G. Principle 7: Rehabilitate all injuries. Substituted aerobic exercise is not specific rehabilitation, and exercise must be directed to restore strength to injured areas. For example, quadriceps exercises particularly to strengthen the VMO are a key to resolving PFSS. Bent and straight leg heel raises may help restore the gastrocnemius-soleus complex to normal function.

XI. Conclusion

A. Running is among the most popular participant sports for adults seeking to maintain overall fitness.

B. The average age of runners has increased, and concerns for medical illnesses and arthritis mimicking injury are appropriate, particularly in older runners.

C. The prospective association of longevity and decreased disability with improved fitness are likely to increase the popularity of running for physical conditioning.

D. Running injuries are multifactorial, with excess mileage and previous injury among the strongest associated factors.

E. Cavus feet have long been suspected of increasing the risk for lower extremity injury, and a recent prospective trial confirmed this.

F. PFSS is the most common running injury, and the knee is the most commonly injured anatomical location.

G. ITB, MTSS, plantar fasciitis, and Achilles' tendinitis are also extremely common injuries in runners.

H. Specific symptoms may lead to concern about high risk injuries.

I. Logical principles that take into account the need to understand and modify the training schedule are key to the successful treatment of running injuries.

References

1. Blair SN et al: Changes in physical fitness and all-cause mortality, *JAMA* 273(14):1093-1098, 1995.
2. Brubaker CE, James SL: Injuries to runners, *J Sports Med* 2(4):189-198, 1974.
3. Clement DB et al: A survey of overuse running injuries, *Phys Sportsmed* 9(5):47-58, 1981.
4. Cowan DN, Jones BH, Robinson JR: Foot morphologic characteristics and risk of exercise-related injury, *Arch Fam Med* 2:773-777, 1993.
5. Crichton KJ et al: Injuries to the pelvis and lower limb. In: Bloomfield J, Fricker PA, Fitch KD, editors: *Textbook of Science and Medicine in Sport,* Melbourne, Australia, 1992, Blackwell Scientific Publications, pp 404-405.
6. Daniels J: Training distance runners—a primer. In: *Sports Science Exchange: Conditioning and Training.* 1989, Gatorade Sports Science Institute. Chicago, IL.
7. Feltner ME et al: Strength training effects on rearfoot motion in running, *Med Sci Sports Exerc* 26(8):1021-1027, 1994.
8. Fields KB, Delaney M, Hinkle JS: A prospective study of Type A behavior and running injuries, *JFP* 30(4):425-429, 1990.
9. Fries JF et al: Running and the development of disability with age, *Ann Intern Med* 121(7):502-509, 1994.
10. Garrick JG: Epidemiology of sports injuries in the pediatric athlete. In Sullivan JA, Grana WA, editors: *The Pediatric Athlete,* Park Ridge, IL, 1990, American Academy of Orthopaedic Surgeons, pp 123-132.
11. Hahn AG: Physiology of training. In Bloomfield J, Fricker PA, Fitch KD, editors: *Textbook of Science and Medicine in Sport,* Melbourne, Australia, 1992, Blackwell Scientific Publications, pp 78-86.
12. Lysholm J, Wiklander J: Injuries in runners, *Am J Sports Med* 15(2):168-171, 1987.

13. MacIntyre J, Lloyd-Smith R: Overuse running injuries. In Renstrom PAFH, editors: *Sports Injuries—Basic Principles of Prevention and Care,* Cambridge, MA, 1994, Blackwell Scientific Publications, pp 130-160.
14. Marti B et al: On the epidemiology of running injuries: the 1984 Bern Grand-Prix study, *Am J Sports Med* 16(3):285-294, 1980.
15. Martire JR: Differentiating stress fracture from periostitis—the finer points of bone scans, *Phys Sportsmed* 22(10):71-81, 1994.
16. McBryde AM: Stress fractures in runners, *Clin Sports Med* 4(4):737-752, 1985.
17. McKelvie SJ, Valliant PM, Asu ME: Physical training and personality factors as predictors of marathon time and training injury, *Percept Motor Skills* 60:551-556, 1985.
18. Nigg BM: Biomechanics as applied to sports. In Harries M et al, editors: *The Oxford Textbook of Sports Medicine,* New York, 1994, Oxford Medical Publications, pp 94-111.
19. Panush RS et al: Is running associated with degenerative joint disease? *JAMA* 255(9):1152-1154, 1986.
20. Robbins SE, Hanna AM: Running-related injury prevention through barefoot adaptations, *Med Sci Sports Exerc* 19(2):148-156, 1987.
21. Schafer W, McKenna J: There's a point to stress, *Runner's World,* pp 75-76, 98, 101-102, Aug 1983.
22. van Mechelen W et al: Is range of motion of the hip and ankle joint related to running injuries? A case control study, *Int J Sports Med* 13(8):605-610, 1992.
23. Walter SD et al: The Ontario cohort study of running-related injuries, *Arch Intern Med* 149:2561-2564, 1989.

CHAPTER 79

Aquatic Sports

Lauren M. Simon, MD, MPH

I. Introduction
   A. The aquatic sports synchronized swimming, diving, and water polo share many of the same medical and orthopedic concerns found in swimmers.
   B. Swimming injuries often depend on age of swimmer, stroke performed, and length of training.[18]
   C. Compared to other sports the risk of injury in swimming is low.[3,23]
   D. Competitive swimmers may swim 8,000-20,000 daily,[6] and the repetitive musculoskeletal stresses place the swimmer at risk for injury.

II. Swimming Stroke Biomechanics
   A. Upper extremity biomechanics.
      1. According to Richardson and associates, the free-style, butterfly, and backstroke have similar shoulder motions divided into two general phases: pull through and recovery.[29,33-36,48]
         a. Pull through is the underwater portion of the stroke subdivided into three phases.
            i. Hand entry: shoulder internally rotated and abducted.
            ii. Mid pull-through: shoulder abducted to 90 degrees.
            iii. End pull-through: shoulder internally rotated and adducted.
         b. Recovery (refer to Figure 79-1) is the above water portion of the stroke divided into three phases.
            i. Elbow lift: shoulder abducted, external rotation.
            ii. Mid recovery: shoulder abducted to 90 degrees and externally rotated.
            iii. Hand entry: shoulder maximally abducted and externally rotated.
      2. Both the adduction/internal rotation of the shoulder in pull-through and the abduction/external rotation of the shoulder in recovery are associated with flexion and extension of the elbow.

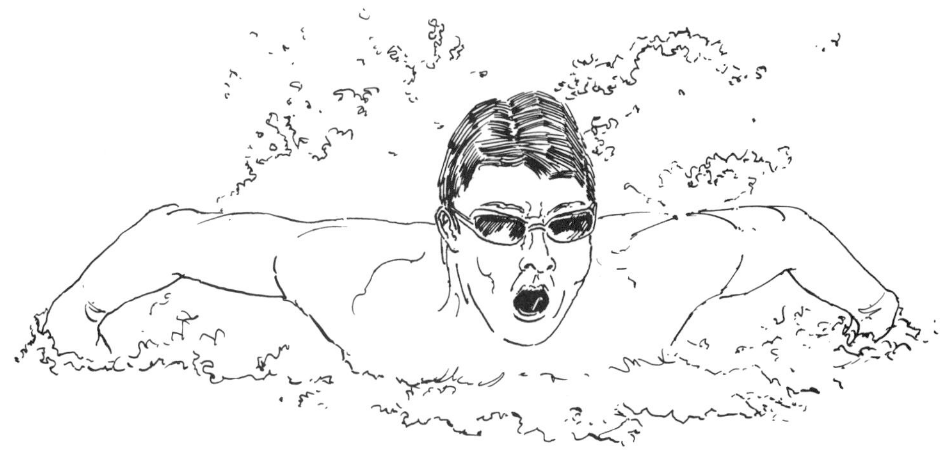

FIGURE 79-1
Swimmer. Butterfly during recovery phase. Body lift enables arms to clear the water.

3. Backstroke and free-style include rotation about the longitudinal axis of the body.
4. Butterfly stroke involves up and down motion instead of rotation.

B. Lower extremity biomechanics.
  1. Knee.
    a. Free-style, backstroke, and butterfly kick knee motion is from extension to 90 degrees of flexion.
    b. Breaststroke kick knee motion is from 130 degrees of flexion to forceful extension. During the breaststroke kick a maximal valgus force is applied to the knees and the feet are dorsiflexed and everted.[34]
  2. Ankle.
    a. Free-style, backstroke, and butterfly kicking motions involve flexion and extension of the ankles.
    b. Breaststroke kicking motion involves dorsiflexion and eversion, which can predispose to compartment syndromes of the lower leg.

III. Orthopedic Concerns in Aquatic Sports
  A. Shoulder.
    1. Shoulder pain is the most common complaint in competitive swimmers.*
    2. Swimmer's shoulder.
      a. Classically, pain caused by impingement of rotator cuff and biceps tendons against overlying undersurface of the acromion and coracoacromial ligament.[6]
      b. The impingement usually occurs at the junction of stroke pull-through and recovery when shoulder is abducted and externally rotated.
      c. Impingement syndrome is also described in synchronized swimming, water polo, diving, and various throwing sports.[32]
      d. Watershed area.[17-19,30,47]
        i. Located 1 cm distal to insertion of biceps and supraspinatus tendons on greater tuberosity of humerus.

*References 7, 11, 15, 17-19, 20, 21, 26, 28, 31, 35, and 36.

ii. In late pull-through with arm adducted there is a "wringing out" of blood supply to supraspinatus,[30] in contrast to hand entry, (abduction forward flexion position) in which angiographic studies demonstrate good supraspinatus blood supply.
iii. Decreased blood supply combined with repetitive microtrauma from swimming strokes may lead to degenerative changes in supraspinatus tendon.

e. Diagnosis and treatment of impingement are discussed in Chapter 34. Additional suggestions for treatment of impingement in aquatic sports are outlined below.
(1) Ice.
(2) Nonsteroidal antiinflammatory medicine.
(3) Stroke modification and variation of strokes.
(4) Swim fins to reduce shoulder strain.
(5) Kickboards: hold board with elbows flexed to avoid reproducing impingement.
(6) Upper arm counterforce brace worn over biceps tendon may relieve symptoms.[6,39]
(7) Strengthen scapular rotators and rotator cuff muscles, especially external rotators, to correct muscle strength imbalance between strong internal and weak external rotators.
(8) Stretch internal rotators.
(9) Physical therapy modalities such as electronic galvanic stimulation or ultrasound.

f. Swimmer's shoulder pain can be divided into four phases.[33]
(1) Pain during workout, not affecting performance.
(2) Pain during and after workout, not affecting performance.
(3) Pain during and after workout, which affects performance.
(4) Pain severe enough to prevent competitive swimming.

g. If swimmer's shoulder is phase 3 or 4, swimmer may need:
(1) Shoulder rest.
(2) Subacromial corticosteroid injection.
(3) Surgery (controversial).

3. Shoulder instability (see Chapter 35).
a. Subluxation or dislocation may be anterior, posterior, or multidirectional.
(1) Cause of shoulder pain in swimmers and other sports.
(2) Anterior subluxation may be associated with anterior glenoid labrum tears, causing painful click in some swimmers.[27]

b. Multidirectional instability.[9,18,24,44,48,50]
(1) Major cause of shoulder pain in competitive swimmers.
(2) Described as symptomatic inferior instability in addition to anterior and or posterior instability.
(3) Flexibility, repetitive shoulder circumduction, and certain stretches may predispose swimmers to this problem.
(4) May coexist with impingement.
(5) Check radiographs for evidence of Bankart lesion of glenoid or Hill-Sachs deformity of humeral head.

c. Apprehension shoulder.
(1) Isolated anterior glenohumeral instability usually from acquired laxity.

(2) Mainly seen in backstroke swimmers from repetitive stretching of anterior capsule.
(3) Anterior subluxation of humeral head occurs during backstroke push-off or flip turns with shoulder maximally abducted and externally rotated.
(4) Treatment.
(a) Strengthen shoulder internal rotators.
(b) Modify backstroke turns.
(c) May need to change stroke.
(d) If conservative therapy fails, may need surgical correction.

4. Other shoulder problems.
a. Bursitis.
b. Scapular winging.
c. Referred neck, clavicular, chest, or lung pain.
d. Suprascapular nerve injury.
e. Thoracic outlet syndrome.

B. Knee.
1. Breastroker's knee.
a. Competitive swimmers have a high incidence of knee pain associated with the breaststroke kick.[10,16,18,37,49]
b. During breaststroke kick a large valgus stress and external rotation force are generated as knee moves from flexion into full extension.
c. Result is medial collateral ligament (MCL) stress, often providing grade I sprain of MCL.
d. Other causes of knee pain associated with breaststroke and other strokes include patellofemoral dysfunction and medial synovial plica syndrome.[33,37,39,49]
e. Treatment.
(1) Ice.
(2) Nonsteroidal antiinflammatory medicine.
(3) Decrease breaststroke distance.
(4) Modify poor breaststroke kick technique.

2. Other causes of swimmer's knee pain.
a. Hypermobile meniscus[33]: rare.
b. Osteochondritis dissecans: may be seen in swimmers and divers.

C. Back and neck.
1. Lumbar back strain.
2. Posterior facet irritation, especially seen in butterfly and breaststroke.
3. Spondylolysis.
a. A cause of low back pain.
b. Stress fracture of pars interarticularis.
c. Seen in breaststrokers, synchronized swimmers, and divers.
d. Associated with hyperextension and accentuated lordosis of spine.
e. May progress to spondylolisthesis.
4. Scoliosis. Some studies show a higher incidence of scoliosis in swimmers than in the general adolescent population.[4]
5. Scheuermann's kyphosis.
a. Occurs in adolescent age group.
b. May be seen in butterfly swimmers.
6. Atlantoaxial instability.
a. Has been found in about 15% of individuals with Down syndrome.
b. Persons with this condition should avoid water polo, breaststroke, butterfly, dive starts, and diving.

7. Additional back and neck problems in divers (See Section VI,).

D. Groin.
1. Pain usually from iliopsoas or adductor strain.
2. Commonly seen in breaststrokers.

E. Foot and ankle.
1. Extensor tendinitis at extensor retinaculum is the most common cause of foot and ankle pain in swimmers.[10,12]
2. Pain and crepitation occur with repetitive neutral to plantar flexion movements in flutter or dolphin kicks.

F. Elbow.
1. Lateral epicondylitis may occur from "elbow up" technique for pull-through strokes in butterfly and free-style.[10]
2. Inflammation of forearm extensors may occur from repeatedly dropping the elbow during stroke.[10,11]

IV. Medical Concerns in Aquatic Sports

A. Asthma (see Chapter 10).
1. Exercise-induced asthma (EIA).
   a. Transient airway obstruction with greater than 10% decrease in FEV_1 or peak expiratory flow rate (PEFR).
   b. Athletes with this condition may participate in competitive swimming.
   c. Premedicate with inhaled $beta_2$-adrenergic agonists or cromolyn sodium.
   d. International Olympic Committee–approved medications for EIA include inhaled albuterol, terbutaline, cromolyn sodium, and oral theophylline.[25]

B. Epilepsy.
1. People with recurrent seizures are at increased risk of drowning.
2. Recommendations for swimming with seizure disorder are controversial. May swim if seizure-free for 6 months with therapeutic drug levels under supervised conditions.[52]

C. Dermatological problems (see Chapter 15).
1. Usually minor in aquatic sports.
2. Common problems are athletes foot, sunburn, warts, rashes.[1,13,16]

D. Nutrition.
1. Swimmers have increased nutritional requirements due to intensity of training.
2. It is not uncommon for swimmers to consume 2500-5000 calories daily.
3. Precompetition meals should be eaten 3-4 hours prior to competition. Easily tolerable, low fat foods should be consumed for pre-meet meal.
4. All day competitions require attention to adequate fluid replacement.[14]

E. Ear, nose, and throat.
1. Otitis externa.
   a. Inflammation of external auditory canal and meatus.[40,41]
   b. May be caused by infection or irritants.
   c. Sources of infection.
      (1) Bacterial: mostly gram-negative organisms, usually *Pseudomonas.*
      (2) Fungal: usually *Aspergillus.*
   d. Predisposing factors.
      (1) Retained moisture in ear canal.
      (2) Removal of protective cerumen manually or by cleaning.
      (3) Damage to canal epithelium by objects such as cotton swabs.[41,46]

e. Signs and symptoms: itching, pain, discharge, swelling of canal, and possible hearing loss.
f. Treatment.
(1) Cleanse ear.
(2) Topical antimicrobial agents with or without hydrocortisone. Cortisporin otic drops are one choice.
(3) Antifungal agents such as 1% tolnaftate for fungal infection.
(4) Ear wick may be needed to instill medicine if excessive ear canal edema.
(5) Ideally, return to pool 7-10 days after initiating treatment, but competitive swimmers may return 2-3 days after beginning treatment.[42]
g. Prevention.
(1) Drying agent use after swimming. Vosol otic drops and white vinegar:alcohol mixture are examples of drying agents.
(2) Molded ear plugs.
2. Rupture of tympanic membrane. May occur from trauma or recurrent otitis media.
3. Rupture of round or oval window of inner ear.
4. Sinusitis and increased nasal secretions are common in aquatic sports.
5. Tympanostomy tubes. Ear plug use recommended for competitive swimmers with tympanostomy tubes.
F. Eye.
1. Chemical conjunctivitis.
a. Chlorinated water results in corneal edema, corneal epithelial defects.
b. The edema causes vision blurring or halo effect.
2. Infective conjunctivitis.
a. Adenovirus types 3 and 4 cause a febrile illness with conjunctivitis and pharyngitis, which may be spread in pool water.[43]
3. Corneal abrasions: may be seen in water polo players.
4. Detached retinas: in diving (rare).
G. Drowning.
1. Drowning is a common cause of accidental death of children in the United States.
2. Drowning is suffocation due to submersion in water. Victims may die of asphyxia secondary to laryngospasm without fluid aspiration or may die of sequel from aspiration.
V. Synchronized Swimming Injuries
A. Most orthopedic and medical concerns in synchronized swimmers are similar to those in swimmers (See Sections III and IV).
B. The upper extremity sculling motion used by synchronized swimmers may contribute to anterior shoulder instability[51] (see Section III).
C. Muscle cramps throughout the body are common in synchronized swimmers and frequently affect calves, toes, and feet.
VI. Diving Injuries
A. Although spring board and platform diving are relatively safe,[22] injuries can occur at different parts of a dive.
B. Components of a dive include board work, take-off, mid-air maneuver, and water entry.
C. Types of injuries.
1. Head: usually occur from hitting diving board or pool bottom.
a. Scalp laceration.
b. Concussion.

c. Rarely, posttraumatic seizure after head injury.
2. Ear and eye: usually occur from improper water entry.
   a. Detached retina.
   b. Ruptured eardrum.
3. Teeth.
   a. Tooth damage usually occurs from hitting board or pool bottom.
   b. May occur from inadvertently biting thigh during a dive.
   c. Chipped or broken teeth are not common injuries in diving.
4. Nose: nasal fracture.
5. Cervical spine.
   a. Neck strain: usually from mid-air twisting maneuver in dive (refer to Fig. 79-2).
   b. Cervical herniated disk with radiculopathy: usually results from hyperflexion of neck instead of neutral position at water entry.[5]
   c. Cervical spine fractures.
      (1) Usually occur in recreational divers diving into shallow water.
      (2) These are preventable injuries.
6. Lumbar spine: injuries usually result from hyperextension of back.[4,5]
   a. Low back strain.
   b. Traumatic spondylolysis (see Section III).
   c. Herniated disk.
   d. Vertebral stress fractures: may occur due to repetitive vertical forces transmitted through diver from diving board.
7. Extremity.
   a. Fingers.
      (1) Lacerations.
      (2) Fractures.
      (3) Abrasions.
   b. Wrist.
      (1) Flat hand water entry involves gripping dorsum and fingers of one hand with opposite hand and fully extending wrists.[5]

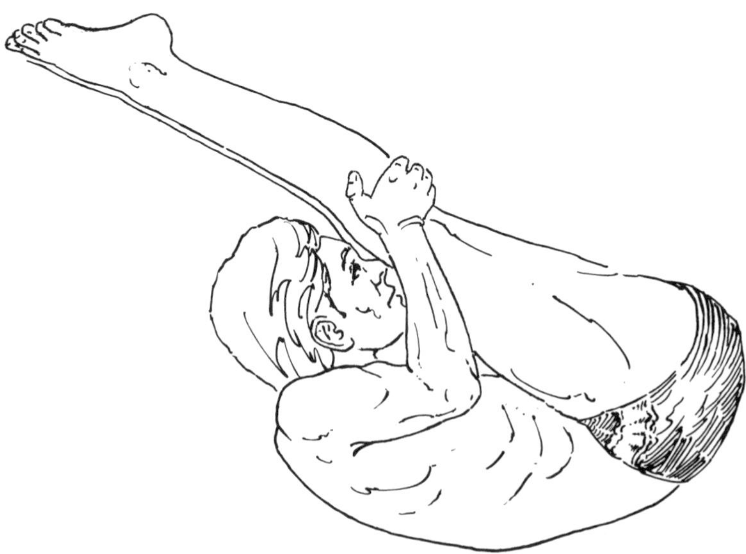

FIGURE 79-2
Diver. Diver in pike position prior to executing a somersault. Divers repeatedly perform maneuvers including twisting and extremes of flexion and extension, which predispose them to injury.

(2) Flat hand entry places stress on distal row of carpal bones. Stress fractures or periostitis of carpal bones may occur.

(3) Ligament and capsular damage can occur to wrist.

c. Elbow: osteochondritis dissecans may occur from overuse syndrome in young divers.

d. Shoulder (also see Section III).

(1) Tendinitis.

(2) Shoulder instability: dislocation of shoulder may occur from failure to hand clasp on water entry, resulting in severe abduction of arms.

VII. Water Polo Injuries

A. Water polo is a contact sport that is a combination throwing and swimming sport (refer to Fig. 79-3).

B. Water polo players use a hand up free-style stroke combined with an "eggbeater" kick. Eggbeater kick combines alternating free-style kick with one leg and breaststroke kick with other leg.

C. Types of injuries.

1. Knee: similar to breaststroker's knee and swimmers knee injuries (See Section III).

2. Thigh: usually occurs from kick to the thigh.

a. Quadricep contusions. Treat as in other sports with early immobilization in 120 degrees of flexion to minimize bleeding and healing time.[2,28]

b. Hamstring contusion.

3. Shoulder.

a. Similar to swimming and throwing injuries (See Section III and Chapter 80).

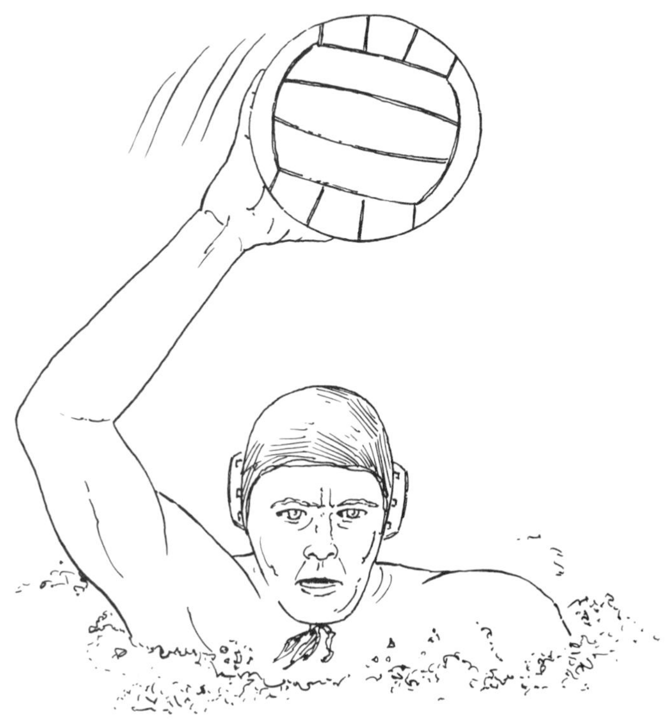

FIGURE 79-3
Water polo player. Water polo injuries include those of swimming, throwing, and contact sports.

4. Elbow: tendinitis.
5. Finger.
   a. Finger injuries are common in water polo (see Chapter 42).
   b. Mallet finger. Rupture of extensor digitorum tendon caused by axial load on extending finger may be seen.
   c. Distal and proximal interphalangeal joint injuries (see Chapter 43).
   d. Ulnar collateral ligament sprain of thumb.
6. Skin (see Section IV, above).
   a. Abrasions.
   b. Lacerations.
   c. Sunburn.
7. Eye: injuries can occur from a finger scratch to the eye or direct trauma.
   (1) Corneal abrasions: treat with anesthetic and eye patch for 24 hours.
   (2) Hyphema.
      (a) Blood in anterior chamber of eye.
      (b) Refer to ophthalmologist.
   (3) Orbital fracture: refer to ophthalmologist.
8. Nose.
   a. Nasal fractures.
   b. Nasal congestion.
   c. Epistaxis.

References

1. Amundson LH: Managing skin problems in athletes. In Mellion MB, editor: *The Team Physician's Handbook,* Philadelphia, 1990, Hanley & Belfus, pp 236-250.
2. Aronen JG, Chronister RD: Quadriceps contusions—hastening the return to play, *Phys Sportsmed* 20(7):130-136, 1992.
3. Backx FJ et al: Sports injuries in school aged children—an epidemiologic study, *Am J Sports Med* 17(2):234-238, 1989.
4. Becker TJ: Scoliosis in swimmers, *Clin Sports Med* 5(1):149-157, 1986.
5. Carter RL: Prevention of springboard and platform diving injuries, *Clin Sports Med* 5(1):185-194, 1986.
6. Ciullo JV: Swimmer's shoulder, *Clin Sports Med* 5(1):115-137, 1986.
7. Dominguez RH: Shoulder pain in swimmers, *Phys Sportsmed* 8:35-42, 1980.
8. Dominguez RH: Water polo injuries, *Clin Sports Med* 5(1):169-184, 1986.
9. Foster CR: Multidirectional instability of the shoulder in the athlete, *Clin Sports Med* 2(2):355-368, 1987.
10. Fowler PJ, Regan WD: Swimming injuries of the knee, foot and ankle, elbow and back, *Clin Sports Med* 5(1):139-148, 1986.
11. Fowler PJ: Upper extremity swimming injuries. In Nicholas JA, Hershman EB, editors: *The Upper Extremity in Sports Medicine,* St Louis, 1990, CV Mosby, pp 891-902.
12. Garrick JG, Requa RK: The epidemiology of foot and ankle injuries in sports, *Clin Sports Med* 7(1):29-36, 1988.
13. Gentile DA, Auerbach PS: The sun and water sports, *Clin Sports Med* 6(3):669-683, 1987.
14. Grandjean AC: Nutrition for swimmers, *Clin Sports Med* 5(1):65-76, 1986.
15. Halpern BC: Shoulder injuries. In Birrer RB, editor: *Sports Medicine for the Primary Care Physician,* ed 2, Boca Raton, FL, 1994, CRC Press, pp 411-433.
16. Hammer RW: Swimming and diving. In Mellion MB, editor: *The Team Physician's Handbook,* Philadelphia, 1990, Hanley & Belfus, pp 559-569.
17. Hawkins RJ, Hobeika PE: Impingement syndrome in the athletic shoulder, *Clin Sports Med* 2(2):391-405, 1987.
18. Johnson JE et al: Musculoskeletal injuries in competitive swimmers, *Mayo Clin Proc* 62:289-304, 1987.
19. Kennedy JC et al: Swimming. In Schneider RC et al, editors: *Sports Injuries: Mechanisms, Prevention and Treatment,* Baltimore, 1985, Williams & Wilkins, pp 368-394.
20. Kennedy JC et al: Orthopedic manifestations of swimming, *Am J Sports Med* 6:309-322, 1978.
21. Kennedy JC, Hawkins RJ: Swimmer's shoulder, *Phys Sportsmed* 2:34-38, 1974.

22. Kimball RJ et al: Competitive diving injuries. In Schneider RC et al, editors: *Sports Injuries: Mechanisms, Prevention and Treatment,* Baltimore, 1985, Williams & Wilkins, pp 192-211.
23. Lanese RR et al: Injury and disability in matched men's and women's intercollegiate sports, *Am J Public Health* 80(12):1459-1462, 1990.
24. Matsen FA, Zuckerman JD: Anterior glenohumeral instability, *Clin Sports Med* 2(2):319-338, 1983.
25. McKeag DB, Hough DO, editors: *Primary Care Sports Medicine,* Dubuque, IA, 1993, Brown & Benchmark, pp 363-367.
26. McMaster WC, Troup J: A survey of interfering shoulder pain in United States competitive swimmers, *Am J Sports Med* 21(1):67-70, 1993.
27. McMaster WC: Anterior glenoid labrum damage: a painful lesion in swimmers, *Am J Sports Med* 14(5):383-387, 1986.
28. McMaster WC: Painful shoulder in swimmers: a diagnostic challenge, *Phys Sportsmed* 14(12): 108-122, 1986.
29. Perry J: Anatomy and biomechanics of the shoulder in throwing, swimming, gymnastics and tennis, *Clin Sports Med* 2(2):265-270, 1983.
30. Rathbun JB, Macnab I: The microvascular pattern of the rotator cuff, *J Bone Joint Surg* 52B:540-553, 1970.
31. Reid DC: Focusing the diagnosis of shoulder pain, *Phys Sportsmed* 22(6):28-44, 1994.
32. Reid DC: *Sports Injury Assessment and Rehabilitation,* New York, 1992, Churchill Livingstone, pp 895-998.
33. Richardson AR: Orthopedic aspects of competitive swimming, *Clin Sports Med* 6(3):639-645, 1987.
34. Richardson AR: The biomechanics of swimming: the shoulder and knee, *Clin Sports Med* 5(1):103-114, 1986.
35. Richardson AB: Overuse syndromes in baseball, tennis, gymnastics and swimming, *Clin Sports Med* 2(2):379-389, 1983.
36. Richardson AB et al: The shoulder in competitive swimming, *Am J Sports Med* 8(3):159-163, 1980.
37. Rovere GD, Nichols AW: Frequency, associated factors and treatment of breaststroker's knee in competitive swimmers, *Am J Sports Med* 13(2):99-104, 1985.
38. Ryan JB et al: Quadriceps contusions, *Am J Sports Med* 19(3):299-304, 1991.
39. Sallis RE: The swimmer. In Birrer RB, editor: *Sports Medicine for the Primary Care Physician,* ed 2, Boca Raton, FL, 1994, CRC Press, pp 223-236.
40. Sarnaik AP et al: Medical problems of the swimmer, *Clin Sports Med* 5(1):47-63, 1986.
41. Schelkun PH: Swimmer's ear—getting patients back in the water, *Phys Sportsmed* 19(7):85-90, 1991.
42. Schuller DE, Bruce RA: Ear, nose, throat and eye. In Strauss RH, editor: *Sports Medicine,* ed 2, Philadelphia, 1991, WB Saunders, pp 189-203.
43. Seiff SR: Ophthalmic complications of water sports, *Clin Sports Med* 6(3):685-693, 1987.
44. Skyhar MJ et al: Instability of the shoulder. In Nicholas JA, Hershman EB, editors: *The Upper Extremity in Sports Medicine,* St Louis, 1990, CV Mosby, pp 181-212.
45. Stanish W: Low back pain in athletes, *Clin Sports Med* 6(2):321-344, 1987.
46. Stricker PR, Green GA: Infections in athletes. In Mellion MB, editor: *Sports Medicine Secrets,* Philadelphia, 1994, Hanley & Belfus, pp 162-166.
47. Stricker PR, Puffer JC: Swimming. In Mellion MB, editor: *Sports Medicine Secrets,* Philadelphia, 1994, Hanley & Belfus, pp 367-372.
48. Tibone JT et al: The shoulder—functional anatomy, biomechanics and kinesiology. In DeLee JC, Drez D, editors: *Orthopaedic Sports Medicine: Principles and Practice,* Philadelphia, 1994, WB Saunders, pp 463-480.
49. Vizsolyi P et al: Breastroker's knee: an analysis of epidemiological and biomechanical factors, *Am J Sports Med* 15(1):63-71, 1987.
50. Warren RF: Subluxation of the shoulder in athletes, *Clin Sports Med* 2(2):339-354, 1983.
51. Weinberg SK: Medical aspects of synchronized swimming, *Clin Sports Med* 5(1):159-167, 1986.
52. Zupanc ML: Therapeutic drug use and epilepsy in sports. In DeLee JC, Drez D, editors: *Orthopaedic Sports Medicine: Principles and Practice,* Philadelphia, 1994, WB Saunders, pp 341-345.

CHAPTER 80

Overhand Throwing Sports

Robert E. Sallis, MD

I. Introduction
   A. Throwing is a central activity in many sports (e.g., baseball, football, water polo, as well as track and field).
   B. In a major league baseball pitcher the margin is minuscule between throwing hard enough to get a major league batter out and yet not so hard as to cause injury.

II. Biomechanics of Throwing
   A. Kinetic energy is generated mainly in legs and torso and is transferred through the throwing arm to the ball. Remaining kinetic energy must then be dissipated.
      1. Injury can occur when muscles improperly generate kinetic energy, when energy is incorrectly transferred through shoulder and elbow to a ball, or when remaining energy is inappropriately dissipated after release.
      2. Correct biomechanics should be maintained during throw to protect thrower from injury.
   B. Four phases occur in the throwing motion; the pain that occurs at each phase often has a distinct cause.
      1. Cocking phase: shoulder abducted to 90 degrees, hyperextended, and maximally externally rotated.
         a. Anterior subluxation may occur at this time because humeral head is forced forward.
         b. Anterior cuff tendinitis may occur secondary to irritation by humeral head.
         c. Dead arm syndrome may occur, and is often associated with an anterior labrum tear.
      2. Acceleration phase: body strides forward and transfers its energy to throwing arm, which is rapidly internally rotated.
         a. Muscle strain of internal rotators (subscapularis, latissimus, and pectoralis major) is common.

b. Impingement syndrome often occurs when supraspinatus rubs against underside of coracoacromial arch.
c. Valgus stress at elbow can lead to strain or tear of ulnar collateral ligament, while compression forces exist at radiocapitellar joint of the lateral elbow.

3. Release and deceleration phase: begins upon ball release, followed by rapid deceleration of humerus when rotator cuff muscles are contracted.
a. Posterior subluxation may occur when humeral head is forced backwards.
b. Posterior cuff tendinitis may occur secondary to irritation by humeral head.
c. Posterior labrum and capsule may be damaged by repeated traction in this area.

4. Follow-through phase: dissipates remaining kinetic energy from arm back through body to trailing leg.
a. Muscle strain occurs when posterior shoulder (usually teres minor and long head of triceps) is repeatedly stressed.
b. Elbow pain may be related to irritation of the olecranon fossa caused by forced elbow extension.

III. Rotator Cuff Injuries

A. Rotator cuff tendinitis.

1. Causes.
a. Generally related to overuse.
b. Glenohumeral instability often contributes.
c. Anatomical factors may worsen because of impingement (acromion shape, degenerative changes).

2. Symptoms.
a. Pain upon throwing.
b. Improves with rest.
c. May have early fatigue or loss of pitching control.

3. Examination findings. Pain upon resisted rotator cuff motion.

B. Impingement syndrome.

1. Causes.
a. Rotator cuff and biceps tendons impinged against acromion and coracoacromial ligament by the humeral head.
b. Often related to similar causative factors as with rotator cuff tendinitis, which can compromise space under coracoacromial arch.
c. Trauma to acromion or acromioclavicular (AC) joint can also narrow space available under arch.

2. Symptoms.
a. Overhead activity exacerbates pain.
b. Symptoms of rotator cuff, biceps tendinitis, or both.

3. Examination findings.
a. Impingement signs positive.
b. Painful arc upon range-of-motion movements (between 80-120 degrees).
c. Pain upon resisted rotator cuff (especially supraspinatus) and biceps motion.
d. Impingement test: symptoms relieved by subacromial injection of lidocaine if caused by impingement.

4. Stages of impingement.
a. Stage 1: athlete usually < 25 years of age.

i. Edema, hemorrhage, and inflammation occur in rotator cuff tendons.
ii. Reversible.

b. Stage 2: athlete usually 25-40 years of age.
   i. Fibrosis, thickened bursae, and tendon scarring occur.
   ii. Irreversible changes.
c. Stage 3: athlete usually > 40 years of age. Tendon rupture and bony changes occur.

C. Rotator cuff tear.
   1. Causes.
      a. Most often caused by chronic rotator cuff tendinitis with impingement.
      b. May occur after episode of trauma or violent activity.
   2. Symptoms.
      a. Rotator cuff tendinitis and impingement pain persist and worsen.
      b. Pain often occurs at night.
      c. Muscle strength is diminished.
   3. Examination findings.
      a. True weakness of rotator cuff. Often difficult to differentiate true weakness from inhibition of strength caused by pain.
      b. Tenderness at supraspinatus tendon and possible palpable defect in cuff over humeral head.
      c. Possible muscle atrophy.

D. Treatment of rotator cuff injury.
   1. Rest from aggravating motion (throwing) and restrict range of arm motion to below the horizontal.
   2. Ice, nonsteroidal antiinflammatory drugs.
   3. Flexibility and strengthening programs.
   4. Graduated throwing program.
   5. Consider corticosteroid injection into subacromial bursa if injury does not respond after 1-2 months.
   6. Consider surgery for chronic impingement or rotator cuff tear.

IV. Biceps Tendon Injury

A. Biceps tendinitis.
   1. Causes.
      a. Overuse.
      b. May be associated with underlying impingement syndrome.
   2. Symptoms: pain over anterior shoulder increases upon resisted elbow flexion or wrist supination.
   3. Examination findings.
      a. Tenderness over long head of biceps tendon at bicipital groove.
      b. Speed and Yergason tests are positive (see Chapter 33 for definition of tests).

B. Subluxation, rupture, or both of biceps tendon.
   1. Causes.
      a. Often results from chronic tendinitis and transverse humeral ligament rupture, which holds tendon in bicipital groove. Chronic tendinitis also makes tendon vulnerable to forceful rupture.
      b. Cortisone injection may weaken tendon and predispose it to rupture.
      c. Rupture occurs upon sudden forceful flexion of arm.
   2. Symptoms.
      a. Snapping sensation in shoulder upon internal and external rotation.

   b. Rupture usually accompanied by extreme local pain and weakness.
  3. Examination findings.
   a. Same as biceps tendinitis.
   b. May have snapping sensation upon external rotation.
   c. Upon rupture of long head, muscle mass moves distally ("Popeye" appearance); weakness occurs upon supination.
 C. Treatment of biceps tendon injury.
  1. Rest, ice, nonsteroidal antiinflammatory drugs.
  2. Therapeutic stretching and exercise.
  3. Tennis elbow strap can be placed on upper arm proximal to widest part of biceps.
  4. Consider cortisone injection (but may predispose to biceps tendon rupture).
  5. Consider surgery.
   a. For athletes who have persistent subluxation (tendon sutured to bicipital groove).
   b. For younger, more athletic patients who have proximal biceps tendon rupture. (Older patients are generally treated conservatively.)
   c. For all distal ruptures.

V. Shoulder Instability
 A. Description.
  1. Laxity is normal glenohumeral translation. Wide variation exists in normal laxity, and laxity is often increased in throwers.
  2. Instability is abnormal translation (i.e., subluxation or dislocation, which results in symptoms).
  3. Glenohumeral instability is a frequent cause of shoulder pain and often coexists with rotator cuff injury, impingement, and glenoid labrum injury.
 B. Pathophysiology.
  1. Repeated overhead throwing stretches static restraints of shoulder (capsule and glenohumeral ligaments).
  2. Dynamic stabilizers (rotator cuff muscles) increase activity to compensate for mild instability.
  3. Dynamic stabilizers fatigue and allow subluxation.
  4. Subluxation leads to increased translation of humeral head, which irritates rotator cuff tendons, labrum, and glenoid.
 C. Causes.
  1. Repeated microtrauma upon overhead throwing as previously described.
  2. Dislocations.
   a. Traumatic (TUBS = traumatic, unidirectional, Bankart labrum lesion, surgical treatment).
   b. Atraumatic (AMBRI = atraumatic, multidirectional, bilateral laxity, rehabilitation, inferior capsule tightening, if surgery needed).
 D. Symptoms.
  1. Generally athlete has pain, but pain is often subtle. Pain is worse during cocking phase with anterior subluxation and during deceleration phase with posterior subluxation.
  2. Shoulder instability frequently occurs concomitantly with other problems.
 E. Examination findings.
  1. Apprehension tests (anterior and/or posterior instability).

2. Sulcus sign (inferior instability).
3. Relocation test (differentiates instability from primary impingement).

F. Treatment of shoulder instability.
1. Treat associated tendinitis, impingement, or labrum injury.
2. Rehabilitaion program includes rotator cuff strengthening and flexibility (to decrease joint instability).
a. Those who have anterior subluxation have weakness of internal rotators and loss of external rotation.
b. Those who have posterior subluxation have weakness of external rotators and loss of internal rotation.

VI. Glenoid Labrum Injury
A. Causes.
1. Recurrent anterior and posterior humeral head translation during throwing motion (such as with instability and subluxation).
2. Indirect trauma may cause injury as well.
B. Symptoms.
1. Pain upon overhead activity, often associated with painful clicking or snapping in shoulder.
2. Symptoms often worse at cocking or follow-through phase of throwing.
C. Examination findings.
1. Tender over glenohumeral joint.
2. "Clunk" test positive (see Chapter 33 for definition of test).
D. Treatment of glenoid labrum injury.
1. Start with conservative treatment (rest, ice, nonsteroidal antiinflammatory drugs).
2. Treat recurrent instability by rehabilitation program.
3. Surgery may be needed if injury does not respond to conservative treatment. (Often use arthroscopic labrum debridement.)

VII. Dead Arm Syndrome
A. Causes.
1. Anterior instability, often with torn anterior labrum.
2. Probably causes transient stretch to brachial plexus.
B. Symptoms.
1. Sudden paralyzing pain and numbness usually during cocking phase of throwing.
2. Frequent lingering feeling of weakness.
C. Examination findings: suggests labrum tear and anterior cuff tendinitis.
D. Treatment: as previously outlined for glenoid labrum injury.

VIII. Effort Thrombosis
A. Causes.
1. Common variant of thoracic outlet syndrome (outlet may be narrowed because cervical rib, abnormal first rib, or hypertrophy of scalene muscles is present).
2. Subclavian or axillary vein becomes acutely thrombosed.
B. Symptoms.
1. Arm swelling and superficial vein prominence, which occur upon throwing.
2. Resolves with rest.
C. Examination findings: usually normal. Exertion will evoke symptoms.
D. Treatment of effort thrombosis.
1. Venogram to confirm diagnosis.
2. Rest, heat, elevation.

3. Warfarin sodium for 3 months.
4. Consider thrombolysis with urokinase.
5. Treat underlying cause (cervical rib, abnormal first rib, hypertrophied callus, or abnormal scalene muscles).

IX. Medial Elbow Injury
  A. Ulnar collateral ligament tear.
    1. Causes.
      a. Valgus stress at elbow when throwing results in microscopic tears within ligament.
      b. Altered pitching mechanics, such as opening up too soon, may contribute.
    2. Symptoms.
      a. Pain at medial elbow, especially during acceleration phase.
      b. May have audible pop with complete rupture during a throw.
      c. May see ulnar nerve irritation.
    3. Examination findings.
      a. Tender at ulnar collateral ligament.
      b. Increased pain at medial elbow upon valgus stress test.
      c. Laxity of ligament can be shown by valgus stress with elbow flexed to 30 degrees to unlock olecranon.
  B. Medial epicondylitis.
    1. Causes.
      a. Flexor and pronator muscles of wrist and portion of ulnar collateral ligament attach at medial epicondyle of elbow.
      b. Increased stress upon repetitive throwing can irritate epicondyle or even lead to avulsion fracture (especially in a young athlete).
    2. Symptoms.
      a. Medial elbow pain; worse upon throwing.
      b. Ulnar nerve irritation may occur.
    3. Examination findings.
      a. Tenderness at medial epicondyle.
      b. Pain increases with resisted wrist flexion or pronation.
  C. Flexor-pronator strain.
    1. Causes: repetitive throwing with stress to flexor-pronator muscles, which attach at medial epicondyle.
    2. Symptoms: pain at medial elbow and proximal forearm; pain increases upon throwing.
    3. Examination findings.
      a. Tender at flexor-pronator muscles of forearm.
      b. Increased pain with resisted wrist flexion or pronation.
  D. Ulnar neuritis.
    1. Causes.
      a. Ulnar groove is bordered by ulnar collateral ligament and medial epicondyle; injury to these structures may thus result in ulnar nerve injury.
      b. Mechanical compromise at the nerve medially may result from traction, friction, or compression.
    2. Symptoms.
      a. Shooting pain, tingling, and numbness down forearm to fourth and fifth fingers.
      b. Grip weakness may occur.
      c. May develop painful popping if nerve subluxates from ulnar groove.
  E. Treatment of medial elbow injuries.

1. Rest from throwing.
2. Ice, nonsteroidal antiinflammatory drugs.
3. Range-of-motion and flexibility programs initiated as pain resolves, followed by progressive resistance exercises to strengthen muscles near elbow.
4. Graduated throwing program. (Should assess throwing mechanics and correct errors.)
5. Cortisone injections can be used with caution to help reduce inflammation around epicondyle.
6. Consider surgery in those who have valgus instability on stress testing or in those who have persistent ulnar nerve irritation or ulnar nerve subluxation.

X. Lateral Elbow Injury: Radiocapitellar Chondromalacia
   A. Causes.
      1. Valgus forces at elbow upon throwing cause strong compression forces at radiocapitellar joint.
      2. Repeated compression forces lead to bony injury. Eventually can result in osteochondritis dissecans and loose bodies.
   B. Symptoms.
      1. Lateral elbow pain upon throwing. Often begins as minimal, then progresses.
      2. Eventually swelling, lack of extension, catching, and even locking may occur if fragments are loose within joint.
   C. Examination findings.
      1. Tender at radiocapitellar joint.
      2. May develop crepitus upon forearm pronation-supination.
      3. Elbow extension restricted as symptoms progress.
   D. Treatment.
      1. Rest, ice, nonsteroidal antiinflammatory drugs.
      2. Consider splinting for short time.
      3. Flexibility and strengthening programs, followed by gradual return to throwing.
      4. Consider surgery for intractable symptoms or to remove loose bodies.

XI. Posterior Elbow Injuries
   A. Inflammation of olecranon fossa (olecranon fossitis).
      1. Causes.
         a. Elbow is forced into full extension during follow-through phase of throwing. This in effect jams olecranon into olecranon fossa.
         b. Can result in inflammation and bony breakdown, which eventually can lead to osteochondritis dissecans and loose bodies.
      2. Symptoms.
         a. Posterior elbow pain upon throwing, especially during follow-through.
         b. Locking or catching may occur.
      3. Examination findings.
         a. Tenderness and swelling around olecranon and fossa.
         b. Lack of full extension associated with pain.
      4. Treatment.
         a. Rest, ice, nonsteroidal antiinflammatory drugs.
         b. Flexibility and strengthening programs, followed by gradual return to throwing.

c. May need surgery to remove loose bodies or spurs, which typically occur at tip of olecranon.

B. Triceps tendinitis.
   1. Cause: overuse upon repetitive throwing.
   2. Symptoms: posterior elbow pain, which is most prominent during deceleration and follow-through phases.
   3. Examination findings.
      a. Tender at distal triceps tendon.
      b. Pain increases upon resisted elbow extension.
   4. Treatment.
      a. Rest, ice, nonsteroidal antiinflammatory drugs.
      b. Flexibility and strengthening.
      c. Gradual return to throwing.

XII. Little League Elbow
   A. Causes.
      1. Repetitive throwing in a skeletally immature athlete.
      2. Muscles and ligaments attach at medial epicondyle near a growth plate. Tensile stresses upon throwing are more likely to injure the weaker growth plate and may lead to avulsion.
   B. Symptoms.
      1. Insidious medial elbow pain, which frequently goes unreported.
      2. Pain progresses upon continued throwing.
   C. Examination findings.
      1. Tenderness at medial epicondyle. May be associated with swelling.
      2. Radiography may show widening or separation at apophyseal line.
   D. Treatment.
      1. Rest and ice. May need to avoid throwing completely until growth plates close.
      2. Gradual return to throwing.
      3. Avoid throwing breaking pitches (curves and sliders).

Acknowledgement

The Medical Editing Department, Kaiser Foundation Research Institute, provided editorial assistance.

Bibliography

Abrams JS: Special shoulder problems in the throwing athlete: pathology, diagnosis, and nonoperative management, *Clin Sports Med* 10:839-861, 1991.

Anderson TE, Ciolek J: Specific rehabilitation programs for the throwing athlete, *Instr Course Lect* 38:487-491, 1989.

Jobe FW, Fanton GS: Nerve injuries. In Morrey BF, editor: *The Elbow and Its Disorders,* Philadelphia, 1985, WB Saunders, pp 497-501.

Jobe FW, Kvitne RS: Shoulder pain in the overhand or throwing athlete: the relationship of anterior instability and rotator cuff impingement, *Orthop Rev* 18:963-975, 1989 [published erratum appears in *Orthop Rev* 18(12):1268, 1989].

Jobe FW, Nuber G: Throwing injuries of the elbow, *Clin Sports Med* 5:621-636, 1986.

Noah J, Gidumal R: Rotator cuff injuries in the throwing athlete, *Orthop Rev* 17:1091-1096, 1988.

Sallis RE: The thrower. In Birrer RB, editor: *Sports Medicine for the Primary Care Physician,* ed 2. Boca Raton, FL, 1994, CRC Press, pp 229-236.

Scheib JS: Diagnosis and rehabilitation of the shoulder impingement syndrome in the overhead and throwing athlete, *Clin Sports Med* 16:971-988, 1990.

CHAPTER 81

Skiing Injuries

Steven D. Stahle, MD

Robert. J. Dimeff, MD

I. Overview
   A. Skiing is a popular, demanding sport.
   B. Between 1960 and 1980 the incidence of skier injuries decreased from 10 per 1000 skier days to 2-4 per 1000 ski days.[3]
   C. Environment, equipment, experience, and type of skiing affect injury and illness in skiers.
   D. This chapter outlines medical and orthopedic injuries of alpine, cross-country, and snowboard skiers.

II. Medical Ski Injuries: Environmental Exposure
   A. Hypothermia.
      1. Defined as a core body temperature of <35°C.
      2. 20% of all ski injuries are cold related.
      3. Mild hypothermia (32°-35°C).
         a. Patient pale, cool with uncontrolled shivering.
         b. Treated with blankets, dry clothes, warm environment, and consumption of warm food and liquids.
      4. Moderate hypothermia (28°-32°C).
         a. Shivering stops; patient may become rigid with deteriorating mental status.
         b. Hypotension, bradycardia, hypoventilation possible.
         c. Treatment: warm environment, heating pad, warm water bottles and lamps and active core rewarming by intubation or facemask, warmed IV fluids.
      5. Severe hypothermia (<28°C).
         a. Patient may be without vital signs; do not pronounce dead until "warm and dead."
         b. Sudden movements and cardiopulmonary resuscitation may trigger fatal cardiac dysrhythmias.
         c. Treat with active core rewarming (intubation, gastric lavage, peritoneal dialysis, etc.).

6. Frostbite.
   a. Tissue appears white to bluish and has little to no sensation.
   b. Treatment: warm water bath for 30 minutes, pain control, tetanus prophylaxis.
   c. Leave blisters intact.
7. Chilblains (frostnip).
   a. Localized itching, swelling, painful erythema of extremities (can appear mottled and waxy) caused by mild frostbite.
   b. Treatment: remove from environment, dry and warm affected area.
8. Prevention: layered clothing, decreased exposure.

B. Altitude syndrome.
1. Acute mountain sickness (AMS).
   a. Usually occurs at 8000 feet and above.
   b. Symptoms usually last 1-3 days and include headache, nausea and vomiting, malaise, and sleep disturbances.
   c. Treatment: self-limiting condition, avoid alcohol, acetazolamide may mimic acclimatization.
2. High altitude pulmonary edema (HAPE).
   a. Related to rapid ascent to >8000 feet, relatively uncommon, can be fatal.
   b. Severe dyspnea, productive cough common. Examination shows tachypnea; rales; pink; frothy sputum; cyanosis.
   c. Treatment is rapid descent, oxygen. Diuretics, steroids, nifedipine may be used.
3. High altitude cerebral edema (HACE).
   a. Presents with severe headache, ataxia, abnormal behavior, hallucinations.
   b. May progress to coma and death.
   c. Treatment is rapid descent. Temporizing treatment includes oxygen, dexamethasone, and hyperbaric chamber.
4. Prevention includes gradual ascent, increased hydration, avoidance of alcohol and sedatives.

C. Sun exposure.
1. Sunburns are very common.
2. Retinal burns, keratosis, and ultraviolet (UV)-induced cataracts are possible.
3. Prevention includes minimizing exposure, UV blocking lotions, glasses or goggles.
4. Treat symptomatically.

III. Orthopedic Ski Injuries

A. Downhill skiing (alpine skiing).
1. Decreased ski injury incidence in 20 years despite an increase in actual total injuries.[14]
   a. Redesigned ski boots and bindings help decrease injury rate (not to anterior cruciate ligament [ACL]).
   b. Improved grooming and instruction have also decreased injury incidence.
2. Injuries occur most often in beginners, frequently when ski bindings are not adjusted properly or fail to release.
3. Overuse injuries.
   a. Not well documented.
   b. Muscles of posture and poling affected.
   c. Treatment is rest, stretching, strengthening, ice, and antiinflammatories.

4. Upper extremity injuries.
   a. Less common than lower extremity injuries.
   b. Usually occurs with falls or collisions.
   c. "Skier's thumb."
      (1) Sprain of ulnar collateral ligament (UCL) at first metacarpophalangeal (MCP) joint. Occurs during a fall with the outstretched hand holding on to the ski pole.
      (2) Diagnosis: comparative examination with unaffected side, stress at zero and 30 degrees of flexion, with radiography.
      (3) Treatment.
         (a) Grade I, II sprains and nondisplaced avulsion fractures: short arm spicacast for 3-6 weeks.
         (b) Grade III sprains: short arm spicacast or possible surgery.
      (4) Stener's lesion: torn proximal end of the UCL lies outside the adductor aponeurosis. May require surgery.
      (5) Prevention: avoid valgus force to thumb (i.e., don't fall).
   d. Shoulder injuries.
      (1) Glenohumeral dislocation is the most common shoulder injury.
         (a) Mechanism is abduction, external rotation.
         (b) Treatment: immediate reduction, immobilization, radiography.
      (2) Acromioclavicular separation.
         (a) Mechanism: fall on point of shoulder, collision.
         (b) Treatment: mostly conservative.
   e. Fractures.
      (1) Less common than lower extremity fractures.
      (2) History, physical examination, and radiography.
5. Lower extremity injuries.
   a. Improved equipment designs have decreased lower extremity injury incidence by 60%.[14]
   b. Incidence of ankle and tibia injuries decreased. Severe knee injuries continue to rise.[6]
   c. Anterior Cruciate Ligament (ACL) injuries.
      (1) Most common injury requiring surgery. 50,000–100,000/year in United States.[7]
      (2) Mechanism.
         (a) "Boot top drawer": during landing the skier hyperflexes the knee while falling backward; the skis, boots, and tibia fall forwards. With quadriceps contracted an anterior force is placed on the tibia, resulting in an anterior drawer and rupture of the ACL.
         (b) The combination of hyperextension, external rotation of the tibia (with the skis acting as a lever), and a valgus load can produce a rupture of the ACL.
      (3) Diagnosis.
         (a) History of one of the above mechanisms with a "pop" and immediate swelling.
         (b) Positive Lachman's test, positive pivot shift.
         (c) Magnetic resonance imaging (MRI) for associated injuries.
      (4) Treatment.
         (a) Immobilization, ice, nonsteroidal antiinflammatory drugs (NSAIDs).
         (b) Range of motion (ROM) exercises, Progressive resistance exercises (PRE) as soon as possible.

(c) Conservative vs. surgical.

d. Medial Collateral Ligament (MCL) sprains.
  (1) Common injury, females >males.[8]
  (2) Mechanism: valgus stress to knee.
  (3) Diagnosis.
    (a) Instability with valgus stress.
    (b) Grade I sprain: 2–5 mm opening.
    (c) Grade II sprain: 6–10 mm opening.
    (d) Grade III sprain: >10 mm opening.
  (4) Treatment.
    (a) Rest, ice, compression, and elevation (RICE), short period of immobilization, bracing, ROM, PRE, functional drills.
    (b) Grade I patients may return to activity as tolerated. Grade II and III patients may require longer brace protection.

e. Meniscal injuries.
  (1) Incidence decreased in acute ACL tears during skiing.[2]
  (2) Diagnosis: positive McMurray's test, joint line tenderness, swelling. MRI helpful.
  (3) Treatment: conservative vs. surgery (surgery for persistent pain, swelling, or mechanical symptoms).

f. Chondral defects.
  (1) Mechanism: direct trauma to knee.
  (2) Diagnosis: localized pain, swelling, positive radiographs, bone scan.
  (3) Treatment: conservative vs. surgery (surgery for persistent pain, swelling, or mechanical symptoms).

g. Fractures.
  (1) Account for 2% of all ski injuries.[7]
  (2) Boot top fracture of tibia/fibula, spiral fractures decreased with the higher, stiffer boot.

6. Accidental death: usually due to head/neck trauma from collision with stationary objects.[5]

B. Cross-country skiing (Nordic skiing).

1. Strenuous cardiovascular sport.
2. One-seventh injury rate of downhill ski injuries.[4]
3. Overuse injuries.
  a. Swedish data suggest >75% of all injuries are overuse injuries.[13]
  b. Classical ski techniques: shin splints, Achilles' tendinitis, and low back pain.
  c. Free-style technique: hip musculature, "skier's toe," triceps, forearm, and wrist.
  d. Treatment: ice, stretch, strengthen, relative rest, antiinflammatories.
4. Upper extremity injuries.
  a. Injury rate similar in downhill skiers.
  b. "Skier's thumb."
  c. Shoulder injuries: glenohumeral dislocation and acromioclavicular separation.
5. Lower extremity injuries.
  a. Increased injuries from lower boot, heel fixation, and faster skis.[13]
  b. Occur mostly on downhill and tracked trails.[1]
  c. Knee injuries.
    (1) MCL injuries >ACL injuries.
    (2) ACL injury.
      (a) Mechanism: similar to downhill.

(b) Diagnosis and treatment as noted.
d. Ankle.
(1) Less protection from lower boot.
(2) Sprains more often than fractures.
e. Fractures.
(1) Accounts for 12% of injuries.[1]
(2) Related to nonrelease bindings, heel fixation devices.
6. Accidental death very rare.
C. Snowboarding injuries.
1. The world's fastest growing winter sport.[4]
2. Technique and equipment.
a. Snowboards: alpine, all-around, free-style.
b. Skier's left foot usually forward.
c. Boots are either soft or hard shell.
d. Bindings are usually nonreleasable.
3. Injury frequency.
a. Usually inexperienced, young males.[9]
b. Forward limb sustains more injuries.[12]
c. Common mechanism: impact > torsional.
d. Lower extremity injuries.
(1) Ankle injuries > knee injuries.[11]
(2) Knee injuries common with hard boot.
(3) Ankle injuries common with soft boot.
e. Upper extremity.
(1) Absorbs most of impact force.
(2) Distal radial fractures commonly due to falls onto outstretched hand.
(3) Fewer thumb injuries than alpine related to lack of ski poles.[12]
f. Deep snow immersion deaths.
(1) Occurs in deep powder, tree wells, and outside groomed areas.
(2) Recent deaths emphasize need for safety education.[10]

References

1. Boyle JJ et al: Cross-country skiing injuries. In Johnson RJ, Mote CD, editors: *Skiing Trauma and Safety. Fifth International Symposium, ASTM STP 860,* Philadelphia, 1985, American Society for Testing and Materials, pp 411-422.
2. Cimino PM: The incidence of meniscal tears associated with acute anterior cruciate ligament disruption secondary to snow skiing accidents, *J Arthroscopy* 10:198-200, 1994.
3. Dimeff RJ: Ski injuries. Presented at American Academy of Family Physicians: Sports Medicine: An in-depth review, Dallas, April 1993.
4. Elmquist LG et al: Nordic and alpine skiing. In Fu FH, Stone DA, editors: *Sports Injuries,* ed 1, Philadelphia, 1994, Williams & Wilkins.
5. Fiore DC: Death on a ski slope, *Phys Sportsmed* 22(2):46-55, 1994.
6. Howe J, Johnson RJ: Knee injuries in skiing, *Clin Sports Med* 1:277-288, 1982.
7. Johnson R: Skiing injuries. Presented at American Academy of Family Physicians: Sports Medicine: An in-depth review, Dallas, February 1995.
8. Johnson RJ, Pope M: Epidemiology and prevention of ski injuries, *Ann Chir Gynaecol* 80(2):110-115, 1991.
9. Jorgsholm P et al: Downhill skiing is developing: snowboard and telemark skiing give new injury pattern, *Lakartidningen* 88:1589-1592, 1991.
10. Kizer KW et al: Deep snow immersion deaths: a snowboarding danger, *Phys Sportsmed* 22(12):49-61, 1994.
11. McLennan JC, McLennan JG: Snowboarding: what injuries to expect in this rapidly growing sport, *J Musculoskeletal Med* 8(11):75-89, 1991.
12. Pino EC, Colville MR: Snowboard injuries, *Am J Sports Med* 17:778-781, 1989.
13. Renstrom P, Johnson RJ: Cross-country skiing injuries and biomechanics, *Sports Med* 8(6):346-370, 1989.
14. Steadman JR, Sterett WI: The surgical treatment of knee injuries in skiers, *Med Sci Sports Exerc* 27(3):328-333, 1995.

CHAPTER 82

Dance

C. Mark Chassay, MD

I. Dance Terminology
   A. Class: avenue by which each dancer becomes better able to meet the challenging physical demands performances can make (classical).
   B. Barre: wooden wall-mounted railing about 3½ feet from floor, which is held by participants to maintain balance. Classes begin here as dancers learn five foot positions (Fig. 82-1) and gradually begin flexibility exercises, which increase in complexity and speed (classical).
   C. Turnout: external hip rotation ideally 180 degrees (classical).
   D. Rolling in: forced eversion and pronation (classical; Fig. 82-2).
   E. Pointe: dancing on toes, starts when dancer is more physically mature (11 or 12 years of age) or consistently performs away from the barre (classical; Fig. 82-3).
   F. Demipointe: extreme plantar flexion, knees flexed about 90 degrees with weight on metatarsal heads (classical; Fig. 82-3).
   G. Plié: extreme plantar flexion, simple knee flexing with weight on metatarsal heads with external rotation of the lower extremities (classical).
   H. Low impact: at least one foot touches the ground at all times (aerobics).
   I. High impact: high energy, explosive movements of all extremities (aerobics).

II. Dance Medicine Team
   A. Instructor.
      1. Makes each dancer aware of physical limitations.
      2. Counsels dancer regarding challenges inherent in physique.
      3. Instructs in proper conditioning, strengthening, and nutrition.
      4. Provides reference regarding proper technique.
   B. Artistic director.
      1. Responsible for proper planning of tour and rehearsal to allow sufficient rest.
      2. Ensures that ideal dance floor is available.
      3. Matches dance requirements with athlete's capabilities.

TABLE 82-1. Overview of most common types of dance

	Classical	Modern	Jazz	Aerobic
Origins	Italian Renaissance Royal feasts/celebrations 15th century	19th century Defiance of ballet	America, later than modern	Late 1980s
Basis	Freedom, grace, ease of movement Aesthetic line	Use of gravity Bonding with nature Defiance of gravity	Sharp, percussive, angular	Choreographed fitness
Particulars	Five foot positions Turnout	Faster Less external hip rotation Knee hyperflexion	No hip rotation High kicks Splits Floor sliding	Abrupt movements Small area
Participants	Mostly female* Begin at 4 years of age Men begin in late teens	Begin at later ages than in ballet	Adolescents Cross-training with ballet	24 million in early 1990s All ages
Footwear	Thin slipper/toe shoe Nonsupportive	None (barefoot)	Lace-up slipper with sole	Supportive, athletic shoe

*Ideal physique includes long arms and legs, small waist, slender neck, and small head.

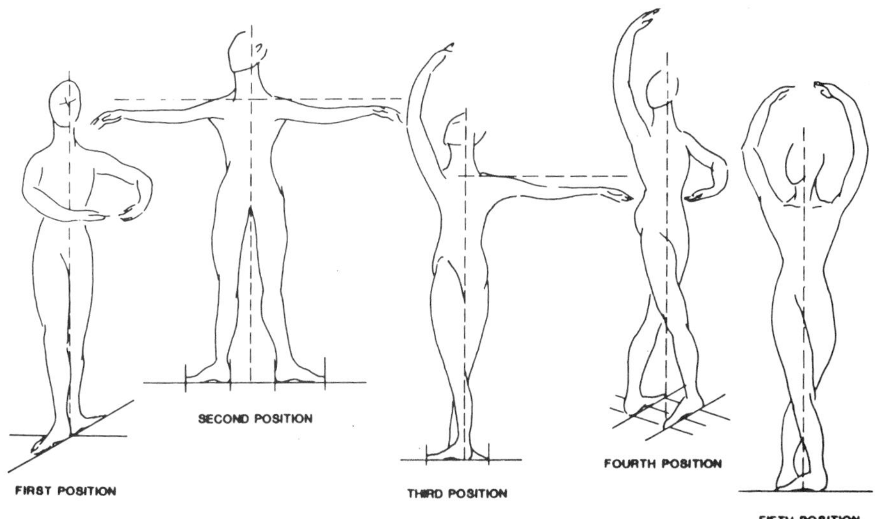

FIGURE 82-1
The basic positions of the arms and legs in classical dance are shown. (Reproduced by permission of the author and publisher from: Nixon JE. Injuries to the neck and upper extremities of dancers. *Clin Sports Med* 1983;2:465. [18])

C. Therapist.
   1. Supervises highly structured rehabilitation program.
   2. Restores injured area.
D. Physician.
   1. Provides prompt diagnosis.
   2. Understands biomechanics of injuries.
   3. Understands psychological demands.

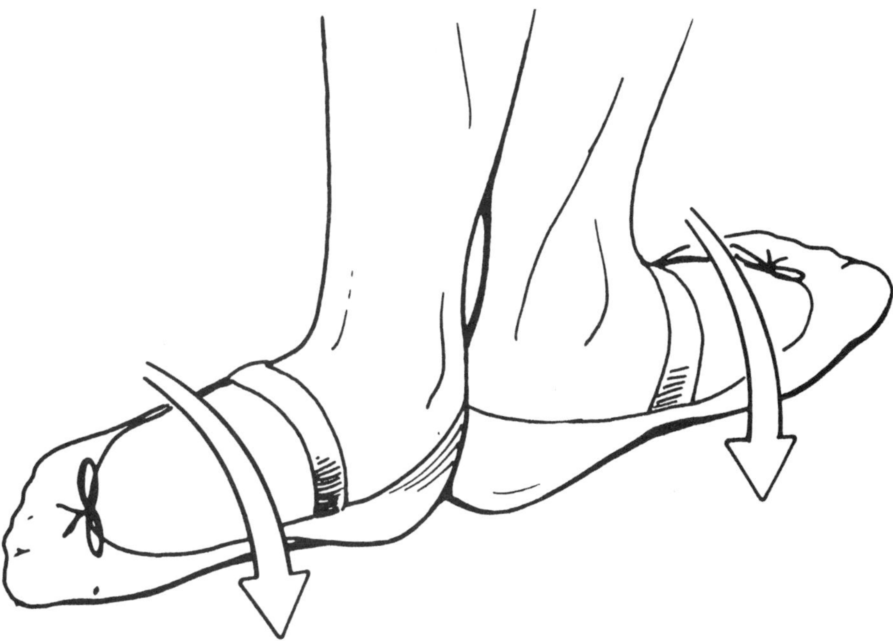

FIGURE 82-2
Rolling-in is a maladaptive technique characterized by extreme pronation and places increased stress on the medial structures of the foot and ankle. (Reproduced by permission of the author and publisher from: Hardaker WT Jr. Foot and ankle injuries in classical ballet dancers. *Orthop Clin North Am* 1989;20:622. [10])

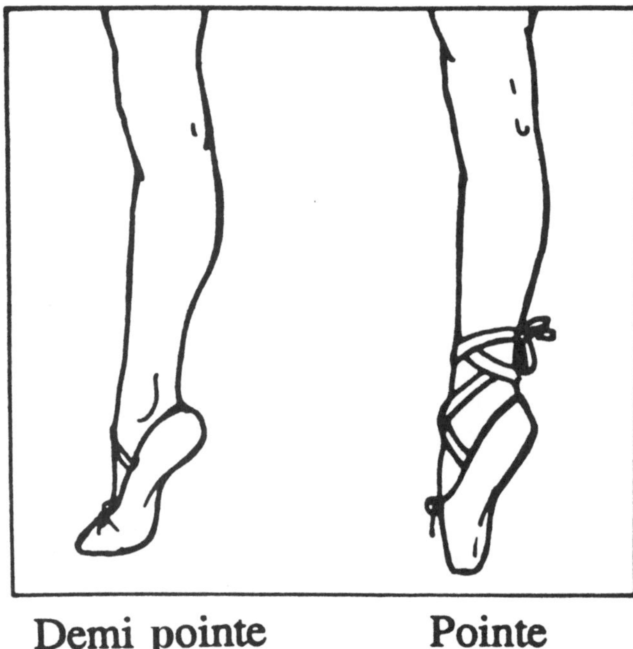

FIGURE 82-3
Relevé positions of demi- and full pointe. (Reproduced by permission of the author and publisher from: Hardaker WT Jr, Vander Woude LM. Dance medicine: an orthopaedist's view. *N C Med J* 1993; 54:71. [13])

III. Medical Concerns
   A. Malnutrition.
      1. "Thin is in" mentality leads to severely restricted dietary intake.
      2. Daily caloric expenditure can approach 5000 kcal (those burned by basal metabolism plus activity).
      3. Carbohydrates fuel of choice for maintaining metabolic balance.
      4. Negative balance of stored carbohydrate is accompanied by fatigue, headache, nervousness, irritability, and loss of concentration and coordination.
      5. Vitamins and minerals: many classical ballet dancers receive <85% of the recommended daily allowance of folic acid, vitamins B_6 and B_{12}, iron, zinc, and biotin. Dancers often view a vitamin pill as a cure-all.
      6. Iron-deficiency anemia reported to affect 15% to 20% of dancers so supplementation may be judicious.
      7. Treatment includes a well-balanced diet as well as proper education regarding nutrition in addition to monitoring percentage of body fat.
   B. Menstrual disorders.
      1. Age: younger, premenarchal girls are at greater risk for development of menstrual disorders than dancers who begin class postmenarche.
      2. Common underlying characteristic is low body fat; 17% body fat is required for menarche, and 22% is required for resumption of menstrual flow after secondary amenorrhea.
      3. Inadequate nutrition.
      4. Low estrogen level.
      5. Physical or mental stress or both affect cortisol levels.
      6. Types:
         a. Delayed menarche.
         b. Primary amenorrhea.

c. Secondary amenorrhea.
d. Irregular cycles.
e. Primary dysmenorrhea.
7. Treatment includes identifying underlying cause.
8. Athletic amenorrhea is diagnosis of exclusion.

C. Eating disorders.
1. Anorexia nervosa.
a. Most serious consequence of "thin is in" mentality.
b. Sevenfold increase occurs in dancers vs. general high school population.
c. Causes are multifactorial.
d. Occurs in 6.5% of professional dance students.
e. Criteria.
i. 20% weight loss by deliberate cachexia.
ii. Amenorrhea.
iii. Distorted body image.
iv. Fat phobia.
v. Signs: bradycardia, hypotension, hair loss.
f. Mortality is high (5% to 15%) even if disease is treated.
g. Treatment begins with psychiatric help to enhance self-esteem as well as to address underlying medical concerns which may appear, such as hypokalemia.
2. Bulimia.
a. Key difference: no amenorrhea or cachexia.
b. Binge eating is followed by purging.
c. Purging can include vomiting, fasting, laxative abuse, and even amphetamine abuse.
d. Difficult to diagnose because of covert acts.
e. Symptom and signs:
i. Depressive mood.
ii. Hypokalemia.
iii. Parotid enlargement.
iv. Dental enamel loss.
v. Anorectal bleeding and hair loss similar to what is seen in anorexia.
f. Treatment includes psychiatry, medicine, nutrition, and, in some instances, dentistry (to address tooth decay secondary to gastric acid exposure).

D. Cardiovascular.
1. Aerobic capacity improves when exercise increases heart rate to 70% of maximum, or target heart rate.
2. Target heart rate (220 − Age) maintained from 20-30 minutes at least three times a week has been shown to decrease morbidity and mortality considerably.
3. All major muscle groups should be used.
4. Echocardiography is known to show greater cardiac volume and thickness measurements in dancers.

E. Vestibulopathy: repetitive jarring trauma in high impact aerobic exercise is associated with a syndrome that includes vertigo, tinnitus, incoordination, and hearing loss due to otolith and cochlea injury.

F. Risk-taking problems.
1. Infectious: close environmental contact can inoculate a whole company.
2. Sex education: abstinence, use of condoms, education.

3. Smoking: no increase over rates in the general age group. Impedes healing and building strong bones.
4. Drugs: education needed on alcohol and marijuana use.

IV. Orthopedic Concerns
A. Prevention: provided by the dance team, which helps to minimize injuries by monitoring dancers. Risk factors include:
1. Technique and training errors.
2. Abrupt changes in time spent in class and in training (fatigue).
3. Abrupt changes in technique.
4. Ill-prepared lifting (mostly by males).
5. Underclassed dancer being asked to go beyond his or her ability.
6. Inappropriate footwear (shock-absorbing soles are required).
7. Inappropriate surfaces (surfaces should combine cushioning with stability).

B. Injuries: causes include demands on physique, techniques used, overuse injury, and even (rarely) traumatic mishaps.
1. Acute trauma: falls, lifting, and sliding into objects.
2. Overuse: major cause of injury. Occurs during:
a. Turn-out.
b. Running.
c. Jumping.
d. Sliding.

C. Rehabilitation and treatment mainstays.
1. Year-round conditioning: flexibility, strength, and stamina.
2. Education of dancer regarding injury and prevention.
3. Provide home care instruction in addition to regular facility care.

D. Neck and back.
1. Neck strain and spasm from lifting partners (trapezius and sternocleidomastoid muscles affected), as well as rhomboid and levator muscle problems. To prevent problems, stress upper body strength in addition to symptomatic treatment.
2. Higher incidence of scoliosis is associated with delayed onset of menses and malnutrition.
3. Spondylolysis of lumbar spine.
a. Related to inability to reach or maintain proper turn-out and overcompensation with lordosis.
b. Characterized by midline pain on lumbar hyperextension.
c. Radiographically oblique view reveals lesion, and bone scan can grade maturity.
d. Treatment: modified activity, restriction to activity that can be completed without pain succeeded by gradual return to normal activity, back rehabilitation with paraspinal, iliopsoas, and abdominal muscle strengthening in addition to treatment mainstays.

E. Upper leg.
1. Chronic tendinitis.
a. Related to chronic overuse.
b. Usually develops from strains.
c. Pain in soft tissue is accompanied by crepitus.
d. Treatment includes mainstays, nonsteroidal antiinflammatory drugs (NSAIDs), and heat.
2. Greater trochanter bursitis.
a. Symptoms are pain and tenderness over lateral aspect of hip over area of greater trochanter.

b. Condition is related to activity-free periods and poor warm-up and flexibility.
c. Treatment includes mainstays, NSAIDs, and, occasionally, ultrasound.

3. Degenerative joint disease of the hip.
   a. Related to chronic overuse.
   b. Sometimes seen in younger dancers.
   c. Characterized by decreased range of motion during rotation, flexion, and abduction.
   d. Treatment includes mainstays and, rarely, surgery.
4. Piriformis syndrome.
   a. Diagnosis is essentially one of exclusion and is associated with overuse.
   b. Related to weak and/or inadequate external rotation.
   c. Caused by entrapment of sciatic nerve.
   d. Characterized by deep pain in the gluteus region, which worsens when climbing stairs, moving from sitting to standing, or increasing activity, and even during prolonged sitting.
   e. Treatment includes flexibility and strengthening of external hip rotators.
5. Tendinitis of sartorius muscle.
   a. Overuse injury frequently seen in dancers.
   b. Related to external hip rotation.
   c. Characterized by tenderness of point and pain during external rotation, full flexion, abduction of hip with resistance, or a combination thereof.
   d. Treatment includes mainstays, ice, as well as inflammation control and analgesia with NSAIDs.

F. Knee.
1. Patellofemoral dysfunction (chondromalacia).
   a. Most common knee ailment.
   b. Related to insufficiency of the vastus medialis in general, to external rotation of the lower leg to compensate for inadequate external rotation of the hips in ballet, and to sliding across floor repeatedly in jazz and modern dance.
   c. Characterized by anterior knee pain related to activity.
   d. Radiography may show change in patellar tracking in merchant or sunrise view.
   e. Treatment is modified activity, mainstays discussed, NSAIDs, lateral support sleeves, and possibly electromechanical stimulation (EMS).
2. Jumper's knee (patellar tendinitis).
   a. Characterized by tenderness at inferior patellar origin.
   b. Chief symptom is pain with jumping and flexion > 90 degrees.
   c. Initial treatment is modified jumping and activity, ice, mainstays, and inferior support sleeve and brace.

G. Lower leg.
1. Stress fracture.
   a. Usually affects distal tibia or fibula.
   b. Caused by overuse, abrupt changes in training or activity.
   c. Characterized by tenderness over site and pain with activity.
   d. Bone scan more of use acutely than plain radiography.
   e. Can develop into overt fracture.

f. Rest for at least 7-10 days until activities of daily living (ADLs) can be completed without pain. Then gradual, pain-free increases in modified activity can be made before returning to full activity.

2. Achilles' tendinitis
   a. Related to chronic overuse.
   b. Mechanism can be mechanical (e.g., tight shoes).
   c. Usually develops from strains.
   d. Characterized by pain in soft tissue (rarely accompanied by crepitus), pain associated with activity and passive dorsiflexion, and increases in tendon width.
   e. Treatment includes an interval of 1-2 weeks of rest in addition to mainstays. Return to modified activity includes pain-free, gradual increase in training and activity. Injections are not appropriate.

H. Ankle.

1. Anterior impingement.
   a. Appears as extreme dorsiflexion (as in demiplié), which causes pain and/or weakness; however, athlete usually complains of decreased depth on plié.
   b. Examination shows tenderness and swelling between lateral malleolus and extensor digitorum and, occasionally, the palpation of exostoses.
   c. Can be mistaken for tight heel cords.
   d. Mechanism is impingement of anterior lip of tibia on neck of talus.
   e. Exostoses can be seen on lateral view radiographs.
   f. Treatment includes NSAIDs, physical therapy, and ankle strengthening during both inversion and eversion. Advanced cases can require surgical removal of osteophytes.
2. Posterior impingement or dancer's heel.
   a. Extreme plantar flexion (as in en pointe, but condition can be seen in extreme dorsiflexion also), which causes pain and/or weakness.
   b. Examination shows tenderness, swelling, and, often, crepitus in posterior ankle.
   c. Can be mistaken for Achilles' tendinitis.
   d. Mechanism is talar impingement in posterior ankle.
   e. Condition exacerbated by os trigonum tarsi problems, enlarged posterior process of calcaneus, and, most commonly, large posterior tubercle.
   f. Treatment includes improving heel traction, NSAIDs, physical therapy, strengthening of ankle during inversion and eversion. Advanced cases can require excision of posterior talar process or os trigonum tarsi.

V. Feet and Toes

1. Dancer's fracture (fracture of fifth metatarsal shaft).
   a. Metatarsal spiral fracture.
   b. Mechanism is inversion injury en pointe.
   c. Radiography shows spiral fracture.
   d. Treatment includes a short period of immobilization, gradual increase in activity, later taping or protection or both.
2. Stress fracture.
   a. Caused by overuse, abrupt changes in use.
   b. Symptoms are tenderness over site and pain with activity.
   c. Bone scan may be needed for diagnosis.
   d. Can be similar to sesamoid disorders.

   e. Treatment is rest for at least 1 week until ADLs can be completed without pain. Rest period required may be longer for second metatarsal base fracture. Then gradually increase modified activity while avoiding pain before returning to normal activity.
3. Morton's neuroma.
   a. Related to constrictive footwear.
   b. Characteristically at interspace between third and fourth toes.
   c. Activity-related pain occasionally radiates, and decreased sensitivity to touch of adjacent toes can occur.
   d. Aggravated by cumulative slamming trauma to foot.
   e. Treatment includes metatarsal pads, local steroid injections, use of orthotics, physical therapy, and surgical removal of neuroma as a last resort.
4. Onychocryptosis (ingrown toenail).
   a. Most frequently caused by incorrect trimming.
   b. Exacerbated or caused by hallux valgus, tight pointe shoes, hypertrophied nail folds.
   c. Inspect for secondary infection or granuloma.
   d. Treatment includes treating infection or granuloma initially, then partial or whole nail excision under local anesthesia if nail is deeply ingrown.

Acknowledgment

The Medical Editing Department, Kaiser Foundation Research Institute, provided editorial assistance.

Bibliography

Belt CR: Injuries associated with aerobic dance, *Am Fam Phys* 41:1769-1772, 1990.

Braun LT: Exercise physiology and cardiovascular fitness, *Nurs Clin North Am* 26:135-147, 1991.

Calabrese LH, Kirkendall DT: Nutritional and medical considerations in dancers, *Clin Sports Med* 2:539-548, 1983.

Frisch RE et al: Delayed menarche and amenorrhea of college athletes in relation to age of onset of training, *JAMA* 246:1559-1563, 1981.

Frisch RE, Wyshak G, Vincent L: Delayed menarche and amenorrhea in ballet dancers, *N Engl J Med* 303:17-19, 1980.

Garner DM, Garfinkel PE: Socio-cultural factors in the development of anorexia nervosa, *Psychol Med* 10:647-656, 1980.

Garrick J: Dance injuries. In Mellion MB, Walsh WM, Shelton GL, editors: *The Team Physician's Handbook,* St Louis, 1986, Mosby, pp 657-662.

Garrick JG, Gillien DM, Whiteside P: The epidemiology of aerobic dance injuries, *Am J Sports Med* 14:67-72, 1986.

Hardaker WT Jr: Foot and ankle injuries in classical ballet dancers, *Orthop Clin North Am* 20:621-627, 1989.

Hardaker WT Jr, Erickson L, Myers M: The pathogenesis of foot injury. In Shell CG, editor: The *Dancer as Athlete,* Champaign, IL, 1986, Human Kinetics Publishers, pp 11-29.

Hardaker WT Jr, Moorman CT III: Foot and ankle injuries in dance and athletics: similarities and differences. In Shell CG, editor: The *Dancer as Athlete,* Champaign, IL, 1986, Human Kinetics Publishers, pp 31-41.

Hardaker WT Jr, Vander Woude LM: Dance medicine: an orthopaedist's view, *N C Med J* 54(2):67-72, 1993.

Hickey M, Hager CA: Aerobic dance injuries, *Orthop Nurs* 13(5):9-12, Sept-Oct 1994.

Kirkendall DT, Calabrese LH: Physiological aspects of dance, *Clin Sports Med* 2:525-537, 1983.

Koszuta L: Low impact aerobics: better than traditional aerobic dance? *Phys Sports Med* 14(7):156-161, 1986.

Maloney MJ: Anorexia nervosa and bulimia in dancers: accurate diagnosis and treatment planning, *Clin Sports Med* 2:549-555, 1983.

Nixon JE: Injuries to the neck and upper extremities of dancers, *Clin Sports Med* 2:459-472, 1983.

Novella TM: Dancers' shoes and foot care. In Ryan AJ, Stephens RE, editors: *Dance Medicine: A Comprehensive Guide,* Chicago, 1987, Pluribus Press, pp 139-176.

Ogilvie-Harris DJ, Carr MM, Fleming PJ: The foot in ballet dancers: the importance of second toe length, *Foot Ankle Int* 16:144-147, 1995.

Ostwald PF et al: Performing arts medicine, *West J Med* 160:48-52, 1994.

Public Participation in the Arts: 1982 and 1985 Compared, Washington, DC, 1987, National Endowment for the Arts, Research Division Note #27.

Richie DH, Kelso SF, Bellucci PA: Aerobic dance injuries: a retrospective study of instructors and participants, *Phys Sportsmed* 13(2):130-140, 1985.

Ryan AJ, Stephens RE, editors: *Dance Medicine: A Comprehensive Guide,* Chicago, 1987, Pluribus Press.

Schneider HJ et al: Stress injuries and developmental change of lower extremities in ballet dancers, *Radiology* 113:627-632, 1974.

Shade AR: Gynecologic and obstetric problems of the female dancer, *Clin Sports Med* 2:515-523, 1983.

Shell CG, editor: The *Dancer as Athlete,* Champaign, IL, 1986, Human Kinetics Publishers.

Speroff L: Can exercise cause problems in pregnancy and menstruation? *Contemp Ob Gyn* 16:57-59, 63-64, 67, 70, Sept. 1980.

Stensland SH, Sobal J: Dietary practices of ballet, jazz, and modern dancers, *J Am Diet Assoc* 92:319-324, 1992.

Teitz CC: Sports medicine concerns in dance and gymnastics, *Clin Sports Med* 2:571-593, 1983.

Vetter WL et al: Aerobic dance injuries, *Phys Sportsmed* 13(2):114-120, 1985.

Vincent LM: *The Dancer's Book of Health,* Kansas City, 1978, Sheed Andrews and McMeel.

Weintraub MI: Vestibulopathy induced by high impact aerobics: a new syndrome: discussion of 30 cases, *J Sports Med Phys Fitness* 34(1):56-63, March 1994.

Werner MJ, Rosenthal SL, Biro FM: Medical needs of performing arts students, *J Adolesc Health* 12:294-300, 1991.

INDEX

B

C

G

J

K

M

Q

T

U

V

W

Y

Z